Handbook of Research on Psychosocial Perspectives of Human Communication Disorders

Sanjeev Kumar Gupta
All India Institute of Speech and Hearing, India

Srinivasan Venkatesan
All India Institute of Speech and Hearing, India

A volume in the Advances in Psychology, Mental Health, and Behavioral Studies (APMHBS) Book Series

IGI Global
DISSEMINATOR OF KNOWLEDGE

Published in the United States of America by
IGI Global
Medical Information Science Reference (an imprint of IGI Global)
701 E. Chocolate Avenue
Hershey PA, USA 17033
Tel: 717-533-8845
Fax: 717-533-8661
E-mail: cust@igi-global.com
Web site: http://www.igi-global.com

Library of Congress Cataloging-in-Publication Data

Names: Gupta, Sanjeev Kumar, 1983- editor. | Venkatesan, S., 1961- editor.
Title: Handbook of research on psychosocial perspectives of human communication disorders / Sanjeev Kumar Gupta and Srinivasan Venkatesan, editors.
Description: Hershey PA : Medical Information Science Reference, [2018] | Includes bibliographical references.
Identifiers: LCCN 2017032792| ISBN 9781522549550 (hardcover) | ISBN 9781522549567 (ebook)
Subjects: | MESH: Communication Disorders--psychology | Communication Disorders--therapy | Caregivers--psychology | Family Relations--psychology | India
Classification: LCC RC428.8 | NLM WL 340.2 | DDC 616.85/50651--dc23 LC record available at https://lccn.loc.gov/2017032792

This book is published in the IGI Global book series Advances in Psychology, Mental Health, and Behavioral Studies (APMHBS) (ISSN: 2475-6660; eISSN: 2475-6679)

British Cataloguing in Publication Data
A Cataloguing in Publication record for this book is available from the British Library.

Advances in Psychology, Mental Health, and Behavioral Studies (APMHBS) Book Series

Bryan Christiansen
Global Research Society, LLC, USA
Harish C. Chandan
Argosy University, USA

ISSN:2475-6660
EISSN:2475-6679

Mission

The complexity of the human mind has puzzled researchers and physicians for centuries. While widely studied, the brain still remains largely misunderstood.

The **Advances in Psychology, Mental Health, and Behavioral Studies (APMHBS)** book series presents comprehensive research publications focusing on topics relating to the human psyche, cognition, psychiatric care, mental and developmental disorders, as well as human behavior and interaction. Featuring diverse and innovative research, publications within APMHBS are ideally designed for use by mental health professionals, academicians, researchers, and upper-level students.

Coverage

- Human Behavior
- Treatment & Care
- Addiction
- Personality Disorders
- Counseling & Therapy
- Neurological Disorders
- Human Interaction
- Developmental Disorders
- Emotional Health
- Cognition

IGI Global is currently accepting manuscripts for publication within this series. To submit a proposal for a volume in this series, please contact our Acquisition Editors at Acquisitions@igi-global.com or visit: http://www.igi-global.com/publish/.

The Advances in Psychology, Mental Health, and Behavioral Studies (APMHBS) Book Series (ISSN 2475-6660) is published by IGI Global, 701 E. Chocolate Avenue, Hershey, PA 17033-1240, USA, www.igi-global.com. This series is composed of titles available for purchase individually; each title is edited to be contextually exclusive from any other title within the series. For pricing and ordering information please visit http://www.igi-global.com/book-series/advances-psychology-mental-health-behavioral/110200. Postmaster: Send all address changes to above address.

Titles in this Series

For a list of additional titles in this series, please visit: www.igi-global.com/book-series

Social, Psychological, and Forensic Perspectives on Sexual Abuse
Rejani Thudalikunnil Gopalan (Gujarat Forensic Sciences University, India)
Information Science Reference • copyright 2018 • 374pp • H/C (ISBN: 9781522539582) • US $195.00 (our price)

Raising Mental Health Awareness in Higher Education Emerging Research and Opportunities
Melissa Martin (State University of New York at Plattsburgh, USA) Jean Mockry (State University of New York at Plattsburgh, USA) Alison Puliatte (State University of New York at Plattsburgh, USA) Denise A. Simard (State University of New York at Plattsburgh, USA) and Maureen E. Squires (State University of New York at Plattsburgh, USA)
Medical Information Science Reference • copyright 2018 • 136pp • H/C (ISBN: 9781522537939) • US $175.00 (our price)

Web-Based Behavioral Therapies for Mental Disorders
Sitwat Usman Langrial (Sur University College, Oman)
Medical Information Science Reference • copyright 2018 • 310pp • H/C (ISBN: 9781522532415) • US $255.00 (our price)

Measuring the Psychological and Electrophysiological Attributes of Human Personality Emerging Research and Opportunities
Sanja Tatalović Vorkapić (University of Rijeka, Croatia)
Information Science Reference • copyright 2017 • 242pp • H/C (ISBN: 9781522522836) • US $130.00 (our price)

Emerging Research in Play Therapy, Child Counseling, and Consultation
Rheta LeAnne Steen (Loyola University New Orleans, USA)
Information Science Reference • copyright 2017 • 436pp • H/C (ISBN: 9781522522249) • US $205.00 (our price)

Workforce Development Theory and Practice in the Mental Health Sector
Mark Smith (Te Pou o te Whakaaro Nui: National Workforce Center for Adult Mental Health, Addiction and Disability, New Zealand) and Angela F. Jury (Te Pou o te Whakaaro Nui: National Workforce Center for Adult Mental Health, Addiction and Disability, New Zealand)
Information Science Reference • copyright 2017 • 378pp • H/C (ISBN: 9781522518747) • US $190.00 (our price)

Improving the Quality of Life for Dementia Patients through Progressive Detection, Treatment, and Care
Jinglong Wu (Okayama University, Japan)
Medical Information Science Reference • copyright 2017 • 353pp • H/C (ISBN: 9781522509257) • US $205.00 (our price)

IGI Global
DISSEMINATOR OF KNOWLEDGE

701 East Chocolate Avenue, Hershey, PA 17033, USA
Tel: 717-533-8845 x100 • Fax: 717-533-8661
E-Mail: cust@igi-global.com • www.igi-global.com

Editorial Advisory Board

List of Reviewers

List of Contributors

Table of Contents

Detailed Table of Contents

challenged by communication disorders struggle to form friendships and make inroads into social groups. Mothers, the primary caregivers in most instances, with their intimate knowledge of their children, are considered the best advocates. This study set out to identify strategies that mothers engage in to pave the way for successful social inclusion of children with communication disorders. An online survey was conducted in different geographical locations. Mothers with children aged 6-13 years who had received speech therapy or are currently receiving speech therapy were invited to participate. Data were analyzed using a mixed methods approach. Outcomes suggest that all mothers believe in social inclusion despite facing a range of inclusion and exclusionary practices. Undeterred by these responses, mothers advocate for social inclusion by engaging in a range of strategies.

Chapter 8
Stress and Anxiety Among Parents of Children With Communication Disorders 141
Kadambari Naniwadekar, All India Institute of Speech and Hearing, India

Parenting is a wonderful and rewarding experience, but in the case of parents of children with communication disorder, this experience is often accompanied with high levels of stress, due to difficulties, frustrations, and challenges that these parents face in everyday life. This chapter was carried out to find the status of stress in parents of children with communication disorder and also to find the levels of stress among mothers as well as fathers, and the level of support system available. The results revealed that most of the parents experience stress and anxiety in bringing up their child with communication disorder, although the stress being more in the mothers. Gender of the child also played a crucial role in determining the levels of stress. The results highlighted the fact that parents of children with autism spectrum disorder have a higher level of stress followed by parents of children with intellectual disability, multiple disability, and hearing impairment.

Section 3
Communication Disorders: Characteristics and Assessment

Chapter 9
Dysphagia in Persons With Communication Disorders... 158
Gayathri Krishnan, All India Institute of Speech and Hearing, India
S. P. Goswami, All India Institute of Speech and Hearing, India

Dysphagia (swallowing disorders) is any difficulty in swallowing that interferes with safe and adequate intake of nutrition and hydration requirements in an individual. It may present itself as a symptom of another underlying medical condition or as a consequence of surgical and pharmacological treatment. While in few, dysphagia resolves itself as a transient phase; in the rest, dysphagia demands immediate treatment. It may be seen as an associated dysfunction in persons with communication disorders (PsWCD) as speech and swallowing functions share many neuro-musculo-skeletal structures at the oral, pharyngeal, and laryngeal level along with their central control processes. This chapter aims at introducing the readers to the signs and symptoms of dysphagia in PsWCD. This is expected to guide the team of professionals working with PsWCDin identification and making appropriate referrals to the concerned professional for effective intervention. This further can accelerate the progress and prognosis of PsWCD towards improved health, development, and quality of life.

Fatigue is a common yet poorly understood topic. The psychological, physiological, social, emotional, and cognitive wellbeing of a person may be affected due to fatigue. Despite a century of research in understanding the effect of fatigue on human systems, there is no concrete explanation as how fatigue affects the perception of speech. Fatigue impairs auditory cognition and the reduced cognitive abilities further increase mental and physical fatigue. Since cognition is markedly affected in individuals experiencing mental fatigue, its consequences are widespread. According to the top-down approach of auditory processing, there is a direct link between cognition and speech perception. Thus, in the present chapter, the influence of fatigue on perception is reviewed. It is noted that the impact of fatigue on cognition and quality of life is different for children and adults. Training in music, meditation, and exposure to more than one language are some of the measures that help to reduce the effect of fatigue and improve cognitive abilities in both children as well as in adults.

This chapter seeks to outline the overarching scenario of behavioral approaches to developmental and childhood speech, language, hearing, and communication disorders. By adopting the dichotomy of skill and problem behaviors, the steps or sequence, procedures, and practices of behavioral assessment and interventions are explained. While doing so, the uniquely Indian cultural underpinnings are highlighted with evidence-based empirical supports for the optimal benefits of the affected individuals. Additionally, two separate segments are focused on guidelines for skill training and problem behavior management along with case illustration on the format for their mapping procedures. The concluding section covers a critique of this approach which continues to hold promise for some more explorations in the contemporary circumstances for the optimum habilitation of these affected individuals.

Persons with aphasia (PWA) face varying difficulties of communication breakdown through different stages of recovery. With speech-language therapy, significant recovery may be seen at unitary levels, but the ultimate success of therapy is evident when the PWA uses all of the units as a whole and is able to communicate optimally to sustain social identities. An individualized intervention program as the focus, a protocol is proposed with seven semi-structured interviews aimed at eliciting discourse incorporating the philosophies of the social model, LPAA, SCA, AphasiaBank Protocol, and Protocol to Measure Participation of Persons with Aphasia. The interviews with the PWA and their communication partners in individual and joint sessions can help the clinician answer questions regarding the PWA's physical abilities, dietary issues, functional independence, personal traits, relationships at home, different social roles played, and subsequently plan a treatment program, and track the holistic recovery of the PWA.

Foreword

Communication disorders cover a wide range of disorders including speech disorder–disorders of voice, articulation, and fluency – language disorders occurring independently are associated with organic, neurological and/or psychological disorders - disorders or delay in language acquisition due to hearing loss, mental retardation, neurological diseases etc. in children, language, dysphagia and dementia occurring due to various deteriorating processes in the human body or neurological diseases – hearing disorders – diseases of the external, middle, inner ear or the auditory pathway. Persons with Communication Disorders often can't express themselves leading to behavioral issues. Hence, the field of communication sciences and disorders is multidisciplinary in nature as it has heavily borrowed from other fields. Therefore, the psychosocial perspectives of Communication Disorders provide an insight into the psychological issues in such persons and their parents/ siblings which in turn should help in a total rehabilitation.

The *Handbook of Research on Psychosocial Perspectives of Human Communication Disorders* has 19 chapters covered in four sections. The first section is on Communication Disorders: Psychosocial Perspectives, the second on Communication Disorders: Siblings and Family, the third on Communication Disorders: Characteristics and Assessment and the fourth on Communication Disorders: Rehabilitation and Intervention. The first section covers topics such as auditory neuropathy spectrum disorders, psychosocial perspectives of persons with aphasia, psychosocial correlates of dissociative motor disorder of impairment or loss of speech and knowledge, and the attitude & practices of primary and secondary school teachers on specific learning disorder. The second section includes topics on 'intertwined lives'-narratives of children with disabilities and their siblings, sibling disposition towards children with special needs, mothers as advocates of social inclusion for children with communication disorders, and stress and anxiety among parents of children with communication disorders. The third section includes chapters on dysphagia, subjective fatigue in children and adults, behavioral approach to speech, language, hearing and communication disorders, discourse elicitation in aphasia, assessment of significant other's burden and their communication strategies to enhance the treatment outcome in aphasia, assessment of cognitive-communicative functions in persons with mild cognitive impairment and dementia of Alzheimer's type. And the fourth section includes socio-cultural models, vocational rehabilitation, speech therapy for children, manual for adult aphasia therapy, and management of the selective mutism.

The field of communication disorders is vast and ever emerging with new methods of assessment and rehabilitation. In a multidisciplinary field, it is essential to provide all interested with state-of-the-art knowledge on all related aspects. This book provides valuable information on psychosocial perspectives of human communication disorders in various domains for students of psychology, communication sciences & disorders, parents and clinicians.

S. R. Savithri
All India Institute of Speech and Hearing, India

Preface

The encouragement and motivation for editing a book on *Handbook of Research on Psychosocial Perspectives of Human Communication Disorders* arose as a consequence of the editors' experiences and active involvement in both research and clinical activities in the area of communication disorders. Communication plays an important role not only in humans but also in the animals. In order to understand and treat effectively, the individuals with communication disorders, in depth knowledge in the area of speech and language acquisition is a prerequisite. Language acquisition is the process by which individuals acquire the capacity to perceive, produce and use words to understand and communicate. Vygotsky's theory of language development, Piaget's stages of cognitive development, Erickson's psychosocial stages, and Bowlby's attachment theory are important to understand the psychosocial perspective of language development in the child.

This book covers need-based issues pertaining to assessment and management of communication disorders. Individuals may demonstrate one or many combinations of speech, language and hearing disorders. It may be developmental or acquired, and may result in a primary disability or can be secondary to other disabilities. The cultural context in defining and discussing speech, language and hearing disorders is also important. The common co-morbid conditions in communication disorders are intellectual disability, borderline intellectual functioning, cerebral palsy, epilepsy, autism, attention-deficit/hyperactivity disorder, and specific learning disabilities. The psychosocial factors are the key components in the cause and may trigger speech, language and hearing issues. Understanding the psychosocial aspects would help to know the associated psychosocial factors and it will also pave the way for the assessment and intervention plan of these clinical conditions.

As per the Census 2011, there are 26.81 million persons with disabilities in India who constitute 2.21% of the total population. Out of total persons with disabilities, 5.07 Million (2.67 Million males and 2.39 Million females) are person with hearing loss and 1.99 million (1.12 million males and 0.87 million females) have speech-related disability (Census of India, 2013). Konadath, Chatni, Lakshmi, and Saini (2017) studied the prevalence rate of communication disorders in Lakshadweep, a group of islands in India, and reported males had higher prevalence of ear-related (53.77% against 46.23%) and speech-language related problems (60.29% against 39.71%). The authors concluded that the prevalence of hearing loss was lesser and the prevalence of speech–language disorders higher compared to the mainland. Among the communication disorders, speech and language disorders were more prevalent. Males were more prone to the communication disorders than females. Sinha et al. (2017) studied the prevalence of communication disorders in a rural population at taluq level of Gujarat, India. The overall prevalence of ear-related disorders was 3.30% (male-1.66%, female-1.63%) and prevalence of speech- and language-related disorder was 0.79% (male-0.60%, female- 0.24%).

Black, Vahratian, and Hoffman (2015) reported that nearly 1 in 12 (7.7 percent) U.S. children age 3-17 have had a disorder related to voice, speech, language or swallowing in the past 12 months. The prevalence of voice, speech, language or swallowing disorders is highest among children aged 3-6 (11.0 percent), compared to children aged 7-10 (9.3 percent) and children aged 11-17 (4.9 percent). World Health Organization (2012) estimated the prevalence of hearing loss. The estimates are based on 42 population-based studies. There are 360 million persons in the world with disabling hearing loss (5.3% of the world's population); 328 million (91%) of these are adults (183 million males, 145 million females); 32 (9%) million of these are children. The prevalence of disabling hearing loss in children is greatest in South Asia, Asia Pacific and Sub-Saharan Africa. Approximately one-third of persons over 65 years are affected by disabling hearing loss. The prevalence of disabling hearing loss in adults over 65 years is highest in South Asia, Asia Pacific and Sub-Saharan Africa.

For most children, the developmental task of acquiring adaptive behaviour such as communication proceeds smoothly. However, children with communication disorders manifest problem/aggressive behavior (e.g., pushing or pulling, screaming, kicking, hitting, biting, throwing articles), attention and social problems due to ineffective means to communicate that have caused concern to parents and caregivers. Early identification, prevention and intervention activities & practices can promote children's healthy cognitive, speech & language, motor, social and emotional development within the home and school environments. It is evident that unless the clinician manages behavioural issues in these children, speech therapy and listening training may not be effective. This publication has covered the chapters on the narrative of children with disabilities, siblings' depositions, behavioural approach and speech therapy for children.

The adults with communication disorders require proper rehabilitation and employment. This book has covered the chapters on socio-cultural models & policy programs and vocational rehabilitation of persons with hearing impairment. The geriatric population also faces communication issues due to neurodegenerative disorders such as aphasia and dementia. This book covers chapters on psychosocial perspectives of persons with late-onset auditory neuropathy spectrum disorder and aphasia, discourse elicitation in aphasia, assessment of cognitive-communication functions in mild cognitive impairment and dementia of Alzheimer's type.

This handbook features 19 chapters authored by leading experts offering an in depth detail of various relevant concepts, characteristics, assessments, and interventions related to communication disorders. Intervention for individuals with communication disorders is influenced by many factors such as nature and severity level of the disorder, age and socio-economic status of the patient, and environmental situations, as well as personal characteristics of both patient and clinician. While making the management plan, clinicians should consider all these points. Maintenance of case history and treatment record is important for future consultation. The objective of treatment plan is to bring improvement in the patient not only in clinical settings but also in his/her personal and social life like home, school/college and work settings. The clinician also needs to encourage the patient to self-monitor and self-correction as needed even in the absence of the clinician. Before starting any intervention plan, clinicians should obtain a baseline data including an audio or video speech/voice sample because it is important to determine the patient's progress and impact of the intervention program (Gupta, 2015). The active involvement of family members throughout the treatment is essential for the better results. Positive and productive patient-clinician and family-clinician relationships are important ingredients for successful intervention. Neither set of elements guarantees success but, both sets do increase the chance of optimal outcomes (Friehe, Bloedow, & Hesse, 2003). Psychological intervention should be used in conjunction with speech and language therapy for the optimum benefit of the persons with communication disorders. Psychological intervention focuses not only on direct one-to-one therapy but also on early identification, assessment, and individualized intervention programs that will help to reduce the manifestation of communication disorders. A multidisciplinary and coordinated team approach involving follow-up from infancy to adulthood is recommended for positive outcomes (Gupta, 2015).

THE ISSUES AND CHALLENGES

There are many issues in the testing and assessment of persons with communication disorders. The conditions of laboratories are not up to the mark in developing countries especially, in the semi-urban and rural areas. The patient and clinician ratio is also a concern. India being a multi-language country, where people speak multiple languages. Language becomes a barrier in testing and assessment. Another issue is use of old and outdated test materials without having recent norms for the population of communication disorders. Sometimes caregivers are biased or unable to report the genuine problems of children with communication disorders. To deal a patient with communication disorder, a multidisciplinary team is required, but all the rehabilitation centers and hospitals do not provide a holistic approach to deal with such persons. Many a time caregivers of patients have a resistant and stigma and due to this they delay the treatment process, in turn, the child gets more severe issues. Dealing with the caregivers/parents of persons with communication disorders is equally important.

SEARCHING FOR A SOLUTION

The field of behavioural and communication sciences are multidisciplinary and have a long-lasting effect on the persons with communication disorders and their family. Therefore, a multidisciplinary approach is essential not only to deal with such persons and their family but also to conduct cutting-edge research in the field of communication disorders. In the assessment of intelligence and personality of communication disorders, systematic process of gathering information about an individual's background, history, skills, knowledge, perceptions, and feelings must be followed. The clinician must focus on gathering information in the following areas such as language, speech, cognition, voice, fluency, and hearing. Early and accurate assessment and psychological intervention in conjunction with speech therapy and listening training are beneficial for the needy population to improve social competency, self-image, self-confidence, depression and anxiety. There is also a continuous need for revalidation of tests for urban and rural population. This publication *Handbook of Research on Psychosocial Perspectives of Human Communication Disorders* has produced 19 chapters and can be used as a basis for further research and clinical practice in the field of communication disorders. This book also offers a range of useful topics for stimulating debate and discussion by researchers and practitioners.

OBJECTIVE OF THE BOOK

The primary objective of the book is to provide a synthesis of the latest research to the academicians, researchers, and practitioners who are working in the area of psychology in association with speech, language and hearing disorders. The secondary objective is to disseminate the contemporary research to the scientific fraternity and clinician for the advancement of the discipline and the benefit of person with communication disorders and their families.

TARGET AUDIENCE OF THE BOOK

A multidisciplinary approach is required to deal effectively for persons with communication disorders. Therefore, the book is helpful for various professionals such as Clinical Psychologists, Audiologists, Speech-Language Pathologists, Special Educators, Occupational Therapists, Physiotherapists, Physiatrists, Otolaryngologists, Neurologists and Paediatricians, who needs recent advancement of psychosocial perspectives of human communication disorders. This book can serve as a complementary textbook for undergraduate and postgraduate courses in the area of Speech-language pathology, Audiology, Clinical Psychology, and Special Education-Hearing Impairment.

ORGANIZATION OF THE BOOK

This book is organized into four sections and 19 chapters. Section 1, which covers Chapters 1-4, elaborates on psychosocial perspectives of communication disorders. Section 2, which covers Chapters 5-8, focuses on communication disorders and siblings and family. Section 3, which covers Chapters 9-14, deals with characteristics and assessment of communications disorders. Section 4 covers Chapters 15-19 and highlights the importance of rehabilitation and intervention in communication disorders. A brief description of each of the chapters is given below.

Section 1: Communication Disorders – Psychosocial Perspectives

Chapter 1 attempts to highlight the enigma of late-onset auditory neuropathy spectrum disorder (ANSD) from a psychosocial perspective. The chapter covers prevalence, onset, characteristics, depression, anxiety, and the psychological problems related to late-onset ANSD.

Chapter 2 focuses on psychosocial perspectives of persons with aphasia. The main thrust areas of the chapter are social life among persons with aphasias, return to work following stroke and aphasia, quality of life, and factors affecting quality of life.

Chapter 3 presents the role of psychosocial factors like stressful life events and adjustment issues in individual with functional voice disorders. This chapter highlights the importance of understanding the individual dynamics, social, and psychological stressors as they are essential to the clinician to devise effective intervention for such persons.

Chapter 4 covers the definitions, issues and challenges, neuropsychological aspects, assessments, diagnosis and treatments for specific learning disorders. The main aim of the chapter is to assess the knowledge, attitudes and current practices pertaining to specific learning disorders, among pre-primary, primary and secondary school teachers in public schools.

Section 2: Communication Disorders – Siblings and Family

Chapter 5 covers the narratives of young children with disabilities and their siblings. This chapter discusses two complex broad themes of a surrogate parenting roles and normative sibling relationships, which at times converge and at times diverge. The findings of this study may encourage healthcare professionals to consider and offer holistic family-centered therapy interventions which recognize and considers sibling relationships as key to communication therapy and family support.

Chapter 6 presents a survey study of sibling disposition towards children with special needs. The study concluded that almost all typically developing siblings were found to have concern and compassion towards their siblings with special needs. However, there are also stray incidences of negative feelings.

Chapter 7 covers a study regarding mothers, the primary caregivers in most instances, with their intimate knowledge of their children, are considered the best advocates. This study set out to identify strategies that mothers engage into pave the way for successful social inclusion of children with communication disorders. An online survey was conducted in different geographical locations. Data were analysed using a mixed methods approach. Outcomes suggest that all mothers believe in social inclusion despite facing a range of inclusion and exclusion in their parenting practices.

Chapter 8 address stress and anxiety among parents of children with communication disorders. The present study was carried out to find the status of stress in parents of children with communication disorder and also to find the levels of stress among mothers as well as fathers, and the level of support system available. The results reveal that most of the parents experience stress and anxiety in bringing up their child with communication disorder, although the stress is more in the mothers.

Section 3: Communication Disorders – Characteristics and Assessment

Chapter 9 analyses the literature regarding dysphagia. Dysphagia may be seen as an associated dysfunction in persons with communication disorders as speech and swallowing functions share many neuro-musculo-skeletal structures at the oral, pharyngeal, and laryngeal level along with their central control processes. The present chapter incorporates the signs and symptoms of dysphagia in persons with communication disorders.

Chapter 10 reviews various studies to examine the influence of fatigue on perception in children and adults. It is revealed that the impact of fatigue on cognition and quality of life is different for children and adults. Training in music, meditation and exposure to more than one language are some of the measures, which help to reduce the effect of fatigue and improve cognitive abilities in both children as well as in adults.

Chapter 11 outlines various approaches to understanding speech, language, hearing, and communication disorders and highlight the importance of behavioural approach in-depth. The chapter also covers the skill training, problem behaviour management, problem behavior mapping, golden rules in management of problem behaviors and common misconceptions about behavioral treatments.

Chapter 12 covers the discourse elicitation in aphasia. The authors identify the role of an individualized intervention program as the focus, a protocol is proposed with seven semi-structured interviews aimed at eliciting discourse incorporating the philosophies of the social model, LPAA, SCA, AphasiaBank protocol and protocol to measure participation of persons with aphasia.

Chapter 13 covers the role of assessment of significant other's burden and their communication strategies to enhance the treatment outcome in aphasia. The author emphasizes, the manner in which significant other's perceive the burden and execute their supportive communication strategies are highly variable and are influenced by many factors like their motivation, emotional attachment, constraints of time and economy, self-confidence and the clinical and individualistic attributes of the PWA.

Chapter 14 highlights the importance of assessments of cognitive-communicative functions in persons with mild cognitive impairment and dementia of Alzheimer's type. The chapter covers the diagnostic criteria, the procedure for clinical diagnosis, cognitive-linguistic deficits, team approach in the assessment of dementia and role of the Speech-Language Pathologist in the assessment.

Section 4: Communication Disorders – Rehabilitation and Intervention

Chapter 15 presents the socio-cultural models and policy programs for rehabilitation of persons with communication disorders. This chapter covers stereotyping and labeling, nomenclature, models and highlights the impact of policy and program with case vignettes.

Chapter 16 discusses the need for vocational rehabilitation in persons with hearing impairment to attain the goal of inclusive development and rights of equal opportunities and participation. It discusses issues and challenges and process of vocational rehabilitation.

Chapter 17 reviews the importance of speech therapy in children with stuttering. Studies were considered for review if (a) they were behavioral intervention of stuttering for children, (b) participants were in the age range of 2-18 years and (c) the outcomes reports on assessed stuttering population. 27 studies were obtained through an electronic search of databases covering two approaches and ten techniques. The analysis of these studies revealed that direct approaches have a stronger evidence base in comparison to the indirect approaches.

Chapter 18 evaluates evidence-based manual for adult aphasia therapy. This chapter provides a brief and comprehensive overview of the manual. It provides information on its contents and an outline about its use in clinical settings. The reader can also develop an understanding of how to assess baseline, document progress and systematically record the outcomes of therapy. Manual for Adult Aphasia Therapy is a clinically valuable therapy material for speech-language pathologists working among patients with aphasia.

Chapter 19 discusses the management of selective mutism. The chapter covers the psychosocial approach to the disorders, the diagnostic criteria, etiology, treatment of the disorders and different types of managements. A brief analysis of two case studies has been given in the chapter.

In conclusion, this book is intended to contribute new horizons in the field of communication disorders and filling the gaps between the two disciplines- behavioural and communication sciences. As a comprehensive collection of latest research findings related to communication disorders, this publication provides researchers, practitioners, academicians, and all the readers with a complete understanding of psychosocial perspectives of human communication disorders.

Sanjeev Kumar Gupta
All India Institute of Speech and Hearing, India

Srinivasan Venkatesan
All India Institute of Speech and Hearing, India

REFERENCES

Black, L. I., Vahratian, A., & Hoffman, H. J. (2015). Communication disorders and use of intervention services among children aged 3-17 years: United States, 2012. NCHS data brief, no 205. Hyattsville, MD: National Center for Health Statistics.

Census of India. (2013). *Disabled population by type of Disability, age, and sex.* Office of the Registrar General and Census Commissioner.

Friehe, M. J., Bloedow, A., & Hesse, S. (2003). Counseling families of children with communication disorders. *Communication Disorders Quarterly*, *24*(4), 211–220. doi:10.1177/15257401030240040701

Gupta, S. K. (2015). Management of communication disorders: A clinical perspective. *International Journal of Psychology and Psychiatry*, *3*(1), 80–93. doi:10.5958/2320-6233.2015.00006.1

Konadath, S., Chatni, S., Lakshmi, M. S., & Saini, J. K. (2017). Prevalence of communication disorders in a group of islands in India. *Clinical Epidemiology and Global Health*, *5*(2), 79–86. doi:10.1016/j.cegh.2016.08.003

Sinha, S. K., Shivaswamy, J., Barman, A., Seth, D., Seshadri, D., & Savithri, S. R. (2017). Prevalence of communication disorders in a rural population at taluq level of Gujarat, India. *Clinical Epidemiology and Global Health*, *5*(2), 73–78. doi:10.1016/j.cegh.2016.08.006

World Health Organization. (2012). *WHO global estimates on prevalence of hearing loss*. Geneva: World Health Organization.

Acknowledgment

We wish to acknowledge the help of all the people involved directly and indirectly in this project and more specifically to the authors, reviewers, and editorial advisory board members who took part in the development process of this book. Without their support, this book would not have become a reality.

We heartily thank each one of the chapter's authors who contributed their time and expertise to this book.

The success of the chapters is attributed to the meticulous work done by the members of the book's Editorial Advisory Board and Board of Reviewers through the double-triple-blind peer review process for improvement of content, coherence, quality, and presentation of the chapters. We thank all the editorial advisory board members as well as reviewers for their valuable input for this book and reviewing the chapters. Some of the contributing authors have also participated in the peer review process: Dr. Malar G and Dr. Prithi Venkatesh Mondreti. We highly appreciate their dual role.

Special thanks to Dr. Purusotham P, Ms. Rachel V, and Ms. Vimala Jayakrishna Kasturi for their support in proofreading of the chapters.

Last but not the least; we thank the IGI Global team, Hershey, PA, for helping us in the completion of this book and timely publication.

Sanjeev Kumar Gupta
All India Institute of Speech and Hearing, India

Srinivasan Venkatesan
All India Institute of Speech and Hearing, India

Section 1

Communication Disorders:

Psychosocial Perspectives

Chapter 1
Late Onset Auditory Neuropathy Spectrum Disorder:
A Psychosocial Perspective

Prashanth Prabhu
All India Institute of Speech and Hearing, India

ABSTRACT

The chapter attempts to understand the enigma of late-onset auditory neuropathy spectrum disorder (ANSD) from a psychosocial perspective. The focus of research has always been on accurate diagnosis and management of individuals with ANSD. However, there are limited studies on the psychological problems faced by individuals with late-onset ANSD. In the present chapter, the studies on late-onset ANSD and the psycho-social problems faced by them are reviewed. They experience serious psychosocial issues which need to be addressed urgently for appropriate management of individuals with ANSD. It is highlighted that a psychologist/psychiatrist should be a part of the rehabilitation team for management of individuals with late-onset ANSD. In addition, the focus of rehabilitation should not be restricted to physiological problems, but the psychological problems should also be addressed. Thus, a patient-centric approach in management would definitely improve the quality of life of some individuals with ANSD.

INTRODUCTION

Auditory neuropathy spectrum disorder (ANSD) is a retro-cochlear pathology in which the outer hair cell functioning is normal but there is an abnormality in the auditory nerve (Berlin et al., 2010; Berlin, Hood, Morlet, Rose, and Brashears, 2003; Deltenre et al., 1999; Roush, Frymark, Venediktov, and Wang, 2011; Starr, Picton, Sininger, Hood, and Berlin, 1996). ANSD was first explained by Starr et al. (1991) as a single case study in detail. The condition was later described in detail on ten subjects and named as auditory neuropathy (Starr et al., 1996). The condition is also described using the terminology 'auditory dys-synchrony' as this would better indicate the pathophysiology of the disorder (Berlin, Hood, and Rose, 2001; Berlin, Jeanfreau, Hood, Morlet, and Keats, 2001).

DOI: 10.4018/978-1-5225-4955-0.ch001

The term 'auditory neuropathy' was not preferred as the eighth cranial nerve (Vestibulocochlear nerve/auditory nerve) itself may not be affected as the pathology can be at inner hair cells (IHC) level or at the level of the synapse of IHC and auditory nerve. In addition, the term auditory neuropathy may lead clinicians not to consider cochlear implant as a management option. It has been shown later that the individuals with auditory dys-synchrony benefit from cochlear implants (Berlin et al., 2003; Peterson et al., 2003). A group of audiologists, neonatologists, medical geneticists, hearing scientists and neurologists had a conference for the development of guidelines on identification and appropriate management of auditory neuropathy. One of the decisions taken in the conference was to replace the current terminology used for describing the clinical condition as auditory neuropathy spectrum disorder (ANSD).

ANSD can affect the functioning of inner hair cells, synapse between the inner hair cells and auditory nerve, or the auditory nerve itself (Starr, Sininger, and Pratt, 2000). Individuals with ANSD may manifest asynchronous firing of the auditory nerve fibers due to demyelinization (Starr, Picton, and Kim, 2001). The demyelinization leads to temporal asynchrony in the firing of the auditory nerve fibers and thus reducing the compound action potential of the auditory nerve. Asynchronization not only affects auditory brainstem responses, but also influences auditory perception dependent on temporal cues (Kraus et al., 2000; Rance, McKay, and Grayden, 2004; Starr, Zeng, Michalewski, and Moser, 2010; Zeng, Kong, Michalewski, and Starr, 2005; Zeng, Oba, Garde, Sininger, and Starr, 1999).

The prevalence of ANSD which is reported in Western countries varies from 11% to 0.5% (Berlin et al., 2000; Cone-Wesson and Rance, 2000; Kraus, Ozdamar, Stein, and Reed, 1984; Rance et al., 1999; Tang, McPherson, Yuen, Wong, and Lee, 2004). There are studies on the prevalence of ANSD on 'at risk' children (Rance et al., 1999) and school-aged hearing impaired children (Tang et al., 2004). Tang et al. (2004) reported that the prevalence was 2.44% in school-going children diagnosed as having hearing impairment. Rance et al. (1999) studied 5199 at-risk children and reported that one in 433 (0.23%) was the prevalence of ANSD and the prevalence was one in nine (11.01%) in children with sensorineural hearing loss of degree greater than the moderate degree. Cone-Wesson and Rance, (2000) concluded from their study that everyone in every 200 children with hearing-impaired will have audiological findings which are consistent with the diagnosis of ANSD. Berlin et al. (2000) assessed the prevalence and reported that one percent out of 1000 children studied with severe to profound hearing loss showed robust otoacoustic emissions in one or both ears and 10% of the children showed robust or OAE of lesser amplitude in one ear at least. In the Indian context, Kumar and Jayaram (2006) reported that one in 183 in individuals who are diagnosed as having sensorineural hearing loss had ANSD. The study was conducted retrospectively and reported that among 11,205 clients (5854 males and 5351 females) who had sensorineural hearing loss, sixty-one of them were identified as having ANSD. Bhat, Kumar, and Sinha (2007) suggested that in children with hearing impairment who going to school, the prevalence of ANSD was 2.47%. They studied 220 children who were of four to 16 years old and reported that ANSD is not an extremely rare disorder.

The onset of symptoms related to ANSD can fall into two different age groups. The symptoms of ANSD can be reported from infancy and childhood or these symptoms may begin to appear in adolescence or early adulthood (Berlin et al., 2010; Kumar and Jayaram, 2006; Sininger and Oba, 2001). Majority of the studies carried out in the Western population suggest that approximately only one out of four individuals with ANSD are over the age of 10 years (Berlin et al., 2010; Sininger and Oba, 2001; Starr et al., 2000). However, as the stark contrast, studies carried out on Indian population have reported that the onset of the symptoms of ANSD was majorly in adolescence (16 to 25 years) referred to as late-onset

ANSD (Kumar and Jayaram, 2006; Prabhu, Avilala, and Manjula, 2012; Shivashankar, Satishchandra, Shashikala, and Gore, 2003).

The characteristics of audiological findings in individuals with ANSD are largely variable. The degree of hearing loss can range from normal to profound degree and majority of the clients show the bilateral symmetrical hearing loss (Sininger and Oba, 2001). The individuals with ANSD may show inconsistent responses during pure tone audiometry and may be difficult to estimate the thresholds. Reverse sloping or peaked audiogram configuration is the most common audiogram configuration noticed in individuals with ANSD (Berlin et al., 2010; Kumar and Jayaram, 2006; Narne, Prabhu, Chandan, and Deepthi, 2014). It has also been noted that individuals with ANSD have speech identification scores that are not proportionate to their degree of hearing loss (Li, Wang, Chen, and Liang, 2005; Starr et al., 1996). In individuals with ANSD, the speech perception abilities depend upon the extent to which the temporal distortions occur at higher levels rather than access to speech information as in individuals with cochlear loss (Rance et al., 2004; Zeng et al., 2005).

BACKGROUND

The uncertain etiology and pathophysiology of ANSD poses a challenge for clinical audiologists in the management of individuals with ANSD. Most researchers argue that the presence of OAE in ANSD patients indicate normal functioning of OHC; which suggests that no further amplification is necessary. In addition, the amplification may damage the preserved OHCs which could lead to hearing loss in patients with ANSD (Starr et al., 1996). The use of powerful hearing aids can lead to an irreversible high-frequency sensory loss. There are many studies which report limited hearing aid benefit in individuals with ANSD (Berlin et al., 2010; Jijo and Yathiraj, 2013; Narne et al., 2014; Starr et al., 1996).

Cochlear implants (CI) are reported to be beneficial in few individuals with ANSD (Mason, De Michele, Stevens, Ruth, and Hashisaki, 2003; Shallop, 2002). The cochlear implants may be beneficial if the lesion is in the inner hair cells and may synchronize the available nerve fibers (Shallop, Peterson, Facer, Fabry, and Driscoll, 2001). However, it may be difficult for patients in a developing country like India to afford CI as the majority of the individuals with late-onset ANSD are from low socio-economic status (Prabhu, Avilala, and Manjula, 2012). Thus, hearing aids are the suggested rehabilitation strategy for management of individuals with ANSD.

Narne et al. (2014) studied hearing aid benefit in 128 individuals diagnosed with ANSD and reported that 89 patients with ANSD did not get benefit with hearing aids and only 26 of them were getting benefit with hearing aids in functional use whereas other 13 of the participants obtained limited benefit with the hearing aid (only for sound detection and awareness). Yuvaraj and Jayaram (2016) studied benefit obtained with hearing aid in 38 individuals diagnosed with late-onset ANSD. They reported that amplitude modulation detection, a test of temporal processing test had a significant association with hearing aid benefit in individuals with ANSD. Jijo and Yathiraj (2013) reported audiological findings and benefit with hearing aids obtained in 64 patients diagnosed as ANSD. They reported that majority of individuals with ANSD did not get benefit with hearing aids and hence they suspected that there may be factors other than peripheral neuropathy which may influence hearing aid benefit in individuals with ANSD. Thus, In India, the options for rehabilitation of individuals with ANSD are limited for those who cannot afford costly cochlear implants and other assistive listening devices.

MAIN FOCUS OF THE CHAPTER

Auditory Neuropathy Spectrum Disorder is a retro-cochlear disorder affecting the speech perception and overall communication. The major focus of studies on ANSD is on audio-vestibular problems and their management. In Indian population, the onset of ANSD is reported to be more during adolescents and adulthood (Jijo and Yathiraj, 2012; Kumar and Jayaram, 2006; Narne et al., 2014; Prabhu et al., 2012; Shivashankar, Satishchandra, Shashikala, and Gore, 2003). Shivashankar et al. (2003) studied 24 patients diagnosed as ANSD and reported that except for one patient who had an onset of ANSD at the age of 44 years, the onset of ANSD was in the first and second decade of life. Similarly, Kumar and Jayaram (2006) reported that the onset was between the ages of 14-24 years in 59% of their 61 patients diagnosed as having ANSD. In addition, Prabhu et al. (2012) also suggested in their study that the onset of ANSD was in the age range of 15-25 years. They suggested using the term late-onset ANSD since the majority of them (47.6%) had an onset of ANSD during puberty. Jijo and Yathiraj (2012) also reported similar findings where the onset of ANSD in Indian context was in the first two decades of life, unlike Western studies. Narne et al. (2014) carried out a large-scale retrospective study in India and reported that the onset of ANSD was at adolescence and adulthood in 82% of their study.

Thus, late-onset ANSD can be a quite debilitating condition as the clients are perfectly normal till adolescence and suddenly exhibit auditory symptoms. This leads to poor communication among the peer group, can lead to social isolation and also decline in academic performance. The problem becomes more serious as there are no clear rehabilitation options for individuals with late-onset ANSD. Most of the clients are suggested to use speech reading and manage without hearing aids, as the hearing aids may worsen the performance and can lead to tolerance problems. All these factors can lead to psychological issues such as stress, depression and anxiety among individuals with late-onset ANSD.

It is well reported in the literature that children with cochlear hearing loss experience emotional difficulties (Stevenson, Kreppner, Pimperton, Worsfold, and Kennedy, 2015; Theunissen et al., 2014). The children and adolescents who are diagnosed with cochlear hearing loss score poorer than normal hearing peers on measures on emotional and behavioral difficulties (Stevenson et al., 2015). However, the studies are limited in the literature which attempts to assess the psychological problems faced by children and adolescents with ANSD (Prabhu, 2016; Prabhu and Jamuar, 2017a; Prabhu and Sneha, 2014). It is essential to assess the individual with ANSD as a whole and provide necessary support. The approach in assessment and management of ANSD should also focus on their emotional or psychological problems. There are few studies which have attempted to document the psychological problems and hearing related handicap in individuals with ANSD (Lima, Mantello, and Anastasio, 2015; Prabhu, 2016; Sebastian, Varghese, and Gowri, 2015). In addition, there are attempts to determine tinnitus related handicap (Prabhu and Sneha, 2014) and dizziness related handicap among patients with ANSD (Prabhu and Jamuar, 2017a).

Prabhu (2016) carried out a study to determine the psychological problems in adolescents and young adults with ANSD using Depression Anxiety Stress Scales (DASS). 20 participants diagnosed with ANSD were considered and the subjective rating scale (DASS) was administered on them. He reported that most of the participants experienced the moderate degree of depression and anxiety. He indicated that this could be because of the lack of definite management options especially in individuals with late-onset ANSD. The study also suggested that the psychological problems were found to be more in females compared to males. He also reported that the poor speech identification scores and the longer onset of hearing loss lead to more severe psychological problems. It is reported in the literature that children and adolescents with cochlear hearing loss score poorer than normal hearing peers on measures on emotional and behavioral difficulties (Stevenson et al., 2015). However, with appropriate use of hearing aids, emotional difficulties are reported to reduce in individuals with cochlear hearing loss (Dawes et al., 2015).

The result of Prabhu (2016) study showed that the psychological problems were seen more in females compared to males. It is also reported in the literature that depression occurs approximately twice as often in women compared men (Murray and Lopez, 1996). The family structure in the majority of the families in India needs women to communicate more with the children they are raised. In addition, the majority of rural India still follows a patriarch system where men go to work and women run the family. Thus, the increased need for effective communication by women could have led to poorer scores in females than males. It was also reported that the severity of depression and anxiety increased drastically with increased duration of onset of the problem. This is expected since they are not getting appropriate management and the condition may progress over time among individuals with ANSD. In addition, ignorance regarding the exact reason for their hearing difficulties could have also lead to these symptoms. Thus, early diagnosis and effective rehabilitation of individuals with ANSD could result in the reduction in symptoms of depression, anxiety and stress. He recommends that there is a need to refer individuals with ANSD also for a detailed psychological assessment and possible rehabilitation.

Lima et al. (2015) reported a 47-year-old woman diagnosed with ANSD. She reported that hearing loss had started since approximately five years and it was progressive in nature. Hearing handicap inventory for adults (HHIA) was administered and showed the moderate degree of handicap. They reported that the ANSD had affected her daily life functioning. She was prescribed a hearing aid and HHIA was repeated after three months of hearing aid use. She reported a slight reduction in hearing handicap with the usage of the amplification device. However, she continued to report discomfort in the presence of intense sounds and noise.

Sebastian et al. (2015) attempted to compare the impact of hearing loss on 10 adults with congenital hearing loss and 10 adults with acquired ANSD. They evaluated the quality of life among the two groups using the quality of life Scale (QOLS) questionnaire (Flanagan, 1978). They reported that adults with ANSD also exhibit psychosocial problems in addition to their auditory problems. They suggested that accepting a hearing loss later in life causes more psychological trauma when compared to individuals with congenital hearing loss. The impaired communication can lead to poor social interaction and isolation from peer group which can affect their overall quality of life (Sebastian et al., 2015). This happens because they have developed a personality and lifestyle, which makes it difficult for them to accept the sudden deprivation of audition at a later stage.

Prabhu (2016) attempted to determine the hearing handicap in 50 individuals with ANSD using the questionnaires hearing handicap inventory for adults (HHIA) and Hearing Handicap Questionnaire (HHQ). He reported that there was significant social and emotional related hearing handicap in those participants. He suggested that lower the speech identification scores, the hearing handicap scores were poor. It was hypothesized that the lack of appropriate rehabilitation option and ignorance regarding the actual cause of the late onset ANSD could have resulted in emotional and social handicap in individuals with ANSD. Thus, he suggested that future research should focus on understanding the pathophysiology of ANSD and design innovative management strategies unique to assist individuals with ANSD.

In addition to auditory problems, individuals with ANSD also experience tinnitus and dizziness which can affect their quality of life. Chandan, Prabhu and Deepthi (2013) determined the prevalence of the tinnitus symptom among individuals with ANSD and they reported that tinnitus is prevalent in 67% of individuals. Prabhu et al. (2012) reported tinnitus as a symptom in 83.3% (25 out of 30) of individuals diagnosed with ANSD. Thus, review of the literature suggests that majority of the individuals with ANSD reported of reduced hearing sensitivity, difficulty in understanding speech, and along with that tinnitus was also one of the major symptoms. There are limited studies which provide information about the effects of tinnitus on person's functioning in daily life and emotional distress in individuals with ANSD.

Prabhu and Sneha (2014) administered self-report tinnitus handicap questionnaire (SR-THQ) on 30 adolescents and adults with ANSD with tinnitus. The result of their study showed that the overall mean percentage of tinnitus handicap in individuals in individuals with ANSD was 59.28%. This suggests that they have a significant tinnitus handicap along with the hearing symptoms. The result also shows significant functional handicap which suggests that tinnitus in individuals with ANSD can affect the routine functioning which is usually ignored. The psychological aspects of tinnitus are usually ignored and the result of the emotional domain of SR-THQ suggested that individuals with ANSD had a handicap of 78.66%. This shows that the persistent tinnitus in individuals with ANSD can lead to emotional problems. The result of the catastrophic domain of SR-THQ suggested that tinnitus was also found to be catastrophic in few individuals with ANSD. They reported that tinnitus affects sleep quality, leads to the reduced concentration at work, lack of social interaction and can cause psychological problems. Hence, it is essential to address tinnitus complaint in individuals with ANSD. They should be counseled regarding the available management strategies. In addition, individuals with ANSD also require psychological intervention to resolve emotional problems.

In addition to tinnitus, vertigo can also be one of the complaints reported by individuals with ANSD. Prabhu and Jamuar (2017b) studied the prevalence of vestibular symptoms in 316 individuals with ANSD. They reported that one in five individuals with ANSD reported of at least one of the vestibular symptom. The vestibular symptoms were more in females and in individuals with earlier onset of hearing loss. However, the research on ANSD has focused on assessment and rehabilitation of auditory symptoms and the vestibular symptoms are usually ignored. Thus, it is also important to assess the effect of vertigo/dizziness on the quality of life of individuals with ANSD. There are limited studies on assessment of handicap because of vestibular problems in individuals with ANSD. Prabhu and Jamuar (2017a) administered the questionnaire dizziness handicap inventory (DHI) on 40 adolescents and adults with ANSD with the complaint of giddiness. They reported that the participants experienced had the moderate degree of dizziness related handicap. They concluded that dizziness affected the quality of life among individuals with ANSD causing emotional problems. They recommend providing appropriate psychosocial support in individuals with ANSD with giddiness.

SOLUTIONS AND RECOMMENDATIONS

There is a very limited literature which addresses the psycho-social problems faced by adolescents and adults with ANSD. It is a common practice to focus on audiological assessment and management of individuals with hearing loss. However, audiologists fail to understand the person and his difficulties in real life situation. Late-onset ANSD can have serious psychosocial issues which are usually ignored. Individuals with congenital hearing loss would know that they have hearing loss but for an individual with late-onset hearing loss, he would have already developed a personality and lifestyle which would fail to integrate hearing loss. This can be a debilitating condition as it completely restricts their communication skills. The personal, social and professional life of the person is drastically affected. The emotional trauma can lead to significant psychological problems in individuals with late-onset ANSD. There are anecdotal reports that many individuals with ANSD are on medicines for depression. They also have high suicidal tendencies as they have suddenly lost their ability to communicate. This tendency further increases as there is no definite rehabilitation option for individuals with ANSD. These serious psychosocial issues need to be addressed urgently for appropriate management of individuals with ANSD. Considering the psycho-social issues, it is highlighted that a psychologist/psychiatrist should be a part of the rehabilitation team for management of individuals with late-onset ANSD. They can provide the necessary psychosocial intervention which is essential for improving the quality of life of individuals with ANSD. In addition, the audiologists should also focus their research on improving hearing aid/cochlear implant strategies to assist in the appropriate rehabilitation of individuals with late-onset ANSD. Counseling, psychoeducation, advocacy, support services, bibliotherapy, and family-centered early intervention services, can be attempted in the management of ANSD. Parent-professional engagements in the management and monitoring process can also further help to optimize outcomes of therapy.

CONCLUSION

The present chapter attempted to understand the enigma of late-onset ANSD from a psychosocial perspective. Most of the literature is focused on assessment and rehabilitation of individuals with ANSD. There are few studies which have attempted to explore their psychosocial problems, hearing handicap, handicap due to tinnitus and vertigo. This is very important because individuals with late-onset ANSD lose their hearing all of a sudden and it ruins their lifestyle. Hearing loss is quite traumatic for them and it affects the material well-being, health and relationship with relatives and spouse. It limits the extent to which they can help others, their civic activities, occupational role, and socialization. Their independence, as well as the quantity of recreation, is also restricted, followed by the deprivation of hearing sense. Thus, professionals need to be sensitive to the emotional problems of individuals with late-onset ANSD. Psychological trauma is as important as their physiological problem and psychological referral to a clinical psychologist may be beneficial to many individuals with ANSD. Thus, the chapter highlights that professionals treating individuals with late-onset ANSD should incorporate patient-centric approach and attempt to treat the patient as a whole than being techno-centric and focusing on accurate diagnosis.

ACKNOWLEDGMENT

The author acknowledges Dr. S. R. Savithri, Director, All India Institute of Speech and Hearing, Mysuru for providing the support.

REFERENCES

Berlin, C. I., Hood, L., Morlet, T., Den, Z., Goforth, L., Tedesco, S., ... Keats, B. (2000). The search for auditory neuropathy patients and connexin 26 patients in schools for the deaf. *ARO Abstracts*, *23*, 23–24.

Berlin, C. I., Hood, L., & Rose, K. (2001). On renaming auditory neuropathy as auditory dys-synchrony. *Audiology Today*, *13*, 15–17.

Berlin, C. I., Hood, L. J., Morlet, T., Rose, K., & Brashears, S. (2003). Auditory Neuropathy/Dys-Synchrony: Diagnosis and Management. *Developmental Disabilities Research Reviews*, *9*(4), 225–231. doi:10.1002/mrdd.10084 PMID:14648814

Berlin, C. I., Hood, L. J., Morlet, T., Wilensky, D., Li, L., Mattingly, K. R., ... Frisch, S. A. (2010). Multi-site diagnosis and management of 260 patients with auditory neuropathy/dys-synchrony (auditory neuropathy spectrum disorder). *International Journal of Audiology*, *49*(1), 30–43. doi:10.3109/14992020903160892 PMID:20053155

Berlin, C. I., Jeanfreau, J., Hood, L., Morlet, T., & Keats, B. (2001). Managing and renaming auditory neuropathy as part of a continuum of auditory dys-synchrony. *ARO Abstracts*, *24*, 137.

Bhat, J. S., Kumar, K., & Sinha, S. K. (2007). Auditory Neuropathy/Dys-synchrony In School-aged Hearing-impaired Children: A South Indian Perspective. *Asia Pacific Journal of Speech, Language and Hearing*, *10*(3), 157–164. doi:10.1179/136132807805297512

Chandan, H. S., Prabhu, P., & Deepthi, M. (2013). Prevalence and characteristics of tinnitus in individuals with auditory neuropathy spectrum disorder. *Hearing, Balance and Communication*, *11*(4), 214–217. doi:10.3109/21695717.2013.821755

Cone-Wesson, B., & Rance, G. (2000). *Auditory neuropathy: A brief review*. Retrieved August 6, 2014, from http://journals.lww.com/co-otolaryngology/Abstract/2000/10000/Auditory_neuropathy__a_brief_review.12.aspx

Dawes, P., Emsley, R., Cruickshanks, K. J., Moore, D. R., Fortnum, H., Edmondson-Jones, M., ... Munro, K. J. (2015). Hearing loss and cognition: The role of hearing AIDS, social isolation and depression. *PLoS One*, *10*(3), e0119616. doi:10.1371/journal.pone.0119616 PMID:25760329

Deltenre, P., Mansbach, A., Bozet, C., Christiaens, F., Barthelemy, P., Paulissen, D., & Renglet, T. (1999). Auditory neuropathy with preserved cochlear microphonics and secondary loss of otoacoustic emissions. *Audiology*, *38*(4), 187–195. doi:10.3109/00206099909073022 PMID:10431904

Flanagan, J. C. (1978). A research approach to improving our quality of life. *The American Psychologist*, *33*(2), 138–147. doi:10.1037/0003-066X.33.2.138

Jijo, P. M., & Yathiraj, A. (2012). Audiological Characteristics and Duration of the Disorder in Individuals with Auditory Neuropathy Spectrum Disorder (ANSD) - A Retrospective Study. *Journal of Indian Speech and Hearing Association*, *26*(1), 17–26.

Jijo, P. M., & Yathiraj, A. (2013). Audiological findings and aided performance in individuals with auditory neuropathy spectrum disorder (ANSD)-A retrospective study. *Journal of Hearing Science*, *3*(1), 18–26.

Kraus, N., Bradlow, A. R., Cheatham, M. A., Cunningham, J., King, C. D., Koch, D. B., ... Wright, B. A. (2000). Consequences of neural asynchrony: A case of auditory neuropathy. *Journal of the Association for Research in Otolaryngology*, *1*(1), 33–45. doi:10.1007101620010004 PMID:11548236

Kraus, N., Ozdamar, O., Stein, L., & Reed, N. (1984). Absent auditory brain stem response: Peripheral hearing loss or brain stem dysfunction? *The Laryngoscope*, *94*(3), 400–406. doi:10.1288/00005537-198403000-00019 PMID:6700356

Kumar, U. A., & Jayaram, M. (2006). Prevalence and audiological characteristics in individuals with auditory neuropathy/auditory dys-synchrony. *International Journal of Audiology*, *45*(6), 360–366. doi:10.1080/14992020600624893 PMID:16777783

Li, F., Wang, H., Chen, J., & Liang, R. (2005). Auditory neuropathy in children (analysis of 14 cases). *Journal of Clinical Otorhinolaryngology*, *19*(1), 19–21. PMID:15830698

Lima, A., Mantello, E., & Anastasio, A. (2015). Monitoring the hearing handicap and the recognition threshold of sentences of a patient with unilateral auditory neuropathy spectrum disorder with use of a hearing aid. *International Archives of Otorhinolaryngology*, *20*(2), 185–188. doi:10.1055-0034-1397338 PMID:27096026

Mason, J. C., De Michele, A., Stevens, C., Ruth, R. A., & Hashisaki, G. T. (2003). Cochlear implantation in patients with auditory neuropathy of varied etiologies. *The Laryngoscope*, *113*(1), 45–49. doi:10.1097/00005537-200301000-00009 PMID:12514381

Murray, C. J. L., & Lopez, A. D. (1996). *The global burden of disease : A comprehensive assessment of mortality and disability from diseases, injuries, and risk factors in 1990 and projected to 2020*. Boston: Harvard School of Public Health: World Health Organization.

Narne, V. K., Prabhu, P., Chandan, H. S., & Deepthi, M. (2014). Audiological profiling of 198 individuals with auditory neuropathy spectrum disorder. *Hearing, Balance and Communication*, *12*(3), 112–120. doi:10.3109/21695717.2014.938481

Peterson, A., Shallop, J., Driscoll, C., Breneman, A., Babb, J., Stoeckel, R., & Fabry, L. (2003). Outcomes of cochlear implantation in children with auditory neuropathy. *Journal of the American Academy of Audiology*, *14*(4), 188–201. PMID:12940703

Prabhu, P. (2016). Evaluation of depression, anxiety, and stress in adolescents and young adults with auditory neuropathy spectrum disorder. *Scientifica*, *2016*, 1–8. doi:10.1155/2016/4378269 PMID:27579218

Prabhu, P., Avilala, V. K. Y., & Manjula, P. (2012). Predisposing factors in individuals with late-onset auditory dys-synchrony. *Asia Pacific Journal of Speech, Language and Hearing*, *15*(1), 41–50. doi:10.1179/136132812805253758

Prabhu, P., & Jamuar, P. (2017a). Evaluation of dizziness handicap in adolescents and adults with auditory neuropathy spectrum disorder. *International Archives of Otorhinolaryngology*, *49*(1), 30–43.

Prabhu, P., & Jamuar, P. (2017b). Prevalence of vestibular symptoms in individuals with auditory neuropathy spectrum disorder-A retrospective study. *Intractable & Rare Diseases Research*, *6*(1), 46–49. doi:10.5582/irdr.2016.01098 PMID:28357181

Prabhu, P. P., & Sneha, P. (2014). Self report tinnitus handicap in individuals with auditory neuropathy spectrum disorder. *Journal of Hearing Science*, *4*(3), 43–50.

Rance, G., Beer, D. E., Cone-Wesson, B., Shepherd, R. K., Dowell, R. C., King, A. M., ... Clark, G. M. (1999). Clinical findings for a group of infants and young children with auditory neuropathy. *Ear and Hearing*, *20*(3), 238–252. doi:10.1097/00003446-199906000-00006 PMID:10386850

Rance, G., McKay, C., & Grayden, D. (2004). Perceptual characterization of children with auditory neuropathy. *Ear and Hearing*, *25*(1), 34–46. doi:10.1097/01.AUD.0000111259.59690.B8 PMID:14770016

Roush, P., Frymark, T., Venediktov, R., & Wang, B. (2011). Audiologic management of auditory neuropathy spectrum disorder in children: A systematic review of the literature. *American Journal of Audiology*, *20*(2), 159–170. doi:10.1044/1059-0889(2011/10-0032) PMID:21940978

Sebastian, S., Varghese, A., & Gowri, M. (2015). The impact of hearing loss in the life of adults: A comparison between congenital versus late onset hearing loss. *Indian Journal of Otology*, *21*(1), 29. doi:10.4103/0971-7749.152857

Shallop, J. (2002). Auditory neuropathy/dys-synchrony in adults and children. *Seminars in Hearing*, *23*(3), 215–223. doi:10.1055-2002-34474

Shallop, J., Peterson, A., Facer, G. W., Fabry, L. B., & Driscoll, C. L. (2001). Cochlear implants in five cases of auditory neuropathy: Postoperative findings and progress. *The Laryngoscope*, *111*(4), 555–562. doi:10.1097/00005537-200104000-00001 PMID:11359119

Shivashankar, N., Satishchandra, P., Shashikala, H. R., & Gore, M. (2003). Primary auditory neuropathy-An enigma. *Acta Neurologica Scandinavica*, *108*(2), 130–135. doi:10.1034/j.1600-0404.2003.00104.x PMID:12859291

Sininger, Y., & Oba, S. (2001). Patients with auditory neuropathy: Who are they and what can they hear? In Y. Sininger & A. Starr (Eds.), *Auditory neuropathy: A new perspective on hearing disorder* (pp. 15–36). Singular Publishing Group.

Starr, A., McPherson, D., Patterson, J., Don, M., Luxford, W., Shannon, R., ... Waring, M. (1991). Absence of both auditory evoked potentials and auditory percepts dependent on timing cues. *Brain*, *114*(3), 1157–1180. doi:10.1093/brain/114.3.1157 PMID:2065245

Starr, A., Picton, T. W., & Kim, R. (2001). Pathophysiology of auditory neuropathy. In Y. Sininger & A. Starr (Eds.), *Auditory neuropathy: A new perspective on hearing disorder* (pp. 67–82). Singular Publishing Group.

Starr, A., Picton, T. W., Sininger, Y., Hood, L. J., & Berlin, C. I. (1996). Auditory neuropathy. *Brain*, *119*(3), 741–753. doi:10.1093/brain/119.3.741 PMID:8673487

Starr, A., Sininger, Y. S., & Pratt, H. (2000). The varieties of auditory neuropathy. *Journal of Basic and Clinical Physiology and Pharmacology*, *11*(3), 215–230. doi:10.1515/JBCPP.2000.11.3.215 PMID:11041385

Starr, A., Zeng, F. G., Michalewski, H. J., & Moser, T. (2010). Perspectives on auditory neuropathy: Disorders of inner hair Cell, auditory nerve, and their synapse. In The Senses: A Comprehensive Reference, (3), 397–412.

Stevenson, J., Kreppner, J., Pimperton, H., Worsfold, S., & Kennedy, C. (2015). Emotional and behavioural difficulties in children and adolescents with hearing impairment: A systematic review and meta-analysis. *European Child & Adolescent Psychiatry*, *24*(5), 477–496. doi:10.100700787-015-0697-1 PMID:25758233

Tang, Y., McPherson, B., Yuen, K. C. P., Wong, L. L. N., & Lee, J. S. M. (2004). Auditory neuropathy/auditory dys-synchrony in school children with hearing loss: Frequency of occurrence. *International Journal of Pediatric Otorhinolaryngology*, *68*(2), 175–183. doi:10.1016/j.ijporl.2003.10.004 PMID:14725984

Theunissen, S. C. P. M., Rieffe, C., Netten, A. P., Briaire, J. J., Soede, W., Kouwenberg, M., & Frijns, J. H. M. (2014). Self-esteem in hearing-impaired children: The influence of communication, education, and audiological characteristics. *PLoS One*, *9*(4), e94521. doi:10.1371/journal.pone.0094521 PMID:24722329

Yuvaraj, P., & Jayaram, M. (2016). Audiological profile of adult persons with auditory neuropathy spectrum disorders. *Journal of Audiology & Otology*, *20*(3), 158–167. doi:10.7874/jao.2016.20.3.158 PMID:27942602

Zeng, F., Kong, Y., Michalewski, H. J., & Starr, A. (2005). Perceptual consequences of disrupted auditory nerve activity. *Journal of Neurophysiology*, *93*(6), 3050–3063. doi:10.1152/jn.00985.2004 PMID:15615831

Zeng, F., Oba, S., Garde, S., Sininger, Y., & Starr, A. (1999). Temporal and speech processing deficits in auditory neuropathy. *Neuroreport*, *10*(16), 3429–3435. doi:10.1097/00001756-199911080-00031 PMID:10599857

KEY TERMS AND DEFINITIONS

Assistive Listening Device: They are special amplification devices which would be beneficial at adverse listening conditions.

Auditory Brainstem Response: Electrical potentials generated from the auditory brainstem. It checks for the integrity of the brainstem.

Cochlear Implants: It is a prosthesis that is inserted surgically inside the inner ear of the patient. It stimulates the auditory nerve directly through electrical stimulation.

Hearing Aids: Amplification device to amplify the soft sounds. It is used as a management strategy for individuals with the sensorineural hearing loss.

Otoacoustic Emissions: Emissions from the outer hair cells of the cochlea obtained from the healthy cochlea.

Tinnitus: The perception of the ringing sensation in the ears.

Vertigo: The sensation of rotation or feeling of spinning sensation.

Chapter 2
Psychosocial Perspectives of Persons With Aphasia

Sunil Kumar Ravi
Shravana Institute of Speech and Hearing, India

Anusha Chilakalapudi
GSR Institute of Craniofacial and Facial Plastic Surgery, India

Krupa Saira George
Samvaad Institute of Speech and Hearing, India

Divya P.
Naseema Institute of Speech and Hearing, India

Shyamala K. Chengappa
All India Institute of Speech and Hearing, India

ABSTRACT

Psychosocial problems are one of the major issues seen in persons with aphasia (PWA), but the severity of these psychosocial problems vary depending upon age, socioeconomic status, nature of job pre-morbidly, family support, emotional factors, and quality of life. The International Classification of Functioning, Disability, and Health (ICF) by World Health Organization in the field of communication disorders, specifically for aphasia and other neurogenic communication disorders, provided clear guidelines and information about the importance of assessment and treatment of PWA in terms of body functions and structures, activities and participation, and environmental and personal factors affecting the quality of life in these individuals. The present chapter is primarily focused on studying the psychosocial aspects in PWA, specifically the quality of life and other psychosocial disturbances in the Indian context.

INTRODUCTION

Traditionally, aphasia has been defined as loss of language and other language-related functions as a result of brain damage caused majorly by cerebrovascular accidents and also the small proportion of other causes such as TBI, tumor, infections and so on. Typically, the deficits in persons with aphasia

DOI: 10.4018/978-1-5225-4955-0.ch002

are limited to language expression and comprehension abilities with or without hemiplegia. Although the research on aphasia has been in place since the early 19th century, much of research was focused on understanding the relationship between neuropathology of brain damage and linguistic deficits. This research on neuropathology and aphasia has been the basis for several classifications of aphasia based on neuroanatomical (Boston classification), linguistic (fluent Vs non-fluent) and psycholinguistic classifications. However, these approaches have focused majorly on linguistic and other related deficits and not much importance was given to psychosocial aspects of persons with aphasia (PWA) till recently. Further, research in the 19th century and early 20th century was also focused on developing several tools/tests and intervention techniques/approaches for assessment and intervention of underlying neuropathology and linguistic deficits in PWA. This research has yielded several test batteries and treatment approaches such as melodic intonation therapy, semantic feature therapy, etc. In recent years, the focus was given on assessing and understanding of functional communication skills in individuals with aphasia and this has led to the development of tests for assessing functional communication in PWA.

However, from the perspective of a PWA, aphasia does not only affect the individual's language or motor abilities, rather it affects multiple domains such as quality of life, psychological, emotions, lifestyle, social life, and so on. Several studies have reported presence of depression and other psychological disturbances due to limited language and motor abilities in PWA and these, in turn, affect the person's quality of life to the greater extent. Psychosocial problems are one of the major issues seen in adults with aphasia, although, the severity of these psychosocial problems vary among PWA depending upon their age, socioeconomic status, nature of job pre-morbidly, family support, emotional factors and quality of life. The International Classification of Functioning, Disability and Health (ICF; World Health Organization, 2001) in the field of communication disorders, specifically for aphasia and other neurogenic communication disorders provided clear guidelines and information about the importance of assessment and treatment of PWA in terms of body functions and structures, activities and participation, and environmental and personal factors affecting the quality of life in PWA. The ICF framework helps us to understand the effects of aphasia on activities and participation which are in turn causing poor quality of life in PWA. The present chapter is primarily focused on understanding the psychosocial aspects in persons with aphasia assessed though Stroke Specific Quality of Life, specifically the quality of life and other psychosocial disturbances in the Indian context. The present chapter also focuses on the importance of assessment, team approach, and review of available tests for assessment and intervention of psychosocial issues in PWA, and applications of ICF model to persons with aphasia in the Indian context.

BACKGROUND

Aphasia

Aphasia has been described as an impairment or loss of language abilities following damage to the nervous system (Benson, 1979). This definition was considered as suitable one by many researchers as it includes the necessary elements like loss of language and brain damage. However, other researchers challenge this definition on the factors like aphasia is not solely language disorder that is caused by brain damage, but there are several other disorders like dementia, closed head injury, right hemisphere damage, and so on. However, the definitions by Darley (1982) and Goodglass and Kaplan (1983) have given the definitions of aphasia in detail focusing on the type of language impairments and other associated symptoms.

Cerebrovascular accident or stroke is one of the major causes of aphasia. Other causes include traumatic brain injury, degenerative disorders, tumors, dementia (Au, Albert, and Obler, 1988), and so on. In India, the prevalence of stroke has been estimated to be around 203 per 1,00,000 population by Sethi (2002), approximately amounting to one million patients. Sudlow and Warlow (1997) have reported that incidence of stroke is approximately 238 and 627 in France and Russia. It is estimated that approximately 20 percent of people who have had an acute stroke will have aphasia (Brust, Shafer, Richer, and Bruun, 1976)

The type and severity of deficits vary depending upon the site of lesion and extent of lesion in individuals with aphasia. The classification model also called as Wernicke-Lichtheim-Geschwind model given by Geschwind, 1965 was taken as the basis for development of several test batteries which in turn classifies aphasic individuals into different types of aphasia. The early classification of aphasia is *fluent* and *non-fluent* types of aphasia. In non-fluent type of aphasia, the speech is slow and hesitant with lack of articulatory precision. Apraxia of speech may also be present in some of the aphasic individuals as an associated symptom. These individuals will have deficits in spontaneous speech, repetition, and naming aspects in varying severity levels with normal or near normal auditory comprehension abilities. In fluent type of aphasia, individual will have a very fluent speech without any hesitations, pauses but have more difficulties in auditory comprehension. The *fluent type* of aphasia includes Wernicke's, conduction, transcortical sensory and anomic aphasia. The *non-fluent type* of aphasia includes global, Broca's, transcortical motor, and mixed aphasia.

Individuals with aphasia exhibit deficits in various components of language, such as phonological impairments, semantic and syntactic impairments and pragmatic impairments majorly. Some of the language deficits include agrammatism, paragrammatism, semantic and phonological paraphasias, etc. depending upon the site and extent of the lesion.

Several tests and batteries are available for assessment of language deficits in individuals with aphasia. Some of them focus on classifying the type of aphasia, some on measuring the severity of aphasia and some on assessing specific language skills in individuals with aphasia. These tests are again classified based on the screening, diagnostic and functional communication assessment tests. Boston Diagnostic Aphasia Examination (BDAE; Goodglass and Kaplan, 1972) and Western Aphasia Battery (WAB; Kertesz, 1982) are the two major diagnostic assessment batteries developed to classify the type of aphasia into various types. Other than these two diagnostic tests, there are other tests to assess individual language functions include Porch Index of Communicative ability (PICA; Porch, 1971), Minnesota Test for Differential Diagnosis of Aphasia (MTDDA; Schuell, 1965).

Although aphasia has been defined as loss of language following brain damage by several authors, these individuals with aphasia are presented with various associated deficits in motor, sensory and cognitive systems with varying severity. Hemiparesis or hemiplegia is commonly associated with Broca's aphasia and the severity of the paralysis range from mild weakness to severe levels. The hemiparesis may affect upper and lower limbs, and also the articulatory system on the affected side. Majority of non-fluent types of aphasics also exhibit apraxia of speech, a motor speech disorder as a co-morbid condition. Individuals with aphasia often exhibit disorders of awareness including motor neglect, inattention and confusional states and sensory deficits such as somatosensory and visual field deficits. Denial of illness is commonly seen in patients with Wernicke's type of Aphasia, whereas, the non-fluent aphasics exhibit more of psychological and emotional disturbances.

Psychosocial Problems in Aphasia

Research studies in western context have reported a close relationship between the effectiveness of communication to psychosocial well-being of the person with aphasia. Language enhances the person's participation in social relations, share experiences and thoughts as it has been described as a method of communicating ideas (Sapir, 1921). In the majority of patients with aphasia following stroke is a sudden onset which limits the language abilities with or without hemiplegia causing limitations in the psychosocial functioning and quality of life of the individual.

Limited language and motor abilities following stroke and aphasia lead to various psychosocial problems, such as depression, frustration, emotional instability, isolation in the social context, changes in the roles and responsibilities in family, difficulties at work and unemployment. These psychosocial and emotional factors have been identified as factors in estimating the prognosis and recovery during and after rehabilitation. Several studies have also reported the higher prevalence of psychological symptoms such as depression due to limitations in their activities, social relations and participation in daily activities which in turn increases dependency on others. Worral and Holland (2003) reported that both external and internal factors have the significant effect on the psychosocial well-being of individuals with aphasia.

One of the major factors affecting psychosocial well-being is limited communication abilities which limit the participation in multiple contexts including family, social, occupational contexts majorly. Individuals with aphasia do exhibit difficulty in communicating their basic needs and carrying out their daily activities and maintaining social communications. Difficulties faced by the communication partners with aphasic speakers will, in turn, increase the psychological disturbances in these individuals.

Social Life Among Persons With Aphasia

Aphasia can cause significant limitations in participation in social activities leading to poor social life and social relationships. One of the major limitations in social life is limited participation in leisure activities such as meeting relatives and friends, attending events, and going out with family members to picnic, etc. due to limited communication abilities and physical impairments. The social life of persons with aphasia is highly correlated with severity of aphasia, communication abilities, emotional health, and age, etc causing severe limitations in the social life of persons with aphasia which, in turn, lead to limited diverse social networks.

Research on the social life among persons with stroke and aphasia have reported significant limitation in social participation in stroke survivors compared to non-aphasic participants, leading to social isolation and exclusion (Cruice, Worrall, and Hickson, 2006; Cruce, Hill, Worrall, and Hickson, 2010; Parr, 2007). Social participation and social life have been shown to be important factors in recovery in individuals with aphasia as these factors contribute significantly to the psychological health, psychosocial well-being, and quality of life (Billings and Moos, 1982; Glass and Maddox, 1992).

In the Indian context, the social life among persons with aphasia differs depending upon several factors such as nuclear/joint family, age, place of living (rural or urban), etc. Social life and participation may be better when the person with aphasia belong to the joint family or from rural areas as more number of family members and friends can significantly improve the social interaction compared to nuclear families or in urban areas. However, the impact of these factors on social life and participation needs to be studied in more detail in the Indian context in view of the varied cultural differences. The cultural factors may also play a significant role in social life of stroke survivors or persons with aphasia which can improve the overall quality of life and life satisfaction.

Return to Work Following Stroke and Aphasia

Individuals with aphasia do exhibit more difficulty in returning to their job due to limited communication abilities and physical abilities which will, in turn, cause emotional disturbances and psychological symptoms in these individuals. Research in the area of returning to work after stroke in western context have shown that stroke patients have improved the overall psychological well-being following return to work (Koch, Egbert, Coeling, and Ayers, 2005; Medin, Barajas, and Ekberg, 2006), however, this is reported to be affected by the job retention and performance at workplace (Possl, Jurgensmeyer, Karlbauer, Wenz, and Goldenberg, 2001). A study on stroke patients in United States by Edwards, Hahn, Baum, and Dromerick (2006) reported that approximately 62% of the patients have experienced difficulty in getting employment following stroke even though they could recover from their motor impairments in 6 months post-stroke which in turn affected the life satisfaction and quality of life among them. Similar findings were also given by Teassell, McRae, and Finestone (2000) for Canadian population, where the authors have reported that only 9% of the stroke population had reported back to their full-time employment and approximately 8% of the stroke population had been employed in part-time jobs. The scenario is no different in the United Kingdom, where 65% of the stroke survivors had been unemployed following stroke and approximately 14% of the stroke survivors had changed their working hours as a result of impairments following stroke (Kersten, Low, Ashburn, George, and McLellan, 2002).

The status of employment after stroke in India is very much similar to the western context, where most of the stroke patients could not return to their work subsequent to stroke and aphasia, although there are no research studies to estimate the effect of stroke on employment in the Indian context. The scenario in India may be more devastating as many of the stroke survivors belongs to the family where the stroke patient himself is a sole earner prior to stroke and losing employment following the stroke will push them into severe financial crisis in the family which will, in turn, cause severe psychosocial problems. Further, a majority of the stroke patients belong to lower and middle socioeconomic status, the unemployment after stroke due to physical and communication deficits can significantly affect their quality of life. The lack of employment following the stroke in India can also be due to non-availability of safe, secure, stable and suitable work environment which will consider the capacity of the stroke patient while returning to their job. In the majority of private organizations, the stroke patients are forced to retire as the employer feels that these individuals cannot return to work due to motor, language and communication deficits.

Although, the United Nations Convention on the Rights of Persons with Disabilities (UNCRPD; 2006) has provided guidelines for people with stroke to return to their work, the implementation of the same has been poor in several parts of the country. The individuals with aphasia should be provided with the suitable employment in the offices and make arrangements for a barrier-free environment to accommodate these individuals. Further studies are required to understand the status of employment following the stroke, factors associated with unemployment in the Indian context and the consequences of unemployment on the quality of life and on psychosocial well-being of persons with aphasia.

Quality of Life in Persons With Aphasia

From the perspective of a PWA, aphasia does not only affect the individual's language or motor abilities, rather it affects multiple domains such as psychological, emotional, lifestyle, social life, etc which will sequentially affect the quality of life of the person with aphasia. Quality of life has been described as an individual's perception about their life in the personal and social contexts and the quality of life depend on the broad range of aspects such as physical and mental health, psychological state, relationships in social context and environmental factors (WHOQoL Group, 1995). A subdomain of quality of life is health-related quality of life (HRQL) and it is mainly focused on the impact of any disease or disorder on quality of life in individuals and it involves assessment of multiple functions including physical health, psychological well being, social and independent functioning. Quality of life may not be same in any two individuals with aphasia, as this is based on person's own perspective of their life. The quality of life may not only give us information about communication or motor deficits, rather it serves as an index for the well-being of the person with aphasia in a holistic manner.

At present, few standard scales are available for assessing the quality of life in individuals with stroke and aphasia in the western context. These questionnaires are divided into aphasia-related, stroke-related and general health-related quality of life scales. Aphasia related quality of life scales include Stroke and Aphasia Quality of Life Scale – 39 (SAQOL-39; Hilari, Byng, Lamping, and Smith, 2003), Aachen Quality of Life Inventory (ALQI; Engell, Hutter, Willmes, and Huber, 2003), and Quality of Communication Life scale (ASHA QCL; Paul et al., 2003).

SAQOL-39 (Hilari et al., 2003) consists of 39 items categorized into physical, psychosocial, communication and energy domains and has been validated on individuals with stroke and aphasia. The four domains of the SAQOL have been majorly affected in individuals with aphasia following stroke and it requires less time compared to other scales. Aachen Quality of Life Inventory (ALQI; Engell et al., 2003) was an adaptation of Sickness Impact Profile and this scale offers the assessment of the quality of life using pictorial stimuli thereby it helps in minimizing the language demands. The scale consists of physical and psychosocial domains and it yields a correlation between the two domains. The physical domain includes items on hemiplegia, and mobility difficulties, whereas the psychosocial domain considers patients emotional and mood state.

Several studies have been carried out on understanding the quality of life among individuals with aphasia since 1990 using scales of quality of life in western context. Few of the studies have also focused on studying the factors affecting the quality of life in individuals with aphasia. Williams et al. (1999) reported that language, upper extremity functioning and social roles were the most affected domains which affect their quality of life. Hilari et al. (2003) have developed Stroke and Aphasia Quality of Life Scale and were used on 95 individuals with long-term aphasia to evaluate the quality of life, acceptability and reliability of the scale and the authors reported the significant decline in the major domains of the scale such as physical, psychosocial, communication and energy. Hobart, Williams, Moran and Thompson (2002) investigated the quality of life after stroke using 36-item Short-Form Health Survey (SF-36) on 177 individuals with stroke. The results revealed the significant effect of stroke on the physical, psychological and social functioning of the individuals following stroke. However, the authors have also reported limited validity for SF-36 scale in assessing the quality of life of stroke survivors due to the limited scoring algorithm.

Similar results were found in a study by Cordini, Oda, and Furlanetto (2005) on Brazilian individuals with aphasia reported that the energy, work, upper extremity function and social roles were the major

Table 1. Summary of Quality of Life scales specifically for persons with stroke

Quality of Life Measurement Scales	Authors	Domains Covered	No. of Items
Stroke and Aphasia Quality of Life Scale – 39 (SAQOL-39)	Hilari, Byng, Lamping, and Smith, 2003	Physical, communication, psychological and energy	39
Aachen Quality of Life Inventory (ALQI)	Engell, Hutter, Willmes, and Huber, 2003	Activity, movement, home management, social interaction, family relationship, ambulation, communication, leisure, self-support, cognition, language	117
WHO Quality of Life questionnaire (WHOQOL-BREF)	WHOQOL Group, 1998	Physical, psychological, social and environment	26
Stroke-Specific Quality of Life Scale (SSQOL)	Williams, Weinberger, Harris, Clark and Biller, 1999	Family roles, language, energy, mood, mobility, thinking, personality, self-care, social roles, upper extremities functioning, vision, and work/productivity	49
Short-Form Health Survey (SF-36)	Ware, Snow, Kosinski, and Gandek (1993)	Physical functioning, role-physical, bodily pain, general health, vitality, social functioning, role-emotional, mental health (these are categorized under Physical and Mental health)	36
Niemi Quality of Life Scale	Niemi, Laaksonen, Kotila, and Weltimo (1988)	Working conditions, activities at home, family relationships, leisure activities	58
Ferrans and Powers Quality of Life Index-Stroke Version	Ferrans and Powers (1985)	Health and functioning, socioeconomic, psychological/spiritual, family	38
Stroke-Adapted Sickness Impact Profile (SA-SIP30)	van Straten, de Haan, Limburg, Schuling, Bossuyt, and van den Bos (1997)	Body care and movement, social interaction, mobility, communication, emotional behavior, household management, alertness behavior, ambulation	30

factors affecting their quality of life. The study also reported vision, mood, personality and family roles as the least affected domains in these individuals.

Sinanović, Mrkonjić, and Zečić, (2012) have investigated the impact of severity and type of aphasia on quality of life in 51 patients with aphasia (divided into 7 types of aphasia) following the stroke after one-year post onset. All the participants were assessed using the SAQOL-39 which consists of 39 questions in four domains, physical (17 questions), communication (7 questions), psychosocial domain (11 questions) and energy (4 questions) domains and each question is rated on a five-point rating scale where 1 indicates minimal or worse result and 5 indicates maximal or best result. The overall results indicated highest scores on the physical domain with an average score of 3.38 followed by psychosocial domain with 3.36 points followed by communication domain with 2.91 points followed by energy domain with 2.86 points. Analysis of scores of each subtype of aphasia indicated lowest scores on quality of life scale for Broca's aphasia and highest scores for anomic aphasia. The severity of aphasia also had the significant effect on the domains of quality of life and also on the overall scores of quality of life in these individuals. The authors have reported that this may be due to the fact that individuals with non-fluent aphasia have severe deficits in communication which may, in turn, cause psychological problems compared to fluent types of aphasia.

Bahia and Chun (2014) have conducted the study on quality of life on Portuguese speaking 11 individuals with aphasia using Stroke Specific Quality of Life (SS-QOL) Scale using structured interview method. Authors have reported the significant decline in QOL following stroke even in individuals with mild severity. The results revealed poor quality of life in non-fluent types of aphasics than influent types of aphasia although it is not significant. Among the domains of SS-QOL, the non-fluent aphasics reported that thinking abilities, social roles and language abilities were the factors majorly affecting their quality of life, whereas, in fluent aphasics, the major factors were personality, social roles and thinking. The study also found that energy, family roles and vision as the least affected domains in non-fluent aphasics and vision, self-care and mobility were the least affected domains in fluent aphasia group.

However, few studies have also reported that there is no correlation between the severities of aphasia to the perception of quality of life among individuals with aphasia. One such study was by Ross and Wertz (2002), who have conducted the study on the perception of quality of life on individuals with aphasia using the brief WHO Quality of Life questionnaire (WHOQOL-BREF: WHOQOL Group, 1998) which consists of 26 questions with each one being rated on a 5-point scale. Although the results of the study have shown the significant decline in quality of life following stroke and aphasia, the authors have not found the correlation between formal language and communication tests and the scores on quality of life questionnaire. Among the domains of quality of life, individuals with aphasia have reported significant difficulties with independence, social relationships, and the environment. Although there exist several scales and questionnaires for assessing the quality of life among individuals with aphasia, Ross and Wertz (2003) and Bose, McHugh, Schollenberger and Buchanan (2009) have argued that there is "no comprehensive, conceptually coherent, psychometrically sound assessment of the quality of life with aphasia exists".

Factors Affecting Quality of Life in Individuals With Aphasia in the Indian Context

The above review of the literature concludes that the quality of life among persons with aphasia depends on several factors such as associated conditions, severity, age, gender, socio-economic status, family support, motivation, medical support, socio-cultural aspects, and other psychosocial aspects in the western context. However, the quality of life among persons with aphasia in the Indian context may be different due to the differences in socio-cultural factors such as the style of living, economic status, family support, medical support, and acceptance of disorder and its consequences. In the Indian context, the majority of persons with aphasia being from middle and lower socioeconomic status and from rural areas, most of the persons with aphasia are far from receiving the medical treatment and rehabilitation due to financial hardship and non-availability of services. The acceptance level and poor awareness about the importance of immediate treatment and rehabilitation of aphasia by the lower socio-economic group who form a major group illiterate population is also a major factor contributing to the quality of life among PWA. In Indian culture, men are always seen as the head of the family and are the sole earners in the family prior to the stroke. However, the family dynamics change when the head of the family has got an attack of stroke in terms of financial stability and other important aspects of life, such as living style, decision making. The non-availability and unaffordability of medical services and rehabilitation services in rural areas play a major role in the poor quality of life for these individuals. Similarly, factors such as family relations, type of family, differences in place of living, age, gender and education levels seem to be more associated with the quality of life of persons with aphasia. As the population of India is diverse in nature in terms of languages, culture, education levels, socioeconomic status, social relationships, there is a great need in understanding the effect of these factors on the overall quality of life of persons with aphasia in the Indian context.

We have studied factors affecting the quality of life in individuals with aphasia following stroke. The study included a total of 35 individuals (21 males and 14 females) with aphasia following stroke in the age range of 35-80 years with 6 months post onset of stroke from the state of Andhra Pradesh, India. Stroke Specific Quality of Life Scale (SS-QOL) which consisted of 49 items in 12 domains, namely, energy, family roles, language, mobility, mood, personality, self-care, social roles, thinking, upper extremities functioning, vision, and work/productivity was administered. The scale was administered to 12 individuals with aphasia and 23 caregivers of persons with aphasia through an informal interview and responses were scored on a five-point rating scale with five being no help needed and one being total help needed and the domain scores and a summary score were calculated.

The results of this study indicated that family, language, mood, and social role domains were severely affected with less than 50% of scores majorly due to limited abilities of communication and motor functioning, followed by energy, mobility, self-care and upper extremity functions. However, stroke and aphasia showed little impact on personality, thinking and vision compared to other domains. The mean scores along with the percentage of the SS-QOL scale are given in Table 2.

The overall results of the present study revealed poor quality of life among persons with aphasia and this is majorly due to the factors such as limited role in family activities (e.g., unable to attend family gatherings due to physical condition), language difficulties (e.g., unable to communicate through speech, difficulty in word finding etc.), mobility issues (e.g., difficulty in walking, climbing stairs, due to hemiplegia), mood disturbances (e.g., discouraged about future, withdrawn from family and friends, lack of confidence), limited social role (e.g., limited social gatherings, reduced social contacts and activities, discontinuation of hobbies), self care (e.g., requiring help/assistance in the majority of self help skills) and not able to return to work/job (Hobart et al., 2016; Bahia and Chun, 2014; Sina nović, et al., 2012; Hilari et al., 2003). The social exclusion of these individuals with aphasia because of the limited communication and mobility, in turn, has led to increased psychosocial problems such as depression and anxiety.

Table 2. Mean scores of individuals with aphasia on SS-QOL domains

Domains of SS-QOL	Maximum Score	Mean Score	Percentage
Energy	15	8.35	55.66%
Family	15	6.94	46.26
Language	25	11.23	44.92%
Mobility	30	16.82	56.06%
Mood	25	12.11	48.44%
Personality	15	12.35	82.33%
Self-care	25	12.94	51.76%
Social role	25	10.94	43.76%
Thinking	15	11.82	78.80%
Upper extremities function	25	14.23	56.92%
Vision	15	13.52	90.13%
Work/Productivity	15	6.76	45.06%
Total	245	138.05	56.34%

Qualitative analysis and personal interview of individuals with aphasia have revealed few specific observations in psychosocial perspectives of individuals with aphasia in the Indian context. Factors such as socioeconomic status, literacy and employment have been found to have the direct impact on the perception of quality of life in PWA. Among the participants of the study, PWA belonging to high socioeconomic status have reported poor quality of life in language, family, energy and social relationships compared to individuals belonging to middle and lower social economic status who reported the significant decline in the domains of work/productivity, mobility, family and upper extremities functioning. Similarly, literates have reported poor quality of life compared to illiterates, especially due to limited language, social relationships and work/productivity. However, these differences were not reported in previous studies carried out in the western context.

ICF FRAMEWORK AND APHASIA

International Classification of Functioning, Disability and Health (ICF) was developed to classify the disabilities in terms of body structure and function, activities and participation, and environmental and personal context. Body structure and function domain categorize the site of lesion and impairments caused due to the lesion, whereas activities and participation domain assesses the individuals' abilities to carry out various activities and about the ability to participate in daily activities of life. Contextual factors explore the environmental (access, mobility arrangements, and communicative access, etc.) and personal factors (age, motivation, personality, education, etc.) which enhance the activities and participation of individuals.

Papathanasiou and Coppens (2013) defined aphasia based on ICF framework as "*an acquired selective impairment of language modalities and functions resulting from a focal brain lesion in the language-dominant hemisphere that affects the person's communicative and social functioning, quality of life, and the quality of life of his or her relatives and caregivers*". Body structure domain of ICF views aphasia as an impairment due to damage to specific areas of the brain related to language and motor functioning, for example, inferior frontal gyrus for Broca's aphasia. However, impairments of body functions associated with aphasia include language, cognitive, sensory and motor impairments such as agrammatism (difficulty in producing syntactically correct sentences), anomia (difficulty with word finding), non-fluent speech (difficulty in producing fluent utterances), alexia (difficulty in reading), agraphia (difficulty in writing), hemiplegia (paralysis or weakness in the right side of the body).

The language, motor and associated problems in individuals with aphasia can also cause significant activity limitations and participation restrictions. These difficulties can be classified under general tasks, communication difficulties, difficulties in carrying out activities of daily living, impaired family relationships and difficulty in maintaining the social life. These difficulties can be seen as losing employment following aphasia due to limited language and motor abilities, social exclusion due to restricted participation in social gatherings, increased dependence on family members and others for activities of daily living and self-care.

Environmental and personal factors have been identified to facilitate the body functions, activities and participation of the individuals with aphasia. Lack of physical and communicative access such as disability friendly access, availability of additional support systems such as alternate communication methods, etc to the individuals with aphasia have been major constraints in the activities and participation of individuals with aphasia. Personal factors and associated psychosocial problems contribute to the prognosis and improvement in individuals with aphasia.

Simmons-Mackie and Kagan (2007) described the various disorders seen in individuals with aphasia using the classification given by ICF framework, i.e., into body function and structures, activities and participation and environmental and personal factors. The authors have classified the brain damage underbody structures domain of ICF and it is coded under the structure of nervous system. Difficulty in formulating and decoding language symbols in individuals with aphasia have been described under body functions which were coded under mental functions, language, verbal memory and attention. Immobility and limited active participation in both personal and social contexts have been described under activities and participation and the environmental factors were described in terms of the support given by others and personal factors included individuals' motivation and emotional stability in general.

Matos, Jesus, and Cruice (2014) explored the outcomes of stroke and aphasia according to ICF classification in Portuguese individuals with aphasia (n=14) and their family members (n=14) and ten speech-language therapists. Results reported significant limitations in body functions and body structures including language and motor movement-related functions. All three groups also reported significant consequences of stroke on activities and participation majorly in community, social and civic life and inter and intrapersonal relations and mobility. The results also revealed poor self-care and motivation in some of the individuals with aphasia. The analysis between individuals, family members and professionals reported similar results on impairments and limitations in individuals with aphasia in daily life.

CONCLUSION

This chapter covered how the language and motor deficits in individuals with aphasia lead to significant decline in quality of life. The chapter also focused on the psychosocial aspects and quality of life in the Indian context using stroke-specific quality of life. It is worth noting that every individual with aphasia does experience limitations in the activities and participation in several activities of daily life and require support from family members and caregivers in activities of daily living and self-care. Although the past research in western context has reported the significant decline in the quality of life among individuals with aphasia, the factors associated with it may differ in the Indian context. The present chapter also reported results of factors affecting quality of life in the Indian context, and it is found that family, language, mood and social role domains were the significantly affected due to limited communication abilities and mobility factors. However, the factors such as personality, thinking and vision do not have any effect on the quality of life in individuals with aphasia in the Indian context. The chapter also reviewed few of the scales available for assessment of the quality of life in stroke survivors and the applications of assessment of the quality of life. It is further recommended that quality of life should be assessed through client-centered approach whenever it is possible as the ratings or description given by proxies may not be the actual feeling or perception of the patient. The chapter also reviewed aphasia disorder in the International classification of functioning, disability and Health (ICF) where each of the disorders associated with aphasia is classified under the body structures and function, activities and participation, and environmental and personal factors.

Traditional assessment test batteries such as Western Aphasia Battery or Boston Diagnostic Aphasia Examination and others will help speech-language pathologists to know the type and severity of aphasia along with few of the associated conditions such as alexia or agraphia, apraxia of speech. However, these communication deficits can affect their quality of life significantly in multiple domains such as family relations, mobility, and social context and so on. Therefore, it is recommended that the assessment of aphasia should also include assessment of the quality of life which will help speech-language pathologists to understand the psychosocial aspects of patients and their family members in detail. This information will help us in planning client-centered rehabilitation for individuals with aphasia in support of family members to improve the overall quality of life. Using ICF classification will enhance the understanding of the deficits in a greater extent and it will help rehabilitation and medical professionals to provide intervention based on deficits in body functions, activities and participation, and modification of environment and personal factors. Speech and Language rehabilitation for people with aphasia includes the use of standard techniques and approaches in treating underlying speech and language impairments and these approaches will, in turn, improve the overall body functions of individuals with aphasia. For example, use of multimodality language stimulation, semantic feature analysis treatment, melodic intonation therapy and constraint-induced language therapy will improve body functions involving language and cognitive functions such as language processing, word finding, spoken language and others. The use of augmentative and alternative communication methods provide a great support to individuals with aphasia to participate in various activities, improve family and social relations, enhancing the job opportunities among others. To summarize, individuals with aphasia do experience poor quality of life due to the underlying deficits in language, communication, and physical impairments. Hence, the goal of speech and language rehabilitation should focus on improving quality of life through a holistic approach which will help the professionals to achieve effective outcomes for individuals with aphasia.

REFERENCES

Au, R., Albert, M. L., & Obler, L. K. (1988). The relation of aphasia to dementia. *Aphasiology*, *2*(2), 161–173. doi:10.1080/02687038808248901

Bahia, M. M., & Chun, R. Y. S. (2014). Quality of life in aphasia: Differences between fluent and non-fluent aphasic augmentative and alternative communication users. *Audiology - Communication Research*, *19*(4), 352–359. doi:10.1590/S2317-64312014000300001353

Benson, D. F. (1979). *Aphasia, alexia, and agraphia* (Vol. 1). Churchill Livingstone.

Billings, A. G., & Moos, R. H. (1982). Stressful life event and symptoms: A longitudinal model. *Health Psychology*, *1*(2), 99–117. doi:10.1037/0278-6133.1.2.99

Bose, A., McHugh, T., Schollenberger, H., & Buchanan, L. (2009). Measuring quality of life in aphasia: Results from two scales. *Aphasiology*, *23*(7–8), 797–808. doi:10.1080/02687030802593189

Brust, J. C., Shafer, S. Q., Richter, R. W., & Bruun, B. (1976). Aphasia in acute stroke. *Stroke*, *7*(2), 167–174. doi:10.1161/01.STR.7.2.167 PMID:1265809

Cordini, K. L., Oda, E. Y., & Furlanetto, L. M. (2005). Qualidade de vida de pacientes com história prévia de AVE: Observação de casos. *Arquivos de Neuro-Psiquiatria*, *54*(4).

Cruce, M., Hill, R., Worrall, L., & Hickson, L. (2010). Conceptualising quality of life for older people with aphasia. *Aphasiology*, *24*(3), 327–347. doi:10.1080/02687030802565849

Cruice, M., Worrall, L., & Hickson, L. (2006). Quantifying aphasic people's social lives in the context of their non-aphasic peers. *Aphasiology*, *20*(12), 1210–1225. doi:10.1080/02687030600790136

Darley, F. L. (1982). *Aphasia*. WB Saunders Company.

Edwards, D., Hahn, M., Baum, C., & Dromerick, A. (2006). The impact of mild stroke on meaningful activity and life satisfaction. *Journal of Stroke and Cerebrovascular Diseases*, *15*(4), 151–157. doi:10.1016/j.jstrokecerebrovasdis.2006.04.001 PMID:17904068

Engell, B., Hütter, B. O., Willmes, K., & Huber, W. (2003). Quality of life in aphasia: Validation of a pictorial self-rating procedure. *Aphasiology*, *17*(4), 383–396. doi:10.1080/02687030244000734

Ferrans, C. E., & Powers, M. J. (1985). Quality of life index: Development and psychometric properties. *Advances in Nursing Science*, *8*(1), 15–24. doi:10.1097/00012272-198510000-00005 PMID:3933411

Geschwind, N. (1965). Disconnexion syndromes in animals and man. *Brain*, *88*(3), 585–585. doi:10.1093/brain/88.3.585 PMID:5318824

Glass, A. T., & Maddox, G. L. (1992). The quality and quantity of social support: Stroke recovery as a psycho-social transition. *Social Science & Medicine*, *34*(11), 1249–1261. doi:10.1016/0277-9536(92)90317-J PMID:1641684

Goodglass, H., & Kaplan, E. (1972). *Boston Diagnostic Aphasia Examination*. Philadelphia: Lea and Febiger.

Goodglass, H., & Kaplan, E. (1983). *The Assessment of Aphasia and Related Disorders* (2nd ed.). Philadelphia: Lea and Febiger.

Hilari, K., Byng, S., Lamping, D. L., & Smith, S. C. (2003). Stroke and aphasia quality of life scale-39 (SAQOL-39). *Stroke*, *34*(8), 1944–1950. doi:10.1161/01.STR.0000081987.46660.ED PMID:12855827

Hobart, J. C., Williams, S. L., Moran, K., & Thompson, A. J. (2016). Quality of life measurement after stroke: Uses and abuses of the SF-36. *Stroke*, *33*(5), 1348–1356. doi:10.1161/01.STR.0000015030.59594.B3 PMID:11988614

Kersten, P., Low, J., Ashburn, A., George, S., & McLellan, D. (2002). The unmet needs of young people who have had a stroke: Results of a national UK survey. *Disability and Rehabilitation*, *24*(16), 860–866. doi:10.1080/09638280210142167 PMID:12450462

Kertesz, A. (1982). *Western aphasia battery test manual*. Psychological Corp.

Koch, L., Egbert, N., Coeling, H., & Ayers, D. (2005). Returning to work after the onset of illness: Experiences of right hemisphere stroke survivors. *Rehabilitation Counseling*, *48*(4), 209–218. doi:10.1177/00343552050480040201

Matos, M. A. C., Jesus, L. M., & Cruice, M. (2014). Consequences of stroke and aphasia according to the ICF domains: Views of Portuguese people with aphasia, family members and professionals. *Aphasiology*, *28*(7), 771–796. doi:10.1080/02687038.2014.906561

Medin, J., Barajas, J., & Ekberg, K. (2006). Stroke patients' experiences of return to work. *Disability and Rehabilitation*, *28*(17), 1051–1060. doi:10.1080/09638280500494819 PMID:16950735

Niemi, M. L., Laaksonen, R., Kotila, M., & Weltimo, O. (1988). Quality of life 4 years after stroke. *Stroke*, *19*(9), 1101–1107. doi:10.1161/01.STR.19.9.1101 PMID:3413807

Papathanasiou, I., & Coppens, P. (2013). Basic concepts and operational definitions. In I. Papathanasiou, P. Coppens, & C. Potagas (Eds.), *Aphasia and related neurogenic communication disorders* (pp. xx–xxii). Burlington, MA: Jones and Bartlett Learning.

Parr, S. (2007). Living with severe aphasia: Tracking social exclusion. *Aphasiology*, *21*(1), 98–123. doi:10.1080/02687030600798337

Paul, D. R., Frattali, C. M., Holland, A. L., Thompson, C. K., Caperton, C. J., & Slater, S. C. (2003). *Quality of communication life scale (QCL)*. Rockville, MD: American Speech-Language-Hearing Association.

Porch, B. E. (1971). *The Porch Index of Communicative Ability*. Palo Alto, CA: Consulting Psychologists Press.

Possl, J., Jurgensmeyer, S., Karlbauer, F., Wenz, C., & Goldenberg, G. (2001). Stability of employment after brain injury: A 7 year follow up study. *Brain Injury: [BI]*, *15*(1), 15–27. doi:10.1080/02699050150209093 PMID:11201311

Ross, K., & Wertz, R. (2003). Quality of life with and without aphasia. *Aphasiology*, *17*(4), 355–364. doi:10.1080/02687030244000716

Ross, K. B., & Wertz, R. T. (2002). Relationships between language-based disability and quality of life in chronically aphasic adults. *Aphasiology*, *16*(8), 791–800. doi:10.1080/02687030244000130

Sapir, E. (1921). *Language: An introduction to the study of speech*. New York: Harcout, Brace and Company.

Schuell, H. (1965). *Differential diagnosis of aphasia with the Minnesota Test*. Minneapolis, MN: University of Minnesota Press.

Sethi, P. K. (2002). Stroke-incidence in India and management of ischemic stroke. *Neurosciences*, *4*(3), 139–141.

Simmons-Mackie, N., & Kagan, A. (2007). Application of the ICF in aphasia. *Seminars in Speech and Language*, *28*(4), 244–253. doi:10.1055-2007-986521 PMID:17935009

Sinanović, O., Mrkonjić, Z., & Zečić, S. (2012). Quality of life and post-stroke aphasic syndromes. *Periodicum Biologorum*, *114*(3), 435–440.

Sudlow, C. L. M., & Warlow, C. P. (1997). Comparable studies of the incidence of stroke and its pathological types. *Stroke*, *28*(3), 491–499. doi:10.1161/01.STR.28.3.491 PMID:9056601

Teassell, R., McRae, M., & Finestone, H. (2000). Social issues in the rehabilitation of younger stroke patients. *Archives of Physical Medicine and Rehabilitation*, *81*(2), 205–209. doi:10.1016/S0003-9993(00)90142-4 PMID:10668776

United Nations. (2006). *Convention on the rights of persons with disabilities*. New York: United Nations.

Van Straten, A., deHaan, R. J., Limburg, M., Schuling, J., Bossuyt, P. M., & van den Bos, G. A. M. (1997). A stroke-adapted 30-item version of the Sickness Impact Profile to assess quality of life (SA-SIP30). *Stroke*, *28*(11), 2155–2161. doi:10.1161/01.STR.28.11.2155 PMID:9368557

Ware, J. E., Snow, K. K., Kosinski, M., & Gandek, B. (1993). *SF-36 Health Survey Manual and Interpretation Guide*. Boston, MA: The Health Institute.

Whoqol Group. (1995). The World Health Organization quality of life assessment (WHOQOL): Position paper from the World Health Organization. *Social Science & Medicine*, *41*(10), 1403–1409. doi:10.1016/0277-9536(95)00112-K PMID:8560308

Whoqol Group. (1998). Development of the World Health Organization WHOQOL-BREF quality of life assessment. *Psychological Medicine*, *28*(3), 551–558. doi:10.1017/S0033291798006667 PMID:9626712

Williams, L. S., Weinberger, M., Harris, L. E., Clark, D. O., & Biller, J. (1999). Development of a stroke-specific quality of life scale. *Stroke*, *30*(7), 1362–1369. doi:10.1161/01.STR.30.7.1362 PMID:10390308

World Health Organization. (2001). *International Classification of Functioning, Disability and Health: ICF*. Geneva, Switzerland: World Health Organization.

Worrall, L., & Holland, A. (2003). Quality of life in aphasia. *Aphasiology*, *17*(4), 329–332. doi:10.1080/02687030244000699 PMID:27005901

KEY TERMS AND DEFINITIONS

Aphasia: Loss of language following brain damage.
Communication: Exchanging of ideas or information through verbal or non-verbal methods.
Hemiplegia: Weakness of paralysis of upper and lower limbs in one side of the body.
Language: A set of arbitrary symbols used for communication.
Psychosocial Health: Defined as balanced mental, social, and emotional state of an individual.
Social Life: Interpersonal relationships with surrounding people in the surrounding context.
Stroke: Death of brain cells due to disruption in the blood flow to the areas of the brain.

Chapter 3
Psychosocial Correlates of Dissociative Motor Disorder of Impairment or Loss of Speech

Shyam Hanumanapura Rajanna
All India Institute of Speech and Hearing, India

Raju Heggadadevanakote Hanumanthaiah
All India Institute of Speech and Hearing, India

ABSTRACT

The present chapter is intended to elucidate the role of psychosocial factors such as stressful life events, adjustment issues in family, social, occupational, and academic setup, personality, and socioeconomic correlates in the individual suffering from functional aphonia/dissociative motor disorder of impairment or loss of speech which is also called as functional voice disorder (FVD). This chapter explores a study carried out by purposively selected (N=32) case files reviews of individuals with FVD who were treated with functional voice therapy. The study results indicated various stressful life events such as marital discord, adjustment difficulties with social, occupational, family, and academic stipulation, and rapidly changing personal and health conditions were significantly associated with FVD. Majority of the cases were belonging to lower socioeconomic status and depressive symptoms were observed. Presence of the persistent role of life events, adjustment issues, and depression influencing development and maintenance along with diagnosis and management techniques are discussed.

INTRODUCTION

Speech is regulated by the operation of voice in humans and speech is the predominant human communication feature which differentiates human being from other creatures in our universe. Various nonorganic voice disorders with varied psychological causes are observed in day to day clinical practice. For these problems, many specialists rely on terms like "psychogenic", "psychosomatic", "somatoform disorder" or "somatization disorder" (Aronson, 1990; Kinz et al., 1988). But these terms were used too inconsistently and their definitions were not clear; it is useful to regard all non-organic voice disorders on

DOI: 10.4018/978-1-5225-4955-0.ch003

a continuum, ranging from "psychogenic aphonia" at the top (i.e. where the role of psychosocial factors in the causality is greatest) via "psychogenic dysphonia" etc. to "professional dysphonia" at the bottom. The latter often stems not only from vocal misuse but also from problems of dissatisfaction at work or from conflicts in private life (Seifert, & Kollbrunner; 2005). The functional voice disorder (FVD) is formerly called as psychogenic aphonia, functional aphonia, conversional aphonia, functional dysphonia, hysterical aphonia or acute sudden voice loss. In this chapter, FVD is referred as dissociative motor disorder of impairment or loss of speech as per the ICD-10 (F44.4; World Health Organization, 1992).

The functional voice disorder is a rather rare disorder with the varying prevalence of 0.4% in general population to 0.98% in a treatment-seeking United States of America's population (Cohen, Kim, Roy, Asche, & Courey, 2012). FVDs are rare; speech-language pathologists, ENT practitioners or general physicians as they refer the individuals who are suspected of having FVD to appropriate professionals such as psychologist, functional voice therapist or psychiatrist depending on accessibility to various setups in different countries for diagnosis and intervention, most of the FVD cases need subsequent management of FVD through therapies and interventions.

In the clinical interviews, clients disclosed that some clients have been taken to faith healers because of lack of awareness of the treatment available for the problem and such cases are more reported from the rural and semi-urban areas. Studies reported that prevalence of FVD is more in adult females than in adult males with the ratio of 5: 1 (Martins et al., 2016). The most frequently diagnosed voice disorder among adults is functional dysphonia (20.5%), acid laryngitis (12.5%), and vocal polyps (12%) (Martins et al., 2016) indicating more cases suffering from FVD among the population with voice disorders. Voice disorders are not mutually exclusive, and overlap is common. Most often FVD co-occurs with the symptoms of the depressive episode which can be elicited through a qualitative clinical interview with the client and family members.

FVD is a condition in which quality of voice, pitch and difference on loudness are inappropriate for gender, age, geographical area and cultural setup is observed is called as a voice disorder (Aronson & Bless, 2009; Lee, Stemple, Glaze, & Kelchner, 2004). Difficulty in speech or voice production or voice disorders resulting from the improper or insufficient use of the vocal mechanism when the physical and mechanical structure of speech or voice production is normal then it is called as FVD. FVD's signs and symptoms include vocal fatigue; muscle tension dysphonia or aphonia (loss of voice); diplophonia; ventricular phonation, breathiness, strained quality of voice (perception of increased effort; tense or harsh as if talking and lifting at the same time), strangled quality voice (like talking with breath held) abnormal pitch, abnormal loudness/volume, asthenia (weak voice) and other signs and symptoms include running out of breath. These signs and symptoms can occur in isolation or in combination. Chronic stressful lifestyle, acute stressful life event, anxiousness, depression and conversion reactions (including conversion aphonia or dysphonia) are the major causal factors of FVDs (Baker, 2003; Rasch et al., 2005). The corresponding relationships between these organic, functional, and psychogenic influences ensure that many voice disorders will have contributions from more than one etiological factor (Stemple, Roy, & Klaben, 2014). Voice quality can also be affected when psychological stressors lead to habitual, maladaptive aphonia and the resulting voice disorders are referred to as FVD (Stemple, Glaze, & Klaben, 2010).

Stressful life events in the individual's life and difficulties in adjustment to the changing life conditions or persistent life situations are the important psychosocial variables which have been studied largely in association with the FVD. Identifying relation between these psychological factors in connection with indispensable exertion to manage FVD is vital. Stressful life events are the unavoidable discrete life experiences which disrupt individual's usual activity, causing a substantial change and creating difficulty in readjustment to the stressors and impacts on the mental health of the individual leading to the difficult or disordered mental state. Instances of living with the disability, sudden loss of the spouse or loved one, difficulty to continue with intimate relationships or sustain the relationship, physical or mental abuse even small incidences like rejection from loved one, extramarital or alleged affairs, failure to seize attention or inability to divert the attention of the loved one can result as a stressful life event (Kotby et al., 2003; Dietrich et al., 2008; Misono et al., 2014). Adjustment difficulty is the consequence of individual's difficulty or lack of ability to resolve or sustain the stressful life events for moving towards comfortable life experience. Patients with voice disorders have difficulty in adjustment with the normal everyday life when compared with the adjustment pattern which they were following premorbidly (Venkatesan, Pushpavathi, & Purushotham, 2011).

Socio-economic factors of an individual which include individual or family income, social status, education and occupational background also exist as stressors in the individual's life. Personality, as defined by the Allport (1937), is the dynamic organization within the individual of those psychophysical systems that determine his/her characteristic behavior and thought. Poor ability to thinking rationally, poor problem-solving capacity, inability to connect with the others in the society, rapid and improper decision making, poor judgment, inability to cope with the difficult situations are the characteristics of individuals with issues in personality (Roy & Bless, 2000; Roy, 2011). Depression is a mood disorder and depressive symptoms include persistent low mood lack of interest in pleasurable activities and lack of sleep and appetite. Depression is the most common mood disorder prevalent in the modern day's civilized society. As the lifestyle, social situations, and values of interpersonal relations and morals are changing the coping skills and adjustment abilities of the individuals are also changing leading to sophistication. However, FVDs have longer history of their existence, with time the occurrence and causes are also getting modified.

FVDs are most often initially reported to a general physician based on the severity and presentation of the difficulty physician refers the cases to the next level that is the speech pathologist and voice therapist. FVD related to the misuse of voice or overuse of the voice is treated by the Speech pathologists and speech therapists. The other cases with functional aphonia which does not have any organic cause or relationship established by the speech pathologist will be referred to the Psychologist/Psychiatrist or functional voice therapist for the further evaluation and management.

Approximately 3 to 5 sessions of 30 to 45 minutes are suggested for the purpose of establishing rapport with the client and take the client into confidence. Functional, behavioral and personality assessments and interventions are carried out depending on the cause, severity and sensitivity of the cases. The first session for the complete and comprehensive case history taking and screening for organic or non-FVD is essential before starting intervention for functional aphonia. In the second session, some projective tests such as Thematic Apperception Test, Rorschach inkblot test, Sentence CompletionTest and assessment of personality of the client using objective tests is needed for the better understanding of the client. Later Therapist can start with the intervention. The commonly used therapeutic techniques are systematic desensitization, relaxation techniques especially the laryngeal musculoskeletal tension reduction technique (Roy & Leeper, 1993), psychoeducation, and supportive psychotherapy (Ruotsalainen et al., 2007).

Technical skills such as observation, interviewing the client and their related individuals are much-needed skills which a therapist must be competent of. Use of appropriate expressions, expertise in the language and communication plays the vital role in engaging client for the intervention of FVD will be additional advantages for the therapist to handle the cases. In the advanced setup, the therapist uses the apparatus such as voice light and biofeedback devices. Previously aversion therapy was applied using electric aversion treatments for the intervention of FVD. As it was eventually harmful in nature, so it is not recommended in clinical practice (Bos-Clark & Carding, 2011).

The rationale behind the present study follows the psychosocial contexts of psychological stressors and adjustment difficulties to manage such stressors which lead to the psychopathology among individuals. Clinician's observation and critical review of literature describe the effect of stressful life events, adjustment difficulties and related psychosocial aspects of FVD. With this note, the present study was aimed to explore the probable relevant psychosocial aspects elucidating the interventional strategies existing for FVD.

METHOD

The main aim of the present study was to identify and assess the psychosocial factors in individuals diagnosed as FVDs/dissociative motor disorder of impairment or loss of speech. The current study was carried out using ex-post-facto research method. Psychosocial factors selected to assess and explore were stressful life events, adjustment difficulties to family, social, occupational and academic conditions and socio-economic status of the participants. A clinical case file review, content analysis, and clinical interview data of 32 individuals diagnosed to have FVDs was selected using purposive sampling method for the present study and existing related literature on etiology, assessment, diagnosis and management of the FVDs was inculcated.

A comprehensive clinical case history was taken by the functional voice therapist and behavioral assessments were done by professional psychologists before the diagnosis of the FVD. However, the cases were initially screened for the organic pathology relating to the voice disorder before referring to the clinical psychology consultation by the speech-language pathologist. The social readjustment rating scale (SRSS) is an inventory of common stressors developed by Thomas Holmes and Richard Rahe in 1967 was used to assess the stressful life events took place in the individual's life. It has 43-items to answer as either 'yes' or 'no' on this scale based on the experience of the stressful event by the respondent in the duration of past one year. The scale provides a schema for interpretation based on the severity of a subject's total scores. The interpretations are done in three grades 'low to moderate' (less than 150 points), moderate to high' (150-299 points), or 'high to very high risk' (300 points or more) of becoming ill in near future. The scale mentions 'life change units' as the measure of individual stress. The clinical interview was done to elicit the information related to the adjustment difficulties individual undergoing in the present condition and SES of the participants. Appropriate qualitative and quantitative analysis was done using content analysis of the interviews and case files. Correlation and mean score was calculated using SPSS program for the statistical analysis of quantitative data. Interpretation and analysis of data were carried out in the present study.

RESULTS

Table 1 shows the socio-demographic characteristics of the sample among which nine (28.1%) were male and 23 (71.9%) were female. 16 (50%) individuals were aged below 18 years, 11 (34.4%) were aged between 18 to 40 years and five (15.6%) were aged above 40 years. 22 (68.75%) of them had studied up to 10th class, nine (28.12%) had studied after 10th class and up to graduation and one (3.12%) had Post

Table 1.

Variables	Sample character	Number(n)	Percentage
Gender	Male	09	28.1%
	Female	23	71.9%
Age group	Up to 18 years	16	50%
	18 to 40 years	11	34.4%
	Above 40 years	05	15.6%
education	Up to 10th class	22	68.75%
	10th to graduation	09	28.12%
	Above graduation	01	3.12%
Socioeconomic status	Lower SES	23	71.87%
	Middle SES	08	25%
	Upper SES	01	3.12%
family type	Nuclear	27	84.3%
	Joint/ Extended	05	15.7%
Resident	Rural	24	75%
	Semi-urban	07	21.88%
	Urban	01	3.12%
marital status	Single	18	56.3%
	Married	10	31.3%
	Separated/ widow	04	12.5%

Graduation. 23 (71.87%) individuals were reported to belong to lower SES (below Rs 20,000), eight (25%) were from middle SES (Rs 20,000-4,00,000) and one (3.12%) was from Upper SES (above Rs 4,00,000). 27 (84.30%) of them were living in the nuclear family and five (15.7%) belonged to the joint/ extended family. 24 (75%) were residing in rural areas, seven (21.88%) of them were from Semi-urban locality and one client was from the urban locality. 18 (56.3%) were single, 10 (31.3%) were married and four (12.5%) of the participants were separated or widow or divorced.

Table 2 shows the characteristics of the samples with FVD. 31 (96.88%) participants were born of non-consanguineous union and 28 (87.5%) participants were not having any family history of medical or psychiatric illnesses showing any impact of consanguinity and family history on FVD. 32 (100%) of the participants were having one or more adjustment issues. 31 (96.88%) were going through stressful life events, 17(53.1%) of them were having depression symptoms, 14 (43.7%) of them were having anxiety symptoms and 30 (93.76%) of them were having emotional difficulty. Seven (21.9%) individuals have shown one of the sensory/motor/behavioral changes, 31 (96.88%) of the cases were having one or more secondary gains after the loss of voice. Nine (28.1%) participants had medical history where as 23 (71.9%) of them were not having any medical emergency in the past. 25 (78.1%) participants reported pain symptoms in chest/throat, remaining seven (21.9%) participants do not reported any sort of pain symptoms in chest or pain suggesting FVD can occur with or without pain in the chest/throat. 31 (96.88%) of the patients with FVD were not professional users of voice, only one case was using her voice for the profession. Vegetative skills were present for 25 (78.1%) cases and 11 (34.4%) of the

Table 2. Functional voice disorder characteristics of the sample

FVD features	Sample character	Number(n)	Percentage
Consanguinity	Absent	31	96.88%
	Present	01	3.12%
Family history	Absent	28	87.5%
	Present	04	12.5%
Adjustment	Absent	32	100%
	Present	0	0%
Stressful life event	Absent	31	96.88%
	Present	01	3.12%
Depression	Absent	15	46.9%
	Present	17	53.1%
Anxiety symptoms	Absent	18	56.3%
	Present	14	43.7%
Emotional difficulty	Absent	02	6.24%
	Present	30	93.76%
*S/M/B changes	Absent	25	78.1%
	Present	07	21.9%
Secondary gain	Absent	01	3.12%
	Present	31	96.88%
Medical history	Absent	23	71.9%
	Present	09	28.1%
Pain symptoms	Absent	07	21.9%
	Present	25	78.1%
Professional voice users	Absent	31	96.88%
	Present	01	3.12%
Vegetative skills	Absent	7	21.9%
	Present	25	78.1%
Swallowing difficulty	Absent	21	65.6%
	Present	11	34.4%
Relapse	Absent	25	78.1%
	Present	7	21.9%

*Sensory/Motor/Behavioral changes

participants were having difficulty in swallowing at the time of FVD. In seven (21.9%) of cases, relapse of FVD was observed.

Table-3 shows the mean, standard deviations and group differences according to age group, education, onset of FVD and presence of depression symptoms. Even though mean score on the SRSS for the overall sample is 148.71 (SD: 20.60) which falls in the interpretation range of 'low to moderate' risk of becoming ill in near future or 30% chance of suffering from stress, significant group differences were

Table 3. Results of life event scales and group difference among participants

Variables	Subgroups	N	Mean	Std. Deviation	t-test
Age group	up to 18 years	16	137.50	17.40	3.460**
	19 to 40 years	11	165.81	14.78	
	above 40	5	153.40	16.75	
	Total	32	149.71	20.60	
Onset	acute	27	147.00	21.24	1.654
	insidious	5	164.40	6.10	
	Total	32	149.71	20.60	
Depression symptoms	absent	15	141.80	19.80	1.928*
	present	17	156.70	19.19	
Education	up to 10th class	9	136.88	17.74	2.161*
	Above 10th class	23	154.73	19.74	

**Significant at 0.01 level
* Significant at 0.05 level

observed in the t-test indicating upper age groups have mild to moderate risk of becoming ill in near future or 50% chance of suffering from stress. The following variables showed the significant difference in Life event scales scores between age groups, education, onset and presence of depression symptoms indicating the difference in the impact of age, education and depression on FVD.

DISCUSSION

Psychological and social factors of FVD are the matter of concern and need to bc understood by the professionals for the effective management and to plan intervention (Wenke et al., 2014). Previous studies reported that comparatively prevalence of FVDs among male and female gender is in the ratio of 1:5 (Baker et al., 2013; Martins et al., 2016). In the present study, nine (28.1%) individuals were male and 23 (71.9%) were female at the ratio of below 1:3. 16 (50%) individuals reported with FVD were below 18 years, 11 (34.4%) were aged between 18 to 40 years and five (15.6%) of the sample were aged above 40 years the t-test results showed the difference of occurrence of FVD between the age group of below 18 years and 19 years to 40 years group. No difference was found between other groups. 22 (68.75%) of the patients had studied till 10th class 9 (28.12%) of them had studied above 10th class up to graduation and one (3.12%) sample had Post graduation suggestive of less educated people are more prone to be affected by FVD. 23 (71.87%) individuals were reported with FVD belong to lower SES. Eight (25%) were from middle SES and one (3.12%) of the sample was from upper SES.

27 (84.30%) of the participants were living in a nuclear family and five (15.7%) belonged to the joint/extended family type. More number of the participants affected by FVD was from nuclear family as the social conditions in the present scenario have more nuclear families. The information on residence of the participants showed that 24 (75%) individuals were residing in rural areas, seven (21.88%) of them were from semi-urban locality and one client was from urban locality. In countries like India education facilities, opportunity to get economic and social independence in rural society is a struggle for

individuals. Coping strategies followed by the rural population can throw the individual to sustain in the stressful conditions. Weak coping skills because of low education and knowledge end up in faulty coping mechanisms leading to FVD. Information in relation with marital status showed that 18 (56.3%) of them were single, 10 (31.3%) were married, and four (12.5%) of the participants were separated or widow or divorced as the LES score of the groups were not showing any significant difference in t-test. It is concluded that marital status does not have any impact on FVD.

Pathologically related characteristics of the individuals with FVD are important to discuss as it is helpful in the understanding of the individual and characteristics of pathology which need to be understood for the management of the FVD. 31 (96.88%) participants were born of non-consanguineous union and 28 (87.5%) participants were not having any family history of medical or psychiatric illnesses indicative of genetic or hereditary factors playing meager or no part on FVD. 32 (100%) of the participants were having one or more adjustment issues indicative of the difficulty to sustain the life situations leading individuals to get susceptible for FVD. 31 (96.88%) were going through stressful life events, 17 (53.1%) of them were having depressive symptoms, 14 (43.7%) of them were having anxiety symptoms and 30 (93.76%) of them were having emotional difficulty, suggestive of stressful conditions in life of individuals with FVD. Seven (21.9%) individuals have shown one of the sensory/motor/ behavioral changes, 31 (96.88%) of the cases were having one or more secondary gains after the loss of voice inculcating previous literature and research findings the dissociative pattern of coping with the stressful life conditions need to understood and the treatment plans or intervention strategies are needed to follow to enhance the coping skills to manage dissociative pattern of coping with the stressors. Nine (28.1%) participants had medical history as it was not having the major impact on FVD. 25 (78.1%) of participants reported pain symptoms in chest/throat, 31 (96.88%) of the patients with FVD were not professional users of voice. Only one case was using her voice for the profession. As major professional voice users tend to have pathology of structural voice disorders in significance pathology of the FVD can be implicit. Vegetative skills were present for 25 (78.1%) cases and 11 (34.4%) of the participants were having difficulty in swallowing at the time of FVD. In seven (21.9%) of cases, relapse of FVD has been observed and the need for relapse prevention is the major concern in the FVD.

IMPLICATIONS

The present chapter elucidates the psychopathological and social constructs of the FVD. It can be referred by the clinical psychology practitioners, functional voice therapists, speech-language pathologists and mental health professionals for the purpose of clinical practice including assessment, diagnosis, interventions, teaching and research purposes. It is useful for the general public for understanding the issues related to FVD and create awareness. The study included in the chapter is an elaborated study which inculcates the cases treated between years 2002 to 2016 in a time period of 15 years is a valuable data in the treatment of FVD.

LIMITATIONS

The chapter was based on the study which was done in a government institute where most often clients belonging to lower and middle socio-economic strata approach for the treatment. Relating to this, drawing inference on the prevalence of FVDs in upper socio-economic strata is not valuable. The sample size which is used in the study was small to generalize the study results. The more statistically significant analysis was not possible as it was a qualitative study and non-parametric tests were used as the data was not normally distributed.

SUGGESTIONS FOR FURTHER RESEARCH

The present study was carried out in a government institute where more clients of lower and middle socio-economic status approach for the treatment. Further research can be done in the various private and multispecialty hospitals for getting clients from the variety of socio-economic strata. The sample size which is used in the study was N=32 which was comparatively small sample further research can be done using the large sample to generalize the study results using systematic empirical research methodology and standardized assessment tools as such it can be statistically analyzed and enhanced significant inferences can be drawn quantitatively. In the present study coping strategies followed by the individuals with FVD was not focused as it was ex-post-facto study an empirical study on coping strategies or coping mechanisms of individuals with FY\VD will be of greater impact for the management of FVD. Research can also be framed to develop a manual or standardize the therapeutic approaches for the dissociative motor disorder of impairment or loss of speech as it can be useful for the future generations.

CONCLUSION

Functional voice disorder of psychogenic nature or dissociative motor disorder of impairment or loss of speech is the difficulty in speech production caused due to the difficulty to sustain the stressful life events, adjustment difficulties and poor coping strategies followed by the individual. Psychosocial aspects such as unbearable unsustainable even sometimes simple or complex adjustment and stressful life circumstances with poor coping skills lack of knowledge in sustaining the life situations leads to the pathological condition of FVD. Understanding the individual dynamics social and psychological stressors encountered by the individual in life is essential for professionals to devise effective intervention.

REFERENCES

Allport, G. W. (1937). *Personality: A psychological interpretation*. Oxford, UK: Holt.

Aronson, A. E. (1990). *Clinical voice disorders-An interdisciplinary approach*. New York: University of Cambridge.

Aronson, A. E., & Bless, D. M. (2009). *Voice Disorders of Structural Origin. In Clinical Voice Disorders* (4th ed.; pp. 24–38). New York: Thieme Med Pub.

Baker, J. (2003). Psychogenic voice disorders and traumatic stress experience: A discussion paper with two case reports. *Journal of Voice*, *17*(3), 308–318. doi:10.1067/S0892-1997(03)00015-8 PMID:14513954

Baker, J., Ben-Tovim, D., Butcher, A., Esterman, A., & McLaughlin, K. (2013). Psychosocial risk factors which may differentiate between women with FVD, Organic Voice Disorder and a Control group. *International Journal of Speech-Language Pathology*, *15*(6), 547–563. doi:10.3109/17549507.2012.721397 PMID:23075157

Bos-Clark, M., & Carding, P. (2011). Effectiveness of voice therapy in functional dysphonia: Where are we now? *Current Opinion in Otolaryngology & Head & Neck Surgery*, *19*(3), 160–164. doi:10.1097/MOO.0b013e3283448f85 PMID:21330925

Cohen, S. M., Kim, J., Roy, N., Asche, C., & Courey, M. (2012). Prevalence and causes of dysphonia in a large treatment-seeking population. *The Laryngoscope*, *122*(2), 343–348. doi:10.1002/lary.22426 PMID:22271658

Dietrich, M., Abbott, K. V., Gartner-Schmidt, J., & Rosen, C. A. (2008). The frequency of perceived stress, anxiety, and depression in patients with common pathologies affecting voice. *Journal of Voice*, *22*(4), 472–488. doi:10.1016/j.jvoice.2006.08.007 PMID:18395419

Holmes, T. H., & Rahe, R. H. (1967). The social readjustment rating scale. *Journal of Psychosomatic Research*, *11*(2), 213–218. doi:10.1016/0022-3999(67)90010-4 PMID:6059863

Kinzl, J., Biebl, W., Rauchegger, H., Weissbacher, S., & Hinterhuber, H. (1988). Funktionelle Aphonie-Ein Konversionssymptom zur Angstabwehr. *Psychosomatik Medizinische Psychologie*, *38*(1), 347–351. PMID:3186903

Kotby, M. N., Baraka, M., El Sady, S. R., Ghanem, M., & Shoeib, R. (2003, October). Psychogenic stress as a possible etiological factor in non-organic dysphonia. Elsevier. doi:10.1016/S0531-5131(03)00858-6

Lee, L., Stemple, J. C., Glaze, L., & Kelchner, L. N. (2004). Quick screen for voice and supplementary documents for identifying pediatric voice disorders. *Language, Speech, and Hearing Services in Schools*, *35*(4), 308–319. doi:10.1044/0161-1461(2004/030 PMID:15609634

Martins, R. H. G., do Amaral, H. A., Tavares, E. L. M., Martins, M. G., Gonçalves, T. M., & Dias, N. H. (2016). Voice disorders: Etiology and diagnosis. *Journal of Voice, 30*(6), 761-e1- e15.

Misono, S., Peterson, C. B., Meredith, L., Banks, K., Bandyopadhyay, D., Yueh, B., & Frazier, P. A. (2014). Psychosocial distress in patients presenting with voice concerns. *Journal of Voice*, *28*(6), 753–761. doi:10.1016/j.jvoice.2014.02.010 PMID:24930373

Rasch, T., Günther, S., Hoppe, U., Eysholdt, U., & Rosanowski, F. (2005). Voice-related quality of life in organic and functional voice disorders. *Logopedics, Phoniatrics, Vocology*, *30*(1), 9–13. doi:10.1080/14015430510006640 PMID:16040435

Roy, N. (2011). Personality and voice disorders. *SIG 3 Perspectives on Voice and Voice Disorders, 21*(1), 17- 23.

Roy, N., & Bless, D. M. (2000). Toward a theory of the dispositional bases of functional dysphonia and vocal nodules: Exploring the role of personality and emotional adjustment. In R. D. Kent & M. J. Ball (Eds.), *The handbook of voice quality measurement* (pp. 461–480). San Diego, CA: Singular Publishing Group.

Roy, N., & Leeper, H. A. (1993). Effects of the manual laryngeal musculoskeletal tension reduction technique as a treatment for functional voice disorders: Perceptual and acoustic measures. *Journal of Voice, 7*(3), 242–249. doi:10.1016/S0892-1997(05)80333-9 PMID:8353642

Ruotsalainen, J. H., Sellman, J., Lehto, L., Jauhiainen, M., & Verbeek, J. H. (2007). Interventions for treating functional dysphonia in adults. *Cochrane Database of Systematic Reviews*, 3. PMID:17636842

Seifert, E., & Kollbrunner, J. (2005). Stress and distress in non-organic voice disorders. *Swiss Medical Weekly, 135*(27-28), 387–397. PMID:16220409

Seifert, E., & Kollbrunner, J. (2006). An update in thinking about nonorganic voice disorders. *Archives of Otolaryngology--Head & Neck Surgery, 132*(10), 1128–1132. doi:10.1001/archotol.132.10.1128 PMID:17043264

Stemple, J. C., Glaze, L. E., & Klaben, B. K. (2010). *Clinical voice pathology: Theory and management* (4th ed.). San Diego, CA: Plural.

Stemple, J. C., Roy, N., & Klaben, B. K. (2014). *Clinical voice pathology: Theory and management.* San Diego, CA: Plural.

Venkatesan, S., Pushpavathi, M., & Purushotham, K. (2011). Adjustment patterns in voice disorders. *Journal of Indian Speech. Language and Hearing Association, 25*(1), 21–30.

Wenke, R. J., Stabler, P., Walton, C., Coman, L., Lawrie, M., O'Neill, J., ... & Cardell, E. (2014). Is more intensive better? Client and service provider outcomes for intensive versus standard therapy schedules for functional voice disorders. *Journal of Voice, 28*(5), 652-e31-e43.

World Health Organization. (1992). *The ICD-10 classification of mental and behavioural disorders: Clinical descriptions and diagnostic guidelines.* Geneva: World Health Organization.

KEY TERMS AND DEFINITIONS

Adjustment Difficulty: Adjustment difficulty is the consequence of an individual's difficulty or lack of ability to resolve or sustain the stressful life events for moving towards comfortable/contended life experience.

Depression: Depression is a mood disorder. It includes persistent low mood, lack of interest in pleasurable activities, and lack of sleep and appetite.

Functional Aphonia: Inability to speak or produce voice even though having normal structural functioning of speech production system. This might have occurred due to inability to sustain psychological stressors or overuse of the voice.

Personality: Personality is an individual's reaction or response system for a given life situation or condition.

Psychotherapy: Psychotherapy is an application of psychological principles and techniques to help an individual to outcome the individual difficulties and increase the wellbeing of the individual. In the present chapter, functional voice therapy is one of the modules of psychotherapy approach used to manage the functional voice disorder.

Socioeconomic Factors: Socioeconomic factors of an individual include individual or family income, social status, education, and occupational background.

Stressful Life Event: Stressful life events are the unavoidable discrete life experiences that disrupt an individual's usual activity, causing a substantial change and creating difficulty in readjustment to the stressors. It impacts on the mental health of the individual leading to the difficult or disordered mental state.

Chapter 4
Knowledge, Attitude, and Practices of Primary and Secondary School Teachers on Specific Learning Disorder

Nandini Jayachandran
Institute for Communicative and Cognitive Neurosciences, India

Mary Iype
Government Medical College Trivandrum, India

Poovathinal Azhakan Suresh
Institute for Communicative and Cognitive Neurosciences, India

Divya Vinod
Institute for Communicative and Cognitive Neurosciences, India

ABSTRACT

Early identification of Specific Learning Disorder (SLD) is essential not only for effective remediation of their problems but would also prevent the problems from aggravating. The role of general education teachers in early identification becomes crucial, as they are the ones who first identify the academic and behavioral issues of school children. The main aims of the study are to assess the knowledge, attitudes, and current practices pertaining to SLD, among pre-primary, primary, and secondary school teachers in public schools from Trivandrum, India, to find whether there exists any relation between years of teaching experience and awareness on SLD and to assess the effect of a short-term training program on the knowledge, attitude, and practices of school teachers. In conclusion, short-term training programs of a multi-disciplinary nature are found to be effective in bringing about improvements with both pre-primary and primary teacher's knowledge factor, but such training is maximally beneficial for improving attitude and practice of teachers in the primary level.

DOI: 10.4018/978-1-5225-4955-0.ch004

INTRODUCTION

Specific Learning Disorder (SLD) is a neuro-developmental clinical condition affecting children during school years, the effects of which persist well into adult life. Though the condition is primarily detected in a given child in terms of well below average skills in the academic areas of reading, writing and mathematics, compared to age and intelligence level, manifestations of SLD has many more shades to it, be it underlying cognitive processing problems or overt behavioral problems or the language deficits or concomitant emotional problems or social skill deficits.

Specific Learning Disorder is not a single disorder, but composed of disabilities in several areas such as receptive and expressive language, basic reading skills as well as comprehension skills, written expression difficulties ranging from copying problems, poor handwriting, spelling errors when writing to dictation to lack of clarity and organization in getting thoughts to writing while asked to do spontaneous writing and poor mathematical calculation and problem solving or mathematical reasoning skills. Moreover, it is highly heterogeneous in clinical presentation, which entails consideration of each child's specific skill deficits and characteristics in assessment as well as management. As there is heterogeneity within each domain and between domains, Lyon et al., (2001) suggests that these disorders should be treated as separate disorders. In same lines, Stanovich (1991), has advocated that domain-specific disabilities be labeled separately, and co-morbidities should be addressed only after initial domain-specific classification is done.

The condition, if remains undetected, may result in chronic poor school performance, class detention and even school dropout leading to low self-esteem, and development of withdrawn aggressive behaviors, anxiety, depression, and even antisocial behaviors. The cornerstone of SLD treatment is remedial education, which should ideally be started early (in primary school years) to take advantage of the higher plasticity of the central nervous system during this period (Karande, 2008).

The field of SLD was initially based on Medical model/framework in terms of minimal brain damage, later shifting to the sensory-motor aspects of learning such as visual, auditory and motor processing skills in the 1950's and 60's and the educational framework focusing on visuomotor processing and discrepancy between scholastic ability and IQ (Karanth, 2008). Since the 1970's there has been a renewed emphasis on SLD as a language based disorder due to several factors such as findings of the high incidence of fluency, articulation disorders and communication disorders among SLD's and due to the emergence of psycho-linguistic studies on the acquisition of language in children (Karanth, 2008; Bashir et al., 1987; Kamhi & Catts, 1989; Scarborough, 1990).

Definitions

The way SLD is conceptually defined is quiet varied with many of the definitions failing to provide explicit criteria to identify the same. The contribution of Venkatesan (2017) in this regard is noteworthy who has systematically compared 23 operational definitions of SLD and has ranked a list of commonly appearing attributes, with processing deficits, exclusionary criteria, poor achievement in academic subjects as expected of age, schooling and IQ, heterogeneity/individual differences, topping the list and average or above average intelligence as a pre-requisite for diagnosis, discrepancy criteria and life-long condition given low priority.

Specific Learning Disability (SpLD) refers to a group of neurodevelopmental disorders that manifest in childhood as persistent difficulties in learning to efficiently read (Dyslexia), write (Dysgraphia), or do simple mathematical calculations (Dyscalculia), despite normal intelligence, conventional schooling, intact hearing and vision, adequate motivation, and socio-cultural opportunity. This hidden disability which affects approximately 5-10% of school going population is currently believed to be the result of a functional problem in brain wiring than an anatomical problem, which is found to be genetically inherited (Shaywitz, 1998; Demonet, Taylor, & Chaix, 2004).

That SLD is largely a clinical diagnosis by exclusion is exemplified in the aforesaid definition too. But the inclusion criteria should essentially have four aspects; 1) academic under-achievement in the absence of Intellectual Disability 2) significant impairment in foundational skills of reading, writing or maths as demonstrated by individually administered standardized measures 3) Both (1) & (2) affects occupational or activities of everyday life 4) substantial deficits in one or more areas of cognitive processing.

One criterion which is gaining ground as a useful indicator, before SLD is diagnosed is Response to Instruction, which is an off-shoot of the recognition that IQ-achievement discrepancy criteria (traditionally used for SLD diagnosis) has to be replaced owing to lack of empirical support for its assumptions like 1) as the discrepancy between IQ-achievement widens severity also increases (Stanovich, Siegel, & Linda, 1994) and 2) the academic performance of students with discrepancy significantly differs from those without discrepancy (Gresham, 2002).

In simple terms, Response to Instruction (RtI) model would mean, a child can be suspected to have SLD if he fails to respond to valid treatment programs (Berninger & Abbot, 1994; Vellutino, Scanlon, & Lyon, 2000; Fuchs & Fuchs, 1998). RtI is not only an early detection system but also a prevention and support system that identifies struggling students and assists them before they fall behind (Gersten et al., 2009). It begins with universal screening and high-quality instruction, with three tiers of intervention.

What Makes the Condition Multi-Dimensional and Controversial?

The field of SLD has evolved through a series of controversies, right from its definition, assessment methods, and criteria for diagnoses, many of which have been clarified with scientific research in the field. It has remained a topic of active research interest largely in the West, over half a century since it was first described by Kirk in 1962, into its possible biological causes, typologies of SLD's, their cognitive, behavioral and academic skill differences, developing sensitive screening and valid identification tools, and development of evidence-based practices.

1. **Low Achievement:** It may be noted that all children who are low achievers educationally would not meet the clinical diagnosis of SLD as per DSM-5; however it is true vice versa, i.e. all SLD's have learning disabilities, as defined educationally (Tannock, 2013).
2. **The Role of Language in SLD:** The connection between language deficits and SLD has been reported since the work of Orton in 1937 (Kamhi & Catts, 1989). Children with Specific Language Impairments in their pre-school were later found to develop SLD signs (Bashir, Wiig, & Abrams, 1987). Several studies provide empirical evidence that a child's skill in developing word reading is closely related to awareness and skill in manipulating phonemes. Though this holds good in less transparent languages like French & English, when it comes to Indian scripts (mostly alpha-syllabaries) and Eastern scripts this relationship does not find much support (Goswami, 1999; Huang & Hanley, 1994; Prakash et al., 1993; Karanth, 2003) owing to greater transparency between orthographic units and phonemes. The speed with which a word is retrieved is linked to reading difficulties. LD's are found to have rapid word retrieval deficits (Korhonen, 1995), naming speed

deficits (Wolf, 1991), difficulties in narrative discourse processing & production (Montague et al., 1990) and problems in comprehending syntagmatic & paradigmatic relations compared to peers (Sharma, 2000).

3. **IQ-Achievement Discrepancy:** The discrepancy between the capacity for general cognitive functioning and achievement, popularly known as IQ-achievement discrepancy has been traditionally used as a convenient way to explain the academic under-achievement of students with average and above average intelligence and accepted in policy in 1977. But the use of this criteria, as the essential criteria in SLD diagnosis, has been disputed due to the following reasons. First, IQ is a gross estimate of a person's cognitive functioning and may not be considered as a measure of learning potential (Reynolds, 1974). Second, there is no clear consensus on how to derive and quantify discrepancy criteria (Stanovich, 1993; Zigmond, 1993). The fact that this criterion is no longer crucial for SLD diagnosis is evident from the abandonment of the same from DSM-5 criteria for SLD diagnosis (APA, 2013).
4. **Cognitive Processing Deficits:** Since 1963, when SLD was first described by Kirk and Weiner, as Minimal Brain Dysfunction, the idea that cognitive processing deficits form the basis of their academic under-achievement, has gathered ample empirical evidence over the years. Low academic achievement is just the tip of the iceberg, with cognitive processing problems lying underneath, mediated by problems in neural circuitry /brain wiring. From the remediation point of view too, accurate assessment of cognitive processing deficits in a given child is very important in formulating remedial programs.

There are two different viewpoints regarding the cognitive factors that contribute or result in academic deficits of SLD. While domain-specific cognitive deficits are core cognitive factors of congenital origin causing SLD, like the phonological deficit theory of dyslexia and defective number module or Number sense deficit of dyscalculia (Pennington & Bishop, 2009; Butterworth, 2005; Wilson & Dehaene, 2007), the domain-general viewpoint is based on the assumption that deficits in domain-general cognitive processing problems like memory, spatial abilities etc., contribute to low basic academic skills. In the case of dyslexia, supportive empirical evidence has been found for deficits in verbal working memory, executive processing, visual learning and semantic memory deficits (Swanson, Zheng, & Jerman, 2009; Rosselli, Matute, Pinto, & Ardila, 2006) and in children with dyscalculia deficits in attention, executive functioning, visual & verbal working memory and processing speed are reported (Fuchs et al., 2006; Geary, 2004; Hitch & McAuley, 1991; Swanson & Jerman, 2006).

Though assessment of cognitive processes has not been considered essential in SLD identification, in 2004, with IDEA putting a renewed emphasis on better approaches for SLD identification, interest in cognitive assessment re-emerged. Currently there is strong support for a combined approach to SLD assessment wherein academic skill deficits need to be demonstrated with standardized tests, use of multiple sources of information (such as teacher and parent reports, class work samples, educational/medical history and RtI) to demonstrate the same and identify specific cognitive & linguistic correlates related to the specific area of under-achievement which will lead to an explanatory diagnosis leading to proper treatment planning (Mather & Gregg, 2006; APA, 2013; Johnson et al., 2010).

5. **Life-long Effects:** SLD is not limited to a particular age or setting (Keogh & Sears, 1991). Though primarily diagnosed during early school years, its effects persist into adult life making it a lifespan disorder (Gerber, 2001). Evidence has been gained from studies on language development of children,

which shows that the growing child continues to master the more subtle syntactic, semantic and pragmatic aspects of language (Karanth, 2008). Another line of evidence comes from persistence of skill deficits over time, which proves that it is much more than a developmental lag with 74% of children first identified in third grade, continuing to remain reading disabled through 9th grade (Francis, Shaywitz, & Steubing, 1994) and 95% of cases diagnosed to have dyscalculia continuing to score in the lowest quartile when re-examined three years later, in their adolescence (Shalev, Manor, Auerbach, & Gross-Tsur, 1998).

6. **Environmental and Contextual Factors:** Though lack of environmental, cultural or social disadvantages is a pre-condition to the diagnosis of SLD, there are a host of conditions like inadequate instruction, poverty, parental illiteracy and lack of stimulation at home, lack of command over instructional language, over-crowded classrooms and the dialectical difference in language which are risk factors contributing to SLD's (Karanth, 2003; Snow et al., 2000). Another contextual aspect affecting SLD is bilingualism and multilingualism, which complicates the clinical picture based on language transparency, for eg., Hindi dyslexics error rates were 10 times more on non-initial vowels and bundled consonants than on initial vowels and ordinary consonants owing to the complex spatial configuration of the same, placing demands on right hemispheric strategies compromised in dyslexics (Nehru, 2001).
7. **Mental Health Aspects:** SLD's may develop secondary emotional and behavioural problems due to continued failure in academic pursuits. So also emotional problems which erupt as an offshoot of family disruptions, poverty etc can also affect academic performance and response to treatment in SLD's. Some Indian studies which have found evidence for psycho-social problems in SLD's find anxiety, self-esteem issues (Mukerjee et al., 1995), self-perception problems (Bhola et al., 1997); perceived peer relations & social competence (Lall, Hirisavae, Kapur, & Subbakrisha, 1997). Significantly high rates of social skill deficits have been found among SLD's, whose severity and number of symptoms increases in more severe SLD's (Gresham & Reschly, 1986; Bruck, 1986).

Ironically it has been found in the Surveys conducted by Office for National Statistics in 1999 & 2004 in the U.K. that SLD's are more prone to have risk factors for mental health problems such as poor general health, exposure to adverse life events, have mothers with mental health needs and poor health, and have families with low educational attainments and higher rates of unemployment, compared to children without SLD's (Meltzer, Gatward, Goodman, & Ford, 2000). About one in 3 children and adolescents with learning disabilities have a diagnosable psychiatric disorder. Thus they are often a socially disadvantaged group, who develop mental health problems not as a consequence of SLD, but because of the increased chances of exposure to poverty, social exclusion and challenging family environments (Emerson & Hatton, 2007).

Neurological Aspects of Specific Learning Disorders

The neurologist's role in the evaluation of a learning disabled child is to look for and diagnose an underlying disorder. Several studies support a genetic component and high rate of occurrence of SLD in twins also points to a genetic predilection (Cardon et al., 1994). Hypothyroidism is to be sought for in the learning disabled. Epilepsy, Neurofibromatosis, Tuberous sclerosis complex, Tourette syndrome and chromosomal disorders may be associated with SLD. Meningitis, encephalitis, traumatic brain injury or cranial irradiation can lead to LD as sequelae. Poor environmental stimulation (Leiva et al., 2001;

Buckingham et al., 2013), low birth weight and malnutrition are known associations (Vohr et al., 1991). Chronic medical conditions like diabetes mellitus and HIV infection are also seen. Above all, intrauterine exposure to toxins and infections; in mild cases may manifest as SLD. Maternal hypothyroidism is one of the well-recognized causes of defective brain development (Haddow et al., 1999). Pesticides can affect brain development in utero or when exposed to early in life (Guillette, 1998). Epileptic encephalopathies may be associated with defective language development or learning disability (Caraballo et al., 2014). Metabolic disorders like phenylketonuria and the urea cycle disorders can be an etiology.

Attention deficit hyperactivity disorder (ADHD) and other psychiatric comorbidities like depression and conduct disorders may coexist in these children (Mayes, Calhoun, & Crowell 2000). They may also have just attention deficit, difficulties with fast, complex social language processes, pragmatic understanding or problems in handling receptive or expressive language. Learning disability may result from peripheral visual or auditory deficits. Children with defects of visual perceptual processing reverse and invert letters like "b" for "d" and words like "was" for "saw". In the initial stages of language acquisition there is a controlled processing of language where each word is painstakingly recognized by the brain; later this gives way to automatic processing. In the dyslexic, this movement from 'controlled processing' to 'automatic processing' does not happen. Defects of auditory perceptual processing render it difficult for the child to process the auditory input to meaningful concepts. The background noises and the tutorial mean almost the same to him or he has to process each sound painstakingly to attach some meaning to it. Memory problems are also seen in dyslexics.

Soft signs seen in these children include lack of concepts of time, difficult to decipher the time on a clock, topographic disorientation, difficulty to orient right and left and poor organizational skills. Discrimination of the top and bottom and today and tomorrow may be difficult.

Neurological Basis of the Etiology

Defects in the temporal auditory processing have been demonstrated in some dyslexics. Defective processing of visual images in the magnocellular part of the lateral geniculate body has been demonstrated in some (Tallal et al., 1993; Lennerstrandt et al., 1993; Livingstone et al., 1991). Dehaene and Cohen have demonstrated a reproducible area called the visual word form area in the left lateral occipitotemporal sulcus using PET studies (Dahaene & Cohen, 2011). There appears to be an association between phonological dyslexia/dysgraphia and damage to perisylvian cortical regions. Attempts to precisely determine the lesion have produced inconsistent results. It has been suggested that posterior perisylvian lesions bordering on the supramarginal gyrus may be the critical neural substrate of phonological dysgraphia (Roeltgen, Sevush, & Heilman, 1983). Dahaene and Cohen demonstrated the triple-code model for arithmetic. They showed that basic arithmetic skills are controlled by three brain regions; the horizontal intraparietal sulcus processes numerical quantities, the left perisylvian language network verbally processes numbers and the ventral occipitoparietal regions processes visual images of numbers (Dahaene et al., 2003). The lateral inferior prefrontal cortex does more complicated mathematics like algebra, geometry, calculus and retrieval of arithmetic facts (Dahaene et al., 2003). In an autopsy series comparing dyslexic to non-dyslexic brain, Kaufmann and Galaburda have demonstrated loss of characteristic architectural organization of the cortical neurons in the left temporal cortex (Kaufmann & Galaburda, 1989).

Reduced verbal automaticity was associated with cerebellar abnormalities, whereas reduced automaticity on motor or motor and verbal tasks was associated with white matter abnormalities (Urion, Huff, &

Carullo, 2015). The decrease in length of the insula has been reported (Logan, 1996). Functional imaging studies suggest a role of the left inferior frontal gyrus in speech perception and rapid auditory processing, as well as in phonological aspects of reading (Fiez & Petersen, 1998; Fiez et al., 1995) Even apparently more complex cognitive functions, such as awareness of time passing, processing of sequences of successive events or duration judgement, also probably necessitate intact temporal coding of information.

Though many neuroanatomic correlates for dyslexia have been demonstrated by many; all the neurophysiological theories underlying dyslexia including the visual perceptual, the phonological, temporal processing defect and hemisphere co-dominance are fragile.

Investigations That Are Essential

A magnetic resonance imaging of the brain to look for cortical dysgenesis, an electroencephalogram, thyroid function test and a thorough physical examination are the baseline. Conditions liked familial microcephaly and SLD has no confirmatory test. Specialized investigations begin with a Karyotype and FISH to look for subtelomeric defects. Chromosomal microarray and the special biochemical assay are done in selected cases.

Treatment

Medical treatment includes atomoxetine or methylphenidate to increase attention. It was formerly believed that these drugs only increase attention and make the child available for learning, however now there is evidence to show that these drugs do increase academic performance. Specific treatment like supplementing thyroxin in hypothyroidism, protein-restricted diet and sodium benzoate in urea cycle disorders and treatment of hyperuricemia in Lesch Nyhan syndrome may be helpful. Specific diet may be useful in other metabolic disorders. Associated ADHD needs medication and psychotherapy. Defective vision and hearing should be promptly corrected. There are conflicting reports of the use of nootropic drugs like piracetam.

Recent research has demonstrated different levels of activity in specific regions of the brain in advanced readers in comparison to poor readers opening up new avenues of research in the quest of a remedial drug, therapy or other intervention.

- **Assessment:** The aim of a comprehensive in-depth assessment is not merely to make a diagnosis but to provide the basis for a deeper understanding of the problem, to identify the student's strengths, and to map out future directions for remedial work. The assessment of SLD requires a comprehensive evaluation of the child using both formal and informal measures to identify the academic skill deficits using standardized measures which are corroborated by information from multiple sources, identify the cognitive processing deficits and relate it to the specific deficits to draw out a treatment plan. As suggested by Witteman, Haries, Bekker, and van Arle (2007), ideally SLD diagnosis should be a three step process with a categorical diagnosis, followed by an explanatory diagnosis and finally treatment planning. A multi-disciplinary approach to assessment would be ideal and in fact essential for SLD, as it is an intrinsic disorder that has medical/biological aspects, cognitive aspects, educational aspects, speech & language aspects, all of which has to be unraveled, the inter-connections understood and worked upon in a collective manner, for best results. A proper workup should be a staged process, wherein a detailed medical & developmental history, followed by evaluations by the multidisciplinary team comprising of a medical specialist, a psychologist, a speech pathologist, a special educator and linguist should be done which would bring out all the missing links in the puzzle of an SLD's problem (Karande & Kulkarni, 2005; Karanth, 2008). This would give a clear road-map for treatment by consensus. Assessment of an SLD child by a psychologist should provide a complete profiling of not only academic but also emotional and social problems, paving the way for specialized instructions & accommodations, which the SLD child is entitled to receive (John et al., 2013).

While identifying SLD children from schools in the community, an initial universal screening by sensitive measures is highly recommended (Gersten et al., 2009). This can be followed by detailed diagnostic testing and confirmation which would go a long way in reducing false positives and inappropriate labeling.

- **Diagnosis:** Currently, this disorder is diagnosed according to the clinical criteria of DSM-5 (APA, 2013) and ICD-10 (World Health Organization, 1992). As per the DSM-5, Specific Learning Disorder is now a single, overall diagnosis, incorporating deficits that impact academic achievement. Unlike the earlier criteria of DSM-IV-TR, the current criteria describe shortcomings in general academic skills and provide detailed specifiers for the areas of reading, mathematics, and written expression.

Another change is the abandonment of IQ-achievement discrepancy and cognitive processing deficits, to be a pre-condition for SLD diagnosis, unless when intellectual disability is suspected. This would simply mean that assessment of cognitive processing problems should be taken up not primarily for diagnosing SLD, but for serving as a basis for intervention planning for the individual child. This, in turn, would make for more efficient use of the specialists time in drawing out individual learning pathways suitable to each child, in collaboration with parents and teachers. Diagnosis relies upon information gathered through multiple sources through a clinical review of the individual's developmental, medical, educational, and family history, reports of test scores and teacher observations, and response to academic interventions (Table 1).

Table 1. Diagnosis made according to the following four criteria

Criteria	Description
a	Persistent difficulty in learning academic skills (including word decoding and fluency, reading comprehension, spelling, Writing difficulties, Number sense & calculation and Mathematical reasoning), for at least 6 months.
b	The affected academic skills are substantially below expectations given the individual's age and result in impaired functioning in school, at work or activities of daily living.
c	Learning difficulties though apparent in the early years is not to be diagnosed until the onset of school years, as in some individuals the disorder is not apparent until the onset of a demand for higher level skills.
d	The academic and learning difficulties occur in the absence of: 1. Intellectual disabilities 2. Visual or hearing impairments 3. Mental disorders (eg: depression, anxiety etc) 4. Neurological disorders 5. Psycho-social difficulty 6. Language differences 7. Lack of access to adequate

DSM-5; APA, 2013.

BACKGROUND

SLD in the Indian Context, Issues and Possibilities

SLD has been slowly gaining attention in our country, as a clinical condition/educationally compromised group which requires timely attention in terms of identification & appropriate remediation, due to the diligent work of a group of professionals from different specialties, who had all the opportunity to work closely with SLD children and took genuine interest to observe and understand them from different angles. We have made strides not only in developing culture specific and valid assessment tools of academic skills (Kapur et al., 2002; Ramaa,1984; Rozario, 2003; Prema, 1998; Ramaa & Gowramma, 2002; Mehta, 2000; Venkatesan, 2006) and behavioral assessment tools (Swarup & Mehta, 1991; Kapur et al., 1995) but also in developing evidence based packages for remediation of SLD in Indian context (Srikanth & Karanth, 2003; Bhasi, 2003; Karibasappa, Nishanimut, & Padakanayya, 2008).

However, the Indian context itself present confounding factors such as bilingualism/multilingualism, overcrowded classrooms, poor awareness among teachers, poor socio-economic conditions, each of which may often violate the necessary pre-conditions/exclusionary criteria for a diagnosis of SLD. For e.g.: DSM-5 diagnostic criteria lists mental disorders like anxiety & depression, psycho-social difficulties, language differences, and lack of access to the adequate instruction to be excluded before a child can be diagnosed. A study by Mukerjee, Hirisave, Kapur, and Subbakrishna (1995) has found SLD children to have high state anxiety, compared to non-SLD matched controls. Kohli et al. (2005) has observed behavioural problems in 70% of the sample while neurotic traits were found in 54% of the sample, in a study of 7-14 yr old SLD's.

Unlike in the Western countries, where a single language is relied upon by people of that country, the Indian scenario has many regional languages, most of which are alpha-syllabaries with differences in script coming into the picture within each State. Hence for proper assessment of SLD in the Indian context, especially in vernacular medium schools, it is necessary to develop standardized assessment tools in their mother tongue. Some effort in this direction has borne fruit with the commendable work by Prema (1998) who has developed a language based reading assessment tool in Kannada, but more has to come in different regional languages to prevent under-detection. When considering intervention of our SLD's academic deficits too, it is important to design intervention materials in vernacular languages as evidence point to the fact that our scripts being highly transparent and consistent, phonological awareness is not as crucial a pre-requisite as in English, for successful reading (Prakash, 2003; Prakash & Rekha, 1992; Prakash et al., 1993).

Parental illiteracy and lack of exposure to literacy-related skills in the home environment have been reported among LD population in Indian context (Suresh & Sebastian, 2003). Another problem is the low general awareness level about the condition in the community, resultant acceptance issues and less constructive action.

When we appraise the knowledge level among teachers in our country, it ranges from mild to moderate level, mostly limited to urban schools. (Lingeswaran, 2013; Saravanabhavan & Saravanabhavan, 2001; 2010). Lack of proper coverage of the topic in the curriculum of teachers training (Chatterjee, 2009), over-crowded classrooms, considerable workload, the dearth of periodic in-service training to upgrade skills in identification & management of SLD (Kamala & Ramganesh, 2013) are some of the important factors pointing to the lack of knowledge and attitudes of teachers in general education stream. Yadav and Agrawal (2008) in a study based on rural primary schools in Allahabad have observed that the situation is far less promising in rural schools. So also even teachers from urban schools are unable to explicate the criteria used in identifying learning and associated problems, though there was a close matching between teachers identified cases of children and standardized diagnostic test of SLD, in a mixed sample of teachers from vernacular and English medium schools (Konanthambigi & Shetty, 2008). This, in turn, results in the delay in proper screening and timely referrals by teachers, for appropriate identification by specialists as well as commencing early intervention.

The level of awareness among school management is also understandably less (Saludes & Artenita, 2009). Consequently, under-achievers are often neglected or ousted as it affects pass percentage and reputation of the school and they refrain from appointing resource teachers and counselors owing to increased costs. Difficulties in accommodating the behavioural excesses of these students in school, interference by parents of other children are also factors the current authors have gathered, while doing this work.

Though inclusive education or mainstreaming is the most viable option in our country, in terms of high costs for specialist assessment & management, relief for these children is not often obtained due to i) Lack of adequate coverage of this area in the training curriculum of Special teachers (Kamala & Ramganesh, 2013). ii) Poor availability of SEN teachers specialized in this area (Karande, 2008). iii) Insensitivity to the need to post SEN teachers to help such children in mainstreamed schools. iv) Reluctance to give admission to such children though it is mandated by law (Afshan, 2009).

In the specific context of Kerala, with high literacy rate among the population, level of aspiration among parents for their ward's academic performance is also high. Hence the vigilance for any sign of below average performance is present, which prompts them to seek facilities for improvement, but the correct understanding of reasons for a child's under-performance is often affected as the teachers fail to make them understand their true problems and convince them to seek the appropriate formal assessment. In a discussion with teachers by the current authors, they report that acceptance issues are a major barrier among parents, which present as resistance to acknowledging the child's academic problems and the tendency to put the blame on teachers.

The Relevance of This Study

Specific Learning Disorder (SLD) is a topic of growing concern worldwide due to the personal, emotional and occupational effects on the affected person as well as the financial implications it has on the family and nation as a whole. In our country, where very few specialists and professionals are available who have ample experience in dealing with SLD children too, prevalence is slated to be at 5-6% (Ramaa & Gowramma, 2002) and at least 5 students have SLD in an average sized class (Thomas, Bhanutej, & John, 2003). The epidemiological study by Suresh and Sebastian (2003) reveals that SLD is observed in 7-8% of the general population in 0-18 age group. However, there is a lack of systematic studies on what percentage among them gets identified correctly and would receive treatment. Efforts to develop evidence-based approaches in the management of SLD, has also taken a back seat (Karanth, 2008; Swaroop & Mehta, 1991).

Background of This Work

In the recent past, research efforts in the field point out that early identification of children at-risk and initiation of remedial measures is the most effective strategy in dealing with SLD as it catches skill deficits before increasing in severity. In this context, the general education teachers of primary school classes who have first-hand information regarding skill deficits of individual children in their classrooms relative to their peers have an important role to play, in this process. Besides, as we go for a formal diagnosis of SLD as per DSM-5, teacher reports form one of the pertinent sources of information, to be considered. At the same time, care should be taken to prevent a false diagnosis of low achievers as SLD, through training efforts to sensitize teachers in the topic of SLD. This is important as there exists a tendency among teachers to over-simplify SLD and low achievement and view them as identical twins, when they are in fact cousins with different parentage but having similar features.

Awareness and knowledge about SLD among teachers would help the parents of affected children go for a diagnostic check-up early enough. Training general education teachers on SLD identification as well as school-level management, would not only lead to increased knowledge level and to well thought out training practices, but also has a secondary effect on curbing incidence rates.

In this study, an effort is made to find out the knowledge, attitudes and practices of general education teachers in this area in a group of urban, unaided schools in Trivandrum, the capital city of Kerala, India known for its high literacy rates as well as health indices. This work is part of a larger project which was taken up with the objective of 'training general education teachers in the identification of SLD from their classrooms (so that they make appropriate specialist referrals) and to equip them with skills to manage the problems of mild severity level at school level with Tier 2 and Tier 3 interventions in collaboration with specialist support'.

Research Questions

1. What is the current awareness level of general education teachers about SLD?
    a. What is their current knowledge level?
    b. What are their attitudes to them?
    c. What are their current practices in identifying and managing them?
2. Is there any relationship between experience gained by teachers in terms of years spent in teaching and the knowledge, attitude and practices of SLD?
3. What are the effects of a short-term training program on the knowledge level, attitudes and practices of SLD children?

METHOD

Procedure

A sample of 65 teachers, from the 1st to 7th standard classes belonging to the Central Board of Secondary Education (CBSE), the Indian Certificate of Secondary Education (ICSE) and State syllabi were administered two multiple-choice questionnaires (which was developed for the purpose by the authors), one which assessed general aspects (with dichotomous i.e., yes/no responses) and the other one assessing specific aspects of SLD with respect to age (multiple choice with 5 choices for each question). The General questionnaire covers the Knowledge, Attitudes and Practice aspects of teachers in SLD. The Specific Questionnaire is comprehensive to cover the cognitive, neurological, and behavioral and speech and language aspects of SLD. This was followed by a three-day intensive training program, into the Neurological, Pediatric, Cognitive, Psychological, Linguistic and Special Educational aspects of SLD, for them.

The training program comprised of didactic lectures, case-studies, case-discussions and discussions, spanning three days, of 6 hours duration each. The aim was to give a clear-cut conceptual understanding of SLD from a multi-disciplinary perspective. Specific Learning Disorder (SLD) has been operationally defined as a neuro-developmental condition diagnosed in school years, manifesting as persistent and substantial difficulties compared to his/her age, in the academic skills of word decoding and fluency, reading comprehension, spelling, writing difficulties, number sense & calculation and mathematical reasoning, for at least 6 months (despite receiving support targeting area of difficulty), in the absence of intellectual disability, sensory issues of vision or hearing, access to adequate instruction, neurological or mental disorders, language differences or psycho-social difficulties. Out of twelve sessions, three sessions were handled by the Psychologist covering behavioral aspects of SLD, Psychological assessment in SLD and interventions in the management of behavioral and cognitive problems of SLD; three sessions by the medical team on Neurobiological aspects of SLD and diagnostic aspects from a Neurological view point, three sessions by Speech-Language Pathologists covering Language deficits in SLD and Speech-Language assessment of SLD, followed by 2 sessions by Linguists covering linguistic analysis of SLD and a single session by the Special Educator who focused on educational aspects of SLD.

A post-assessment was done following the program, using the aforementioned questionnaire to assess the effect of training in their knowledge, attitude and practice regarding SLD's. This paper discusses the results & analysis of the General Questionnaire.

Sample Details

Out of the total sample of 65 teachers, 4 were avoided as their questionnaires were incomplete.

Tools

A questionnaire comprising of 32 open-ended items, stratified into three domains of knowledge, attitude and practices in the area of SLD, was developed by the Principal author and Co-authors based on extensive literature survey on Specific Learning Disorders. The questionnaire consisted of 11 items, grouped into knowledge (addressing the cognition and speech, language aspects of SLD), 6 items measuring Attitudes towards SLD's and 5 items addressing current Practices in the identification of SLD as well as management. The 8 questions comprising of medical /neurological aspects of SLD coming under the knowledge domain has been treated separately in the analysis, to avoid unequal distribution of questions among sub-domains of neurological and cognitive and speech-language aspects. All the items except,

Table 2. Sample details of the present study

Category of Teachers	Number	Teaching Experience (Number of Years)	
		Mean	SD
Pre-primary	21	15.38	8.42
Primary	20	10.05	6.98
Middle-school	20	11.10	7.36

two questions from Knowledge Module (No's: 17 &18), one from Attitude Module (No: 32) and two questions from Practice domain (31 & 32), are dichotomous in nature, with Yes/no option. A score of one was assigned to each correct response. Incorrect answers and unanswered items were scored zero, for the dichotomous items. For the rest of the questions with multiple options, the scoring is as follows; a) Highly agree(5), Agree(4), Neutral(3), Disagree(2), Highly disagree(1); b) 4 option questions (No: 31)- option (b)=3, (a)=2, (c)=1, (d)=0 ; and 5 option question (No: 32)- (a)=0, (b)=3, (c)= 4, (d)=1, (e)=2. For question number 17, the options are scored as (a) & (b) =o, (c)=2 and (d)= 1 and for number 5 (0=no answer/nil; 1 for partially correct answer and 2 for correct answer), both items being in the knowledge domain. Thus the maximum obtainable score in the Knowledge category (excluding items in the Neurological part) is a score of 16 and in the Neurology part is the score of 8.

While administering the questionnaire to the teachers no specification of the domain was done and a mixed order of item presentation was adhered to, to make it as informal as possible. Questionnaires were filled in by participants themselves, with examiners available to help, as and when doubts regarding the meaning of questions, arose. Content validity was established by getting the tool rated by experts in the field. The maximum possible score in Knowledge is 16, Attitude is 10 and Practice is 10; the grand total being 36.

RESULTS

This study was aimed to find out the current knowledge level, attitudes and practices in identification and management of SLD among Primary and Secondary school teachers in the general education stream and the effect of a training program on SLD for them. The teachers were grouped into three based on the classes they engaged as, Pre-primary, Primary & Middle school. The questions were on the teacher's knowledge about SLD, their attitude towards them & the practical options they would choose for an SLD child. Statistical analyses were done using SPSS software, as per the research questions. Questions 1 & 4 of the questionnaire has been omitted, from the analysis.

To answer the Research Question 1, the comparison of the mean scores of the pre-primary, primary & middle school teachers were supplemented with one-way ANOVA regarding their pre-training scores to ascertain the level of understanding of teachers on SLD, prior to the training. Table 3 & 4 indicates the results of the teachers.

The mean scores on knowledge were 8.71 for the Pre-primary teachers, 9.20 for the Primary teachers & 10.10 for the Middle school teachers. The results indicate no significant variation between the three groups of teachers on their knowledge about SLD before the training and the percentage range of mean knowledge scores are 50% in Pre-primary, 56% in Primary group and 62% in the Middle school group.

Table 3. The mean and standard deviation scores of the three groups of teachers before training

Variables	Knowledge		Attitude		Practice		Total	
	Mean	SD	Mean	SD	Mean	SD	Mean	SD
Pre-primary	8.71	2.34	7.24	1.30	7.57	1.50	23.52	3.54
Primary	9.20	2.28	6.70	1.03	7.25	1.48	23.15	3.10
Middle school	10.10	2.79	7.80	1.24	8.10	1.77	26.00	3.87

Figure 1. The mean scores of the three groups of teachers (pre-primary, primary, and middle school) on knowledge, attitude, and practice and total score before training

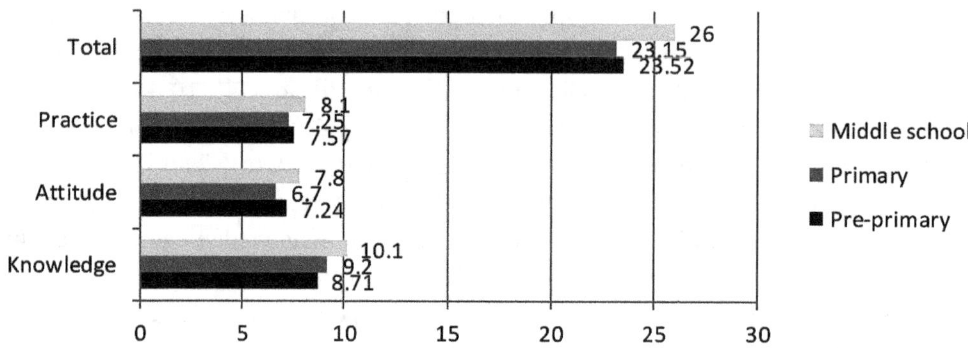

Table 4. One-way analysis of variance on the knowledge, attitude, practice and total scores before training with regard to the three groups of teachers

Variables	Source	Sum of Squares	Df	Mean Sum of Squares	F
Knowledge	Total sum of squares	20.157	2	10.078	
	Sum of squares between groups	357.286	58	6.160	1.64
	Sum of squares within groups	377.443	60		
Attitude	Total sum of squares	12.102	2	6.051	4.22*
	Sum of squares between groups	83.210	58	1.435	
	Sum of squares within groups	7.373	2	3.686	1.46
Practice	Total sum of squares	146.693	58	2.529	
	Sum of squares between groups	154.066	60		
	Sum of squares within groups	156.46	62	2.52	
Total	Total sum of squares	96.441	2	48.221	3.90*
	Sum of squares between groups	717.788	58	12.376	
	Sum of squares within groups	814.230	60		

* Significant at p>0.05

The mean scores on attitude were 7.24 for the Pre-primary teachers, 6.70 for the Primary teachers & 7.80 for the Middle school teachers. The results indicate significant variation between the three groups of teachers on their attitude towards SLD children before the training.

The mean scores on practice were 7.57 for the Pre-primary teachers, 7.25 for the Primary teachers & 8.10 for the Middle school teachers. The results indicate no significant variation between the three groups of teachers on their approach to LD children before the training.

The mean total scores (knowledge, attitude & practice together) were 23.52, 23.15 & 26 for the Pre-primary, Primary & Middle school teachers respectively. The results indicate significant variation between the three groups of teachers on their overall idea about LD, before the training.

To summarize, it has been found that there is the significant difference in secondary/middle school teacher's attitude and overall idea regarding SLD compared to primary school teachers, prior to training.

To explore which group of teachers show the significant difference in attitude scores, Duncan's test was done (refer Table. 5), which has shown the significant difference in scores between Primary and Secondary school teachers, with latter having better attitude scores compared to Primary teachers.

To answer RQ 1 regarding what is the current level of knowledge, attitude and practice of teachers in each category a percentage analysis were also computed, with respect to each question in the questionnaire (refer Table 6).

Regarding the questions in Knowledge Module, in the first one (Question 2) which examined whether it is a curable condition, Pre-primary teachers reported the highest percentage of awareness (81%) compared to both Primary & Middle school teachers (both 65%). This may be attributed to their experience of getting young learner's problems corrected when identified early.

However, for the second question on whether SLD's are mentally challenged (Question 3) it was revealed that deeper knowledge about SLD, is lacking in all three groups, with relatively better knowhow among Pre-primary (33%) & Middle school teachers (25%). In case of primary school teachers,

Table 5. Pre-training attitude total score comparison using Duncun's Test[a,b]

Section Code	N	Subset for Alpha = 0.05	
		1	2
1-4	20	6.70	
Preprimary	21	7.24	7.24
5-7	20		7.80
Sig.		.157	.140

Means for groups in homogeneous subsets are displayed.
a. Uses Harmonic Mean Sample Size = 20.323.
b. The group sizes are unequal. The harmonic mean of the group sizes is used. Type I error levels are not guaranteed.

Table 6. Percentage of correct responses in questions on knowledge

Variables	Question	% of Correct Response by Pre-Primary Teachers		% of Correct Responses by Primary Teachers		% of Correct Responses by Middle School Teachers	
		Fully	Partially	Fully	Partially	Fully	Partially
Question 1	2	81%		65%		65%	
Question 2	3	33%		15%		25%	
Question 3	5		9.5%	15%	35%	15%	35%
Question 4	9	76.2%		75%		85%	
Question 5	14	47.6%		60%		55%	
Question 6	17	14.3%	4.8%	30%		60%	5%
Question 7	18	33.3%	52.4%	15%	75%	20%	
Question 8	19	23.8%		15%		45%	
Question 9	22	38.1%		40%		40%	
Question 10	24	52.4%		40%		40%	
Question 11	29	71.4%		80%		70%	

only 15% got the correct response, which might be because at primary level more attention is paid by teachers into the academic deficits.

When asked to give their definition of SLD (Question 5), again the superficial knowledge about SLD is evident specifically in the Pre-primary teachers, among whom only 9.5% could define it at least partially correct. The Primary teachers showed a better idea with15% defining it fully correct and 35% defining partially correct. A similar trend has been observed among Middle school teachers as well, with 15% being fully correct and 35% partially correct. Probably the teachers at the Pre-primary level, lacks knowledge or cannot differentiate the specific telltale signs of SLD as it presents in Pre-primary classes.

The language processing deficits in SLD (Question 9) is acknowledged by more than 75% of teachers in all groups, with the highest percentage of correct answers among Middle school teachers (80%). This shows that generally, teachers are aware of the language related issues in SLD.

The teachers, in general, demonstrated fairly good idea on language delay as a pre-cursor of SLD (Question 14), with the highest percentage of correct answers reported by Primary teachers (60%) followed by those in Middle school (55%), with Pre-primary teachers scoring the least at 47.6%. This may be due to the fact that teachers in the Primary group are more likely to notice language delays and deviances, as deficits. The similar trend observed among Middle school children may be because such deficits become more pronounced at this age, compared to primary years.

While assessing their idea regarding the prevalence of SLD (Question 17), 60% of the Middle school teachers were fully correct in their assessment (with 5% being partially correct), while it came down to 30% among primary school teachers. Surprisingly only about 14.3% of Pre-primary teachers responded correctly, with 4.8% giving partially correct responses. This again may be a pointer to the lack of recognition of SLD features in the pre-primary stage.

Presence of behavioral issues such as inattention and lack of persistence to complete goal-directed activities in SLD (Question 18), has been acknowledged by the highest number of teachers in the Pre-primary group (33.3%), compared to both Primary (15%) & middle school teachers (20%). So also the majority of the sample gave at least partially correct responses, with 52.4% among Pre-primary teachers and 75% in the primary group. This would mean that while pre-primary teachers suspect learning issues based on behavioral features, the other two groups consider it only as a partial indicator of the problem.

The role home environment plays in causing SLD (Question 19) has been reported to the contrary by 45% of Middle school teachers, followed by 23.8% in Pre-primary and 15% of primary teachers. This shows that the Middle school teachers consider the home environment, to play a role in causing SLD.

While both 40% of Middle school teachers, as well as primary teachers, believe that SLD's have a high expectancy of failure due to repeated failures (Question 22), only 38.1% of the Pre-primary teachers, feel the same. This may be because of erring and correcting at lower classes, is a normal practice which is seldom taken seriously, while in higher classes repeated failures lead to lower confidence levels and expectancy of failure.

While more than 50% of Pre-primary teachers felt that reading and writing disorder would essentially co-exist (Question 24), only about 40% each of Primary teachers and Middle school level, felt so. This may be because at primary and higher levels, due to their experience with such children, teachers ought to see children, develop reading or writing problems alone, as well.

The perception that unrecognized hearing deficit can result in SLD (Question 29) is quite high in all groups, with the highest percentage of Primary teachers (80%), followed by Pre-primary (71.4%) and Middle school level (70%).

While more than 50% of those teaching in Middle school feel that it is better for SLD's to learn in the special school setting (Question 6), only about 23.8% in Pre-primary and 22.7% from Primary feels so. This might be because at lower class less the possibility of the correction in classroom setting is better, compared to higher age-group where the demands of the curriculum are hard to be met even with specialized classroom interventions.

While about 80% of primary teachers showed partial agreement on the role of teachers in identifying and managing SLD (Question 8), more than 60% of Pre-primary and 55% of Middle school teachers also shared the same opinion, indicating that as group teachers feel that they have a role in SLD.

That SLD's have better chances of improvement when compared to other language disorders (Question 10), is quite high in among the three teacher groups, with 100% agreement in the Middle school students, followed by more than 90% agreement in Pre-primary and Middle school sections. This would mean that they have rightly understood that given appropriate interventions, SLD has the better prognosis.

The agreement to the fact that provision of extra-time for exams would help SLD's (Question 11), is quite high among all three teacher groups, with 85% agreement in the Pre-primary school students, followed by more than90% agreement in Primary and Middle school sections.

While the majority of Middle school teachers (70%) feel that giving exemptions for SLD during exams is justifiable (Question 15), only 47.6% of Pre-primary teachers and 40% of Primary teachers, believes so, which may be because the latter group of teachers feels that there is more scope for correction in younger age group, due to which exemptions may not be a requirement.

In general the teachers feel that the current curriculum does not allow sufficient flexibility for SLD students (Question 16), which is least agreed by Primary teachers and Middle school ones; but about 38.1% of Pre-primary teachers believed in inherent flexibility, which may be because as the academic load is less in here, the teachers find it easier to implement changes in instructional methods to accommodate the needs of SLD's as well.

The majority of teachers in this study, with about 95% of Pre-primary, 90% of Primary teachers and 85% of Middle-level ones, believe that mainstreaming would benefit SLD's (Question 7).

The group in general also acknowledges the essential role Resource teachers play in teaching SLD's (Question 12), with more than 90% agreement among both Pre-primary and Middle school teachers and 75% of Primary teachers, believing so. The slight reduction in the latter group may be because they feel that adapting classroom teaching methods to accommodate the needs of SLD's too, can handle the problem.

Table 7. Percentage of correct responses in attitude

Variables	Question	% of Correct Response by Pre-Primary Teachers		% of Correct Responses by Primary Teachers		% of Correct Responses by Middle School Teachers	
		Fully	Partially	Fully	Partially	Fully	Partially
Question 1	6	23.8%		20%		55%	
Question 2	8	38.1%	61.9%	20%	80%	45%	55%
Question 3	10	90.5%		90%		100%	
Question 4	11	85.7%		90%		90%	
Question 5	15	47.6%		40%		70%	
Question 6	16	38.1%		10%		20%	

Table 8. Percentage of correct responses in practice module

Variables	Question	% of Correct Response by Pre-Primary Teachers		% of Correct Responses by Primary Teachers		% of Correct Responses by Middle School Teachers	
		Fully	Partially	Fully	Partially	Fully	Partially
Question 1	7	95.2%		90%		85%	
Question 2	12	90.5%		75%		100%	
Question 3	13	61.9%		45%		70%	
Question 4	31	33.3%	66.7%	35%	65%	45%	50%
Question 5	32	38.1%	52.4%	15%	60%	30%	65%

The benefits of provision of scribe facility for SLD's with writing problems is welcomed most by Middle school teachers (more than 70%), followed by Pre-primary (61.9%). However, only 45% of Primary teachers, agree the same, which might reflect the fact that (Question 13) their writing problems are perceived to be correctable with appropriate remediation.

While more than 45% of the Middle school believe intimating parents for specialist referral, when they notice a child as having learning problems (Question 31), a mild reduction of 35% of Primary school and 33% are found among Pre-primary teachers is observed, which may be due to the fact that these problems are considered as passing problems or they have difficulty in convincing parents of a need for referral, who often are found to have acceptance issues.

When it comes to taking constructive steps like building rapport and counseling for the child with students who exhibit disturbed behavior in class (Question 32) too, more than 38% of pre-primary school teachers do so, while a slight reduction is seen among middle school teachers. A marked reduction is observed in primary school teachers which may be because in general teachers are not aware as to how to handle such disturbed behaviors in classroom situation.

To answer Research Question 2, regarding the relationship between experience gained by teachers in terms of years spent in teaching with the knowledge, attitude and practices of SLD, a correlation analysis was done (refer Table 9).

It has been found that for the Primary school teachers a significant correlation of (r=0.52, significant at 5%) was obtained, as the years of experience increased an increase in combined scores on SLD awareness was also found to increase. No such trends were observed in the case of Pre-primary or Middle school

Table 9. Correlation between the years of experience and the total score before training for the pre-primary, primary and middle school teachers

Category	Factors	Mean	SD	'r'
Pre-primary teachers	Years of experience	15.38	8.42	0.04
	Total score	27.38	5.06	
Primary teachers	Years of experience	11.18	7.71	0.52*
	Total score	27.23	5.04	
Middle school teachers	Years of experience	10.86	7.34	-0.02
	Total score	29.82	5.97	

*Significant at p>0.05

teachers. To explore which component or components of knowledge, attitude and practice contributed to this relationship among primary teachers, a correlation analysis was done which revealed that both the practice score and attitude score show a significant positive correlation at p <.05 level, which indicates that as they get more experienced in the teaching process they develop favorable attitudes and more effective practices in the management of SLD's (refer Table 10).

To answer Research Question 3, on the effectiveness of the training module was further analysis was done using paired sample t-test of the scores of the teachers to the questionnaire before and after training. This was done separately for knowledge; attitude, practice & total for each of the three teacher groups (refer Table 10).

The result of the comparisons of scores on knowledge before and after training is depicted in table 10. It has been found that both for Pre-primary (M (before training) =8.56; SD=2.61; M (after training) =11.13; SD=1.67) and Primary school teachers (M (before training) = 9.07; SD=2.25; M (after training) =11.87; SD=1.25) a significant improvement (p<.001) has been found in the knowledge on SLD. However, such a trend is absent among Middle school teachers, in the current sample. This might be due to the fact that though there was no significant difference between the scores of the three groups of teachers prior to training, the Middle school teachers were better informed on knowledge aspects of SLD (M=10.18, SD=2.61), compared to Pre-primary (M=8.56, SD=2.61) and Primary teachers (M=9.50, SD=2.41), even prior to training.

The result of the comparisons of scores on attitude before and after training is depicted in Table 12. In the case of the scores on attitude towards SLD, a significant improvement in attitude towards SLD

Table 10. Correlation between the years of experience of Primary school teachers and the score in knowledge, attitude, and practice

Variables	(1)	(2)	(3)	(4)
(1)Years of experience	1			
(2)Knowledge score	0.10	1		
(3)Attitude score	-0.04	0.28*	1	
(4)Practice score	-0.16	0.03	0.30*	1
Mean	12.23	9.33	7.25	7.64
SD	7.85	2.51	1.26	1.61

*Significant at p>0.05

Table 11. Comparison of the score on knowledge before and after training with regard to the three groups of teachers

Variables	Before Training		After Training		't'
	Mean	SD	Mean	SD	
Pre-primary	8.56	2.61	11.13	1.67	-3.79**
Primary	9.07	2.25	11.87	1.25	-4.91**
Middle school	10.33	2.92	11.40	1.68	-1.49

Significant at 1%**

Figure 2. Comparison of the score on knowledge before and after training with regard to the three groups of teachers

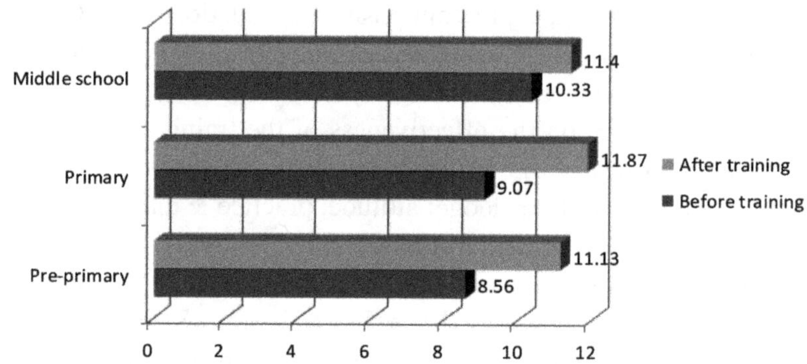

Table 12. Comparison of the score on attitude before and after training with regard to the three groups of teachers

Variables	Before Training		After Training		't'
	Mean	SD	Mean	SD	
Pre-primary	7.13	1.36	7.06	1.18	0.15
Primary	6.67	1.11	7.60	1.12	-3.50**
Middle school	8.20	0.94	7.87	1.25	-0.45

Significant at 1%**

Figure 3. Comparison of the score on attitude before and after training with regard to the three groups of teachers

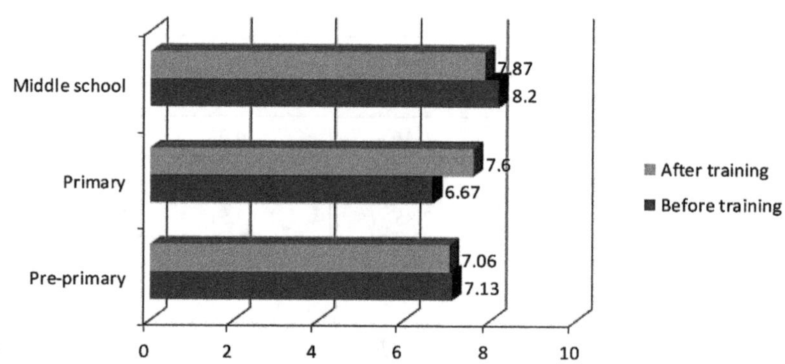

(p<.001) is found among Primary school teachers, which indicates a more favorable attitude towards SLD children through the training.

However, no significant improvements in attitudes have been found in both Pre-primary teachers (M (before training) =7.13, SD= 1.36; M (after training) =7.06. SD =1.18) and among the Middle school teachers (M (before training) =8.2, SD= 0.94; M (after training) =7.87, SD=1.25).

The result of the comparisons of scores on practice before and after training is depicted in table 6, Here again it has been found that significant improvement (p<.001) has been observed in practice

Table 13. Comparison of the score on practice before and after training with regard to the three groups of teachers

Variables	Before Training		After Training		't'
	Mean	SD	Mean	SD	
Pre-primary	7.63	1.54	8.13	1.71	-0.98
Primary	7.27	1.53	9.00	0.85	-4.25**
Middle school	8.00	1.96	8.60	0.91	-1.26

Significant at 1%**

Figure 4. Comparison of the score on practice before and after training with regard to the three groups of teachers

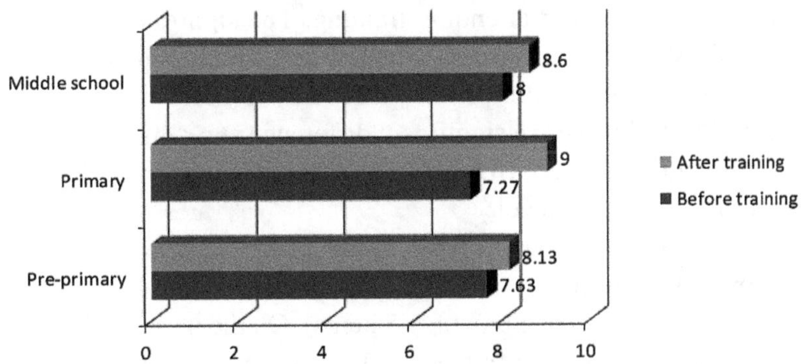

scores of Primary teachers, after training (M (before training) =7.27, SD=1.53 & M (after training) = 9.00; SD=0.85). The teachers in primary level handle children from class1 to 4, which is the stage when early detection of SLD is possible. So the importance of the practical application is most crucial for this group. A positive improvement in this scale promises better identification & referral to children in need.

However the score on practice was seen to have no significant improvement in the case of Pre-primary teachers (M (before training = 7.63; SD=1.54); M (after training) =8.13; SD=1.71), as well as Middle school teachers (M (before training = 8; SD=1.96); M (after training) =8.60; SD=0.91).

The significant improvement perceived in the sample has been established through paired sample t-test which points to the effectiveness of the training program on the sample (refer Table 14).

The result of the comparisons of the total scores before and after training is depicted in Table 14, which shows that there is the significant improvement in both the Pre-school and Primary groups of teachers,

Table 14. Comparison of the total score before and after training with regard to the three groups of teachers

Variables	Before Training		After Training		't'
	Mean	SD	Mean	SD	
Pre-primary	23.31	3.95	26.31	2.85	-2.84*
Primary	23.00	3.16	28.47	1.85	-6.80**
Middle school	26.53	3.78	27.87	2.00	-1.67

Significant at 1%**, Significant at 5%*

Figure 5. Comparison of the total score before and after training with regard to the three groups of teachers

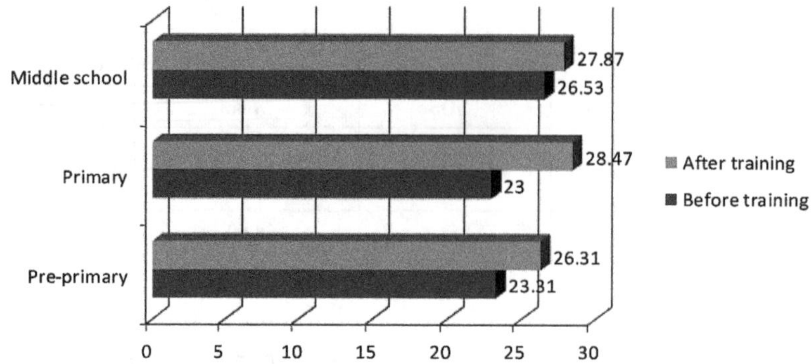

but not in Middle school teachers, after attending training. The significant improvement perceived in the sample has been established through paired sample t-test which points to the effectiveness of the training program on the sample. Both in Pre-primary teachers (M (before training) =23.31; SD=3.95; M (after training) =26.31; SD=2.85) where a significant difference at $p<.01$ has been found and in case of Primary school (M (before training) =23; SD=3.16; M (after training) =28.47; SD=1.85) a significant improvement has been found at $p<.05$ level.

To probe into the questions that yielded the maximum change in their level of understanding; paired sample t-test was performed on an item level. The questionnaire consisted of 22 items, grouped into knowledge (11 items), attitude (6 items) & practice (5 items). On the item level analysis of attitude questions, no significant change was observed in any single item. In the case of items addressing practice only one item was perceived to have a significant (5% level of significance) change in the sample.

Considering the questions addressing knowledge of the sample, the significant change was perceived in 8 out of the 11 questions. Paired sample t-test of knowledge questions before and after training is depicted in Table 15.

The results show that Questions 5, 14, 17,18, 24 & 29 have contributed to the difference in scores prior to training at $p<.001$ level and Questions 3 & 9, at $p<.005$ level.

DISCUSSION

The analysis of the results of the current study reveal that level of knowledge as well as their practices with SLD, is comparable among the Pre-Primary, Primary and Secondary school teachers. This finding draws support from the study by Lingeswaran (2013) who found the low fund of knowledge among Primary school teachers, in our country, on SLD. Saludes and Artenita (2009), has also claimed that educators have low knowledge and awareness of the condition. Lopes and Crenitte (2013) go a step further to reveal that elementary teacher's knowledge about SLD is largely superficial. The finding that secondary school teacher's attitude and overall idea regarding SLD is better compared to Primary school teachers, prior to training, indicates that they have a realistic perception of SLD's problems and have a favorable attitude. This finding is supported by the observation by Shari and Vranda (2015) that only 5% of primary school teachers have adequate knowledge of SLD.

The Secondary school teachers have more positive attitudes and general idea regarding SLD compared to Primary school teachers in this study finds support from the study by Elias (2014) who found

Table 15. Comparison of the score before and after training on each question of knowledge regarding the sample

Variables	Before Training		After Training		't'
	Mean	SD	Mean	SD	
Question1	0.59	0.50	0.75	0.44	-2.06*
Question2	0.16	0.37	0.27	0.49	-1.63
Question3	0.39	0.64	1.31	0.71	-7.79**
Question4	0.82	0.74	1.08	0.56	-1.99
Question5	0.51	0.51	0.92	0.27	-5.14**
Question6	0.37	0.49	0.88	0.99	-3.48**
Question7	3.82	1.09	4.31	0.68	-3.12**
Question8	0.29	0.58	0.39	0.49	-1.00
Question9	0.47	0.50	0.67	0.48	-2.11*
Question10	0.45	0.50	0.75	0.44	-3.45**
Question11	0.76	0.42	0.98	0.14	-3.71**

Significant at 1%**, Significant at 5%*

Secondary school teachers to have a reasonable idea on dyslexia, though training on specific aspects may be required to fine-tune their knowledge. This trend may be because Secondary teachers are more likely to note academic skill deficits in their students, which is both glaring and would result in serious gaps in achievement, often of persistent nature.

The finding that the more experienced the teachers are i.e., the number of years of teaching experience the better is the knowledge, positive attitudes and practices specifically among Primary school teachers, finds support from the observation of Venkatesan and Purusotham (2007) that SLD features in primary school years present as academic deficits of writing and arithmetic difficulties. Since primary school years is the formative stage of the very same academic skills which are affected in SLD's, greater exposure gives them better knowledge about the same, translating into positive attitudes and practices. It was also found that there was a positive relation between better scores in attitude and better score in practice among Primary teachers which means that the better their attitudes to SLD the better they were in adopting methods in identifying and managing SLD's.

In the subsequent analysis of the effectiveness of the training module, it has been found that the score on knowledge is seen to have significantly improved in the case of Pre-Primary and Primary school teachers. This finding is supported by the studies by Lopes and Crenitte (2013) and Daniel, Gupta, and Sagar (2013) who made the similar finding that that primary school teachers report significant improvement in knowledge prior to focused training on Learning Disabilities and child psychiatric disorders. Deepthi et al. (2015) also seconds this finding with their observation that structured training programs are effective in increasing knowledge level of SLD among primary school teachers.

The finding that improvement in attitude scores and practice scores were limited to Primary teachers indicates a more favorable attitude towards SLD children through the training, which might be a reflection of the improvement in knowledge on SLD, which has instilled in them the confidence that with timely identification & appropriate interventions and accommodations, SLD can be managed at the school level. This finding gets support from Woodcock's (2013) evidence that primary teacher trainees were found to have the moderately higher positive attitude to SLD students compared to their secondary counterparts. Interestingly though the Middle school teachers have a higher mean score than their Pre-Primary & Primary school counterparts they did not seem to have a significant improvement in their attitude scores which might be due to an already existing favorable attitude prior to the training.

The absence of improvement among Pre-Primary teacher's practice scores might be due to the fact that Pre-Primary teachers handle first-time school goers & the symptoms relating to LD might not be noticeably pronounced at this stage, hence the practical applicability is also minimal. So also, at the middle school level teachers might have understood the fact that SLD's require special assistance in addition to classroom interventions for effective management.

The finding that significant improvement in the overall scores was found in Pre-Primary and Primary teachers alone, might be due to the fact that in general Middle school teacher's attitude to SLD was more favorable even before training and hence training effects became minimal. So also those teachers in the lower classes might have understood the scope and access they have for early identification of SLD's.

It has also been found that the questions in the knowledge domain contributed to the maximum change in their level of understanding prior to training with a majority of them viz., 8 out of 11 questions producing the significant difference between pre & post scores. This again reiterates the findings from previous studies by Antony et al. (2013) that educational programs are quite effective in improving knowledge and attitudes of teachers to SLD's. Lopes and Crenitte (2013) also claim that orientation programs can cause alterations in teacher's conception of learning disorders.

This indicates that imparting training programs focusing on factual knowledge on SLD would definitely improve the knowledge level of SLD among teachers. This would, in turn, reflect favorable attitude changes and give them a better orientation to practical remediation aspects.

FUTURE RESEARCH DIRECTIONS

Training programs intended to improve knowledge level can be made more intensive with hand–on–experience to teachers, in the identification of SLD's from their own classrooms, with the help of professionally prepared checklists. A gender-matched sample could probe whether there is the significant difference between gender in knowledge, attitudes and practices of SLD as well as in training effects.

CONCLUSION

The teachers in the pre-primary, primary and secondary school have no significant variation in either the knowledge level or practices about SLD. But Secondary/Middle school teachers have better attitudes and overall idea regarding SLD, compared to Primary school teachers. The Primary school teachers show improvement in their overall idea of SLD as they gain more teaching experience, which will reflect in changes in attitudes and practical management of SLD. Imparting short-term intensive multi-disciplinary training programs, on Specific Learning Disorders for Primary school teachers improves the knowledge level about the condition, creates positive attitudes and paves the way for better practices of early identification and appropriate referrals. Such training programs would also benefit Pre-Primary teachers by improving their factual knowledge on SLD. This would result in the identification of at-risk children leading to prevention of SLD.

IMPLICATIONS

Short-term intensive in-service training programs designed focussing on factual aspects of SLD, should be a regular practice for Pre-primary and Primary school teachers of the general education classrooms, to improve awareness of SLD leading to more positive attitudes towards them and adopting informed practices like timely identification, appropriate specialist referrals and classroom management strategies. This would also sensitize the teachers to a more realistic perception of their problems and seek appropriate classroom intervention strategies. It would also go a long way in reducing stress levels of affected children and their parents' in-turn would be a cost-effective way to tackle SLD in our country.

REFERENCES

Afshan, Y. (2009, February 26). Fresh concessions for dyslexic students. *The Hindu*. Retrieved from http://www.hindu.com/2009/02/26/stories/2009022659340400.htm

American Psychiatric Association. (2013). *Diagnostic and statistical manual of mental disorders* (5th ed.). Arlington, VA: American Psychiatric Publishing.

Antony, F., Venkatesan, S., Jayarama, G., & Gupta, S. K. (2013). Impact of an educational program about learning disability on primary school teachers. *Periyar University Journal of Psychology*, *1*(1), 83–87.

Bashir, A. S., Wiig, E. H., & Abrams, J. C. (1987). Language disorders in childhood and adolescence: Implications for learning and socialization. *Pediatric Annals*, *16*(2), 145–156. doi:10.3928/0090-4481-19870201-08 PMID:3562098

Berninger, V. W., & Abbott, R. D. (1994). Redefining learning disabilities: Moving beyond aptitude–achievement discrepancies to failure to respond to validated treatment protocols. In G. R. Lyon (Ed.), *Frames of reference for the assessment of learning disabilities: New views on measurement issues* (pp. 163–184). Baltimore, MD: P.H. Brookes.

Bhasi, S. (2003*). Remediation for arithmetic disorders-A neuropsychological perspective* (Unpublished doctoral dissertation). Department of Clinical Psychology, NIMHANS, Bangalore.

Bhola, P., Hirisave, U., & Kapur, M. (1997). Self perception and learning environment in children with scholastic skill disorder. In R. Hegde, S. Malhotra & L. P. Shah (Eds.), Research endevours in child and adoloscent psychiatry in India. Goa: Indian Association for child and Adolescent Mental Health.

Bruck, M. (1986). Social and emotional adjustments of learning disabled children: A review of the issues. In S. J. Ceci (Ed.), *Handbook of cognitive, social, and neuropsychological aspects of learning disabilities* (pp. 361–380). Hillsdale, NJ: Erlbaum.

Buckingham, J., Wheldall, K., & Wheldall, R. B. (2013). Why poor children are more likely to become poor readers: The school years. *Australian Journal of Education*, *57*(3), 190–213. doi:10.1177/0004944113495500

Butterworth, B. (2005). The development of arithmetical abilities. *Journal of Child Psychology and Psychiatry, and Allied Disciplines*, *46*(1), 3–18. doi:10.1111/j.1469-7610.2004.00374.x PMID:15660640

Caraballo, R. H., Cejas, N., Chamorro, N., Kaltenmeier, M. C., Fortini, S., & Soprano, A. M. (2014). Landau–Kleffner syndrome: A study of 29 patients. *Seizure*, *23*(2), 98–104. doi:10.1016/j.seizure.2013.09.016 PMID:24315829

Cardon, L. R., Smith, S. D., Fulker, D. W., Kimberling, W. J., Pennington, B. F., & DeFries, J. C. (1994). Quantitative trait locus for reading disability on chromosome 6. *Science*, *266*(5183), 276–279. doi:10.1126cience.7939663 PMID:7939663

Chatterjee, M. (2009). *Indian teachers still not trained to tackle dyslexia.* Retrieved from http://www.daijiworld.com/news/news_disp.asp?n_id=65148

Dahaene, S., & Cohen, L. (2011). The unique role of the visual word form area in reading. *Trends in Cognitive Sciences*, *15*(6), 254–262. doi:10.1016/j.tics.2011.04.003 PMID:21592844

Daniel, L. T., Gupta, S., & Sagar, R. (2013). Effect of educational module on knowledge of primary school teachers regarding early symptoms of childhood psychiatric disorders. *Indian Journal of Psychological Medicine*, *35*(4), 368. doi:10.4103/0253-7176.122228 PMID:24379497

Deepthi, G., Padmavathi, N., Philip, R. R., & Kavitha, R. R. (2015). Effect of structured teaching program on knowledge regarding specific learning disabilities among primary school teachers. *International Journal of Psychiatric Nursing*, *1*(1), 69–72. doi:10.5958/2395-180X.2015.00017.1

Dehaene, S., Piazza, M., Pinel, P., & Cohen, L. (2003). Three parietal circuits for number processing. *Cognitive Neuropsychology*, *20*(3-6), 487–506. doi:10.1080/02643290244000239 PMID:20957581

Démonet, J. F., Taylor, M. J., & Chaix, Y. (2004). Developmental dyslexia. *Lancet*, *363*(9419), 1451–1460. doi:10.1016/S0140-6736(04)16106-0 PMID:15121410

Elias, R. (2014). *Dyslexic Learners: An Investigation into the Attitudes and Knowledge of Secondary School Teachers in New Zealand* (Unpublished dissertation). University of Auckland, New Zealand.

Emerson, E., & Hatton, C. (2007). *The Mental Health of Children & Adolescents with Learning Disabilities in Britain.* Retrieved on May 5, 2017, from http://www.lancaster.ac.uk/staff/emersone/FASSWeb/Emerson_07_FPLD_MentalHealth.pdf

Fiez, J. A., & Petersen, S. E. (1998). Neuroimaging studies of word reading. *Proceedings of the National Academy of Sciences of the United States of America*, *95*(3), 914–921. doi:10.1073/pnas.95.3.914 PMID:9448259

Fiez, J. A., Raichle, M. E., Miezin, F. M., Petersen, S. E., Tallal, P., & Katz, W. F. (1995). PET studies of auditory and phonological processing: Effects of stimulus characteristics and task demands. *Journal of Cognitive Neuroscience*, *7*(3), 357–375. doi:10.1162/jocn.1995.7.3.357 PMID:23961866

Francis, D. J., Shaywitz, S. E., & Steubing, K. K. (1994). Measurement of change: Assessing behavior over time and within a developmental context. In G. R. Lyon (Ed.), *Frames of reference for the assessment of learning disabilities: New views on measurement issues* (pp. 29–58). Baltimore, MD: Paul H. Brookes.

Fuchs, L. S., & Fuchs, D. (1998). Treatment validity: A unifying concept for reconceptualizing the identification of learning disabilities. *Learning Disabilities Research & Practice*, *13*, 204–219.

Fuchs, S. L., Fuchs, D., Compton, L. D., Powell, R. S., Seethaler, P. M., Capizzi, A. M., ... Fletcher, J. M. (2006). The cognitive correlates of third – grade skill in arithmetic, algorithmic computation and arithmetic word problems. *Journal of Educational Psychology*, *98*(1), 29–43. doi:10.1037/0022-0663.98.1.29

Geary, D. C. (2004). Mathematics and learning disabilities. *Journal of Learning Disabilities*, *37*(1), 4–15. doi:10.1177/00222194040370010201 PMID:15493463

Gerber, P. J. (2001). Learning disabilities: A life-span approach. In D. P. Hallahan & B. K. Keogh (Eds.), *Research and global perspectives in learning disabilities* (pp. 167–180). Mahwah, NJ: Erlbaum.

Gersten, R., Chard, D. J., Jayanthi, M., Baker, S. K., Morphy, P., & Flojo, J. (2009). Mathematics instruction for students with learning disabilities: A meta-analysis of instructional components. *Review of Educational Research*, *79*(3), 1202–1242. doi:10.3102/0034654309334431

Goswami, U. (1999). The Relationship between Phonological Awareness and Orthographic Representation in Different Orthographies. In M. Harris & G. Hatano (Eds.), *Learning to Read and Write: A Cross-Linguistic Perspective*. New York: Cambridge University Press.

Gresham, F. M. (2002). Responsiveness to intervention: An alternative approach to the identification of learning disabilities. In R. Bradley, L. Danielson, & D. Hallahan (Eds.), *Identification of learning disabilities: Research to practice* (pp. 467–519). Mahwah, NJ: Erlbaum.

Gresham, F. M., & Reschly, D. J. (1986). Social skill deficits and low peer acceptance of mainstreamed learning disabled children. *Learning Disability Quarterly*, *9*(1), 23–32. doi:10.2307/1510398

Guillette, E. A. (1998). An anthropological evaluation of preschool children exposed to the toxic effects of pesticides in Mexico. *Environmental Health Perspectives*, *106*(6), 347–353. doi:10.1289/ehp.98106347 PMID:9618351

Haddow, J. E., Palomiki, G. E., Allan, W. C., Williams, J. R., Knight, G. J., Gagnon, J., & Klein, R. Z. (1999). Maternal thyroid deficiency during pregnancy and subsequent development of the child. *The New England Journal of Medicine*, *341*(8), 549–555. doi:10.1056/NEJM199908193410801 PMID:10451459

Hitch, G. J., & McAuley, E. (1991). Working memory in children with specific arithmetical learning difficulties. *British Journal of Psychology*, *82*(3), 375–386. doi:10.1111/j.2044-8295.1991.tb02406.x PMID:1954527

Huang, H. S., & Hanley, J. R. (1994). Phonological awareness and visual skills in learning to read Chinese and English. *Cognition*, *54*(1), 73–98. doi:10.1016/0010-0277(94)00641-W PMID:7851080

John, A., Sadasivan, A., Sukumaran, B., Bhola, P., David, N. J., & Manickam, L. S. S. (2013). Practice Guidelines: Learning Disabilities. *Indian Journal of Clinical Psychology*, *40*(1), 65–88.

Johnson, E. S., Humphrey, M., Mellard, D. F., Woods, K., & Swanson, H. L. (2010). Cognitive processing deficits and students with specific learning disabilities: A selective meta-analysis of the literature. *Learning Disability Quarterly*, *33*(1), 3–1. doi:10.1177/073194871003300101

Kamala, R., & Ramganesh, E. (2013). Knowledge of Specific Learning Disabilities among Teacher Educators in Puducherry, Union Territory in India. *International Review of Social Sciences and Humanities*, *6*(1), 168–175.

Kamhi, A. G., & Catts, H. W. (Eds.). (1989). *Reading Disabilities: A Developmental language Perspective*. Boston: Allyn & Bacon.

Kapur, M., Barnabas, I., Reddy, M. V., Rozario, J., & Uma, H. (1995). Developmental psychopathology checklist for children (DPCL): A preliminary report. *Nimhans Journal, 13*, 1–9.

Kapur, M., John, A., Rozario, J., & Oommen, A. (2002). *NIMHANS index of specific learning disabilities. In Psychological Assessment of Children in the Clinical Setting* (pp. 88–126). Bangalore: Department of Clinical Psychology, National Institute of Mental Health and Neurosciences.

Karande, S. (2008). Current challenges in managing specific learning disability in Indian children. *Journal of Postgraduate Medicine*, *54*(2), 75. doi:10.4103/0022-3859.40765 PMID:18480515

Karande, S., & Kulkarni, M. (2005). Specific learning disability: The invisible handicap. *Indian Pediatrics*, *42*(4), 315–319. PMID:15876592

Karanth, P. (2003). *Cross-linguistic study of acquired reading disorders: Implications for reading models, disorders, acquisition, and teaching*. New York: Kluwer Academic/Plenum Publishers. doi:10.1007/978-1-4419-8923-9

Karanth, P. (2008). Learning disability and language learning. In K. Thapa, G. M. Aalsvoort, & J. Pandey (Eds.), *Perspectives on Learning Disabilities in India* (pp. 80–94). New Delhi: Sage Publications.

Karibasappa, C. N., Nishanimut, S. P., & Padakannaya, P. (2008). A remedial teaching programme to help children with mathematical disability. *Asia Pacific Disability Rehabilitation Journal*, *19*(2), 76–90.

Kaufmann, W. E., & Galaburda, A. M. (1989). Cerebrocortical microdysgenesis in neurologically normal subjects: A histopathologic study. *Neurology*, *39*(2), 238–244. doi:10.1212/WNL.39.2.238 PMID:2915796

Keogh, B. K., & Sears, S. (1991). Learning disabilities from a developmental perspective: Early identification and prediction. In B. Y. L. Wong (Ed.), *Learning about learning disabilities* (pp. 485–503). San Diego, CA: Academic Press. doi:10.1016/B978-0-12-762530-0.50023-0

Kirk, S. A. (1962). *Educating exceptional children*. Boston: Houghton Miffin.

Kirk, S. A., & Weiner, B. B. (1963). *Behavioural Research on Exceptional Children*. Washington, DC: The Council for Exceptional Children.

Kohli, A., Malhotra, S., Mohanty, M., Khehra, N., & Kaur, M. (2005). Specific learning disabilities in children: Deficits and neuropsychological profile. *International Journal of Rehabilitation Research. Internationale Zeitschrift fur Rehabilitationsforschung. Revue Internationale de Recherches de Readaptation*, *28*(2), 165–169. doi:10.1097/00004356-200506000-00011 PMID:15900188

Konathambigi, R. J., & Shetty, M. (2008). Teacher identification of learning problems. In K. Thapa, G. M. Aalsvoort, & J. Pandey (Eds.), *Perspectives on Learning Disabilities in India*. New Delhi: Sage Publications.

Korhonen, T. T. (1995). The persistence of rapid naming problems in children with reading disabilities: A nine-year follow-up. *Journal of Learning Disabilities*, *28*(4), 232–239. doi:10.1177/002221949502800405 PMID:7738435

Lall, A., Hirisavae, U., Kapur, M., & Subbakrisha, D. K. (1997). Perceived peer relations, social competance in children with specific disorders of socialistic skills. *Nimhans Journal, 15*(2), 133–137.

Leiva, P. B., Inzunza, B. N., Pérez, T. H., Castro, G. V., Jansana, M. J., Toro, D. T., ... Ivanovic, M. D. (2001). The impact of malnutrition on brain development, intelligence and school work performance. *Archivos Latinoamericanos de Nutricion, 51*(1), 64–71. PMID:11515234

Lennerstrandt, G., Ygge, J., & Jacobsson, C. (1993). Control of binocular eye movements in normals and dyslexics. *Annals of the New York Academy of Sciences, 682*, 232–239. PMID:8323115

Lingeswaran, A. (2013). Assessing knowledge of primary school teachers on specific learning disabilities in two schools in India. *Journal of Education and Health Promotion, 2*(1), 30. doi:10.4103/2277-9531.115807 PMID:24083280

Livingstone, M. S., Rosen, G. D., Drislane, F. W., & Galaburda, A. M. (1991). Physiological and anatomical evidence for a magnocellular defect in developmental dyslexia. *Proceedings of the National Academy of Sciences of the United States of America, 88*(18), 7943–7947. doi:10.1073/pnas.88.18.7943 PMID:1896444

Logan, W. J. (1996). Neuroimaging and functional brain analysis. In J. H. Beitchman, N. J. Cohen, M. M. Konstantareas, & R. Tannock (Eds.), *Language learning and behavior disorders: Developmental, biological and clinical perspectives*. Cambridge, UK: Cambridge University Press.

Lopes, R. C. F., & Crenitte, P. A. P. (2013). Analytical study of teacher's knowledge about learning disorders. *Revista CEFAC, 15*(5), 1214–1226. doi:10.1590/S1516-18462012005000091

Lyon, G. R., Fletcher, J. M., Shaywitz, S. E., Shaywitz, B. A., Torgesen, J. K., Wood, F. B., & Olson, R. (2001). Rethinking learning disabilities. In C. E. Finn, A. J. Rotherman, & C. R. Hokanson (Eds.), *Rethinking Education for a New Century* (pp. 259–287). Washington, DC: Thomas B. Fordham Foundation and the Progressive Policy Institute.

Mather, N., & Greg, N. (2006). Specific learning disabilities: Clarifying, not eliminating a construct. *Professional Psychology, Research and Practice, 37*(1), 99–106. doi:10.1037/0735-7028.37.1.99

Mayes, S. D., Calhoun, S. L., & Crowell, E. W. (2000). Learning disabilities and ADHD: Overlapping spectrumn disorders. *Journal of Learning Disabilities, 33*(5), 417–424. doi:10.1177/002221940003300502 PMID:15495544

Mehta, H. (2000). *A Low Cost Diagnostic Test of Mathematics Disability (TMD) in Children aged 7 to 10 Yrs* (M.Ed Dissertation). Mumbai: SNDT Womens University.

Meltzer, H., Gatward, R., Goodman, R., & Ford, T. (2000). *Mental Health of Children & Adolescents in Great Britain*. London: The Stationary Office. doi:10.1037/e622732007-001

Montague, M., Maddox, C. D., & Dereshiwsky, M. I. (1990). Story grammar and comprehension and production of narrative prose by students with learning disabilities. *Journal of Learning Disabilities, 23*(21), 190–197. doi:10.1177/002221949002300310 PMID:2313193

Mukerjee, S., Hirisave, U., Kapur, M., & Subbakrishna, D. K. (1995). Anxiety, self-esteem in children with specific disorders of scholastic skills. *Nimhans Journal, 17*(2), 117–121.

Nehru, R. (2001). *Distorted grapheme representation: A new hypothesis to explain reading disorders.* Poster presentation at the 5th British Dyslexia Association International Conference, York, UK.

Pennington, B. F., & Bishop, D. V. (2009). Relations among speech, language, and reading disorders. *Annual Review of Psychology, 60*(1), 283–306. doi:10.1146/annurev.psych.60.110707.163548 PMID:18652545

Prakash, P. (2003). Early reading acquisition. In P. Karanth & J. Rozario (Eds.), *Learning disabilities in India: Willing the mind to learn* (pp. 63–65). New Delhi: Sage Publications.

Prakash, P., & Rekha, B. (1992). Phonological awareness and reading acquisition in Kannada. In A. K. Srivastava (Ed.), *Researches in child and adolescent psychology* (pp. 47–52). New Delhi: NCERT.

Prakash, P., Rekha, D., Nigam, R., & Karanath, P. (1993). Phonological awareness, orthography and literary. In R. J. Scholes (Ed.), *Literary and language analysis.* Hillsdale, NJ: Lawrence Erlbaum Associates.

Prema, K. S. (1998). *Reading Acquisition Profile in Kannada* (Doctoral dissertation). Mysore: University of Mysore.

Ramaa, S. (1984). *Diagnosis and remediation of dyslexia* (Doctoral dissertation). Mysore: University of Mysore.

Ramaa, S., & Gowramma, I. P. (2002). A systematic procedure for identifying and classifying children with dyscalculia among primary school children in India. *Dyslexia (Chichester, England), 8*(2), 67–85. doi:10.1002/dys.214 PMID:12067188

Reynolds, C. R., & Willson, V. L. (1974). Critical measurement issues in learning disabilities. *The Journal of Special Education, 18*(4), 451–476. doi:10.1177/002246698401800403

Roeltgen, D. P., Sevush, S., & Heilman, K. M. (1983). Phonological agraphia: Writing by the lexical-semantic route. *Neurology, 33*(6), 755–765. doi:10.1212/WNL.33.6.755 PMID:6682519

Rosselli, M., Matute, E., Pinto, N., & Ardila, A. (2006). Memory abilities in children with subtypes of dyscalculia. *Developmental Neuropsychology, 30*(3), 801–818. doi:10.120715326942dn3003_3 PMID:17083294

Rozario, J. (2003). Assessment of Learning Disabilities. In P. Karanth & J. Rozario (Eds.), *Learning Disabilities in India: Willing the Mind to Learn* (pp. 51–61). New Delhi: Sage Publications.

Saludes, M. C., & Artenita, D. (2009). *The knowledge and perceptions on learning disabilities in the cities of region XI of the Philippines and a region in New York City, N.Y., U.S.A.* The 19th Asian Conference on Mental Retardation, Singapore. Retrieved from www.gtid.net/acmr19/pdf/11.pdf

Saravanabhavan, S., & Saravanabhavan, R. C. (2001). Attitudes toward disabilities across cultures. *Educational Theory and Practice, 23*(2), 49–60. doi:10.7459/ept/23.2.04

Saravanabhavan, S., & Saravanabhavan, R. C. (2010). Knowledge of learning disability among pre-and in-service teachers in India. *International Journal of Special Education, 25*(3), 133–139.

Scarborough, H. S. (1990). Very early language deficits in dyslexic children. *Child Development, 61*(6), 1728–1743. doi:10.2307/1130834 PMID:2083495

Shalev, R. S., Manor, O., Auerbach, J., & Gross-Tsur, V. (1998). Persistence of developmental dyscalculia: What counts? Results from a three year prospective follow up study. *The Journal of Pediatrics*, *133*(3), 358–362. doi:10.1016/S0022-3476(98)70269-0 PMID:9738716

Shari, M., & Vranda, M. N. (2015). Knowledge of primary school teachers in identifying children with learning disabilities. *Disability, CBR and Inclusive Development*, *26*(3), 68–76. doi:10.5463/DCID.v26i3.443

Sharma, A. (2000). *Language Skills in Children with Learning Disability* (Unpublished Masters Dissertation). Mangalore University.

Shaywitz, S. E. (1998). Dyslexia. *The New England Journal of Medicine*, *338*(5), 307–312. doi:10.1056/NEJM199801293380507 PMID:9445412

Snow, C. E., Burns, M. S., & Griffin, P. (Eds.). (2000). *Preventing Reading Difficulties in Young Children. US National Research Council Report*. Washington, DC: National Academy Press.

Srikanth, N., & Karanth, P. (2003). Speech language pathologists and remediation of reading disabilities. In P. Karanth & J. Rozario (Eds.), *Learning Disabilities in India: Willing the Mind to Learn* (pp. 150–165). New Delhi: Sage Publications.

Stanovich, K. E. (1991). Discrepancy definitions of reading disability: Has intelligence led us astray? *Reading Research Quarterly*, *26*(1), 7–29. doi:10.2307/747729

Stanovich, K. E. (1993). A model for studies of reading disability. *Developmental Review*, *13*(3), 225–245. doi:10.1006/drev.1993.1010

Stanovich, K. E., Siegel, L. S., & Linda, S. (1994). Phenotypic performance profile of children with reading disabilities: A regression-based test of the phonological-core variable-difference model. *Journal of Educational Psychology*, *86*(1), 24–53. doi:10.1037/0022-0663.86.1.24

Suresh, P. A., & Sebastian, S. (2003). Epidemiological and neurological aspects of learning disabilities. In P. Karanth & J. Rozario (Eds.), *Learning Disabilities in India: Willing the Mind to Learn* (pp. 30–43). New Delhi: Sage Publications.

Swanson, H. L., & Jerman, O. (2006). Math disabilities: A selective meta-analysis of the literature. *Review of Educational Research*, *76*(2), 249–274. doi:10.3102/00346543076002249

Swanson, H. L., Zheng, X., & Jerman, O. (2009). Working memory, short-term memory, and reading disabilities: A selective meta-analysis of the literature. *Journal of Learning Disabilities*, *42*(3), 260–287. doi:10.1177/0022219409331958 PMID:19255286

Swarup, S., & Mehta, D. H. (1991). *Behavioural Checklist for Screening Learning Disabled*. Mumbai: SNDT Women's University.

Tallal, P., Miller, S., & Fitch, R. H. (1993). Neurobiological basis of speech: A case for the prominence of mental processing. *Annals of the New York Academy of Sciences*, *682*(1 Temporal Info), 27–47. doi:10.1111/j.1749-6632.1993.tb22957.x PMID:7686725

Tannock, R. (2013). Rethinking ADHD and LD in DSM-5: Proposed changes in diagnostic criteria. *Journal of Learning Disabilities*, *46*(1), 5–25. doi:10.1177/0022219412464341 PMID:23144062

Thomas, S., Bhanutej, K., & John, S. (2003). Dealing with Dyslexia. *The Week*, *21*, 36–42.

Urion, D. K., Huff, H. V., & Carullo, M. P. (2015). MRI in assessing children with learning disability, focal findings, and reduced automaticity. *Neurology*, *85*(7), 604–609. doi:10.1212/WNL.0000000000001849 PMID:26180142

Vellutino, F. R., Scanlon, D. M., & Lyon, G. R. (2000). Differentiating between difficult-to-remediate and readily remediated poor readers: More evidence against the IQ-achievement discrepancy definition of reading disability. *Journal of Learning Disabilities*, *33*(3), 223–238. doi:10.1177/002221940003300302 PMID:15505962

Venkatesan, S. (2006). *Mimeograph on Development and Standardisation of Appraisal of Kids with Specific Handicaps in Arithmetic and Reasoning Activities (AKSHARA)*. Mysore: All India Institute of Speech and Hearing.

Venkatesan, S. (2017). Analysis of attributes in the official definitions for learning disability. *The International Journal of Indian Psychology*, *4*(2), 46–57.

Venkatesan, S., & Purusotham, P. (2007). Historical analysis on course and clinical presentations of children with learning disabilities in India. *Disabilities and Impairments*, *21*(2), 99–107.

Vohr, B. R., Coll, C. G., Lobato, D., Yunis, K. A., O'Dea, C., & Oh, W. (1991). Neurodevelopmental and medical status of low-birthweight survivors of bronchopulmonary dysplasia at 10 to 12 years of age. *Developmental Medicine and Child Neurology*, *33*(8), 690–697. doi:10.1111/j.1469-8749.1991.tb14946.x PMID:1717327

Wilson, A. J., & Dehaene, S. (2007). Number sense and developmental dyscalculia. In D. Coch, G. Dawson, & K. Fischer (Eds.), *Human behavior, learning and the developing brain: Atypical development*. New York: Guilford Press.

Witteman, C. L. M., Harries, C., Bekker, H. L., & Van Aarle, E. J. M. (2007). Evaluating psychodiagnostic decisions. *Journal of Evaluation in Clinical Practice*, *13*(1), 10–15. doi:10.1111/j.1365-2753.2006.00689.x PMID:17286717

Wolf, D. F. (1991). *The effects of task, language of assessment, and target language experience on foreign language learners performance on reading comprehension tests* (Doctoral dissertation). University of Illinois at Urbana-Champaign.

Woodcock, S. (2013). Trainee teachers attitudes towards students with specific learning disabilities. *Australian Journal of Teachers Education*, *38*(8), 16–29.

World Health Organization. (1992). *The ICD-10 classification of mental and behavioural disorders: Clinical descriptions and diagnostic guidelines*. Geneva: World Health Organization.

Yadav, D., & Agarwal, V. (2008). A baseline study of learning disabilities: Its prevalence, teacher awareness and classroom practices. In K. Thapa, G. M. Aalsvoort, & J. Pandey (Eds.), *Perspectives on Learning Disabilities in India* (pp. 221–238). New Delhi: Sage Publication.

Zigmond, N. (1993). Learning disabilities from an educational perspective. In G. R. Lyon, D. B. Gray, J. F. Kavanaugh, & N. A. Krasnegor (Eds.), *Better understanding learning disabilities: New views from research and their implications for education and public policies* (pp. 251–272). Baltimore, MD: Brookes.

KEY TERMS AND DEFINITIONS

Early Detection: Early detection is defined as awareness of commonly appearing signs of SLD in the form of delayed language, poor listening and comprehension, slow letter recognition, slowness in blending letters to words, poor reading comprehension, spelling errors in writing, difficulty in spontaneous writing, slowness and frequent errors in mathematical calculations, and difficulty with word problem solving as well as behavioral features of restlessness, lack of concentration, etc., and skill in detecting the same during early school years, both those who at-risk (2nd Standard or below) and those from 3rd to 5th standard.

IQ-Achievement Discrepancy: The substantial difference between a person's measured general intelligence level and his/her scores in one or more areas of academic achievement.

Language Learning: The capacity to acquire receptive and expressive oral and written language skills such as listening and oral comprehension skills and expressive skills.

Primary School Teachers: General education teachers teaching students in the Central Board of Secondary Education, the Indian Certificate of Secondary Education or State Boards, from 1st to 4th standard.

Response to Instruction (RtI): An approach to identify SLDs by providing targeted assistance (for at least 6 months) in areas of difficulty to students having features of the same or who are underachieving and diagnosing them as SLDs if they fail to make sufficient progress.

Secondary/Middle School Teachers: General education teachers teaching students in the Central Board of Secondary Education, the Indian Certificate of Secondary Education or State Boards, from 5st to 7th standard.

Specific Learning Disorder (SLD): Is operationally defined as a neuro-developmental condition diagnosed in school years, manifesting as persistent and substantial difficulties compared to his/her age in the academic skills of word decoding and fluency, reading comprehension, spelling, writing difficulties, number sense and calculation, and mathematical reasoning for at least 6 months (despite receiving support targeting area of difficulty) in the absence of intellectual disability, sensory issues of vision or hearing, access to adequate instruction, neurological or mental disorders, language differences, or psycho-social difficulties.

Teacher's Training: Teacher's training refers to training in the form of lectures, discussion, and hands-on exposure imparted by experts/specialists in the field of specific learning disorder aimed at improving knowledge level, positive attitude, and realistic understanding of general education teachers, special education teachers, or teacher educators.

Chapter 5
"Intertwined Lives": Narratives of Children With Disabilities and Their Siblings

Shyamani Hettiarachchi
University of Kelaniya, Sri Lanka

Gopi Kitnasamy
Cerebral Palsy Lanka Foundation, Sri Lanka

Dilani Gopi
National Center for Cerebral Palsy and Developmental Disorders, Sri Lanka

Fathima Shamra Nizar
National Center for Cerebral Palsy and Developmental Disorders, Sri Lanka

ABSTRACT

Sibling relationships are complex and unique, often spanning a range of deep emotions. The experiences of children with disabilities and their siblings are arguably seldom documented, particularly in the Global South. The aim of this chapter was to uncover the narratives of young children with disabilities and their siblings in Sri Lanka. Ten dyads of children with disabilities and their siblings and one quartet of siblings were included in this study. Opportunities were offered to the participants to engage in conversation aided by kinetic family drawings. An interview guide was used to support this process. The participant data were analyzed through the lens of the "lived experience" of family dynamics in the tradition of interpretative phenomenological analysis. This chapter will discuss the two complex broad themes of a surrogate parenting role and normative sibling relationships, which at times converge and at times diverge.

INTRODUCTION

Siblings play a pivotal role in the lives of children with disabilities, in its best form, enabling powerful transformative bonds, assuming roles as parents, as well as taking on the roles of teachers and friends (Davidoff, 2006). The relationship between a child with disabilities and his/her sibling may be complex, given the level of dependence or independence, family dynamics and the socio-cultural realities the fam-

DOI: 10.4018/978-1-5225-4955-0.ch005

ily has to contend with. Siblings of children with disabilities are often on the periphery of discussions; their views not always taken into account, particularly in the Global South, where children are meant to be 'seen and not heard'. The experiences and views of children with disabilities and their siblings are often not documented or taken into account when deciding on intervention and management to support children with disabilities and their families (Young, 2007), even when therapy is family-centered. This chapter aims to document the lived experiences of children who have siblings with disabilities.

BACKGROUND

While socio-economic background, family size and the severity of the disability, the attitude and expectations of the parents and the temperament of the child are said to influence the reaction of a sibling of a child with cerebral palsy, for instance, the type of disability is considered less pertinent (Gallagher & Powell, 1989). That said, the type and severity of cerebral palsy or disability may, in fact, require a high-level of care, which could influence the quality of life of the child individually as well as the family as a whole.

According to Zetlin (1986), five types of sibling relationships exist. The first relationship type is of warmhearted feelings and widespread involvement, with the role of surrogate parent or best friend adopted by some towards their sibling with a disability. The second and third are of warmhearted feelings but moderate or minimal involvement respectively. The fourth type of relationship is one of the resentful feelings and minimal involvement and the fifth characterized by no involvement. It is possible that siblings move between these relationship types with age and maturation.

An early view proposed by psychologists was the assumption that the presence of a child with disabilities at home disrupted or damaged the family unit (Kutner, 2016). More contemporary research has suggested that while there may be an increase in the levels of family stress or in siblings experiencing stress (Nunez & Rodriquez, 2005; Stoneman, 2005), having a child with disabilities may not result in disruption or damage but rather promote creativity and personal growth (Kutner, 2016). Growing up with a sibling with a disability could result in a range of mixed emotions, challenges and opportunities (Gallagher & Powell, 1989). Among the negative consequences and conflicting emotions uncovered within the literature are feelings of jealousy due to the attention received by their brother or sister (Boyse, 2009; Kutner, 2016; Schleichkorn, 1993) and as a result anger and resentment at the lack of attention received by them (Boyse, 2009; Russell, Russell, & Russell, 2003). In addition, children with siblings with disabilities may feel socially ostracized by peers resulting in loneliness (Russell et al., 2003) or be concerned that their sibling may not act in socially acceptable ways (Cuskelly & Gunn, 2006; Dew, Baladin, & Llewellyn, 2008). The child may also be worried and scared that they may lose their sibling or feel guilty for the negative feelings they carry towards their sister or brother or for being spared the same difficulties (Boyse, 2009). They may require reassurance for harboring feelings of their sibling's difficulties being their fault (Kutner, 2016), and therefore a possible risk factor for sibling adjustment issues (Sharpe & Rossiter, 2002, cited in Lobato & Kao, 2005)

The suggestion within the literature is that young kindergarten children may, in fact, require reassurance that they were not the causative agent of their sibling's disability (Kutner, 2016). Other concerns include worrying about their sibling, embarrassment at what their sibling is unable to do and pressure to be skilled at tasks that their sibling finds challenging, resentment that they have to take care of their sibling which may take time off activities they would wish to engage in, fear that they will lose their sibling and a sense of guilt around the negative feelings they may have towards their sibling with disabilities (Cogher, Savage, & Smith, 1992; Dormans & Pelligrino, 1998; Finnie, 1997; Kutner, 2016; Sharpe & Rossiter, 2002; Schleichkorn, 1993).

As older children may require explaining their sibling's disability to their friends, they may need adequate social skills to understand and formulate their explanations. Facing the community and dealing with possible perceived notions of stigma is said to bring about a sense of embarrassment and resentment of having to constantly explain their sibling's difficulties to others (Moore, Howard, & McLaughlin, 2002; Russell et al., 2003). This coupled with having to care for their sibling, which may result in them foregoing things they want to do or go places they wish to, is said to add to feelings of resentment (Boyse, 2009).

In contrast, the positives reported include a greater valuing among siblings of children with disabilities of difference and diversity (Valtolina, 2004) as well as patience, kindness and supportiveness, compassion and helpfulness, empathy, insight and a sense of dependability and loyalty stemming from standing up for their sibling with disabilities (Cogher et al., 1992; Dormans & Pelligrino, 1998; Finnie, 1997; Kutner, 2016; Sharpe & Rossiter, 2002; Schleichkorn, 1993).The literature also suggests that many identify having a sibling with a disability as an opportunity for personal growth (Kutner, 2016) associating positive feelings about caring for a brother or sister. Among the positive attributes noted are patience supportiveness, kindness, warmth, compassion, and helpfulness (Beilby, Byrnes, & Young, 2012; Boyse, 2009; Russell et al., 2003). Siblings are reported to be able to be joyous about any achievement, however small, achieved by their brother or sister (Dallas, Stevenson, & McGurk, 1993).

The lack of systematic support to deal with the emotional load of having a child with cerebral palsy, for instance, could impact on members of the family unit, including siblings (Finnie, 1997). This may, in fact, equip siblings of children with disability to act as facilitative role models who could take on a central role within family-centered intervention (Mophosho, Widdows, & Taylor Gomez, 2010). Of the many roles adopted by siblings of children with disabilities is that of an older sibling, regardless of his/her chronological age on birth order within the family (Beilby et al., 2012; Dallas et al., 1993). This may result in increased maturity (Dormans & Pellegrino, 1998) with greater responsibility placed on his/her shoulders (Cogher et al., 1992).

For instance, a study undertaken by Mophosho and colleagues (2010) evaluated the relationships between adolescent children and their siblings with cerebral palsy, which included 4 children between 9-18 years with their sibling with cerebral palsy. The thematic analysis of the interview data exploring perceptions of the lived experiences of both sets of participants revealed the emergent themes of acceptance, helpfulness, wishing, responsibility, friendship, and resilience. The authors conclude that siblings of children with cerebral palsy should be included within family intervention as agents able to offer a pivotal facilitative role as 'role models' for their siblings with disabilities.

There is a body of evidence suggesting that female siblings are expected to take on a share of the care responsibilities foregoing their free time (McHale, Simeonsson, & Sloan, 1984; Rani, Chakravarthy, & Reddy, 2016). A study on siblings of children with learning disabilities in Andhra Pradesh, India, arguably similar in culture to Sri Lanka, found that a large part of caregiver duties was assigned to older sisters, seen as 'natural support systems' (Rani et al., 2016). The authors argue that these care responsibilities deter girls from accessing age-appropriate activities, with pressure to engage with their sibling with learning disability in contrast to male siblings. From a cultural perspective, the lack of a social security system in India (which is similar to other resource-poor countries) speaks to the need to develop natural support resources in the form of siblings, who are seen as 'natural future guardians' (Rani et al., 2016) of children with disabilities.

In isolation or in combination, these factors arguably make navigating sibling relationships very complex, suggesting the value of exploring child perceptions to influence the family-centred intervention process. However, much of our understanding of the experiences of siblings of children with disabilities comes from the Global North, which arguably consists of particular social networks and support systems, not to mention government-funded support mechanisms. Given the socio-economic, cultural and political realities of the Global South, it is important for researchers, policy makers and healthcare professionals to better understand the complex, nuanced nature of sibling relationships vis-à-vis culture and disability rights.

METHOD

The study undertaken was qualitative in nature, incorporating spoken narratives with artwork. The objectives of this study were:

- To explore and document the narratives of children with disabilities on their lived experience in Sri Lanka.
- To explore and document the narratives of young siblings of children with disabilities on their lived experience in Sri Lanka.

Participants

Ten dyads of children with disabilities and their siblings without disabilities and one quartet of siblings were included in the study. The participants ranged from 5 years to 16 years, from a diverse ethnic and religious background including from a Sinhala, Muslim and Tamil ethnicity and Buddhist, Christian, Hindu and Islamic faith background. All participants were from one district, Gampaha.

Study Setting and Procedures

The children were seen at their homes or at special centers that the children accessed. The participants were recruited through professional connections with specialist centers. Ethical approval was sought and received from the Ethics Review Committee of the Faculty of Medicine, University of Kelaniya, Sri Lanka. Written information and written consent was sought from the participants' parents prior to data collection.

Study Design and Data Collection Tools/Procedures

The research study, which is a qualitative study aimed to explore and document the lived experiences of young children with disabilities and their siblings using semi-structured interview sand art work. The meeting with each participant began with a few questions to build a comfortable rapport, following which, the participants were invited to draw a picture of their family. This procedure was borrowed from the Art therapy technique of kinetic family drawings (Marijcke, Veltman, & Brown, 2003). This led to a semi-structured interview in which the family picture or portrait was used as a starting point which offered opportunities for projection and adequate distance when reflecting in-depth on sibling relationships and the family context. The discussion was continued with the use of an interview guide. The interview guide included 6 topic areas based on the literature on siblings with disabilities (family life, you (the participant), sibling relationships, communication, school and support) and potential questions. Each interview lasted on average 30 minutes.

The researchers conducted the interviews in English, Tamil or Sinhala or using alternative and augmentative communication (AAC) systems; generally low-tech communication boards and multi-modal response methods of facial expression, gesture, vocalization and low-tech AAC systems, as per the communication mode of the participants. In addition, the participants were offered opportunities for artwork, particularly of family portraits. This art therapy technique was used by the first researcher who is a drama therapist and speech and language therapist by profession, to offer opportunities for projection and adequate distance, using the drawings and storyline to generate deeper reflection on their sibling, and their family context.

As recommended by Strauss and Corbin (1990), field notes were made following the interviews, which added useful information in the context of the interviews. Of the possible recording methods available such as note taking during or after the interview (Green & Thorogood, 2004), audio recording (Burns & Grove, 2009) or video recordings (Radcliffe, 2004), we chose to audio record the interviews. This permitted the researchers to gain verbatim descriptions without the intrusion of a video camera in the room.

Data Analysis

All interviews and descriptions of artwork which were audio recorded were subsequently transcribed verbatim. The data was translated into Sri Lankan English in an attempt to capture and maintain the authenticity of the participant voices.

The qualitative interviews and narratives on the artwork were analyzed using the key principles of *Interpretative Phenomenological Analysis* (Smith, Flowers, & Larkin, 2009) and aspects of *Kinetic Family Drawing Technique from Art Therapy* (Burns & Kaufman, 1972). 'Kinetic family drawings', is a technique used widely to explore child perceptions in the family context (Marijcke, Veltman, & Browne, 2001; 2003), which offers a glimpse of the phenomenological world of the children. The confidentiality of all the participants was maintained by assigning pseudonyms for each.

Following careful and repeated readings of the transcripts of the participant interviews, the transcripts were coded using the data as a guide. Themes were then identified based on the patterns observed across the transcripts for each emergent theme. This led to the interpretation and identification of subordinate themes and sub-themes, rooted in the participants' narratives.

RESULTS

Surrogate Parenting Role[1]

Protector

Apparent within the narratives of the siblings of children with disabilities is the multiple responsibilities taken on as protector and carer in a role as a surrogate parent to their brother or sister with disabilities. The surrogate parenting role imbibed by some of the siblings was evident whether their brother or sister with disabilities was older or younger. Sajini[2] (14 years old) with a younger sister with cerebral palsy and epilepsy (Surani, 5 years) narrated at length and candidly her experience of 'looking out' for her sister. She said, *'I look out for her. We all do. Sometimes, I notice people in the village looking at her. I stare back at them.'* In conversation, I asked Sajini what it is she feels when people in her village 'look' at her sister. Sajini went on to explain that she feels people are judging her sister, looking at her and through association, at the family, with pity, which she found difficult to bare.

I can see that they are feeling sorry for nangi[3]. They don't say it but they look at her and I can see that they are thinking 'ah pau[4] look at that little girl'. If they say anything to her, I promise you I will hit them. I get very angry. ... sad ... she is my sister, no? No one in our village will dare to say anything. I will not let anyone in my neighborhood say anything to my family....They will not get away if they do.

Sajini's words capture a sense of anger at feeling judged and her use of anger as a defense against this perceived societal view. While the literature suggests that siblings of children with disabilities carry feelings of jealousy and anger that little attention is paid to them (Boyse, 2009; Russell et al., 2003; Kutner, 2016), Sajini's anger is projected outward on behalf of her sister and family. Inherent within the view expressed by Sajini is a sense of perceived societal pity and 'shame' connecting to the charity model and tragic model of disability (Goodley, 2016), which presents a view of persons with disabilities as objects of pity by mainstream society due to karmic explanations of disability or 'tragic' causative factors, which irritates and angers her. The valuing or devaluing or judgment of human worth through the lens of ableism (Campbell, 2009) results in projections of 'shame' and 'pity' on persons with disabilities. Arguably, Sajini's coping mechanism to deal with societal pity is through anger and defensiveness.

Describing her drawing of her family, Sajini said that she placed her sister in the middle, with her parents to one side and her older brother and herself to the other side of her young sister. *'She is in the middle of our family. We all look after her.'*

This role of the surrogate parent in the form of protector was taken on by young siblings as well. Madhavi, at 8 years old, had already taken on this role for her older brother Raghavan, who is 16 years old, with cerebral palsy. Her mother reported how Madhavi is very close to her older brother and is always 'looking out' for him. On request, Madhavi went on to explain the family portrait she drew, as *'my father, mother, older brother and I'*. She said *'Anna[5] needs help with bathing, going to the bathroom and eating. I am not allowed to help yet because I am small. But I ask my mother and grandmother if they gave Anna his food or if they put the TV for him. I can understand Anna. He tells in the sign language.'* While Boyse (2009) contends that children with siblings with a disability may be angry that little attention is paid to them. Madhavi's reaction suggests the reverse of this, with her angry a result of her sibling not being paid attention to.

This is also in contrast to the assertion by Mophosho and colleagues (2010) that older siblings of children with disabilities, specifically with cerebral palsy, are generally better adjusted than younger siblings to having a sibling with a disability. Madhavi, in fact, appears to show empathy and a sense of responsibility far beyond her years, reflecting maturity and acceptance of diversity (Dormans & Pellegrino, 1998; Valtolina, 2004). As Cogher et al. (1992) suggests, as Raghavan requires much physical care, the sibling may be given more responsibilities, which in Madhavi's case, according to her own words and that of her mother, appears to be that Madhavi is taking on responsibilities out of her own volition and sense of 'duty' towards protecting her brother.

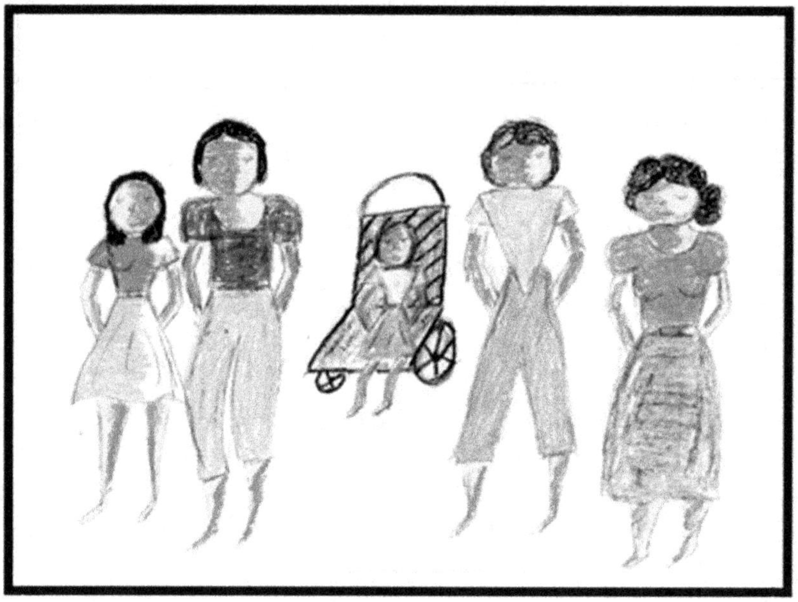

Figure 1. Sajini's drawing of her family

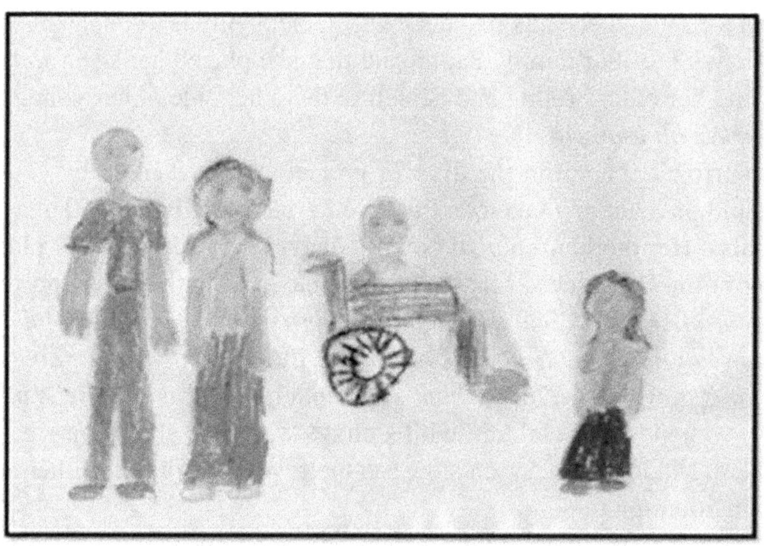

Figure 2. Family portrait by Madhavi

However, the role of substitute carer with qualities of protection and caring was also taken over by children with disability in the care of usually younger siblings. Azeema (6 years) bemoaned the fact that her older sister, Farzana (8 years) with a diagnosis of learning disabilities and visual difficulties, was not at her school to 'help her'. As she put it, *'I would like my sister to come to my school as she will be able to help me. ... She is going to another school. I wish she can come to mine.'* Asked why she would like her sister at her school, Azeema reported that *'my Akka*[6] *helps me'. She helps me to put the books in order* *into my bag.'*Proceeding to talk about her picture she declared, *'I am in the middle (points to the girl in a pink shirt). My older sister is next to me in red.'* Interestingly, in her family portrait, Azeema draws herself as the bigger of the two with her older sister Farzana portrayed to a side, smaller in dimensions.

Caregiver Role

The two sisters, Selvi (13 years) and Bawani (10 years) discussing their experiences, talked about taking on the role of 'helping' their sister. Selvi and Bawani had taken turns to care for their sister Sankeetha when they were all attending the same school. Echoing the concerns about not being able to go to the same school anymore, Bawani noted that *'if she is near me, that will be good. I can look after her'.* Adding to this, Selvi, the younger of the two sisters commented that she too *'likes to help'.* She recounted how she would go in search of her sister during the interval to see if she is alright and take her to the toilet. Explaining her picture titled 'my family', Selvi said *'Sankeetha is between us. I am in the corner.'* She had placed her younger sister between the two older sisters; Bawani and herself, suggesting a sense of protection.

Akin to Selvi's account, Bawani too shared her experiences of taking turns with Selvi to support Sankeetha during the interval at school. She said, *'it is a little difficult ... but we take turns to help her because she is our sister, no?'* She too described her picture, also titled 'my family' saying *'I put my sister next to me. I can look after her.'*While there was a propensity for this role of 'caregiver' to be adopted exclusively by female siblings, similar to accounts in previous literature (Orsmond & Seltzer, 2000; Rani et al., 2016), possibly indicating a cultural bias, the chosen dyads had very few male siblings without a disability.

At one level, it appears that both older sisters are taking on the role of surrogate carer, engaging in very personal care of their younger sister with disabilities. Although there is a general belief that older siblings are able to better adjust to their sister's or brother's disability (Gallagher & Powell, 1989), older

Figure 3. Azeema's portrait of her family

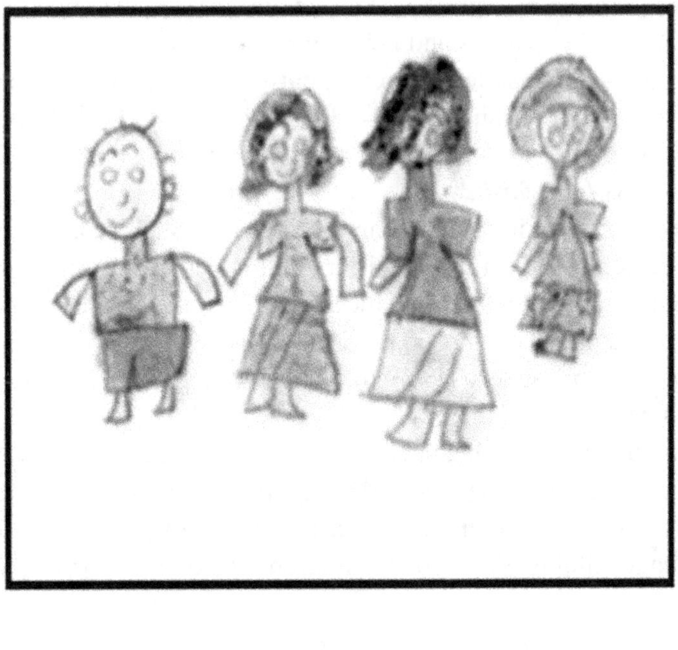

Figure 4. Selvi's drawing titled 'My family'

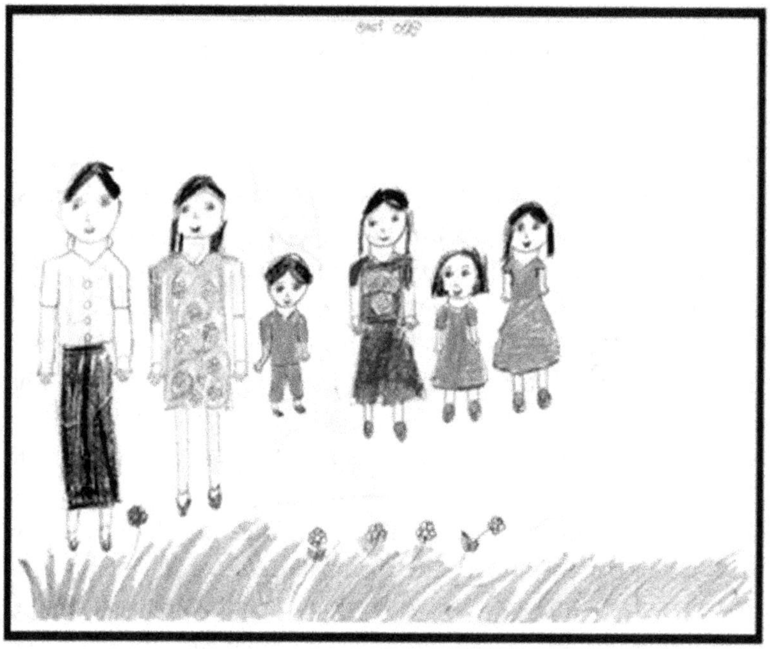

and younger siblings of the current study appeared to take on the role of protector, suggesting a comparable level of adjustment. At another level, indicating the complexity of sibling relationships, while acknowledging the support she got at her previous school, Sankeetha reported that she likes her siblings as they *'play with me'* and that she wants to *'become friendly with them'*. However, she added that she *'does not like to go home because parents and siblings hit (her) and (her) younger brother steals (her) things'*, and *'they disturb (her) while studying.'*

Nevertheless, in her drawing, Sankeetha had included her sisters but did not include herself in the family portrait. She did go on to explain that she likes to go to Galle Face[7] and go shopping to buy chocolate as well as talk with her parents and help them with cooking.

Ishan, a 12-year old boy with dyskinetic cerebral palsy with athetoid movements recounted similar concerns. Talking about his relationship with his older sister, he said, *'I like my sister when she gives me her phone to play games but I don't like her not helping me sometimes, hitting me and when Akka[8] does not give me food unless I ask for it.'*

Refusing to explain his drawing in detail, Ishan displayed his picture saying only *'This is my family'*. His picture appears to depict his parents, older sister and himself and is titled 'My Family'.

This role of the caregiver was assumed by all the siblings without disabilities to varying degrees. This role of siblings as surrogate parents has been reported on in the literature before (Beilby et al., 2012; Davidoff, 2006). Dallas and colleagues (1993) argue that siblings of children with disabilities take on an older sibling's role, irrespective of their age.

One specific explanation for this within the local context may be a cultural role, as in South Asia, and certainly, in Sri Lanka, children are socialized and culturally expected to take care of their aging parents; older siblings are meant to take care of their younger siblings. It may well be that irrespective of age, of whether an older or younger sibling, these young children took on a surrogate parent role for their sister

Figure 5. Bawani's drawing titled 'My family'

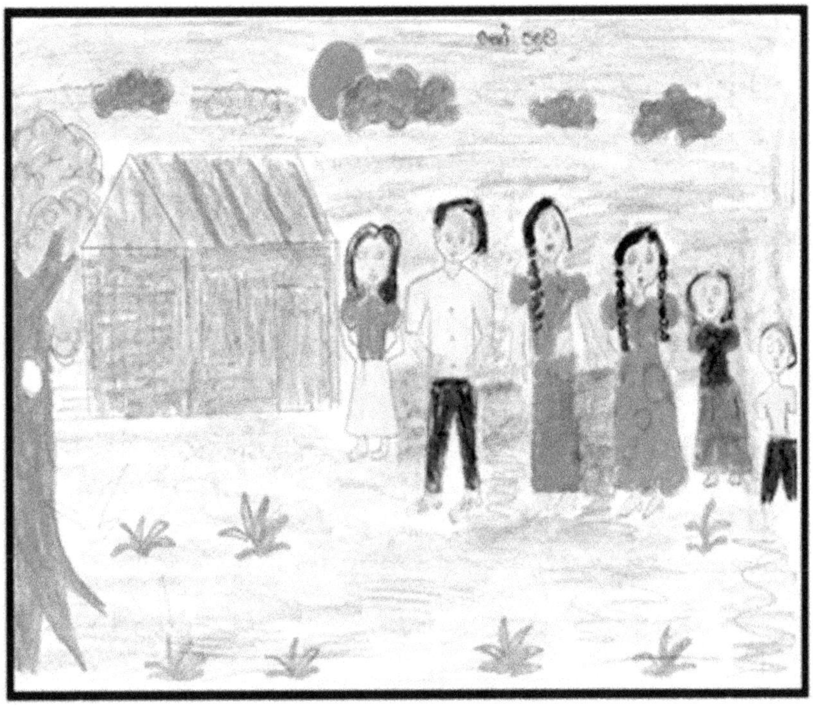

Figure 6. Sankeetha's family portrait

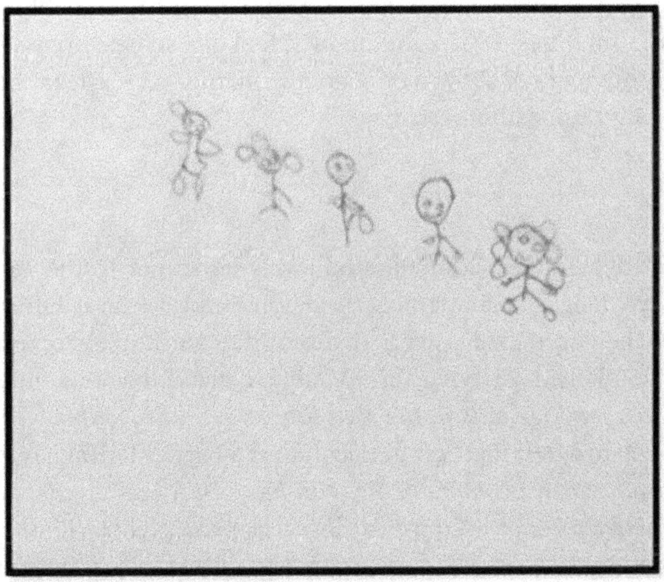

Figure 7. Ishan's drawing titled 'My family'

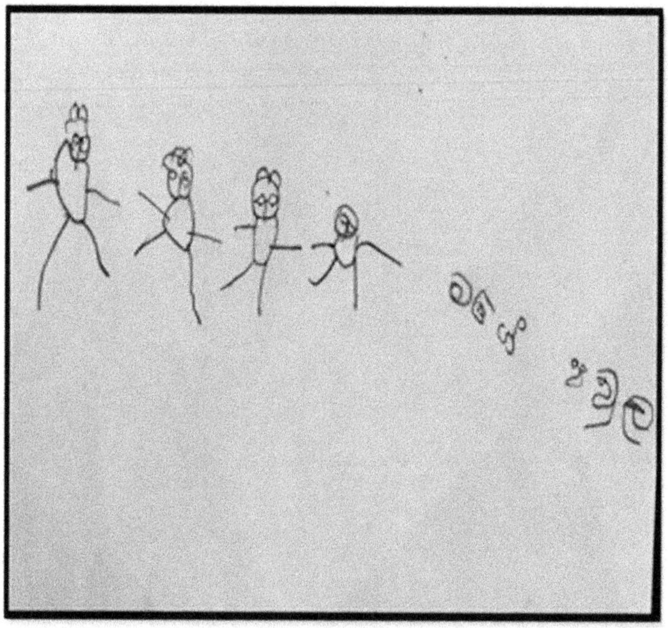

or brother with disabilities, potentially viewed as 'younger' in their care needs. So, this may be reflective of a cultural pattern of caring, be it an older or younger sibling towards a child with disabilities.

As Rani and colleagues (2016) state, the reliance on building a strong bond with siblings without disabilities to ensure the long-term welfare of the child with disability arguably places tremendous pressure on children without disabilities. If they did, in fact, feel this sense of pressure, the siblings without disability in the current study did not show it or state it explicitly (at least, for now), instead, adopting a hands-on active role in care responsibilities.

Interpreter

Many of the children with disabilities within the study were either non-verbal or had a limited verbal expression, which posed a challenge to communication at home and at school. Often acting as an interpreter in conversations between their brother or sister with disabilities and adults, some of the siblings discussed how they enabled conversations. Clarifying this, Madhavi stated that she understands her brother the best. *'I ask what (do) you want? He tells in the sign language. …Sometimes, I have to translate for my grandparents.'* She went on to assert that communication is a barrier to Raghavan accessing mainstream school as *'the normal teacher can't communicate with him. They can't understand him. That's why he goes to the center. It is better for him.'* A similar view was proposed by Sunila (13 years) whose sister Anila (8 years), diagnosed with dyskinetic cerebral palsy with athetoid movements, uses a few single words, smiling and facial expression to communicate at home and a low-tech communication book at times at the special school she attends. Sunila explained how Anila calls her to play and how often, she is the sole person to understand her sister, taking on the role of interpreter. Explaining this, she said:

My sister says about 5 to 6 words, ow (yes), amma (mother), ak (for sister) haa (yes), nae (no) and bae (can't). My sister stays happily smiling. I am the only one who understands her sometimes. I explain what she is trying to say to my parents.

However, unlike for Raghavan where Madhavi was the key person who understood him, Sunila conceded that not only her but her grandfather too was equally able to understand Anila. Taking on the role of the interpreter was seen as part of the *'duty'* of an older sister by Sajini. The remit of an older sibling, she explains, is to ensure that a younger sibling, in this case, Dilrukshi, have her *'voice heard'*.

I am much older than her, no? I must help to make her voice heard. I am usually able to understand what nangi[9] *is trying to say when her face changes or she makes a sound. People don't understand her because they don't understand her sounds or her face. It is my duty to help, no?*

Advocate

Particularly with brothers or sisters who are non-verbal, the siblings also took on the role of an advocate; 'voicing' the needs, feelings, and concerns of their siblings with disabilities. Madhavi explained how she speaks with her grandparents, who often look after them, questioning as to why sometimes their caregiver commitments have not been fulfilled. She said, I ask my grandmother *'why you (did you) not put the TV for him?'*, suggesting that she is always looking out for her brother. In conversation, Madhavi's mother explained how sensitive Madhavi is to Raghavan's needs, in her view, more than her, the grandparents or her husband, contending that all the adults get 'told off' for any presumed lapses in Raghavan's care.

The role adopted by these siblings typified by warmhearted feelings and intensive contact similar to a surrogate parent or best friend is identified by Zetlin (1986) as one of five types of sibling relationships observed among children with developmental disorders and their siblings. Cogher and colleagues (1992) found that commensurate to the requirement of physical support, siblings of a child with a disability may be afforded more responsibility. What was evident within the current study was how more of the siblings whose brother or sister with disabilities appeared to require more physical care, adopted the role of surrogate caregiver.

While Madhavi was very compassionate towards her brother, there was also a role reversal in her taking on the role of 'supervising' the care received by her brother as well as being 'his voice'. While taking on the role of advocate, the siblings without disabilities acted as facilitative role models for their siblings with disabilities (Mophosho et al., 2010). Dormans and Pellegrino (1998) argue that being a sibling of a child with a disability could result in greater maturity, acceptance of diversity and a greater sense of responsibility. The siblings in this study certainly took on roles of caregiver and advocate, beyond that which would be expected of their age.

Sajini, talking about her sister Dilrukshi described her personality and her needs as follows:

She is very vicious. She does not like anyone touching her head. She starts to cry. Shouts. Even though she is small, she is very vicious. ... But because her nerves have not developed, she cannot speak. So, I need to speak to her; make sure she gets everything she wants ... because people outside the family don't understand her.

Her words allude to a perceived lack of agency for her sister and therefore a need to help bridge this through her role as an advocate for her sister's needs outside the family home, although she concedes that her sister *'gets her own way'* at home.

In the discussion, she also raised concerns about the lack of support agencies, particularly for education suitable for her sister. Making this point, she went on to say that,

... the nursery center where my sister goes to is to be taken away. That's such a shame. It is the only school in this village for children like my sister. I don't know what will happen in the future to her. I have asked my mother to speak to the school to explain this. I would have liked to have gone and spoken myself but I am busy with my O/L examination at present. ... I would have otherwise. ... I have spoken to the Manager in the past

Implicit within Sajini's words is the suggestion that the role of an advocate is one that she has taken on in the past and a role which she regrets not being able to fulfill at the moment.

Boyse (2009) notes that siblings of children with disabilities show qualities of compassion, helpfulness, and loyalty, the latter a result of standing up for their sister or brother and confronting challenges. The acceptance and appreciation of difference and diversity could also result in friendship and a sense of loyalty and dependability towards their brother or sister, also possibly due to frequently speaking-up for their sibling. The literature suggests that this may also offer opportunities to develop empathy for others with a disability, great insights into coping and resilience (Boyse, 2009; Mophosho et al., 2010).

NORMATIVE SIBLING RELATIONSHIPS

Playmates

Siblings form a lifelong special bond, sharing a common childhood journey of experiences often navigating a similar familial emotional landscape. At its best, siblings share positive experiences and memories. The love they shared for each other was evident throughout the narratives of children with disabilities and their siblings. In all of the sibling dyads consulted, all the children reported enjoying diverse types of play and having their siblings as their playmates. Bawani spoke in a soft muted voice about her love and care of her sister. As she disclosed, *'I love her. I play with her. Teach her',* combining a 'teaching role' as part of her responsibility as an older sibling. Their younger brother Thiru, who at just 5 years old, enjoyed the company of all his sisters as, *'like playing ... akkas*[10] *... pee thaara (duck) game'.* Describing his two drawings, he stated that it is *'my sister Sankeetha ...me'* about the first drawing, and *'my sister and I'* about the second drawing, making reference only to his sister who has motor difficulties, who in the drawing is the larger of the figures.

Having seen the drawings of his two older sisters, Thiru went on to draw a picture of his family, displaying all four of his older sisters and himself saying, *'my sister Selvi. My sister Bawani. My sister Sankeetha. (The) sun.'* In this drawing, Thiru had brought his oldest sister Selvi to the forefront, moving his other two sisters Bawani and Sankeetha, with motor difficulties, to the background.

The children enjoyed each other's company, whether with or without disabilities, playing games, similar to children without disabilities. Children who are older took on the role of 'teaching' their younger siblings, suggesting normative relationships. As Bawani suggested, *'I want to teach her. Play*

Figure 8. Thiru's portraits of his sister and himself

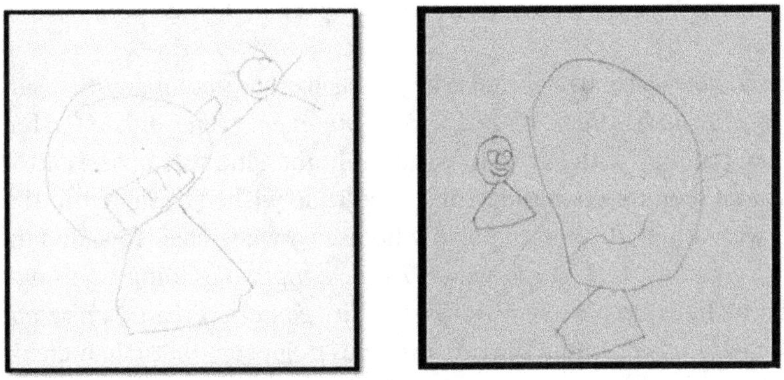

Figure 9. Thiru's drawing of his sisters

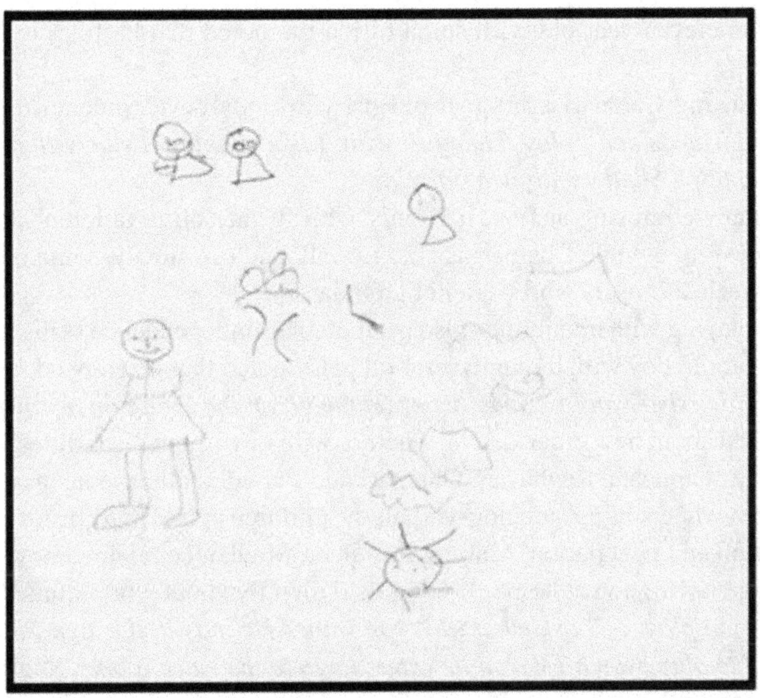

together with her. Athuru mithuru[11]'. Many of the children with or without disabilities shared their joy of playing with their siblings, in games that ranged from PlayStation to cricket, dolls and more traditional children's games like 'athuru mithuru', again suggesting typical, often gendered play, arguably denoting 'traditional' sibling relationships. Pubudhu also talked about playing with his sister and taking on the role of teaching her letters and words. Although Pubudhu has spina bifida, he appears to consider motor play. Making this point clear, he said,

We play haengi muththang[12]. We play the 'teacher' game. I teach her the letter 'a', mother, father, grandmother, butterfly, hoppers[13]. I tell my nangi[14] to come to play … I teach her.

Sunila too discussed how she and her sister enjoyed each other's company. She said, *'we play together. My nangi calls me to play with dollies. She also calls me to carry her outside'.* Her sister Anila smiled when asked if she likes to play with her older sister at home. She was observed to enjoy using a paint app on an IPad at school, pointing to indicate the friend she wished to share the IPad with.

Ishan (12 years) with athetoid cerebral palsy who uses a wheelchair revealed that at home, he likes to *'play car, bike, race games. … I like to watch TV … eat pizza'.* Going on to name all his friends at school, he noted that he likes *'to play cricket, Ludo, play games on the tab, share food'* and to *'have a chat and be together with them'.* In the play mentioned, it appears that Ishan engages in physical play with his older sister at home (race games) and with his friends at school (cricket), uninhibited by his motor difficulties. Likewise, Sankeetha, who in spite of her fears of getting hit by her siblings, commented on how she likes to *'play ball, watch television'* at home with her siblings. At a school with her friends, she enjoyed doing *'handwork with them, draw with them … play … play in the swimming pool'.* Similarly, Udhara, an eleven-year old with spina bifida too noted that he likes to *'play ball … with a friend close to home.'*

Describing her drawing, Chamari, a 5;0-year-old girl with global developmental difficulties exclaimed, *"I like playing. (My) friends don't play. They just wait. I like running. I run with my friends. I play but with him (points to a boy). Shall we draw a ball?'*

Although seemingly confusing at first, it is only with further observation at the end of the school day that it became clear that while Chamari is able to walk and run slowly, some of the friends she was referring to were wheelchair users who were not ambulatory.

Explaining how playing with his siblings also promoted his independence skills, describing his drawings, Amal, a 4;3-year old boy with diplegic cerebral palsy noted that he enjoyed *'(I like) going (to the) park … with mum, older sister and younger sister let me go on the swing on my own. I like it.'*

The children talked about how older sisters, whether with or without disabilities, direct and dominate joint play. In the play, it appears, Raghavan, Chamari and Pubudhu all have agency in initiating and directing the play. Even when siblings are non-verbal, the children spoke in terms of an equal partnership within communication and negotiation. Making this clear, Madhavi explained how she and her brother love playing on their Play Station at home. When asked directly about who initiates play, she said, *'No, my brother tells (me) to play. … I ask what (do) you want? He tells in the sign language. He use[15] the sign language to tell to play, watch TV or if he wants to go to the wash room'.* Raghavan, responding to yes/no questions reported that he enjoys Play Station, particularly the game 'Need for Speed', which he plays with his father and his sister, claiming that he is always the 'winner'.

Nevertheless, some of the older children who have younger siblings with disabilities recounted how their brother or sister had his/her own way, directing the nature of play. Anila, at just 8 years old, though not clear to strangers, is said to be able to indicate her needs. As her sister Sunila put it, *'My sister likes to go to hotels for meals on her birthday…we released some birds. She likes going to the temple and releasing birds to freedom. We then went to the hotel as she is the one who told us. … She also lets me know when she wants to carried outside'.* Sunila's explanation suggests that her younger sister is able to let her needs be known, with clear agency.

Figure 10. Chamari's drawing depicting her friends

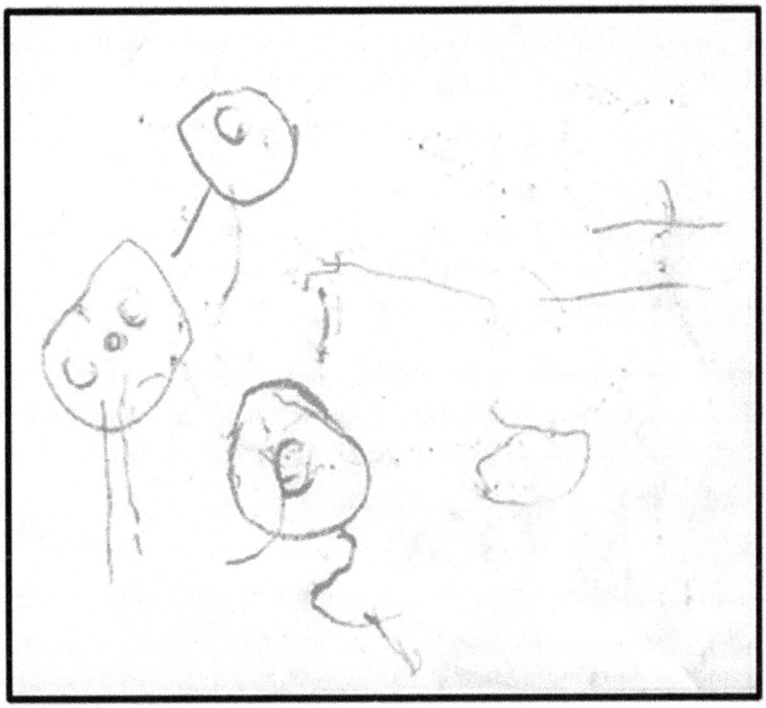

Figure 11. Amal's drawings

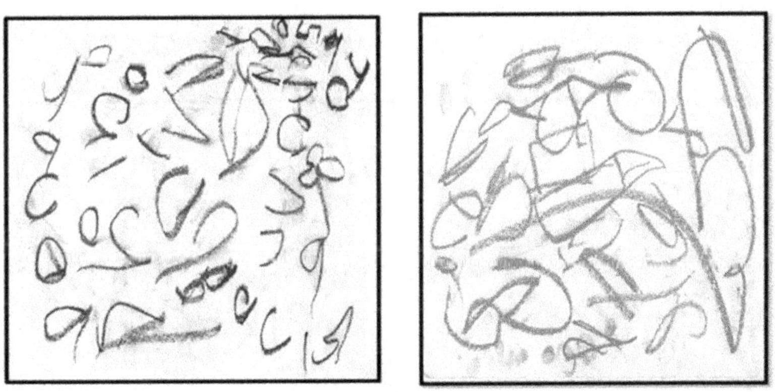

Love and Friendship

The children with disability and their siblings without disability were comparable in their need for and reported enjoyment of friendships. The close bond often seen between them was evident in many of the dyads with a sibling with or without disability viewed as a 'best friend', in-line with Zetlin's (1986) first type of sibling relationships. The close friendships enjoyed between the siblings was evident in how some dyads referred to each other. For Azeema, her older sister, Farzana, is her closest friend and beloved older sister. She noted with admiration that *'She is my best friend. My older sister. She helps me'*. Farzana, the older of the two sisters diagnosed with a learning disability and visual difficulties, drew the following picture, saying *'thangachchi'*[16].

Finnie (1997) referring specifically to children with cerebral palsy notes that families are unsupported in dealing with the emotional impact of having a child with a disability, which can affect family members including siblings. While the impact on siblings may be complex, nuanced and subtle, the current findings indicate close bonds as per Davidoff's (2006) assertion in previous literature, with affection and love apparent between them. The findings appear to be more comparable with the notion of a dual reaction of positive and negative effects on siblings of children with disabilities (Gallagher & Powell, 1989).

Chamari with global developmental delay, while describing her second picture, talked about how Amal (also with diplegic cerebral palsy) is her friend. She said, *'he (points)...friend...he gives me flowers. ... I am drawing flowers'*.

Chamari's friend Amal, discussing opportunities to meet with friends noted how he goes to church every Sunday with his older sister and parents. Narrating his Sunday ritual and his drawing, he recounted that, *'I go to church...my mother...my sister ... the church... friends... a fan'*.

Similarly, talking about his friendships, Udhara also drew a picture. He described how he goes every Sunday to his local temple with his family and how he looks forward to meeting his friends at Sunday school. He started off the conversation saying, *'(I like) going (to the) temple ... park ... with mum, (my) nanda*[17] *and sudu nona*[18] *... playing ...see saw...friends'*. Talking about meeting his friends he noted, *'I go (to the temple) with my friend. We meet our friends there. ...we pray ...we play'*.

As a whole, the children depicted their relationships as positive, closely resembling the affection, roles adopted and interest within normative sibling relationships. The finding of friendship between children with disabilities and their siblings confirms Davidoff's (2006) view that sibling relationships are important as children with disability take on the role of informal teacher, surrogate parent or friend.

Figure 12. Farzana's picture of 'thangachchi' (my younger sister)

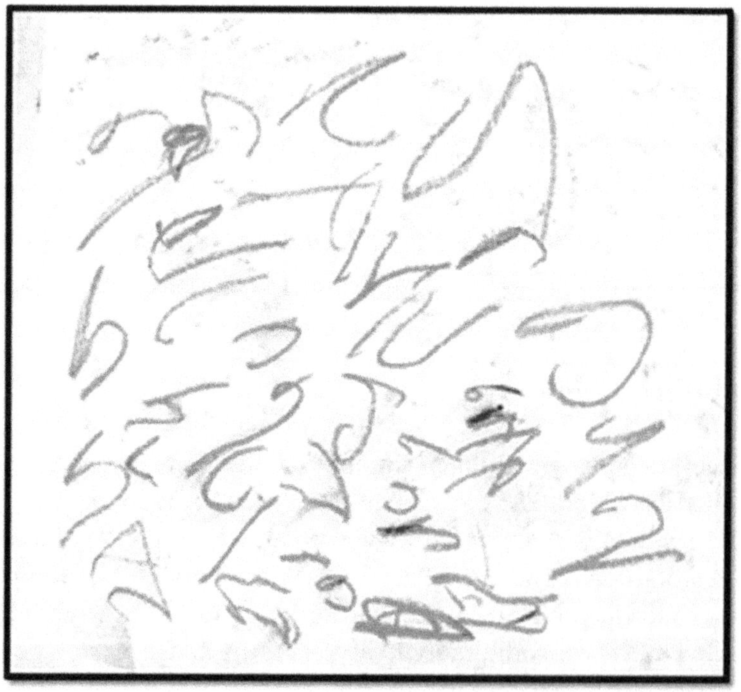

Figure 13. Chamari's drawing described as 'friends'

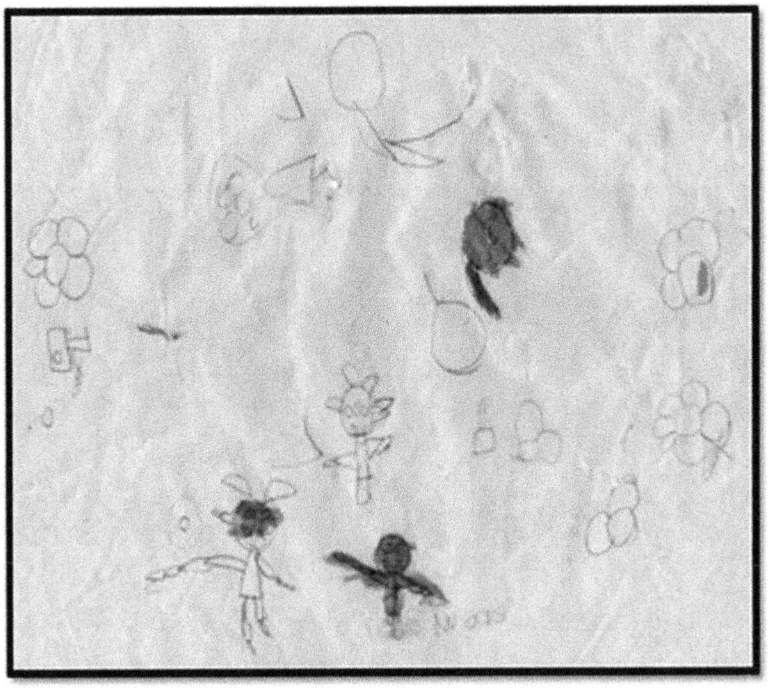

Figure 14. Amal's depiction of his family at church

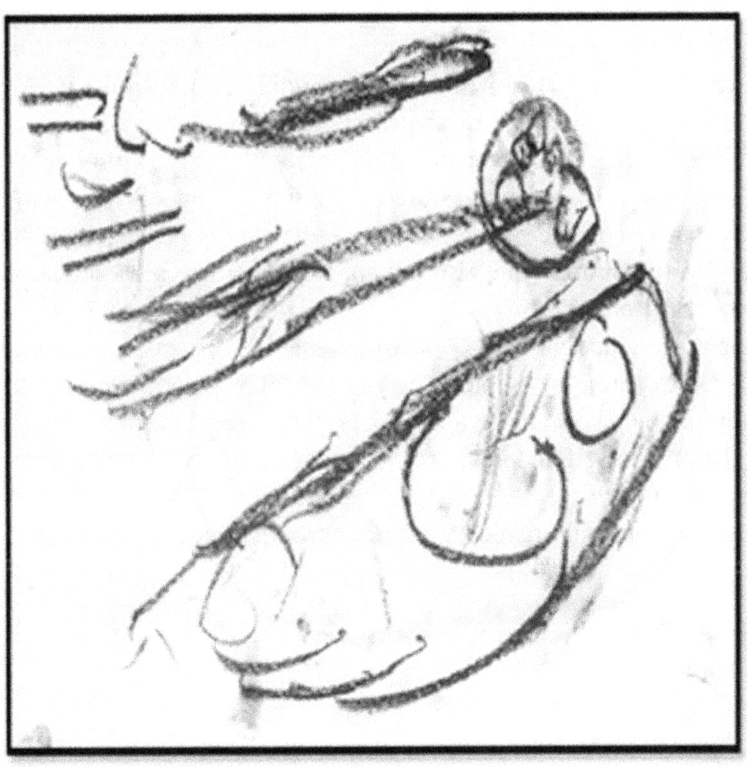

Figure 15. Udhara's drawing

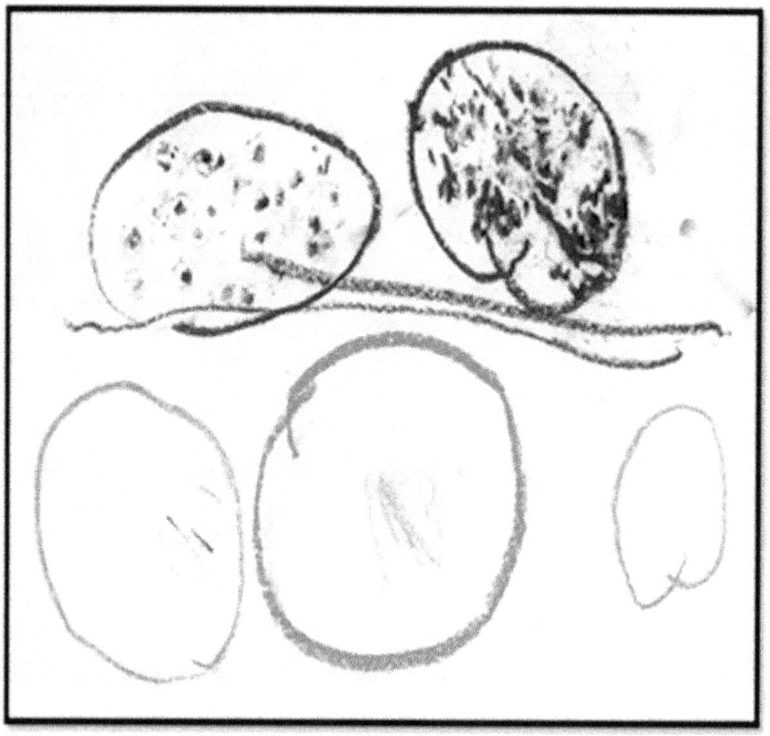

Dreams

All the children shared their dreams for the future, responding to questions of 'What would you like to become when you grow up?' unhindered by any thought or stigma related to disability. The responses ranged from dancer, pilot, racing car driver to the teacher and even to 'jobs' reserved for the imagination. Indicating his dream job, Raghavan gestured and then responded to closed questions to express his wish to have a job connected with racing cars and at the center as a teacher. His sister expressed her dream *'to be a dancer'* in the future while also talking about her brother's dream saying *'anna wants to be a racing car driver or a teacher'.*

Ishan who is in the same school as Raghavan articulated his dream of becoming a pilot, not viewing his motor difficulties as inhibiting his choice. Similarly, Malki, who is 6 years old with a learning disability, drew her future plans of becoming a doctor. When describing her picture, she spoke candidly, using few words but making herself understood clearly. She responded to the question on her future work saying *'doctor (pause)...hospital'.*

In contrast to the others, unencumbered by a sense of reality, indicating her imagination and playfulness, Sankeetha said that she wants *'to become Dora',* the Disney cartoon character when she is older.

Figure 16. Malki's depiction of her future work as 'a doctor'

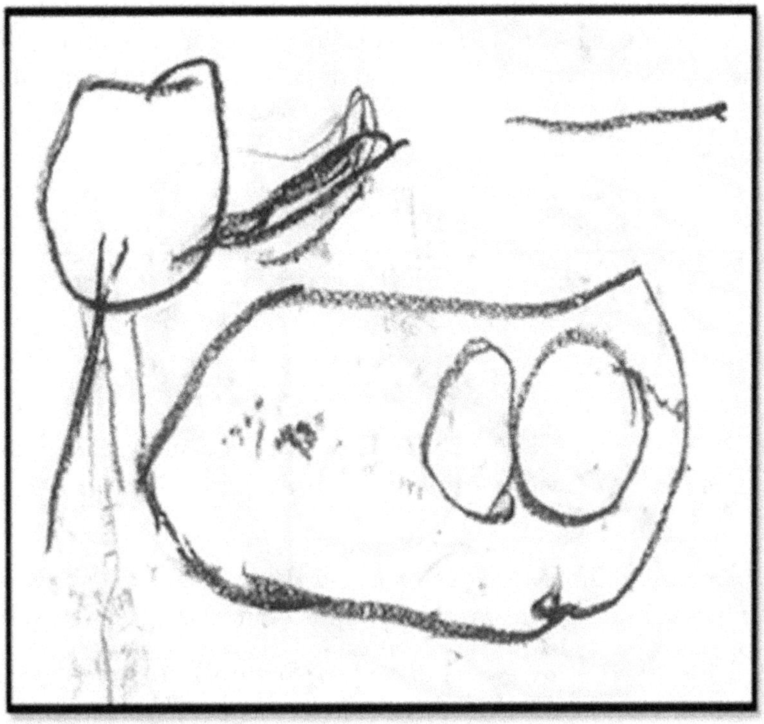

CONCLUSION

The narratives of the children with disabilities and their siblings without disabilities revealed a range of complex roles and emotions navigated through by these young siblings, as per previous literature. Overall, the child dyads and group of siblings shared their views candidly, detailing aspects of normative sibling relationships of play and friendship. The siblings without disabilities explained the complex roles navigated within the family, adopting a surrogate caregiver role, imbibing qualities of protector, caregiver, interpreter, and advocate. In spite of the arguably many challenges faced by children with disabilities in accessing education, employment, and community events, the children with disabilities, commensurate with their siblings without disabilities, allowed themselves to dream of the future and of a comparable future with equal opportunities to become what they hoped to. The findings of this study may encourage healthcare professionals to consider and offer holistic family-centered therapy interventions which recognize and consider sibling relationships as key to communication therapy and family support.

LIMITATIONS OF THE STUDY

One limitation of this study concerns the representativeness of the participants, who were from one geographical area in a large city (Gampaha). It also comprised of more children with cerebral palsy and therefore an over-representation of children with motor difficulties compared to children experiencing sensory, cognitive or mental health difficulties. An attempt was made to include children who are diverse in their language use, gender and socio-economic background, even though all the participants were from one geographical area. Many of the children with cerebral palsy were non-verbal or used limited clear speech. The available AAC systems were not always able to capture the complexity of the children's thoughts and views, requiring more preparation in terms of icons offered and communication options available.

We only had the opportunity to collect one round of data and limited observation. In follow-up studies, an ethnographic approach will be favored with a broader group of clients who are representative of gender, ethnicity, type of disability, language and socio-economic background together with opportunities to observe sibling relationships within the family setting.

REFERENCES

Beilby, J. M., Byrnes, M. L., & Young, K. N. (2012). The experiences of living with a sibling who stutters: A preliminary study. *Journal of Fluency Disorders*, *37*(2), 135–148. doi:10.1016/j.jfludis.2012.02.002 PMID:22531288

Boyse, K. (2009). Siblings with Siblings with Special Needs. *Your Child Development & Behavior Resources*. Retrieved September 14, 2017, from http://www.med.umich,edu/yourchild/topics/specneed.htm

Burns, N., & Grove, S. K. (2009). *The Practice of Nursing Research: Appraisal, Synthesis, and Generation of Evidence*. St Louis, MO: Saunders Elsevier.

Burns, R. C., & Kaufman, S. H. (1972). *Actions, Styles, and Symbols in Kinetic Family Drawings (KFD): An Interpretive Manual*. New York: Brunner/Mazel.

Campbell, F. K. (2009). *Contours of ableism: The production of disability and abledness*. London, New York: Palgrave Macmillan. doi:10.1057/9780230245181

Cogher, L., Savage, E., & Smith, M. F. (1992). *Cerebral palsy. The child and young person*. London: Chapman & Hall Medical.

Cuskelly, M., & Gunn, P. (2006). Adjustment of Children who have a sibling with Down syndrome: Perspectives of Mothers, Fathers and Children. *Journal of Intellectual Disability Research*, *50*(12), 912–925. doi:10.1111/j.1365-2788.2006.00922.x PMID:17100952

Dallas, E., Stevenson, J., & McGurk, H. (1993). Cerebral-palsied children's interactions with siblings-I. Influence of severity of disability, age and birth order. *Journal of Child Psychology and Psychiatry, and Allied Disciplines*, *34*(5), 621–647. doi:10.1111/j.1469-7610.1993.tb01062.x PMID:8340436

Davidoff, L. (2006). The sibling relationship and sibling incest in historical context. In P. Coles (Ed.), *Sibling relationships* (pp. 17–48). London: Karnac Books, Ltd.

Dew, A., Baladin, S., & Llewellyn, G. (2008). The psychosocial impact in siblings of people with lifelong physical disability: A review of the literature. *Journal of Developmental and Physical Disabilities*, *20*(5), 485–507. doi:10.100710882-008-9109-5

Dormans, J. P., & Pelligrino, L. (Eds.). (1998). *Caring for children with cerebral palsy: A team approach*. Baltimore, MD: Paul H. Brookes Publishing Co.

Finnie, N. R. (1997). *Handling the young cerebral palsied child at home* (3rd ed.). London: Butterworth-Heinemann.

Gallagher, P. A., & Powell, T. H. (1989). *Topics in early childhood special education: Families in special education*. PRO-ED, Inc.

Goodley, D. (2016). *Disability Studies. An Interdisciplinary Introduction (2nd ed.)*. London: SAGE Publications Ltd.

Green, J., & Thorogood, N. (2004). *Qualitative Methods for Health Research*. London: Sage.

Kutner, L. (2016). When A Sibling Is Disabled. *Psych Central*. Retrieved September 14, 2017, from https://psychcentral.com/lib/when-a-sibling-is-disabled/

Lobato, D. J., & Kao, B. T. (2005). Brief Report: Family-based group intervention for young siblings of children with chronic illnesses and developmental disability. *Journal of Pediatric Psychology*, *30*(8), 678–682. doi:10.1093/jpepsy/jsi054 PMID:16260437

Marijcke, W., Veltman, M., & Browne, K. D. (2003). Trained raters' evaluation of kinetic family drawings of physically abused children. *The Arts in Psychology*, *30*(1), 3–12. doi:10.1016/S0197-4556(02)00230-7

Marijcke, W. M., Veltman, B. A., & Browne, K. D. (2001). Identifying childhood abuse through favorite kind of and kinetic family drawing. *The Arts in Psychotherapy*, *28*(4), 251–259. doi:10.1016/S0197-4556(01)00110-1

McHale, S. M., Simeonsson, R. J., & Sloan, J. (1984). Children with handicapped brothers and sisters. In E. Schopler & G. Mesibov (Eds.), *The effect of Autism on the family* (pp. 327–342). New York: Plenum. doi:10.1007/978-1-4899-2293-9_19

Moore, M., Howard, V., & McLaughlin, T. (2002). Siblings of children with disabilities: A review and analysis. *International Journal of Special Education*, *17*, 49–64.

Mophosho, M., Widdows, J., & Taylor Gomez, M. (2010). Relationships between adolescent children and their siblings with cerebral palsy: A Pilot Study. *Journal on Developmental Disabilities*, *15*(3), 81–87.

Nunez, B., & Rodriguez, L. (2005). *Los hermanos de persons con discapacidad: una asignatura pendiente*. Buenos Aires: Asociacion AMAR.

Orsmond, G. I., & Seltzer, M. M. (2000). Brothers and sisters of adults with mental retardation gendered nature of the sibling relationship. *American Journal of Mental Retardation*, *105*(6), 486–508. doi: PMID:11958202

Radcliffe, D. (2004). *Video and Audio Methods in Qualitative Research* [On-Line Booklet]. Retrieved September 14, 2017, from http://www.don.ratcliffs.net/video/

Rani, K. R., Chakravarthy, K.N.V.V.S.S.S., & Reddy, D.C.S. (2016). Perceptions and problems of other siblings in a family having mentally retarded children. *IOSR Journal of Humanities and Social Science*, *21*(1), 7-12.

Russell, C., Russell, C., & Russell, M. (2003). We're here too: Supporting 'sibs' of children with special needs. *Exceptional Parent*, *33*, 36–39.

Schleichkorn, J. (1993). *Coping with Cerebral Palsy. Answers to Questions Parents Often Ask* (2nd ed.). PRO-ED, Inc.

Sharpe, D., & Rossiter, L. (2002). Siblings of Children with a Chronic Illness: A Meta-Analysis. *Journal of Pediatric Psychology*, *2*(8), 699–710. doi:10.1093/jpepsy/27.8.699 PMID:12403860

Smith, J. A., Flowers, P., & Larkin, M. (2009). *Interpretative Phenomenological Analysis: Theory, Method and Research*. London: Sage.

Stoneman, Z. (2005). Siblings of children with disability: Research themes. *Mental Retardation*, *43*(5), 339–350. PMID:16131231

Strauss, A., & Corbin, J. (1990). *Basics of qualitative research. Grounded theory procedures and techniques*. Sage.

Valtolina, G. G. (2004). *L'altro fratello. Relazione fraternal e disabilita*. Milano: FrancoAngeli.

Young, S. (2007). The forgotten sibling. *Australian and New Zealand Journal of Family Therapy*, *28*(01), 21–27. doi:10.1375/anft.28.1.21

Zetlin, A. G. (1986). Mentally retarded adults and their siblings. *American Journal of Mental Deficiency*, *91*(3), 217–225. PMID:3799727

KEY TERMS AND DEFINITIONS

Cerebral Palsy: A non-progressive neurological condition that affects posture and movement.

Drama Therapy: The use of drama and theatre techniques to support the exploration and expression of feelings, encouraging personal growth and better mental health within a therapeutic setting.

Global South: Countries formerly known as "Third World" or "developing countries."

Learning Disability: A cognitive impairment that affects the learning of new skills and independence.

Normative: Behaviors or relationships deemed typical for a child's/person's age.

Phenomenology: A qualitative research approach that aims to uncover and document the lived experiences of participants.

Siblings: A familiar relationship of a brother or sister who is older or younger.

Surrogate: A person taking on a role of another or substituting for another.

ENDNOTES

1 The participants' responses have been presented verbatim, including any errors of syntax.
2 All participant names have been changed to pseudonyms in this article to maintain confidentiality.
3 Meaning 'younger sister' in Sinhala.
4 Meaning 'shame' in Sinhala.
5 Meaning 'older brother' in Tamil.
6 Meaning 'older sister' in Tamil and Sinhala.

7 An ocean-side urban park.
8 Meaning 'older sister' in Sinhala.
9 Meaning 'younger sister' in Sinhala.
10 Meaning 'older sisters' in Tamil (and in Sinhala).
11 A children's game.
12 Hide & Seek.
13 A type of food.
14 Meaning 'younger sister' in Sinhala.
15 The grammatical structures used by the participant were maintained for authenticity here, even if there is a syntactic error.
16 Younger sister in Tamil.
17 The word aunt in Sinhala.
18 Meaning 'white lady', a reference in Sinhala to his younger sister.

Section 2

Communication Disorders:

Siblings and Family

Chapter 6
Sibling Disposition Towards Children With Special Needs

Prithi Venkatesh Mondreti
All India Institute of Speech and Hearing, India

Malar G.
All India Institute of Speech and Hearing, India

ABSTRACT

The background research leading to this chapter probed into the nature of disposition and dominant patterns of feelings displayed b typically developing siblings towards children with special needs arising out of communication disorders. The resultant findings may contribute of facilitation of constructive relationship between them. A survey type of research design was adopted for the purpose of collecting relevant data from primary caregivers of 34 children with communication disorders resulting from either sensory impairments, or neurodevelopmental disorders. An emotional-behavioral rating scale including 10 common dispositions of siblings towards children with special needs had been developed for the purpose following review of relevant literature. The caregiver-participants were to rate the frequency of manifestation of the emotions of behaviors described on a four-pointing rating scale of never, sometimes, often or always. Other relevant information like number of siblings, order of birth, gender of children with special needs, as well as educational and socio-economic status of the caregivers were collected. Analysis of the data revealed feelings of concern and care predominantly prevalent among siblings of children with special needs. Nevertheless, there is scope for further shaping the positive dispositions into constructive behaviors that support optimal development of children with special needs.

INTRODUCTION

In contrast to conventional models for disability rehabilitation that were based on legal perceptions and medical remedies, the contemporary emphasis is on processes that are founded on human rights and grounded in the community. Thus the growing child with differential abilities is no longer viewed as one who is disabled or different, but as one who is in need of special provisions like early identification, timely intervention with appropriate strategies and need-based technology that leads to an independent

DOI: 10.4018/978-1-5225-4955-0.ch006

and productive life assimilated in the social milieu. In this context, along with the professional provisions from expert rehabilitators, the integral involvement of family and local community becomes equally important. Fostering a healthy and supportive relationship between children with special needs and their family, which is their immediate social environment, is essential for having a conducive and constructive life. Traditional family set-ups are led by adult members like parents, grandparents, uncles and aunts who are mature with a natural inclination to take care of needs of children with special needs in the family. Budding members like siblings and cousins are also an integral part of the family whose acceptance and support make more sense and are better appreciated by children with special needs. However, young growing children may not have necessary maturity to stand up to these expectations. This chapter is based on an independent survey undertaken to investigate the existing trends in attitudes and behaviors of typically developing siblings of children with communication disorders with an intention of discerning means for enhancing sibling participation in their development.

BACKGROUND

Importance of Family in Development of Children

The word 'family' might seem to be a simple, single word, but it has multifaceted implications attached to it according to the perspective in which it is being described. The plainest definition describes it as a group consisting of biological parents and their offspring living together as a unit. Further, deliberations may vary according to the economic, cultural, social and several other aspects depending on the context under consideration; but the common aspect among the members in every family is their mutual love, affection and significance of those people who belong to their family (Blessing, n.d.).

Children imbibe their natural behaviors from their families. Research indicates that the development of positive behaviors in a young child is significantly influenced by how well his or her family functions. Childhood dependency on caregivers not only helps children in fulfillment of immediate life needs, but in the long run also helps them imbibe the characteristics and values observed in the family. These in turn help children develop the ability to handle demands and crises in life drawing from the psychological resources gained from early family experiences (Mahalihali, n.d.).

For a child born into a family, it becomes the first social institution executing the primary role of fostering a healthy environment where the members are committed to each other and communicate frequently and fluently without impinging into each others' freedom or space. Thereby family becomes the field for initial social exposure for a child that shapes his/her self-worth, attitudes, values and behavior; thus playing a crucial role promoting skills, morals and values among children (Swindoll, n.d.).

The family further espouses the complex psychosocial development of young children to mature and function as integrated persons in their own right in the larger society outside the family. Through the care and attention tendered during their early years, families enhance the ability in children to discriminate between social, asocial and anti-social trends, strengthen their resolute to encounter and manage adversities, and thus enable them to establish stronger ties with people outside the family. Eventually, a conducive family environment wherein children's material, psychosocial and emotional requirements are met helps them turn out to be both socially and psychologically well-adjusted adults (Rupured and Quick, 1989).

Ultimately as indicated by Family Pediatrics Report (Schor, 2003), "*Families are the most central and enduring influence in children's lives regardless of their education, composition, income and values*". The report further emphasizes that the interpersonal relationship within the family has far reaching consequences in the development of children and that those children who are raised by two parents who are both responsible and dedicated usually perform well in school.

Role of Family in the Educational Growth and Development of Children

The role of the family in the overall development of the children is inevitable and all-pervasive in all domains of psychosomatic growth and learning. Scientific literature accentuates the fact that positive parental inclinations and involvement are dependable and decisive contributors to the education of children. As the age-old adage righty alludes to, parents are the first and foremost educators of children. And most of the learning that children imbibe from parents are caught rather than taught. Parental interest in children's education is a primary indicator that effectively conveys their value for education and ultimately translates into a greater appreciation for education on the part of children themselves (Henderson and Mapp, 2002).

Research evidences have shown positive associations between parent involvement and academic achievement. As per education policy and practice of department of National Education Association in the USA (2008); parent, family and community involvement in education correlates with higher academic performance and school improvement. The policy furthermore states that when school, parents, families and communities work together for supporting the learning of children, it augments the prospects to earn higher grades, attend school more regularly, stay in school longer and enroll in higher level programs. The report also highlights the fact that a stronger school-family-community partnership fosters higher educational aspirations and more motivated students. While studies have shown that parental engagement may positively impact student academic attainment, it is necessary to distinguish between two notions there being involving parents in schooling, in comparison to engaging parents in learning. It is the engagement of the parents in the learning which has shown the greatest positive impact.

International research (Emerson, Fear, Fox, and Sanders, 2012) has shown that parental engagement has a positive impact on student's achievement resulting in higher grades and test scores, lower dropout rates, higher rate of successful completion of classes and increased enrolment in advanced and higher-level programs like commencing post-secondary education and higher graduation rates. In spite of overwhelming research endorsement of the positive impact of parental involvement in education of children, there are also a few discordant notes like that of Catsambis and Beveridge (2001); Fan and Chen (1999); Izzo, Weissberg, Kasprow, and Fendrich (1999); Shumow and Lomax (2001) who reported that parents interaction with school and other parents had little effect. Findings also suggest that their efforts to contact school or involve in children's homework might even have a negative influence, especially at high school level. Even though not explicated, the result could also have been influenced by other factors like tendency among adolescent, high school students to resist parent dominance and influence.

Family Perspectives of Rearing Children With Special Needs

Families are the backbone for all children for ensuring a successful and secure future, it holds true for children with special needs also. Having children with special needs entails additional responsibilities on parents and family. Family members have to absorb the added demands on time and financial resources. However, it is not always over with expense of the material resources, rearing children with special needs are also said to have a draining effect on the psycho-emotional reserves of the family. In intense situations with the prospect of having to raise children with severe developmental and/or multiple problems, researches have generated evidences to the fact where parents are under severe duress and stress leading them to extreme despair (Baker-Ericzén, Brookman-Frazee, and Stahmer, 2005).

Empirical evidences endorse the fact that parents of children with special needs experience more stress as compared to children without special needs. It is not just the diagnosis that leads to the disadvantageous condition, but rather the precarious state of affairs and obligatory adjustments required on part of parents having children with special needs that lead to the deplorable circumstances. Children's maladaptive behavior has been identified as a major factor that leads to increased burden and stress. Other factors like constant demand for personal care and medical attention add to the pressures of rearing a special child and have been frequently associated with negative family impact, stress and burden (Neely-Barnes and Dia, 2008).

In general family management also, parents of children with special needs report increased stress as compared to parents of typically developing children. This is because they may be unable to divert their attention to other aspects of family functioning like spending quality time with other family members and allocating time and financial resources to their healthy siblings. Comparison of children with special needs to the typically developing children in terms of achievement, responsibility and short as well as long-term contributions to the household, and negligence of sibling health and development are other significant factors leading to family pressures and discordance. As parents confront immense challenges in bringing up children with special needs, the other family members who have to share these challenges are the siblings of children with special needs (Baker-Ericzén et al., 2005; Dyson, 1997).

Nevertheless, the possible predicaments faced in rearing children with special needs could be transformed to potential prospects through the positive disposition of diverse members of the family and their cohesive efforts in resolving the problems posed by the presence of disabilities. Effective cognitive appraisal and self-efficacy in parents have been acknowledged as constructive factors that help them in tackling adverse implications encountered in raising children with special needs. Lustig (1972) through his survey of 116 caregivers of children with mental retardation found that when families were able to accept the disability in a positive way, they perceived themselves as competent enough to handle the requirement of the special child more effectively. A positive acceptance of the child's special needs has given the parents an increased sense of purpose, personal growth, improved relationships, social networks, increased spirituality, tolerance, sensitivity followed by a more positive future outlook, as reported. Thus families' acceptance or rejection of special needs in their children determines the quality of life of parents and families.

Prospects of Growing Up With Children With Special Needs

From the perspective of typically developing siblings in the family, having siblings with special needs is found to serve as a source of impediment as well as a chance for improvement. Having siblings with special needs has been reported to extend constructive opportunities to develop worthy qualities like patience, kindness and supportiveness, acceptance of differences, compassion and helpfulness, empathy, dependability and loyalty as a result of standing up for their brother or sister. They also can make use of their opportunity to develop productive skills for home and man management, and can serve as supportive human resources to their parents (Partridge, 2017). But it is not a rosy path that they take in the process of developing these virtues.

Ms. Smith (2016), a mother of four including a child with special needs reports from experience that the typically developing siblings come face to face with wide-ranging complex problems-beginning from feeling ignored of parental attention or their problems being minimized before the critical problems of sibling with special need, followed by developing impressions that they are asked to help too much, or expected to grow and mature too early within home. The issues also extend outside home in the form of isolation in peer group, or in extreme situations intolerance and cynicism faced in the social milieu.

Empirical evidences also reinstate the difficulty in coping with a sibling with special needs reporting that the typically developing siblings often grow up in a situation of considerable stress. This stress could be due to lack of cognitive and emotional maturity to deal with their experiences. They may have a mixed feeling, on one hand, the child may feel loving and protective towards their brother or sister, but at the same time, they may feel resentment, embarrassment, guilt, sorrow and fear. The young siblings may lack skill and understanding to deal with those feelings without any other means available to vent out. This in turn can lead to low self-esteem, shame and sense of worthlessness. As a consequence, they may face depression and anxiety, and in extreme situations repulsive feelings like jealousy, anger, resentment, embarrassment and even retrospective guilt for such emotional retorts. However, it is necessary to mention that if the siblings are adequately and appropriately supported by the parents, their self-esteem and sense of competence are enhanced. They may also develop a range of positive qualities like compassion, tolerance and maturity (Strohm, 2008).

To conclude, for overall development of children with special needs, parents play a crucial role, but the role of the siblings cannot be ignored as they also contribute in helping the special child grow and flourish as a wholesome human being. Nevertheless, on condition that parents interact with them and involve them in a constructive manner, help them to come into terms and accept the disabling condition, and develop adequate coping mechanisms and problem-solving skills (Strohm, 2008).

Need for the Study

Constructive involvement of typically developing siblings in the rearing and rehabilitation of children with special needs will be possible only if their psychological perspectives towards their special siblings are identified and acknowledged appropriately. Knowledge of psychological perspectives, both positive and negative disposition, can help parents to undertake effective measures to overcome sibling discordance and its associated problems among the typically developing children and groom them into helpful human resources. In view of the above, a need was felt to survey the existing status of sibling disposition towards children with special needs in their family. The investigators were interested in carrying out this exercise in the oriental world where families are known for their traditional, close-knit bonding.

METHOD

The present study adopted a survey research design in order to describe, explain and interpret the complimentary and contradictory dispositions demonstrated by siblings of children with special needs.

Participants

- **Primary Participants – Typically Developing Siblings:** The primary participants were typically developing siblings of children with special needs. They were identified through purposive sampling reaching out to as many caregivers as possible having children with and without special needs, and caregivers of only 34 such siblings consented for their participation in the study. These typically developing children had siblings with communication disorders like autism spectrum disorders, hearing impairment, or intellectual disability. Majority of these typically developing siblings (92%) were from middle socio-economic strata; while the rest (8%) were from below poverty line. The participant-siblings were predominantly natives of the south-Indian states of Kerala and Karnataka. Seventy-one percent were from Karnataka, while another 23% were from Kerala. Two children were from north-India.

- **Secondary Participants/Sources of Information – Caregivers of Children With and Without Special Needs:** The primary participants were children in early and late childhood, an age considered immature for objective reflections about their own dispositions and emotions. Hence, the prime caregivers of these children were included in the study as secondary sources of information to express their reflections about their typically developing children's outlook and reactions towards their siblings with special needs. Thus, the study included 34 caregivers having more than one child along with the children with special needs who consented to participate in the study after being informed about the purpose and process of the research study. It was only primary female caregivers, that is, mothers who agreed to share information about their typically developing children's attitude and approach towards their children with special needs. Of these participant mothers, 32 had one child with special needs along with other typically developing children, while two of them had two children with special needs each. All these participant mothers were young adults in the age group of 18 to 35 years. Substantial numbers among these mothers were literate with secondary (41%) or post-secondary (35%) education, while only one lacked literacy skills. Another 20% had pursued higher education, with 8% having professional training in the field of education. These participant-mothers served as secondary participants providing information about reactions of their typically developing wards towards their siblings with special needs.
- **Passive Participants – Children With Special Needs:** Children with special needs were considered as passive participants of the study, as the study involved collecting data on reflections of their typically developing siblings towards them. Eighteen of these children were with sensory impairment that is, hearing impairment; while 16 others had neuro-developmental disabilities like autism spectrum disorder or intellectual disability. The equal number that is seventeen children each were from the early and late phases of childhood. Twenty of them were male children and the other fourteen were female children.

Research Tool

After review of relevant literature (De Caroli and Sagone, 2013; Strohm, 2008), the investigators had identified six positive and four negative dispositions and consequent behavioral development that were frequently observed among typically developing siblings of children with special needs. Statements were framed so as to record whether these reflections and reactions occurred among the siblings surveyed. A four-point frequency scale of 'Always' 'Often' 'Sometimes' and 'Never' was incorporated to record the intensity of occurrence. If it was a positive statement, the occurrences were awarded a score of 3, 2, 1, and 0 respectively. If it was negative statement, the scoring was vice versa.

The first draft of the questionnaire was provided to six experts working in the field of special education, with a minimal qualification of post graduation and more than 10 years of work, for validation of the content and structure of the tool. Those items which received 80% consent from the evaluators were retained. Evaluators' suggestions for improvement of the tool were also incorporated. Consequent to revision of the tool following evaluator feedback, it was translated into languages of the caregiver participants, namely Kannada and Malayalam, apart from the original English version by special educators with expertise in the language along with not less than five years of work experience. Later they were verified by another pair of language experts with more than 10 years of experience in the field of special education.

Data Collection and Analysis

The questionnaire was distributed to the participants after explaining the purpose of this study and seeking oral consent from them. In the presence of the researcher they had to fill in their responses. The filled in questionnaires was collected and the cumulative score for each participant was calculated.

RESULTS AND DISCUSSION

Before commencing the analysis, the data was subjected to Shapiro-Wilk test for normality in order to perceive the nature of sample distribution. The resultant statistic of 0.965 with a non-significant significance of 0.343 indicated that the sample scores were normally distributed. The findings led to further subjection of data to parametric statistical measures.

Affective Tendencies Among Siblings of Children With Special Needs

Initially, the general tendency of disposition towards siblings with special needs was appraised by computing the mean and standard deviation. The results and findings have been presented in Table 1.

As per the results, siblings of children with special needs are disposed with moderately positive feeling towards their siblings with special needs. This is inferred from the fact that the response format has two responses 'never' and 'sometimes' indicating low levels of affections, while the other responses 'often' and 'always' indicated high levels of affections towards the sibling with special needs. Thus a maximum possible mean score of 30, across 10 items with the highest positive frequency receiving a maximum score of three, would have implied best possible affections, while scores below 15 will imply low levels of affections. From the results on the table, it could be inferred that the affections are positive but a moderate 70% (21 out of 30). Among the siblings, two siblings were found to exhibit maximum level of positive affections with full score of 30. However, it is of concern that one sibling had revealed very low affections towards his/her sibling with special needs with a minimum score of 8. Nevertheless, it is of consolation that the response was from an immature sibling of tender age of four, wherein the psychological perspectives towards their brother/sister with special need is yet to mature. Whereas, both the siblings who displayed optimal affections were at the thresholds of adolescence, thus having matured

Table 1. Descriptive analysis of the affective tendencies among siblings

N	Minimum	Maximum	Mean Score	Std. Deviation
34	8.00	30.00	20.8235	5.67542

Table 2. Relationship of age, ordinal position and number of siblings with sibling disposition

Personal and Familial Traits of Children With Special Needs		
Age	**Ordinal Position**	**Number of Siblings**
-0.025	-0.043	0.153

dispositions. The positive emotions of typically developing adolescent children for their sibling with special needs could be due to the fact that they have not experienced parental favoritism or negligence as reported (Powel and Gallagher, 1993).The elder siblings, as inferred from the results, showed more positive feelings towards their sibling with special needs. This may be due to the fact that they have experienced an enriching feeling while taking care of their siblings who are in need of assistance and they consider it as a natural part of their sibling relationship as noted by other researchers (Dervishaliaj and Murati, 2014). The low affection exhibited by one of the siblings could be due to the order of birth, as reported in a study by Ewen (2010, as cited in Martirosyan, 2013), which stated that younger born children tend to be more competitive and sometimes even rebellious.

Impression of Personal and Familial Traits of Children With Special Needs on Sibling Disposition

In order to investigate the relationship between factors like age, ordinal position and number of siblings of children with special needs on the affections they received, diverse statistical measures were used depending on the nature of data involved. For numerical data like age and number of siblings Pearson's correlation was employed, while for ordinal data of child's birth position Spearman's rho was used to speculate the nature of their relationship. The results have been presented in the Table 2.

From the results in the Table 2, it is evident that younger children with special needs who are lower in birth rank and with more than one sibling were recipients of more positive affections. More detailed discussions follow.

- **Relationship of Sibling Disposition With Age of Child With Special Needs:** The chronological age of children with special needs was correlated with the affective score of the sibling. Negative correlation of -0.025 reveals that younger the age of children with special needs tender the affection towards them. However, as the correlation coefficient even though positive is very low and statistically insignificant, it does not help in arriving at concrete conclusions.
- **Relationship of Sibling Disposition With Ordinal Position of Children With Special Needs:** For the purpose of analysis, the ordinal position of child with special needs was ranked as three if he/she was the elder child, as 2 if he/she was the middle child and 1 if he/she was the youngest child. It is vital to note here that none of the children with special needs had more than two siblings. A statistically insignificant negative score of -0.043 hints that, if younger than the other siblings and lower in the birth order, the child with special needs is treated more affectionately. In other words, older children tend to be more concerned and caring towards their younger siblings with special needs. Similar findings were reported in a study conducted by Unruh (1992) wherein it was found that older female siblings had more motherly feelings towards their siblings with special needs, wherein they engaged in care-giving related activities.

- **Relationship of Sibling Disposition With Number of Siblings in the Family:** A positive correlation of 0.153, even though low and statistically insignificant reveals that more the number of siblings, better the treatment by them. The low co-efficient could be because only two of the children with special needs covered in the survey had more than one sibling. However, the positive reflections might have been influenced by the companionship to share responsibilities between the typically developing siblings. Similar to previous research observations by Dew, Balandin and Lewellyn (2008), which show that typically developing siblings display positive dispositions towards having a brother/sister with disabilities regardless of age and the number of siblings. This study also lends tentative directions regarding influence of sibling characteristics like age, number, etc. on the nature of reactions.
- **Relationship of Sibling Disposition With Gender of Children With Special Needs:** Further analysis was carried out to probe the influence of gender of the child with special needs in drawing affections of siblings. Independent sample t-test was used to compare between disposition towards male and female children with special needs, and the results have been presented in Table 3.

As inferred from the results in Table 3, male children with special needs are found to receive more preferential treatment in the family as it is generally found in traditional Indian families. However, the lack of significance in the difference might indicate that more progressive social changes are observed towards gender equality over a period of time. Fielder, Simpson and Clark (2005) reported that culture, traditions, interests and environmental contexts all have an effect on sibling relationships. But as Al-Kubaisi (2000; as cited in Jaradat, n.d.) states, attitudes related to social situation and events tend to change for the better due to exposure to contemporary development.

- **Consideration of Nature of Disability:** The passive participants included 18 children having special needs arising out of the sensory impairment of hearing loss and the remaining 16 children had neurodevelopment disorder like intellectual disability or autism spectrum disorder. The impact of nature of disability on sibling affections was explored with the help of independent sample t-test, the results of which have been presented in Table 4.

The insignificant t-values eliminate chances of concrete evidences regarding influence of nature of disabilities on sibling disposition. However, comparison of mean values hints that children with neurodevelopmental disorders like intellectual disability or autism might tend to draw more affection from their siblings. However, children with hearing impairment also do not lag much behind in receiving sibling attention, with mean difference of just one score which is also statistically insignificant. The positive feeling towards children with neurodevelopment disabilities could have been because of sympathy aroused due to their immature behaviors and lack of self-reliance. In case of children with hearing impairment, they physically look as able as any other child, drawing natural sense of sibling competitiveness towards them.

Table 3. Influence of gender on the affection towards children with special needs

Gender of Children With Special Needs	N (df = 32)	Mean Score of Affection	Standard Deviation	Mean Difference	t	Sig.
Male	20	21.30	5.98	1.92	0.973	0.080
Female	14	19.38	4.71			

Table 4. Influence of nature of disability

Nature of Disability	N (df = 32)	Mean	Standard Deviation	Mean Difference	t	Sig.
Sensory (Hearing) Impairment	18	20.3889	6.43647	0.92	-0.468	0.139
Neurodevelopment Disorders	16	21.3125	4.84037			

Moreover, as Alemayehu (2000) and Tekleweldeab (2006) suggest through their findings, difficulties in communicating with children with hearing impairment might have also led to alienation from siblings.

IMPLICATIONS AND RECOMMENDATIONS

The field of study though restricted in size and locale, has led to insightful findings which point towards further directions. The results could be taken as a forerunner for more detailed and extensive survey, followed with programs for integrated family-based rehabilitation including siblings taking into consideration suggestions of practitioners like Meyer (2001) who extended useful tips to cultivate proactive disposition in siblings so as to bear a positive outlook and play a constructive role in bringing up children with special needs.

According to Meyer (2001), typically developing siblings according to their developmental phase and level of maturity should be helped to acquire informative knowledge about the nature of special needs in their siblings and its implications so that they are able to understand and accept them better. They could also be helped to connect and network with other siblings of children with special needs so that they find companionship to share their feelings and experiences. Caregivers should also take care that they develop and maintain good communication with their typically developing children and set aside devoted time for them, in spite of their burdens in taking care of their wards with special needs. In the longer run, such healthy relationships may nurture the typically developing siblings into trustworthy partners in sharing their special needs responsibilities. As siblings mature, it is also necessary that parents discuss and involve them in planning for the future of the family especially in terms of obligations towards the siblings with special needs.

CONCLUSION

Post-survey impressions are as expected in traditional Indian society where, family bonds are still stronger and warmer; so as to display constructive care and concern for children with special needs even at the tender age of preschool phase. The child's younger age, lower order of birth and complex nature of the disability are found to strengthen the sibling relationships. If these positive feelings are further strengthened, siblings could be enabled to become responsible and dutiful stakeholders in families' responsibility of bringing up the child with special needs. As Reagon, Higbee, and Endicott (2006) opine the role of typically developing siblings in the life of children with special needs is more crucial for the development of social competence. Thus it becomes vital that sibling relationships be positive given that they are the most frequently available play partners. They further suggest that positive support, effective coping strategies, open discussion, planning and sensitivity can facilitate more positive relationships between typically developing children and their siblings with special needs. To conclude, as McHale, Sloan, and Simeonsson (1986) suggest positive relationships, less conflict, effective coping strategies, and minimal perceived parental favoritism in the family environment could lead to better understanding among their siblings about children with special needs and in turn, could contribute to positive demeanor and helpful interactions.

ACKNOWLEDGMENT

The reported study was a non-funded, independent survey undertaken by the authors in the premises of All India Institute of Speech and Hearing, Mysuru. They express their gratitude to Prof. S. R. Savithri, Director, AIISH and Prof. M. Pushpavathi, Head of the Department of Special Education for extending permission for carrying out the survey and publication of this chapter based on the survey. They thank all participant-caregivers for consenting and cooperating by offering their valuable inputs.

REFERENCES

Baker-Ericzén, M. J., Brookman-Frazee, L., & Stahmer, A. (2005). Stress levels and adaptability in parents of toddlers with and without autism spectrum disorders. *Research and Practice for Persons with Severe Disabilities*, *30*(4), 194–204. doi:10.2511/rpsd.30.4.194

Blessing, M. (n.d.). *Meaning of family*. Retrieved from http://family.lovetoknow.com/about-family-values/meaning-family

Catsambis, S., & Beveridge, A. (2001). *Neighborhood and school influences on the family life and mathematics performance of eighth-grade students*. Retrieved from http://www.csos.jhu.edu/ crespar/techReports/Report54.pdf

De Caroli, M. E., & Sagone, E. (2013). Siblings and disability: A study on social attitudes toward disabled brothers and sisters. *Procedia: Social and Behavioral Sciences*, *93*, 1217–1223. doi:10.1016/j.sbspro.2013.10.018

Dervishaliaj, E., & Murati, E. (2014). Families of children with developmental disabilities: Perceptions and experiences of adolescent siblings of children with developmental disabilities. *European Scientific Journal*, *10*(2), 129–142.

Dew, A., Balandin, S., & Llewellyn, G. (2008). The psychosocial impact on siblings of people with lifelong physical disability: A review of the literature. *Journal of Developmental and Physical Disabilities*, *20*(5), 485 507. doi:10.100710882-008-9109-5

Dyson, L. L. (1997). Fathers and mothers of school-age children with developmental disabilities: Parental stress, family functioning, and social support. *American Journal of Mental Retardation*, *102*(3), 267–279. doi:10.1352/0895-8017(1997)102<0267:FAMOSC2.0.CO;2 PMID:9394135

Emerson, L., Fear, J., Fox, S., & Sanders, E. (2012). Parental engagement in learning and schooling: Lessons from research. A report by the Australian Research Alliance for Children and Youth (ARACY) for the Family-School and Community Partnerships Bureau, Canberra.

Fan, X., & Chen, M. (1999). Parental involvement and students' academic achievement: A meta-analysis. Arlington, VA: National Science Foundation, National Center for Education Statistics. ED430048.

Fiedler, R., Simpson, L., & Clark, M. (2005). *Parents and families of children with disabilities*. Englewood Cliffs, NJ: Pearson Prentice Hall.

Henderson, A. T., & Mapp, K. L. (2002). *The impact of school, family and community connections on student achievement*. Annual Synthesis 2002, Southwest Educational Development Laboratory. Retrieved from https://www.sedl.org/connections/resources/evidence.pdf

Izzo, C. V., Weissberg, R. P., Kasprow, W. J., & Fendrich, M. (1999). A longitudinal assessment of teacher perceptions of parent involvement in children's education and school performance. *American Journal of Community Psychology*, *27*(6), 817–839. doi:10.1023/A:1022262625984 PMID:10723536

Jaradat, N. A. (n.d.). *Attitudes of intellectual disability children's siblings toward intellectual disability*. Retrieved from http://www.zu.edu.jo/MainFile/Profile_Dr_UploadFile/Researcher/Files/ResearchFile_4051_7_50.pdf

Lustig, D. C. (1997). Families with an adult with mental retardation: Empirical family typologies. *Rehabilitation Counseling Bulletin*, *41*(2), 138–157.

Mahalihali, K. (n.d.). *Family influences on the development of a child's behavior*. Retrieved from http://www.kon.org/urc/v5/mahalihali.html

Martirosyan, A. (2013). *Sibling relationships in families with a child with special needs: A case study of a Norwegian family with a child with Down syndrome and her three siblings* (Unpublished Master's dissertation). University of Oslo, Norway.

McHale, S., Sloan, J., & Simeonsson, J. (1986). Sibling relationships of children with autism, mentally retarded, and nonhandicapped brothers and sisters. *Journal of Autism and Developmental Disorders*, *16*(4), 399–413. doi:10.1007/BF01531707 PMID:3804956

Meyer, D. (2001). Meeting the unique concerns of brothers of sisters of children with special needs. *Insights*, *51*, 28–32.

National Education Association USA. (2008). *Policy brief: Parent, Family, Community Involvement in Education*. Retrieved from www.nea.org/assets/doc/PBII_Parent Involvement08.pdf

Neely-Barnes, S. L., & Dia, D. A. (2008). Families of children with disabilities: A review of literature and recommendations for interventions. *Journal of Early and Intensive Behavior Intervention: JEIBI*, *5*(3), 93–107. doi:10.1037/h0100425

Olika, R. E. L. (2013). *Attitudes hearing impaired children face from hearing people* (Unpublished master's dissertation). University of Oslo, Norway.

Partridge, L. (2017). *Siblings of children with special needs*. Retrieved from http://extendedfamilycare.com/pittsburgh/siblings-of-children-with-special-needs/

Powel, T. H., & Gallagher, P. A. (1993). *Brothers and sisters: A special part of exceptional families*. Baltimore, MD: Paul H. Brookes.

Reagon, K., Higbee, T., & Endicott, K. (2006). Teaching pretend play skills to students with autism using video modeling with siblings as model and play partners. *Education & Treatment of Children*, *29*, 517–528.

Rupured, M., & Quick, S. (1989). *Family vitality: Characteristics of strong families. Publication H.E. 7-138*. University of Kentucky Cooperative Extension Service.

Schor, E. L. (2003). Family pediatrics report of the task force on the family. *Pediatrics*, *111*(6), 1541–1571. PMID:12777595

Shumow, L., & Lomax, R. (2001). *Parental efficacy: Predictor of parenting behavior and adolescent outcomes*. Paper presented at the Annual Meeting of the American Educational Research Association, Seattle, WA.

Smith, J. D. (2016). *On parenting: Eight things siblings of children with special needs struggle with*. Retrieved from https://www.washingtonpost.com/news/parenting/wp/2016/12/20/8-things-siblings-of-children-with-special-needs-struggle-with/?utm_term=.faaa29548765

Strohm, K. (2008). Too important to ignore: Siblings of children with special needs. *Australian e-Journal for the Advancement of Mental Health*, *7*(2), 1–6. doi:10.5172/jamh.7.2.78

Swindoll, C. R. (n.d.). *Characteristics of a healthy family*. Retrieved from http://www.lifeway.com/Article/eight-characteristics-of-a-healthy-family

Unruh, A. (1992). Siblings of children with special needs. *School of Occupational Therapy*, *59*(3), 151–158. PMID:10120258

KEY TERMS AND DEFINITIONS

Children With Special Needs: Children with special needs include those children with communication disorders arising out of hearing loss, autism spectrum disorders, or intellectual disability.

Disability: Sensory disability of hearing loss as well as neurodevelopmental disabilities of autism spectrum disorders or intellectual disability.

Disposition: Attitudes and behaviors of siblings towards children with special needs.

Negative Disposition: Negative feelings, anger, immature behavior, and temper tantrums.

Positive Disposition: Positive feelings, love, concern, compassion, and protection.

Siblings of Children With Special Needs: Brothers or sisters who could be elder or younger in the birth order to children with special needs.

Survey Research Design: Gathering of information about complimentary and contradictory dispositions demonstrated by siblings of children with special needs with use of an emotional-behavioral scale.

Chapter 7
Mothers as Advocates of Social Inclusion for Children With Communication Disorders

Shalini Felicity Wickremesooriya
Institute of Professional Studies, Sri Lanka

ABSTRACT

Social inclusion is based on acceptance and belonging irrespective of any status, disability, or disadvantage. The ability to communicate empowers humans in their quest for social inclusion. However, children challenged by communication disorders struggle to form friendships and make inroads into social groups. Mothers, the primary caregivers in most instances, with their intimate knowledge of their children, are considered the best advocates. This study set out to identify strategies that mothers engage in to pave the way for successful social inclusion of children with communication disorders. An online survey was conducted in different geographical locations. Mothers with children aged 6-13 years who had received speech therapy or are currently receiving speech therapy were invited to participate. Data were analyzed using a mixed methods approach. Outcomes suggest that all mothers believe in social inclusion despite facing a range of inclusion and exclusionary practices. Undeterred by these responses, mothers advocate for social inclusion by engaging in a range of strategies.

INTRODUCTION

Although human needs and abilities may vary, all humans experience a deep need to forge associations with one another through social inclusion. Inclusion arises from the idea of valuing human beings and not merely tolerating them (Frazee, 2002). Each individual is considered to have a special place in the fabric of a diverse community which works at fostering active engagement (Taylor, 2007). Social inclusion for individuals with disabilities means that they must have "access to respect, access to a sense of oneself as a whole person and access to identity as a valued contributor, a bearer of rights, knowledge and power", within communities (Frazee, 2002, p. 4). Communication, a basic human right, facilitates social inclusion. Friendships are formed, relationships are built, independence is gained, choices are

DOI: 10.4018/978-1-5225-4955-0.ch007

made, emotions are expressed, and learning is achieved through communication (Jones, 2002). Children with communication disorders are challenged by this task and require advocacy to equalize the power base. Mothers, usually the parent who spends the most time with children, are in a unique position to engage in advocacy for social inclusion (Ewles, Clifford, and Minnes, 2014). As children observe their mothers and become partners, they learn the art of self-advocacy (Knight and Oliver, 2007).

BACKGROUND

Social Inclusion

Inclusion is built on the belief that every individual must be an active member of their community (Diamond and Hong, 2010). The concept of a "society for all" was first formulated at the World Summit for Social Development in Copenhagen in March of 1995 (UNDESA, 1995). This was followed by the Millennium Declaration, which considers social inclusion as a stepping stone to global peace (UNDESA, 2000). In September of 2015, world leaders agreed that inclusion be a core objective in the 2030 Agenda for Sustainable Development (UNDESA, 2016). Goal 10:2 of the 2030 agenda focuses on empowering and promoting "social, economic and political inclusion of all, irrespective of age, sex, disability, race, ethnicity, origin, religion or economic or other status" while Goal 4 emphasizes inclusive education and Goal 16 inclusive societies and institutions (UNDESA, 2016).

Social inclusion is based on the premise that every individual regardless of ability, status or any other classification has equal dignity and is worthy contributors to society (Lombe, 2007). It has been described as a "…connection to the network of community development, it is to become more than a speck of dust, to have a forename and surname, with one's own distinctive features, skills and abilities, able to receive and give stimulus, to imitate and be imitated, to participate in a process of changing one's own life and collective life" (Busatto, 2007, p. 4). Hence, social inclusion is to have a voice that is heard, accepted, and respected (Taylor, 2007) as individuals negotiate with one another to be part of a community.

Social Inclusion of Individuals With Disabilities

Research suggests that the skills of children with disabilities are enhanced when they experience inclusion (Antia, Jones, Luckner, Kreimeyer, and Reed, 2011; Frankel, Gold, and Ajodhia, 2010). Furthermore, inclusion is socially rewarding, as friendships that would normally elude disabled children in segregated settings take shape. The children feel cared for, honored, and cherished by other human beings, thereby fulfilling a deep human need (Finke, McNaughton, and Drager, 2009). Inclusion also nurtures independence as it encourages growth and discovery (Stahmer, Akshoomoff, and Cunningham, 2011). It frees individuals to acquire a high self-worth (Diamond and Hong, 2005) and improves wellbeing, happiness, self-esteem, and mental health (Mahar, Cobigo, and Stuart, 2013; Forrester-Jones et al., 2006).

Social inclusion can take place in a private setting such as home or a public setting such as community center (Simplican, 2015). Social inclusion can also be viewed as a process or an outcome (Frazee, 2002). The process affects almost all societal activities and depends on the active participation of individuals with and without disabilities. It means that individuals without disabilities remove barriers and create a welcoming atmosphere with open communication (Hess, Molina, and Kozleski, 2006). It requires actively encouraging children with disabilities to participate, to let their voices be heard, and to engage in discovering self with the knowledge that the community supports them (Frazee, 2002). When social inclusion is viewed as an outcome, society will reflect greater equality and higher levels of tolerance (UNDESA, 2016). Negative attitudes, stereotypes, and stigmas will be nonexistent (Power, 2013). Inclusion will be reflected in the organization of the community; the variety of opportunities provided for children with disabilities to be socially active within the community will be abundant (Frazee, 2002).

Inclusion challenges the long-held views of deficit within a person and draws attention to society's role in supporting individuals with disabilities. Inclusion gave rise to the social model movement that was introduced in the publication Fundamental Principles of Disability (UPIAS, 1976, cited in Slee, 2011). The social model discourages communities and establishments from maintaining exclusionary practices that are "oppressive, discriminatory and disabling" and encourages a closer look at their response to individuals with disabilities (Mittler, 2000, p. 3). The social model, therefore, seeks to minimize the effects of disability by considering the needs of a population and dismantling offensive physical and attitudinal obstructions (Tregaskis, 2004).

Global statistics highlight that while 10% of the world's population is disabled, two-thirds of people with disabilities live in developing countries (UNDESA, 2009). Studies in various countries indicate that the concept of social inclusion and exclusion is multidimensional and dependent on the context (UNDESA, 2016). A study in the Caribbean revealed that individuals with disabilities such as physical impairments are more accepted, than individuals with mental, psychological, or developmental disabilities such as autism (Thomas, 2009). A study of Arab caregivers has revealed that Arab fathers feel ashamed of their children with disabilities (Crabtree, 2007). Another study in the Bahamas revealed that negative constructs regarding disability were passed down through generations and need to be changed for successful inclusion (Johnson and Harris, 2014). A study in New Zealand indicated that teachers were challenged in their progression towards inclusion due to negative attitudes of parents within school communities (Stark, Gordon-Burns, Purdue, Rarere-Briggs, and Turncock, 2011). According to a study in Pakistan, cultural beliefs in this part of the world encouraged individuals with disabilities to remain in their homes and therefore discouraged social inclusion (Mehmood, Bhatti, and Ali, 2015). A similar view is reported from China where children with disabilities are considered *shazi* or idiots, and therefore excluded (McCabe, 2007). A study conducted in Bosnia, Herzegovina, and Bulgaria reports that parents with children with disabilities were actively engaged in setting up parent organizations and formulating practices for advocacy (Bećirević and Dowling, 2010).

When discussing social inclusion, it is imperative that the discussion touch upon social exclusion. Social exclusion is a conscious process and a state of mind in which one actively pursues the goal of shutting out people from full participation in mainstream society. It is also a personal experience that cannot be ignored (UNDESA, 2010). Several studies have focused on exclusion (Russell, 2003; Connors and Stalker, 2007) and reported that social exclusion causes psychological and emotional trauma for the individuals concerned and even their families (UNDESA, 2009).

The social relational model of disability identifies two types of barriers that affect personal identity: "barriers to doing" which consider material effects and "barriers to being" which consider psycho-emotional effects (Thomas, 2004). Communities that define the individual with the disability, subscribe to the concept of ignoring the human being and highlighting the disability (Lyons, 2005). Barriers to doing include lack of physical access to public spaces and lack of access to tools and opportunities that enable communication (UNDESA, 2009). Barriers to being are witnessed when individuals with disabilities are denied their rights to participate in the socioeconomic and cultural systems because of fear and ignorance (UNDESA, 2009).

Attitudes are often a part of a bigger picture and not merely the point of view of a single individual (McGeown, 2012). Attitudes are shaped by parental views, media, and witnessed behaviors (Siraj-Blatchford, 2004). Social exclusion of individuals with disabilities occurs because disability is often accompanied with negative constructions and labeling (Nielsen, 2012). When attitudes are negative, bias can set in as early as birth (Siraj-Blatchford, 2004). Individuals with disabilities are considered victims when society's response includes pity, embarrassment, guilt, and condescension. Some people fear individuals with disabilities and steer clear of any contact, essentially practicing exclusion (Danforth, 2008). The deep-rooted practices of exclusion that pervade many societies need to be addressed for communities to be more inclusive (Slee, 2004).

A sincere effort and a long-term political commitment at the highest level are required to remove barriers and bring about laws, policies, institutions, attitudes, and behaviors that showcase true social inclusion (UNDESA, 2016). It has been suggested that five levels of inclusion—visibility, consideration, access to social interaction, rights, and resources—be considered in incremental stages to promote social inclusion (Therborn, 2007). Early childhood educators are called upon to encourage inclusion among the youngest members of society by crushing negative perceptions, misperceptions, repressive discourse and biased behaviors among students (MacNaughton, 2005). The inclusion-exclusion gap can also be narrowed through parent advocacy (Cook, Tankersley, Cook, and Landrum, 2000; Westwood and Graham, 2000).

Parent Advocacy

Advocacy belongs to the family of conflict resolution. It refers to the act of enabling an individual or a group of people to advance a certain viewpoint through the use of resources and information (Dalrymple, 2005). Most people need advocacy at some point in their lives. Advocacy at the basic level is communication which attempts to convince others to bring about change (Thackeray and Hunter, 2010). It is a relationship between the advocate, who actively seeks to help others speak for themselves, and the person or persons being supported (Lewington and Clipson, 2004).

Most parents engage in advocacy on behalf of their children either continuously or at some point in their lives (Ryan and Cole, 2009). However, parent advocacy is especially important for children with communication disorders since they often cannot "speak up" for themselves (Knight and Oliver, 2007). These children require a voice or voices, other than their own, to fight for their rights. Parents, often feel a moral obligation to advocate on behalf of their children with disabilities (Wang, Mannan, Poston, Turnbull, and Summers, 2004). Advocacy in relation to parents with children with disabilities is described as action taken by parents on behalf of their child to ensure that children receive sufficient support, adequate care, and child rights (Ewles et al., 2014). Successful advocates support children with disabilities to become active participants rather than assume the role of passive victims (Knight and Oliver, 2007). They also advocate not merely for their children but for others as well (Wang et al., 2004).

Parents, with their unique knowledge of their children, are the first and best advocates of children with disabilities (Webster, Cumming, and Rowland, 2016). Hence, it has been suggested that parents develop their advocacy skills within the first few years of their child's life (Wang et al., 2004).

It has been reported that parents' cognitive levels and coping styles determine levels of success (Neely-Barnes and Dia, 2008). Parents need to assume a realistic attitude towards disability, maladaptive behaviors, and care needs to effectively advocate for their children. They also require knowledge and understanding to positively impact their own perceptions regarding disability (Johnson and Harris, 2014; Woodgate, Ateah, and Secco, 2008) and to be aware of the current policies that affect their children

(Wakelin, 2008). Parents need to learn the skill of advocacy through education, support, and mentorship (Hess et al., 2006), be more direct in their requests and be prepared to educate others regarding the unique characteristics of their children and their contributions to the world (Woodgate et al., 2008). Parents who adjust their thinking and consider themselves capable of coping with the demands of advocacy experience better outcomes (Lustig, 2002).

Historically, parents of children with disabilities have banded together to support one another and to advocate on behalf of their children in a variety of ways: protests, meetings, rallies, and through the media (Carter, 2013). Parents have advocated as individuals via telephone conversations, letters and informing professionals about their child's unique wants and capabilities (Wang et al., 2004, p.148). They have participated in studies to advocate for their children (Hess et al., 2006). They have raised funds for research and been the driving force behind incorporating organizations that cater to the needs of individuals with disabilities (Carter, 2013). Some parents have raised awareness about the intrinsic benefits of living with an individual with disability: personal and spiritual growth, tolerance, sensitivity, and a shedding of negative beliefs on disability (Scorgie and Sobsey, 2000). Further, they have advocated for improved services and to create changes in systems at community and country level (Wang et al., 2004) by enacting laws, creating public awareness, educating the public and directing more funds for disability services (Black and Baker, 2011).

While advocacy targeted at a large sector of society has yielded benefits, parents with children with disabilities struggle to cope with the unexpected demands on time, emotions, and finances that come with having a child with a disability (Baker-Ericzén, Brookman-Frazee, and Stahmer, 2005). They are left with little or no time to engage in day-to-day advocacy with smaller, more intimate communities (Carter, 2013). Mothers, often the primary caregivers of children with disabilities (Ryan and Cole, 2009; Cole, 2004) are reported to experience higher levels of stress and anxiety than fathers (Pozo and Sarriá, 2014). Because mothers are less likely to be engaged in paid employment (Shearn and Todd, 2000), they feel isolated from adult interaction, experience loneliness and a sense of being undervalued (Ryan and Cole, 2009). Parents report that they feel embarrassment (Gray, 2002), guilt (Hotschild, 1979) shame (Williams, 2001) and hurt (Ryan, 2010) whilst out in public. Hence, some parents opt to avoid social activities (Schaff, Toth-Cohen, Johnson, Outenn, and Benevides, 2011) thus limiting opportunities for advocacy in social settings. However, other research suggests that despite being exhausted and emotionally drained while engaging in advocacy activities (Wang, et al., 2004), more and more families are embracing differences and living lives that are 'normal' for them (Rehm and Bradley, 2005). For mothers who venture outside, they are called upon to act as mediators between their child and the social world as they negotiate, facilitate and manage social encounters (Read, 2000). Mothers who seek to actively advocate for their children with disabilities, are in terms of the social field of self-advocacy, persons with valued capital (McKeever and Miller, 2004). Her insider knowledge, hands-on experience and skills acquired become an asset to many. However, the experience of advocacy can either be considered a stressor or a success depending on the perception of the role of an advocate and subsequent outcomes (Nachshen and Jamieson, 2000). Fear of being in the spotlight can also discourage parents from engaging in advocacy (Resch et al., 2010) whilst the level of assertiveness needed for successful advocacy might conflict with cultural norms (Kalyanpur, 2000).

Parents, caregivers, and professionals seek to encourage children with disabilities to engage in self-advocacy (Stuntzner and Hartley, 2015). It is a skill that individuals with disabilities ought to cultivate to ensure that their needs are met in a variety of social settings (Fabian, 2007). Successful advocacy is witnessed when those attempting advocacy possess information concerning their options and rights and are supported by persons who can help them consider their options (Hess et al., 2006). It is a developed ability which can be learned by engaging with adults as they seek to advocate for children (Stuntzner and Hartley, 2015). It is also empowering; because knowing how to negotiate effectively will ensure full inclusion and participation in life events (Goodley, 2005).

Communication Disorders

The ability to communicate develops from the moment a child is born. The individuals in a child's life, especially mothers, play a vital role in shaping and encouraging the development of communication (Vernon-Feagans et al., 2008). As parents and caregivers respond to the first vocalizations, they give meaning to the sounds, thus encouraging the child to communicate (Sun and Fernandes, 2014). Mothers who talk with their children in appealing and interesting ways, irrespective of their education and socioeconomic levels, aid in the rapid development of communication (Vernon-Feagans et al., 2008).

Some infants and toddlers are challenged in their communication development due to neuromotor, cognitive, genetic, sensory, or social disabilities, they may display slow development with babbling, delays in producing first words, an inability to understand language, or a lack of clarity in speech (Davidoff, 2017). These features may indicate a delay or disorder (RCSLT, 2009). Delays arise when speech and language develop in the expected sequence but at a slower pace. Late language development is not a lifelong condition and is usually correctible with speech therapy (LeComer, 2006). Communication disorders may be considered primary or secondary disorders. The disorder is considered a primary disorder in the absence of another identifiable disorder or social cause (Lindsay, Dockrell, Desforges, Law, and Peacey, 2010). It is considered a secondary disorder when accompanied with another disorder (Berkman et al., 2015). There is also a subgroup of children who have communication disorders due to socioeconomic disadvantage (Locke, Ginsberg, and Peers, 2002). Communication disorders may also be acquired disorders or developmental disorders. Acquired disorders manifest as a result of injury sustained after birth. Developmental language disorders are believed to be present at birth but made manifest in the course of child development (Berkman et al., 2015).

Other terms used to describe communication disorders (Haynes, Moran, and Pindzola, 2006) include: speech and language impairments (RCSLT, 2009), specific speech and language difficulties (Lindsay and Dockrell, 2000), specific speech and language impairments (IASLT, 2007), and specific developmental disorders of speech and language (World Health Organization [WHO], 2007). These diagnostic terms have been advocated for by professional bodies such as the Royal College of Speech and Language Therapists in the UK (RCSLT, 2009), the Irish Association of Speech and Language Therapists (IASLT, 2007), the American Association of Speech and Audiology (ASHA, 1993), the American Psychiatric Association (APA, 2000), and United Nations organizations (WHO, 2007).

Communication disorders refer to a broad range of problems including disfluency of speech, articulation and phonological difficulties, voice disorders, the inability to express thoughts effectively when speaking, deficits in understanding, and difficulties using language in social situations (Gillam, Marquardt, and Martin, 2011). Some professionals consider deficits in listening, reading, speaking, and writing to be evidence of communication disorders (Wegner, Grosche, and Edmister, 2003). The inability to effectively convey meaning (Gillam et al., 2011), "*receive, send, process, and comprehend concepts or verbal, nonverbal and graphic symbol systems*" (ASHA, 1993, pp.40-41) and difficulties with "*fluency, forming sounds and words, formulating sentences, understanding what others say, and using language socially*" (Bercow, 2008, p. 13) are all characteristics of communication disorders.

Variations in terminology, definitions, assessment tools, and procedures present distortions to statistics globally and therefore need to be considered with caution (Lindsay et al., 2010; Martin and Miller, 2003). It has been reported that approximately 1% of five-year old's entering school in 2007 in the UK were diagnosed with communication disorders (Bercow, 2008). An American survey states that approximately 7.7% of children between the ages of 3 and 17 are diagnosed with communication disorders (Black, Vahratian, and Hoffman, 2015) while a study in Australia reveals that 13% of school-aged children were identified with communication disorders (McLeod and McKinnon, 2007). It was estimated that 5% of children between the ages of 5 and 6 were communication impaired in Ireland (IASLT, 2007). Another study (CERI, 2004) conducted in three countries reveals that students with communication disorders in mainstream schools in Canada amounted to 1.5%, Finland 3.12%, and Turkey 0.01%. The 2011 census in India reveals that 7.5% of the disabled population of 2.21% are considered to have speech difficulties (Census of India, 2011). It is reasonable to assume these statistics have changed, since some were recorded more than 10 years ago. However, given the diverse interpretations and other factors involved, it is difficult to predict accurately. The dilemmas discussed and additional reasons such as scarcity of researchers, denial by families, and absence of culturally and linguistically suitable assessment tools result in a lack of statistics from the Asian and African continents (Wickremesooriya, 2012).

Social communication develops as early as the first year of a child's life, when the child learns to watch adult interactions, participate in social exchanges, and communicate actively with sounds, gestures, and facial expressions (Weatherby, 2006). Social communication, a seemingly easy and natural process for many children, can challenge children with communication disorders (Beitchman and Brownlie, 2010). Hence, these children face hardships in everyday society where spoken language is the predominant medium of social interaction (Olusanya, Ruben, and Parving, 2006). Challenged children can develop unconventional, inappropriate, or socially deviant behaviors (Weatherby, 2006). They may even isolate themselves as they become frustrated with the listeners or themselves (Martin and Miller, 2003). Due to breakdowns in communication, there is the need to constantly negotiate the right to communicate, to be heard, and to be accepted (Bray, 2006). Children with communication disorders are bullied more often than their peers (Beitchman and Brownlee, 2010). Research reveals that approximately 36% of students with communication disorders are at risk of being bullied as compared to 12% of their peers who do not display communication difficulties (Conti-Ramsden, Botting, Simkin, and Knox, 2004). These reasons prevent them from forming meaningful social relationships (Brinton and Fugiki, 2006). However, some children with communication disorders feel a compulsion to forge their own identities, regardless of peer response, to gain acceptance and be included (Slee, 2011).

METHOD

The study is based on combining the concepts of inclusion, parent advocacy, child rights and the social model of disability. The focus group is children with a primary diagnosis of communication disorders. These included stuttering, expressive language delays, receptive language deficits, pragmatic disorder and articulation and phonological disorders.

The objective of this study is to be informed about the different ways that mothers advocate for the social inclusion of their children with communication disorders within their communities. Communities include the people they meet during their day to day excursions such as, neighbourhood, school, public transit, therapy clinics, recreational facilities and shops. The purpose of the study is to empower a wider audience of mothers to be successful advocates, thereby promoting social inclusion.

Research Questions

Developing questions is an important aspect of research since it narrows down the objective of the research through specific questioning (Creswell, 2005).

The research questions targeting a global audience were:

1. What do mothers believe regarding a child's right to social inclusion?
2. What do mothers believe are the outcomes of social inclusion for a child with communication disorders and the community?
3. What responses do mothers and children receive when they attempt to engage in conversation with community members?
4. Where do mothers and children experience social exclusion and exclusion?
5. Who includes and excludes the mothers and children?
6. What are the different approaches that Mothers use to enable Social Inclusion?

Tools

The survey methodology is employed to study the characteristics of a population. Surveys involve gathering information from groups of people about the existing conditions in the social and economic world at a particular time. They describe existing conditions that can be compared with existing standards or shown as a connection between particular happenings (Cohen, Manion, and Morrison, 2000). It is carried out in an organized and methodical manner, using well-defined concepts, methods, and procedures (Groves et al., 2011). Since a survey can be administered via face-to-face contact, telephone, mail, or the web (Bajpai, 2011), it is suitable for a large and dispersed population base (Groves et al., 2011). The mixed mode approach is currently gaining popularity in the social sciences (Query and Wright, 2003). This approach combines two survey methods in a bid to ensure maximum coverage with minimal costs and fewer non-response errors (Dillman, Smyth, and Christian, 2009).

The online survey method chosen for this study has many advantages. Online surveys can reach a relatively large dispersed population at a lower cost and in less time (Yun and Trombo, 2000). Virtual communities enable researchers to gain access to people who share specific interests, attitudes, beliefs, and values about a problem, issue, or activity (Wright, 2005) and reduce research costs significantly (Biemer and Lyberg, 2003). More respondents are willing to share information on their own time via online surveys (Groves et al., 2011) especially if the topic is of personal interest (McDonald and Adam, 2003). In addition, anonymity and confidentiality can be guaranteed for online surveys when seeking opinions on one or numerous topics (Nardi, 2015), while expecting quick responses (McDonald and Adam, 2003).

The online survey method is, however, considered unsuitable for respondents who are not technically savvy (Couper, 2000). Other cited disadvantages to the use of online surveys include: the perception of effort and time needed to complete the survey resulting in a low return rate (Crawford, Couper, and Lamias, 2001), misunderstandings, and bias that may develop due to the wording of questions (Bajpai, 2011).

Data Collection

The life of a survey can be broken down into several stages; the planning stage, the design and development stage and the implementation stage. Each stage consists of a systematic step by step process.

The planning stage involves reviewing existing research, considering resources available to facilitate the study, identifying the target population, deciding on data collection pathways, and choosing methods of analysis (Cohen et al., 2000). As in most research activity, the first step is to engage in a literature review. Existing research on advocacy for children with communication disorders was sparse. However, a broader search regarding inclusion and advocacy unearthed studies directed at educational services (Wang et al., 2004), professional services (Resch et al., 2010; Bailey et al., 2005) or concerning children with autism (Wright and Taylor, 2014; Ryan and Cole, 2009; Ryan, 2005; Gray, 2002). Hence, it was soon evident that this study can enhance the current body of information and spur on further research. Resource availability was limited for this exploratory study. Hence, it was determined to keep costs low and manageable. Since the objective of the study was to study global perspectives, the target population was to be drawn from as many continents as possible. Mothers whose children had received speech therapy within the last 12 months or were currently receiving therapy, and whose primary disorder is communication, between the ages of 6 and 13, were identified as probable respondents. Children within this age range were selected because mothers are more involved with children during the early years as they advocate for their children to receive sufficient support, adequate care, and child rights (Wright and Taylor, 2014; Ewles et al., 2014). The disorders included stammering, articulation and phonological difficulties, voice disorders, expressive and receptive language difficulties and pragmatic disorder. A period of four weeks was set aside for data collection. The online survey mode was selected primarily because it can be sent out to a wider audience quickly and at a low cost (Yun and Trombo, 2000). Data analysis was conducted using a mixed method approach combining qualitative and quantitative data analysis methods (Thomas, 2003). Since the questions were a combination of closed, open-ended and semi-structured questions both quantitative and qualitative analysis was required.

The design and development phase included designing a data collection instrument and piloting the survey. The survey method used a questionnaire to collect pertinent information (Bajpai, 2011). Existing studies that conducted surveys to understand parent advocacy were studied. These included the Parent advocacy scale (Nachshen, Anderson, and Jamieson, 2001) which focuses on membership and roles in advocacy organizations, the amount of advocacy undertaken by the parent, the focus and personal views regarding advocacy; Parent advocacy in special education (Burke and Hodapp, 2016) which concentrates on educational settings; the Advocacy activities scale (Malec, Brown, and Moessner, 2010) which seeks to measure involvement in activities directed at advocating for individuals with acquired brain injury and Advocacy by parents of young children with special needs (Wright and Taylor, 2014) which considers settings in which advocacy takes place, perceived gains and processes. None of these studies were directed at parent advocacy for social inclusion by engaging directly with community members either as individuals, pairs or small groups, and none involved children with communication disorders. Therefore, none of the questions were deemed suitable for this study. The questions that were selected were derived through formal and informal conversations with focus groups consisting of Speech and Language Therapists/Pathologists, academics in the field and mothers of children with communication disorders. These conversations were via online communities and through face-to-face encounters.

A perusal of literature helped identify guidelines that ought to be followed when structuring and wording a survey questionnaire. Questions were framed using simple language, sensitive to the needs of the respondent population (Groves et al., 2011). Overlapping questions (q) were included (q: 2 and 3, q: 4 and 5, q: 7 and 8) to gauge respondent understanding. A combination approach with a mix of closed (q: 1-5, 10) and open-ended (q: 6-9) questions was opted for because closed questions are readily answered and answers to open-ended questions supply further views on the topic (Bajpai, 2011). The wording, font size, and format were selected carefully, because words and presentation often influence answers (Christian and Dillman, 2004). Questions were organized in a logical format with clear headings and numbers so respondents could complete the survey easily (Bajpai, 2011). Adequate space was provided for answers to the open-ended questions to prompt detailed responses (Christian and Dillman, 2004). A limited number of questions (10) were chosen so that mothers for whom time and energy are precious commodities could complete the surveys (Myers, Mackintosh, and Goin-Kochel, 2009) and because shorter web-based surveys usually have a higher response rate (Weimiao and Yan, 2010). Since it is an exploratory study, and because the study wished to gather global perspectives rather than compare data, questions that focused on age, level of education of the mother, race/ethnicity, marital status and income group are not included. However, the respondents were required to state their country of residence. Factor analysis of the items highlighted six categories: mothers' views regarding rights of child (q:1), mothers' beliefs regarding outcomes of social inclusion for the children (q:2, 3) and the community (q:4, 5), social exclusion experiences, people and places (q:6, 7), social inclusion experiences, people and places (q:8), different approaches that mothers engage in to enable communication between their children and community members, (q: 9) and factual information (q:10). On completion of its design, the questionnaire was piloted with a select group of respondents, who were not part of the actual sample used for the final survey, for errors and clarity (Dillman et al., 2009). The feedback was utilized to reframe two questions (q:7, 8). These questions, originally designed as open-ended questions, were redesigned as multiple-choice questions with space to include examples of experiences and an "other" option to provide respondents with an opportunity to write as many relevant responses. The questionnaire was then ready to be tested for sensitivity, validity and reliability (Wong, Ong, and Kuek, 2012). Sensitivity deals with the ability to measure variability in responses (Zikmund, 2003). This study opted for a 6 stem Likert scale as part of the questionnaire and semi-structured questions, to ensure that sensitivity to responses is maintained. Validity concerns accuracy of measurement. It may be considered as face validity; construct validity, content validity and criterion validity (Bolarinwa, 2015). The validity of this survey was conducted by engaging a panel of experts to scrutinize the efficiency of the measures that represent the theories under consideration. Reliability is the degree to which the survey will elicit the same information each time it is administered (Wong et al., 2012). Hence, reliability requires following the rules of designing a survey. This study as described above followed a series of design guidelines to preserve reliability. The finalised questionnaire was then ready for circulation (Appendix).

The implementation stage involved identifying possible respondents, contacting those respondents, and conducting the survey. It was decided that the author would reach out to the global community via a SLP/T Facebook group of which the author is a member, through telephone and in person. The Facebook group were invited to select at least five of their clients whose primary disorder is communication disorders and contact the mothers, requesting them to participate in the survey. The invitation email designed by the author, set out the objectives of the study. This was shared with the group to email it out to the mothers. Once a mother agreed to participate, she received the URL by email on a Monday, with an explanation on the process of accessing and completing the survey. Email reminders were sent out twice on subsequent Mondays. The survey was available for two weeks after the second email.

RESULTS

This section focuses on data analysis, the process of sorting and interpreting data to report results and arrive at conclusions. Survey data enables the constructing of quantitative and qualitative descriptors (Cohen et al., 2000). Since closed, open-ended and semi-structured questions were included in the survey, a mixed method; quantitative and qualitative, approach to analysis was selected (Onwuegbuzie and Leech, 2006). Quantitative analysis focuses on presenting and interpreting data that has been compiled into numbers, measurements, and frequencies (Thomas, 2003). Qualitative analysis seeks to find meaning and hidden ideas in words (Spencer, Ritchie, Lewis, and Dillon, 2003).

The number of respondents were counted, and the response rate was calculated by dividing the number of people who submitted the survey (n=48) by the number of people contacted (n=58). Hence, the survey response rate is 82.76%. This exceeded the general expectation of 70% (Nulty, 2008).

The closed questions (q:1-5, q:10) were considered first. Data collected was organized on spreadsheets and frequency counts recorded. Next relative frequency statistics were obtained for each category. A pie chart and a 2D-stacked bar chart enabled presenting data in a visual format under two headings: geographical dispersion and the mothers' views on social inclusion.

A mixed methods analysis was applied to the data received from the open-ended (q:6, 9) and semi-structured questions (q:7, 8) to locate patterns, themes, and relationships that reflect the objectives of the study (Wellington and Szczerbinski, 2007). Responses for the open-ended questions (q:6, 9) were recorded on a spreadsheet and then organised into groups that echoed the same response. A validation group, independent from the study, evaluated the data analysis for consistency and accuracy. Frequency counts were recorded, and relative frequency statistics obtained. The data was then displayed on a table (q:6) and a clustered bar chart (q:7). Responses for the semi-structured questions (q:7, 8) were also organised on a spreadsheet, patterns located, frequency counts documented, and relative frequency statistics obtained. This data too was scrutinized by the validation group. The data was then presented on 3D stacked column charts.

Data concerning the geographical locations of the respondents were analyzed first (q:10) to study the geographical diversity of the respondents. The data was organized on a pie chart with the percentages rounded to the nearest tenth (Figure 1).

Figure 1. Geographical areas of survey respondents

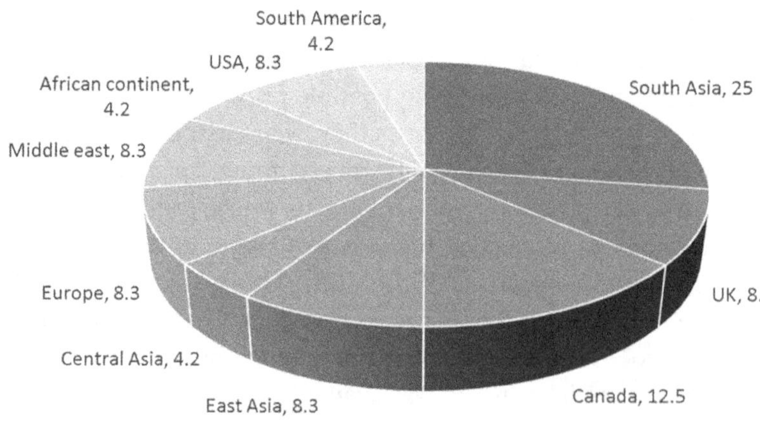

The respondents represented all continents. The highest representation was from South Asia (25%; n=12) followed by Canada (12.5%; n=6), USA, Middle East, Europe, East Asia, United Kingdom (each 8.3%; n=4) and South America, Africa and Central Asia (each 4.2%; n=2 each).

Research Question 1: What Do Mothers Believe Regarding a Child's Right to Social Inclusion?

This question focused on rights of children. It is an important question for mothers because a mother's failure to know that her child has a right to social inclusion will prevent her from advocating on behalf of her child. Given the fact that data was collected at a global scale this was of vital importance since understanding of rights can differ according to the geographical location. The question (q:1) was designed to gain responses at five levels: agree, somewhat agree, neutral, somewhat disagree, disagree. Relative frequency statistics were obtained, and data was then organized in a 2D-stacked bar chart (Figure 2) along with findings for the other closed questions (q:2-5). As per the results, all respondent mothers (100%; n=48) believe that social inclusion is the right of every child.

Research Question 2: What Do Mothers Believe Are the Outcomes of Social Inclusion for a Child With Communication Disorders and the Community?

This question was -directed at mothers' views on social inclusion and its impact on the child (q: 2,3) and the community (q: 4,5). The closed questions (q:2-5) were designed to gain responses at five levels: agree, somewhat agree, neutral, somewhat disagree, disagree. Frequency counts were recorded, and relative frequency statistics were obtained for each question by calculating the total number of responses and then dividing the number in each category by the total. The data was then organized in a 2D-stacked bar chart (Figure 2) with questions organized in chronological order from bottom to top.

The questions (q:2,3) that focused on the benefits to the child indicated that all mothers (100%; n=48) agreed with the statement, "social inclusion helps my child to build friendships and be part of a

Figure 2. Mothers' beliefs regarding social inclusion

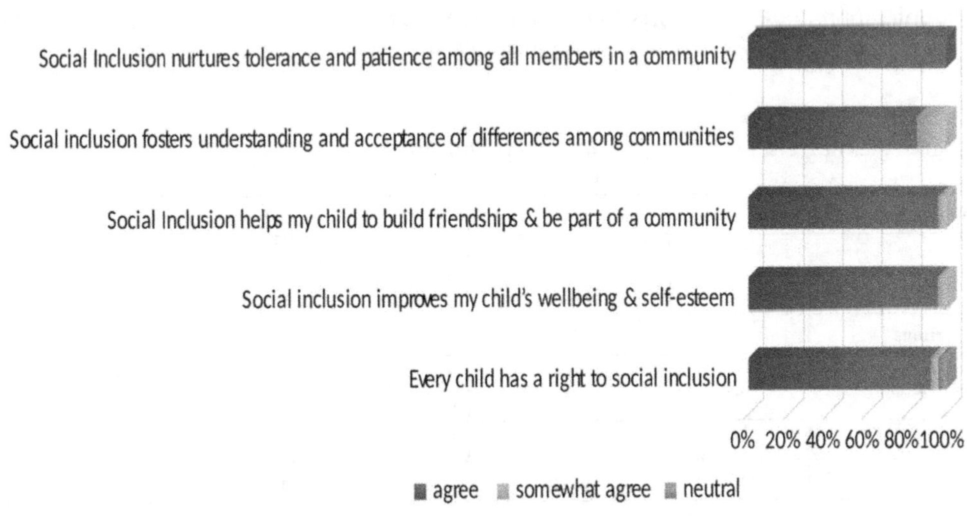

community", while majority of mothers (95.83%; n=46) agreed with the statement "Social inclusion improves my child's wellbeing and self-esteem" and the rest (4.17%; n=2) somewhat agreed with this statement. The questions (q:4,5) that focused on the benefits to the community showed the following results. The majority (95.83%; n=46) agreed that social inclusion fosters understanding and acceptance of differences, while a minority (4.17%; n=2) stated that they somewhat agreed. Most mothers (79.17%; n=38) also agreed that social inclusion nurtures tolerance and patience among all members in a community whilst a few somewhat agreed (16.67%; n=8) and a minority (4.17%; n=2) remained neutral.

Research Question 3: What Responses Do Mothers and Children Receive When They Attempt to Engage in Conversation With Community Members?

This question was answered through responses received for q:6. The practices were identified by sifting through the data and identifying patterns. Two categories emerged; inclusion practices and exclusion practices. Data was organized on a table for comparison (Table 1). Thereafter, frequency counts were recorded, and relative frequency statistics calculated.

The variety of inclusion practices was less than the variety of exclusion practices by a ratio of 4:6. "Welcome us" was the most frequently encountered inclusive practices (58.33%; n=28). This was followed closely by "support us" and "consider our feelings," each scoring 54.17% (n=26). The practices "appreciate and encourage us" was recorded by a minority (4.17%; n=2).

The most frequently encountered exclusion practice was "make rude remarks". This practice was encountered by less than half of mothers (41.57%; n=20). "Avoid us" (37.5%; n=18) and "ignore us" (33.33%; n=16) were the other exclusion practices that were experienced by a significant number of participants. A minority group reported "ask inappropriate questions regarding the disability" (8.32%; n=4), "stare" (4.17%; n=2), and "appear helpless and uneasy" (4.17%; n=2).

The comments that accompanied mothers' views regarding inclusion and exclusion practices provide insight to their experiences. Of the mothers who encountered inclusion one commented; "Some people appear helpless. They want to be nice but do not know how. So, when I introduce my daughter and she smiles and says hello very softly, there is a look of relief on their faces. Once the ice is broken they chat easily with Sarah, showing patience and understanding. She thrives in such situations". Another mother added that, "even if Rick stumbles, because he is a stutterer, people wait patiently. That is very supporting for him". "People appreciate our efforts to be friendly and encourage Tash with positive comments like, you are so polite", described another mother. Of the mothers who experienced exclusion one explained,

Table 1. Practices experienced whilst out in the community

Inclusion Practices	n	%	Exclusion Practices	n	%
Welcome us	28	58.33	Make rude remarks	20	41.57
Support us	26	54.17	Avoid us	18	37.5
Consider our feelings	26	54.17	Ignore us	16	33.33
Appreciate and encourage us	2	4.17	Ask inappropriate questions regarding the disability	4	8.32
			Stare	2	4.17
			Appear helpless and uneasy	2	4.17

"I am disappointed in humans especially when they see Marie struggling to articulate and they totally ignore her or ask me – what is wrong with her? People can be ignorant of how intrusive they are. This upsets both of us, and for days we stay away from talking to others because we are hurt". Another mother commented that "Some people cross the street to avoid us. Ajith loves to talk to people and they don't understand him because he has a cleft lip and palate. So, they either stare at him or avoid us. He is also bullied by people, young and old, who comment on his facial abnormality. These encounters are hurtful. But thank God, Ajith still reaches out and tries to socialise wherever we go." One mother reported that, "when we are in the elevator people turn their back on us because my son who is 8 years old drools a lot."

Research Question 4: Where Do Mothers and Children Experience Social Inclusion and Exclusion?

By analyzing responses for q:7 and 8, it was possible to identify places that include and exclude children with communication disorders (Figure 3). Frequency counts were recorded, and relative frequency statistics calculated. This combined data was arranged on a 3D-stacked column chart for ease of analysis.

As displayed by the chart, total inclusion (100%; n=48) is experienced in segregated settings such as special schools and therapy clinics. More than half of the sample (54.17%; n=26) reported that they felt included in public places such as malls whilst half (50%; n=24) were included at recreation facilities such as swimming pools. More than half (54.17%; n=26) of the respondents, however, reported that they experienced exclusion in mainstream schools.

Sample quotes regarding mothers' views on places that include and exclude are as follows. A Mother's comment regarding special schools; "We tend to interact more with the special needs community. That is where we feel more at ease, even more than our closest family". Another commented regarding public places, "very rarely have we felt exclusion by people even though my son has severe stammering. But because he is in a wheelchair we are excluded due to inaccessible places". A comment regarding rec-

Figure 3. Places that include and exclude

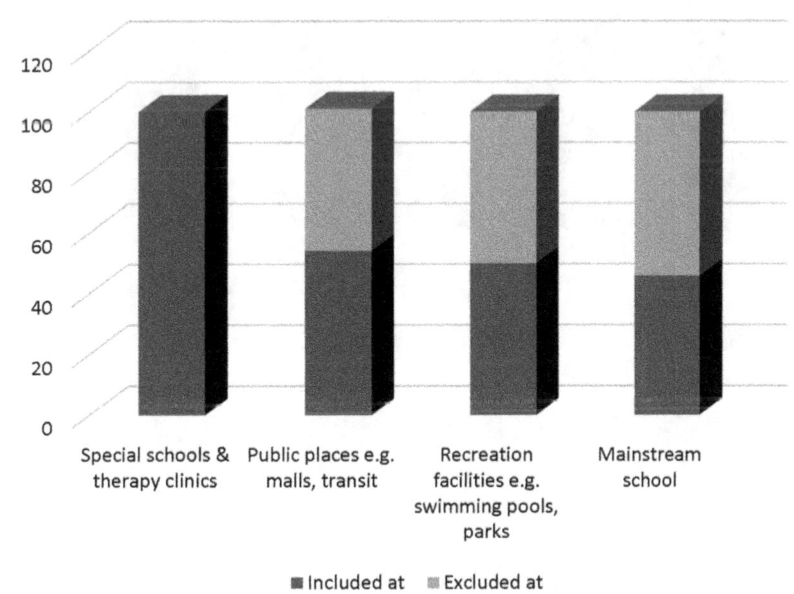

reational facilities, "We feel accepted at recreation facilities. Because people are busy having fun, they don't focus on Moira's voice". One mother added regarding exclusion in a mainstream school, "Akemi feels ignored by the students in school. Because she takes time to respond they think she is daft".

Research Question 5: Who Includes and Excludes Mothers and Children?

By analyzing q:7 and 8, it was possible to identify those who included and excluded mothers and children with communication disorders. Frequency counts were recorded, and relative frequency statistics was calculated to enable presenting the data in a 3D-stacked column chart (Figure 4).

As per the chart, most of the mothers (91.67%; n=44) reported that they felt included by family, friends, and other families with children with disabilities. Inclusion by religious communities ranked second (75%; n=36), followed by neighbors (54.17%; n=26) and strangers (29.17%; n=14).

Sample quotes from mothers reveal relationships. Regarding family members, one mother commented, "it took a long time for our family to understand ways of including Mani. But now they are her ardent supporters". Another mother added, "our friends have been more supportive than family. I am truly grateful for this". "Most of our friends are families with children with special needs. So, we are included. This makes life easy" commented one mother regarding other families with special needs children. Regarding religious communities, "according to our religion the speech defect is karma. So, our religious community pity Kavi. That is not exactly inclusion". Regarding neighbours, "our neighbours keep to themselves. When we meet them, they are polite to Mariam but don't really talk to her.

Figure 4. People that include and exclude

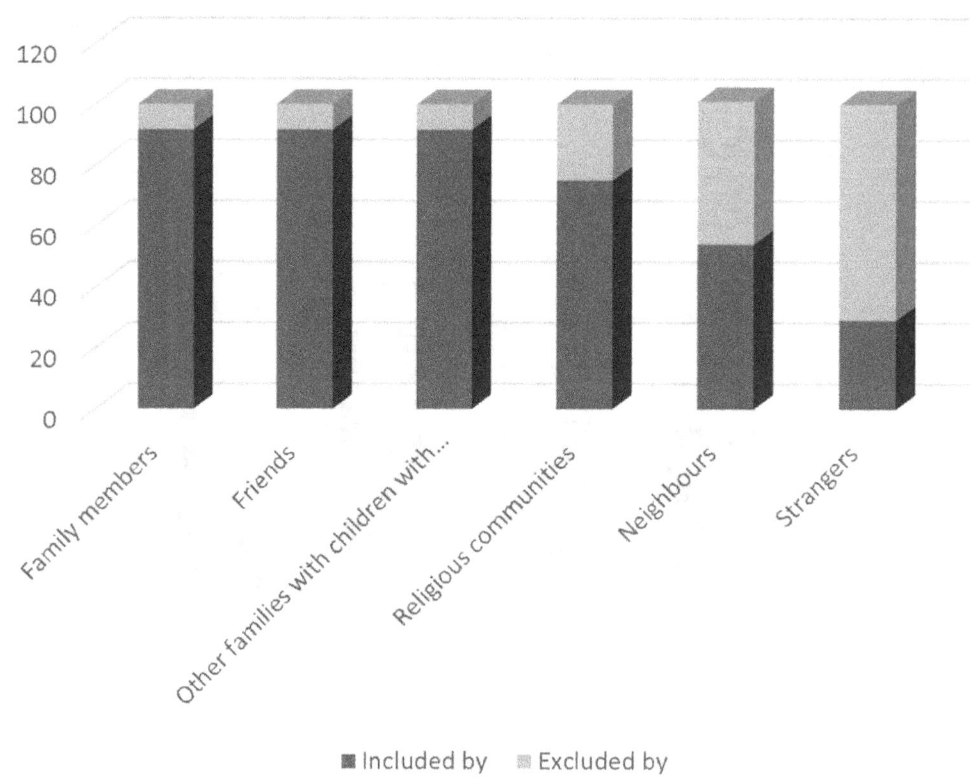

Some even avoid eye contact." Regarding strangers, "we are culturally shy from striking conversations with strangers. But when we are forced to engage in conversation, Justine is unsure and shy, and most strangers pretend that she is not there".

Research Question 6: What Are the Different Approaches That Mothers Use to Enable Social Inclusion?

Sifting through the responses provided for q: 9, patterns were identified, and data was categorised. This led to unravelling eight approaches. The approaches were then quantified; frequency counts were recorded, and relative frequency statistics calculated, and data was arranged on a progressively decreasing proportion beginning from the top (Figure 5).

It is noted that most of the mothers (75%; n=36) acquired knowledge regarding their child's disability and practiced social inclusion by engaging with people regardless of race, culture, religion, or ability. Other approaches included: attempting advocacy with a positive attitude (66.67%; n=32), viewing every opportunity as a time for practice (50%; n=24), and using a consistent approach (50%; n=24). Developing communication skills to facilitate three-way communication between the child-stranger-self (41.67%; n=20) and persisting in a non-confrontational manner (37.5%; n=18) were other popular approaches. A few mothers (4.16%; n=2) considered letting people know about the child's disability.

Sample comments from mothers are as follows. Regarding knowledge acquisition; "I followed an online course and joined an online community that discusses speech problems. It has helped our whole family". Regarding engaging with all people; "I really don't care what people think of me. I want my child not to feel less just because he has a speech disorder and goes for therapy. I make sure that we talk to as many people as we meet every day". Regarding a positive attitude; "I try to be friendly and easy going when trying to engage other people in conversation with Liza. Even if some people ignore her or appear puzzled by her words I push on with a smile even though my heart is breaking". Regarding using every opportunity; "Whether it be the supermarket, bus stop, doctor's office, playground or any place it doesn't matter, I make sure that Prasad speaks to people. I am spending so much on therapy, what is the use if he doesn't get a chance to practice?" Regarding developing skills to enable three-way communication; "This was so difficult for me. People kept ignoring Nana and speaking to me. I used to

Figure 5. Approaches for social inclusion

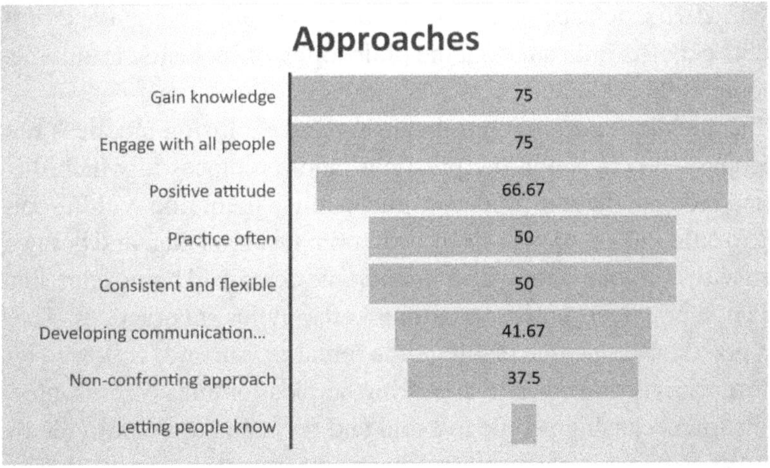

come home and bawl like a kid in frustration. But as I kept doing it and thinking of all the things that went right and wrong I mastered the technique with time. This is so important". Regarding persisting in a non-confrontational manner; "I have a strong personality. So, often I want to shake people for not acknowledging Tami. I learned the hard way by making many mistakes". Of the two mothers who considered letting people know about the disability one stated that; "Letting people know in a matter of fact way has helped Chantelle develop a positive self-image. When parents apologise for a kid's disability it diminishes the child's self-esteem. I was determined not to let that happen. It has worked for us and I would encourage other mothers to try it".

DISCUSSION

The study set out to identify approaches that mothers use to promote social inclusion for children with communication disorders. All continents were targeted to reach an appropriate number of mothers representing this population and to be informed of the different approaches the mothers engage in. Online surveys were sent out with these respondents in mind.

Responses were received from 11 geographical areas covering all continents, thus demonstrating that online surveys are suitable for reaching dispersed populations (Sullivan-Bolyai et al., 2014). The response rate exceeded the norm. This may be attributed to two factors; personalizing the first contact with each possible respondent and addressing potential respondent's concerns, primarily surrounding confidentiality of information and anonymity, immediately.

Analysis of the closed questions designed to gauge mothers' views on social inclusion indicated that all mothers believe that every child has a right to social inclusion (Diamond and Hong, 2010). This contrasts with a study highlighting how fathers feel ashamed of their children with disabilities (Crabtree, 2007). The mothers also agreed or somewhat agreed that social inclusion improves their children's well-being, helps build friendships, and enables them to be part of a community, similar to other studies (Finke et al., 2009; Mahar et al., 2013; Forrester-Jones et al., 2006). All the mothers also agreed that society benefits from social inclusion for children with disabilities, because inclusion helps nurture qualities such as patience, tolerance, understanding, and acceptance of differences. This interpretation furthers the view that inclusion is valuing human life and not merely tolerating it (Busatto, 2007; Frazee, 2002). However, some mothers were neutral regarding nurturing of tolerance and patience among all members of a community, indicating the existence of deep-rooted practices of exclusion that pervade some societies (Mehmood et al., 2015; McCabe, 2007; Slee, 2004). The high percentage of those who believe in social inclusion and its benefits indicates that the philosophy of inclusion is embraced by those who are either partially or completely excluded.

The answers to the questions pertaining to inclusion and exclusion practices revealed three themes: the practices, the people who engage in the practices, and the places in which the practices occurred. The practices reported indicate that the process of inclusion is in motion within societies. The public are consciously seeking to cultivate relationships by welcoming, supporting, and being considerate to mothers and their children with communication disorders. Some described being appreciated and encouraged. The number of exclusion practices, however, outnumbered inclusion practices. The most frequently experienced exclusion practice was people making rude remarks. This was followed by avoiding, ignoring, asking inappropriate questions, staring, and appearing helpless or uneasy. This indicated a prevalence of fear and negative constructs causing people to avoid and perhaps ignore individuals with disabilities as demonstrated in earlier studies (Danforth, 2008; Thomas, 2004). It also points to negative attitudes and bias that exist within communities' due to ignorance, fear, and indifference (UNDESA, 2009).

When considering places, it is interesting to note that while full inclusion is experienced in segregated settings like schools and therapy clinics, less than half of those who are present in school settings experienced inclusion. Approximately half of the respondents felt included in public places and recreation facilities. By focusing on people, the analysis reveals that inclusion happens mostly with family members, friends, and other families with children with disabilities. The analysis, therefore, highlights that inclusion takes place in familiar communities and settings while exclusion occurs in mainstream society.

It is evident that mothers and their children with communication disorders live in communities that both include and exclude. However, as this study reveals mothers who believe in social inclusion engage in many positive approaches to enable engagement and conversation between their children and community members as they go about their everyday lives. These approaches can be broadly classified into three groups; mothers preparing for the task (by acquiring knowledge and developing communication skills), cultivating attitudes (by attempting advocacy with a positive attitude, viewing every opportunity as a time for practice, practicing social inclusion by engaging with people regardless of race, culture, religion, or ability and persisting in a non-confrontational manner) and setting themselves up for success (by using a consistent approach and being flexible and informing people about their child's disorder). The most often practiced approach is to gain knowledge regarding the disability. These mothers understand that knowledge changes perceptions and empowers one to advocate successfully (Johnson and Harris, 2014). The next most frequently used strategy involves engaging with all people irrespective of differences. This method of inclusion is intended to break down barriers and unite many (UNDESA, 2016). Since an optimistic attitude leads to better outcomes (Lustig, 2002), mothers attempt advocacy with a positive attitude, seizing every opportunity and employing a flexible, yet consistent approach. Some mothers also feel the need to develop special communication skills to facilitate three-way communication between the child-stranger-self (Hess et al., 2006) while a few mothers inform people about their children's communication disorders (Ryan, 2010). By acknowledging the presence of the disorder, these mothers are demonstrating to their children that, instead of being labeled and shamed, they can actively seek inclusion by divulging their limitations (Knight and Oliver, 2007). These approaches imply, as shown in a previous study (Ryan, 2010), that mothers who opt to invest much time and effort when they go out into the community with their children, facilitate inclusion.

According to the findings of this study, inclusion, and exclusion practices are prevalent in the 11 geographical locations. Exclusion in public, overt and covert, as demonstrated through words and actions, is more common than exclusion in more intimate, familiar settings. Hence, effort needs to be directed at changing the hearts and minds of people who hold adamantly to damaging views and bias. Parent advocacy within communities whilst engaging in daily activities, as discussed in this study, is an ideal way to chip away at the barriers and ensure that children with communication disorders are heard, accepted, and respected.

IMPLICATIONS

The results, although with a global coverage, represent a small fraction of the target population. Further, being a global study, many variables, such as culture, education, resources and religion, could have contributed to the mothers' motivation and choice of approaches. These variables were not considered in this exploratory study. Therefore, it cannot be concluded that the outcomes are a complete representation of the population under scrutiny. However, the study is a stepping stone to uncovering and understanding the role of mother advocates as they attempt to seek social inclusion for children with communication disorders within their communities whilst going about their everyday life.

The findings reveal that most mothers consider inclusion a right. They, therefore, seek to obtain this right for their children in varying degrees. Despite exclusion being witnessed mothers actively seek social inclusion by engaging in different approaches. While the literature review revealed some strategies that mothers engage in, new strategies emerged through this study. These include: engaging with all people irrespective of differences, seizing every opportunity to practice advocacy, employing a consistent approach while being flexible and letting people know about the disability.

The information collected about advocacy approaches will prove a contribution to the global knowledge base. It also encourages other researchers to study the phenomenon from varied perspectives including but not limited to smaller geographical areas and different communities. Dissemination of these findings will further enable and empower mothers to advocate for inclusion.

FUTURE RESEARCH DIRECTIONS

This study focuses on families with children with communication disorders and discusses a mother's role in advocacy for the child. The decision to focus on mothers was taken due to their extensive involvement with rearing children. However, most children belong to families consisting of two parents. Hence, future research focusing on father's and/or combined parental roles in advocacy may pave the way for creating a family-centered approach to advocacy. It will also start a discussion regarding joint parent advocacy for children with communication disorders thereby influencing the direction of and methods for promoting social inclusion on a global scale. Further, the study focuses on mothers reporting their experiences. The views of the third parties involved in the conversation are unknown. Neither is it clear of the children's views regarding their mothers' attempts of social inclusion. These gaps warrant further study since the mothers' perspectives are now known through this and other research (Ryan, 2005, 2008; Gray 2002).

CONCLUSION

Social inclusion for children with communication disorders and the role of mothers as advocate is addressed through this study. The detailed empirical evidence is used to support the argument that mothers who consistently advocate on behalf of their children with communication disorders enable social inclusion. The online survey methodology ideally suited to meet the objective of this research. The mixed methods approach to analysis provided a broader perspective on the topic under focus. This ensured a cohesive data analysis. The evidence points to the conclusion that all mothers desire social inclusion despite encountering exclusionary practices in places and with people at varying degrees. The mothers, using their intimate knowledge of their children, have designed, tested, and practiced a range of approaches. They have thus demonstrated that social inclusion is achievable through an unwavering commitment to advocacy and continuity with creative solutions that can be replicated in most settings.

ACKNOWLEDGMENT

A special 'thank you' to the Mother-Son duo, Linda and Thomas, who inspired me to research the topic of social inclusion from a mother's perspective. My sincere gratitude is also extended to all clinicians, mothers and children who willingly participated in the study. Appreciation is also extended to fellow researchers who extended their time and shared their knowledge and expertise and to the reviewers for their valuable suggestions. This exploratory research received no specific grant from any funding agency in the public, commercial, or not-for-profit sectors.

REFERENCES

American Psychiatric Association (APA) (Ed.). (2000). Diagnostic and statistical manual of mental disorders, fourth edition, text revision (DSM-IV-TR).Washington, DC: American Psychiatric Association.

American Speech-Language-Hearing Association (ASHA). (1993). Definitions of communication disorders and variations. *ASHA. Supplement*, *35*(c10), 40–41. PMID:8097650

Antia, S. D., Jones, P., Luckner, J., Kreimeyer, K. H., & Reed, S. (2011). Social outcomes of students who are deaf and hard of hearing in general education classrooms. *Exceptional Children*, *77*(4), 489–504. doi:10.1177/001440291107700407

Bailey, D. B., Hebbeler, K., Spiker, D., Scarborough, A., Mallik, S., & Nelson, L. (2005). Thirty-six-month outcomes for families of children who have disabilities and participated in early intervention. *Pediatrics*, *116*(6), 1346–1352. doi:10.1542/peds.2004-1239 PMID:16322157

Bajpai, N. (2011). *Business research methods*. New Delhi, India: Pearson Education.

Baker-Ericzén, M. J., Brookman-Frazee, L., & Stahmer, A. (2005). Stress levels and adaptability in parents of toddlers with and without autism spectrum disorders. *Research and Practice for Persons with Severe Disabilities*, *30*(4), 194–204. doi:10.2511/rpsd.30.4.194

Bećirević, M., & Dowling, M. (2010). *Inclusion or illusions? Policies and practices for children with disabilities and their families in Bosnia and Herzegovina and Bulgaria* (Unpublished doctoral dissertation). The Open University, London, UK.

Beitchman, J., & Brownlie, E. (2010). Language development and its impact on children's psychosocial and emotional development. In Encyclopedia of language and literacy development (rev. ed.; pp. 1-8). Montreal, Quebec: Centre of Excellence for Early Childhood Development and Strategic Knowledge Cluster on Early Child Development.

Bercow, J. (2008). The Bercow report: A review of services for children and young people (0-19) with speech, language and communication needs. Nottingham, UK: DCSF Publications.

Berkman, N. D., Wallace, I., Watson, L., Coyne-Beasley, T., Cullen, K., Wood, C., & Lohr, K. N. (2015). *Screening for speech and language delays and disorders in children age 5 years or younger: A systematic review*. Rockville, MD: Agency for Healthcare Research and Quality.

Black, A. P., & Baker, M. (2011). The impact of parent advocacy groups, the Internet, and social networking on rare diseases: The IDEA League and the IDEA League United Kingdom example. *Epilepsia, 52*(2), 102–104. doi:10.1111/j.1528-1167.2011.03013.x PMID:21463291

Black, L. I., Vahratian, A., & Hoffman, H. J. (2015). Communication disorders and use of intervention services among children aged 3–17 years: United States (DHHS Publication No. 2015–1209). Washington, DC: U.S. Government Printing Office.

Bolarinwa, O. A. (2015). Principles and methods of validity and reliability testing of questionnaire used in social and health science researches. *The Nigerian Postgraduate Medical Journal, 22*(4), 195–201. doi:10.4103/1117-1936.173959 PMID:26776330

Bray, M. (2006). Language and communication in young people with learning difficulties. In J. Clegg & J. Ginsborg (Eds.), *Language and social disadvantage: Theory into practice* (pp. 106–121). London, UK: John Wiley and Sons Ltd.

Brinton, B., & Fugiki, M. (2006). Social intervention for children with language impairment: Factors affecting efficacy. *Communication Disorders Quarterly, 28*(1), 39–41. doi:10.1177/15257401060280010501

Burke, M. M., & Hodapp, R. M. (2016). The Nature, Correlates, and Conditions of Parental Advocacy in Special Education. *Exceptionality, 24*(3), 137–150. doi:10.1080/09362835.2015.1064412

Busatto, C. (2007). *Solidary governance for creating inclusive societies*. Paper presented at the Expert Group Meeting on Creating Inclusive Society: Practical Strategies to Promote Social Integration, Paris, France.

Carter, I. (2013). Advocacy for children with disabilities: Issues and strategies. In *Special needs parenting: Working together for success, monograph II*. Retrieved March 13, 2017, from http://www.adoption.ca/uploads/Image/Monograph2-Irene-FINAL.pdf

Census of India. (2011). *Measurement of Disability through census, National Experiences*. Office of the Registrar general and Census Commissioner, New Delhi, India. Retrieved October 27th, 2017, from https://unstats.un.org/unsd/demographic-social/meetings/2016/bangkok--disability-measurement-and-statistics/Session-6/India.pdf

Center for Educational Research and Innovation (CERI) (Ed.). (2004). *Equity in education: Students with disabilities, learning difficulties and disadvantages*. Paris: OECD Publication Service.

Christian, L. M., & Dillman, D. A. (2004). The influence of graphical and symbolic language manipulations on responses to self-administered questions. *Public Opinion Quarterly, 68*(1), 58–81. doi:10.1093/poq/nfh004

Cohen, L., Manion, L., & Morrison, K. (2000). *Research methods in education*. London, UK: Routledge. doi:10.4324/9780203224342

Cole, B. A. (2004). *Mother–Teachers: Insights into Inclusion*. London: David Fulton.

Conti-Ramsden, G., Botting, N., Simkin, Z., & Knox, E. (2001). Follow-up of children attending infant language units: Outcomes at 11 years of age. *International Journal of Language & Communication Disorders*, *36*(2), 207–219. doi:10.1080/13682820010019883 PMID:11344595

Cook, B. G., Tankersley, M., Cook, L., & Landrum, T. J. (2000). Teachers' attitudes toward their included students with disabilities. *Exceptional Children*, *67*(1), 115–135. doi:10.1177/001440290006700108

Couper, M. P. (2000). Web-based surveys: A Review of Issues and Approaches. *Public Opinion Quarterly*, *64*, 464–494. doi:10.1086/318641 PMID:11171027

Crabtree, S. A. (2007). Maternal perceptions of care-giving of children with developmental disabilities in the United Arab Emirates. *Journal of Applied Research in Intellectual Disabilities*, *20*(3), 247–255. doi:10.1111/j.1468-3148.2006.00327.x

Crawford, S. D., Couper, M. P., & Lamias, M. J. (2001). Web surveys: Perception of burden. *Social Science Computer Review*, *19*(2), 146–162. doi:10.1177/089443930101900202

Creswell, J. W. (2005). *Educational research: Planning, conducting, and evaluating quantitative and qualitative research* (2nd ed.). Upper Saddle River, NJ: Pearson Education.

Dalrymple, J. (2005). Constructions of child and youth advocacy: Emerging issues in advocacy practice. *Children & Society*, *19*(1), 3–15. doi:10.1002/chi.828

Danforth, S. (2008). John Dewey's contributions to an educational philosophy of intellectual disability. *Educational Theory*, *58*(1), 45–62. doi:10.1111/j.1741-5446.2007.00275.x

Davidoff, B. E. (2017). AAC with energy-earlier. *ASHA Leader*, *22*(1), 48–53. doi:10.1044/leader.FTR2.22012017.48

Diamond, K. E., & Hong, S. Y. (2010). Young children's decisions to include peers with physical disabilities in play. *Journal of Early Intervention*, *32*(3), 163–177. doi:10.1177/1053815110371332

Dillman, D. A., Smyth, J. D., & Christian, L. M. (2009). *Internet, mail and mixed-mode surveys: The tailored design method*. Hoboken, NJ: Wiley.

Ewles, G., Clifford, T., & Minnes, P. (2014). Predictors of advocacy in parents of children with autism spectrum disorders. *Journal on Developmental Disabilities*, *20*(1), 73–82.

Fabian, E. S. (2007). Counselor advocacy for access: Addressing the challenges of disability. In C. C. Lee (Ed.), *Counseling for social justice* (pp. 75–94). Alexandria, VA: APA.

Finke, E. H., McNaughton, D. B., & Drager, K. D. (2009). All children can and should have the opportunity to learn: General education teachers' perspectives on including children with autism spectrum disorder who require AAC. *Augmentative and Alternative Communication*, *25*(2), 110–122. doi:10.1080/07434610902886206 PMID:19444682

Forrester-Jones, R., Carpenter, J., Coolen-Schrijner, P., Cambridge, P., Tate, A., Beecham, J., ... Wooff, D. (2006). The social networks of people with intellectual disability living in the community 12 years after resettlement from long-stay hospitals. *Journal of Applied Research in Intellectual Disabilities*, *19*(4), 285–295. doi:10.1111/j.1468-3148.2006.00263.x

Frankel, E. B., Gold, S., & Ajodhia, A. (2010). International preschool inclusion: Bridging the gap between vision and practices. *Young Exceptional Children*, *13*(5), 2–16. doi:10.1177/1096250610379983

Frazee, C. (2002). *Thumbs up! Inclusion, rights and equality as experienced by youth with disabilities* (Working paper).Toronto, Canada: Laidlaw Foundation.

Gillam, R. B., Marquardt, T. P., & Martin, F. N. (2011). *Communication sciences and disorders: From science to clinical practice* (2nd ed.). Sudbury, MA: Jones and Bartlett Publishers.

Goodley, D. (2005). Empowerment, self-advocacy, and resilience. *Journal of Intellectual Disabilities*, *9*(4), 333–343. doi:10.1177/1744629505059267 PMID:16330487

Gray, D. E. (2002). Everybody just freezes. Everybody is just embarrassed: Felt and enacted stigma among parents of children with high functioning autism. *Sociology of Health & Illness*, *24*(6), 734–749. doi:10.1111/1467-9566.00316

Groves, R. M., Fowler, F. J., Couper, M. P., Lepkowski, J. M., Singer, E., & Tourangeau, R. (2011). *Survey methodology* (2nd ed.). Toronto, Canada: John Wiley and Sons Inc.

Haynes, W. O., Moran, M. J., & Pindzola, R. H. (2006). *Communication disorders in the classroom: An introduction for professionals in school settings*. London, UK: Jones and Bartlett Publishers International.

Hess, R., Molina, A., & Kozleski, E. B. (2006). Until somebody hears me: Parental voice and advocacy in special education decision-making. *British Journal of Special Education*, *33*(3), 148–157. doi:10.1111/j.1467-8578.2006.00430.x

Hothschild, A. (1979). Emotion work, feeling rules and social structure. *American Journal of Sociology*, *85*(3), 551–575. doi:10.1086/227049

Irish Association of Speech and Language Therapists (IASLT). (2007). *Specific speech and language impairment in children: Definition, service provision and recommendations for change*. Dublin, Ireland: Author.

Johnson, S., & Harris, O. (2014). Special educator attitudes toward children with communication disorders in the Caribbean. *Caribbean Educational Research Journal*, *12*(2), 133–148.

Jones, J. (2002). *Fact sheet: Communication*. Birmingham, UK: British Institute of Learning Disabilities.

Kalyanpur, M., Harry, B., & Skrtic, T. (2000). Equity and advocacy expectations of culturally diverse families' participation in special education. *International Journal of Disability Development and Education*, *47*(2), 119–136. doi:10.1080/713671106

Knight, A., & Oliver, C. (2007). Advocacy for disabled children and young people: Benefits and dilemmas. *Child & Family Social Work*, *12*(4), 417–425. doi:10.1111/j.1365-2206.2007.00500.x

LeComer, L. (2006). *A parent's guide to developmental delays: Recognising and coping with missed milestones in speech, movement, learning and other areas*. Stillwater, OK: New Forums Press Inc.

Lewington, W., & Clipson, C. (2004). *Advocating for equality*. London, UK: Independent Advocacy Campaign, Scope.

Lindsay, G., & Dockrell, J. (2000). The behaviour and self-esteem of children with specific speech and language difficulties. *The British Journal of Educational Psychology*, *70*(4), 583–601. doi:10.1348/000709900158317 PMID:11191188

Lindsay, G., Dockrell, J., Desforges, M., Law, J., & Peacey, N. (2010). Meeting the needs of children and young people with speech, language and communication difficulties. *International Journal of Language & Communication Disorders*, *45*(4), 448–460. doi:10.3109/13682820903165693 PMID:20565326

Locke, A., Ginsberg, J., & Peers, L. (2002). Development and disadvantage: Implications for the early years and beyond. *International Journal of Communication Disorders*, *37*(1), 3–15. doi:10.1080/13682820110089911 PMID:11852457

Lombe, M. (2007). *Presentation.* In Expert Group Meeting on Creating and Inclusive Society: Practical Strategies to Promote Social Integration, Paris, France.

Lustig, D. C. (2002). Family coping in families with a child with a disability. *Education and Training in Mental Retardation and Developmental Disabilities*, *37*(1), 14–22.

Mahar, A. L., Cobigo, V., & Stuart, H. (2013). Conceptualizing belonging. *Disability and Rehabilitation*, *35*(12), 1026–1032. doi:10.3109/09638288.2012.717584 PMID:23020179

Malec, J. F., Brown, A. W., & Moessner, A. (2010). Two new measures for assessing advocacy activities and perceived control after acquired brain injury. *Disability and Rehabilitation*, *32*(1), 33–40. doi:10.3109/09638280902980936 PMID:19925274

Martin, D., & Miller, C. (2003). *Speech and language difficulties in the classroom* (2nd ed.). London: David Fulton Publishers.

McCabe, H. (2007). Parent advocacy in the face of adversity: Autism and families in the People's Republic of China. *Focus on Autism and Other Developmental Disabilities*, *22*(1), 39–50. doi:10.1177/10883576070220010501

McGeown, J. (2012). *Out of the shadows: A qualitative study of parents' and professionals' attitudes and beliefs about children with communication disability in Uganda and how best to help them* (Unpublished master's thesis). University College London, UK.

McKeever, P., & Miller, K. L. (2004). Mothering children who have disabilities: A Bourdieusian interpretation of maternal practices. *Social Science & Medicine*, *59*(6), 1177–1191. doi:10.1016/j.socscimed.2003.12.023 PMID:15210090

McLeod, S., & McKinnon, D. H. (2010). Support required for primary and secondary students with communication disorders and/or other learning needs. *Child Language Teaching and Therapy*, *26*(2), 123–143. doi:10.1177/0265659010368754

Mehmood, Z., Bhatti, A. G., & Ali, S. H. (2015). Schools as an agent of socialization for disabled children: A study of disabled children of special education institutes in Jalapur Pirwala. *Journal of Social Sciences*, *9*, 333–342.

Mittler, P. (2000). *Working towards inclusive education: Contexts.* London, UK: David Fulton Publishers.

Myers, B. J., Mackintosh, V. H., & Goin-Kochel, R. P. (2009). My greatest joy and my greatest heartache: Parents own words on how having a child on the autism spectrum has affected their lives and their families lives. *Research in Autism Spectrum Disorders*, *3*(3), 670–684. doi:10.1016/j.rasd.2009.01.004

Nachshen, J. S., Anderson, L., & Jamieson, J. (2001). The parent advocacy scale: Measuring advocacy in parents of children with special needs. *Journal on Developmental Disabilities*, *8*, 93–105.

Nardi, P. M. (2015). *Doing survey research. A guide to quantitative methods* (3rd ed.). London: Routledge.

Neely-Barnes, S. L., & Dia, D. A. (2008). Families of children with disabilities: A review of literature and recommendations for interventions. *Journal of Early and Intensive Behavior Intervention: JEIBI*, *5*(3), 93–107. doi:10.1037/h0100425

Nielsen, K. E. (2012). *A disability history of the United States*. Boston: Beacon Press.

Nulty, D. D. (2008). The adequacy of response rates to online and paper surveys: What can be done? *Assessment & Evaluation in Higher Education*, *33*(3), 301–314. doi:10.1080/02602930701293231

Olusanya, B. O., Ruben, R. J., & Parving, A. (2006). Reducing the burden of communication disorders in the developing world: An opportunity for the Millennium Development Project. *Journal of the American Medical Association*, *296*(4), 441–444. doi:10.1001/jama.296.4.441 PMID:16868302

Onwuegbuzie, A. J., & Leech, N. L. (2006). Linking research questions to mixed methods data analysis procedures. *Qualitative Report*, *11*(3), 474–498.

Power, A. (2013). Making space for belonging: Critical reflections on the implementation of personalized adult social care under the veil of meaningful inclusion. *Social Science & Medicine*, *88*, 68–75. doi:10.1016/j.socscimed.2013.04.008 PMID:23702211

Pozo, P., & Sarriá, E. (2014). Prediction of stress in mothers of children with autism spectrum disorders. *The Spanish Journal of Psychology*, *17*, 1–12. doi:10.1017jp.2014.6 PMID:25012691

Read, J. (2000). *Disability, the Family and Society: Listening to Mothers*. Buckingham, UK: Open University Press.

Rehm, R. S., & Bradley, J. F. (2005). Normalization in families raising a child who is medically fragile, technology dependent and developmentally delayed. *Qualitative Health Research*, *15*(6), 807–821. doi:10.1177/1049732305276754 PMID:15961877

Resch, J. A., Mireles, G., Benz, M. R., Grenwelge, C., Peterson, R., & Zhang, D. (2010). Giving parents a voice: A qualitative study of the challenges experienced by parents of children with disabilities. *Rehabilitation Psychology*, *55*(2), 139–150. doi:10.1037/a0019473 PMID:20496968

Royal College of Speech and Language Therapists (RCSLT). (2009). Resource manual for commissioning and planning services for SLCN: Speech and language impairment. London, UK: RCSLT.

Ryan, S. (2005). "People don't do odd, do they?" Mothers making sense of the reactions of others towards their learning-disabled children in public places. *Children's Geographies*, *3*(3), 291–306. doi:10.1080/14733280500352920

Ryan, S. (2010). 'Meltdowns', surveillance and managing emotions; going out with children with autism. *Health & Place, 16*(5), 868–875. doi:10.1016/j.healthplace.2010.04.012 PMID:20462783

Ryan, S., & Cole, K. R. (2009). From Advocate to Activist? Mapping the Experiences of Mothers of Children on the Autism Spectrum. *Journal of Applied Research in Intellectual Disabilities, 22*(1), 43–53. doi:10.1111/j.1468-3148.2008.00438.x

Schaff, R. C., Toth-Cohen, S., Johnson, S. L., Outenn, G., & Benevides, T. W. (2011). The everyday routines of families of children with autism: Examining the impact of sensory processing difficulties on the family. *Autism, 15*(3), 373–389. doi:10.1177/1362361310386505 PMID:21430016

Scorgie, K., & Sobsey, D. (2000). Transformational outcomes associated with parenting children who have disabilities. *Mental Retardation, 38*(3), 195–206. doi: PMID:10900927

Shearn, J., & Todd, S. (2000). Maternal employment and family responsibilities: The perspectives of mothers of children with intellectual disabilities. *Journal of Applied Research in Intellectual Disabilities, 13*(3), 109–131. doi:10.1046/j.1468-3148.2000.00021.x

Simplican, S. C. (2015). *The capacity contract: Intellectual disability and the question of citizenship*. Minneapolis, MN: University of Minnesota Press. doi:10.5749/minnesota/9780816693979.001.0001

Siraj-Blatchford, I. (2004). Quality teaching in the early years. In A. Anning, J. Cullen, & M. Fleer (Eds.), *Early childhood education: Society and culture* (pp. 137–148). London, UK: SAGE Publications Ltd.

Slee, R. (2004). Inclusive education: A framework for reform? In V. Heung & M. Ainscow (Eds.), *Inclusive education: A framework for reform* (pp. 58–66). Hong Kong: Hong Kong Institute of Education.

Slee, R. (2011). *The irregular school: Exclusion, schooling and inclusive education*. New York, NY: Routledge.

Spencer, L., Ritchie, J., Lewis, J., & Dillon, L. (2003). *Quality in qualitative evaluation: A framework for assessing research evidence*. London, UK: National Center for Social Research.

Stahmer, A. C., Akshoomoff, N., & Cunningham, A. B. (2011). Inclusion for toddlers with autism spectrum disorders. *Autism, 15*(5), 625–641. doi:10.1177/1362361310392253 PMID:21486899

Stark, R., Gordon-Burns, D., Purdue, K., Rarere-Briggs, B., & Turncock, K. (2011). Other parents' perceptions of disability and inclusion in early childhood education: Implications for the teachers' role in creating inclusive communities. *He Kupu, 2*(4), 4–18.

Stuntzner, S., & Hartley, M. T. (2015). Balancing self- compassion with self-advocacy: A new approach for persons with disabilities. *Annals of Psychotherapy and Integrative Health*, 12-28. Retrieved from http://www.annalsofpsychotherapy.com/

Sun, I. Y. I., & Fernandes, F. D. M. (2014). Communication difficulties perceived by parents of children with developmental disorders. *Communication and Developmental Disorders, 26*(4), 270–275. PMID:25211685

Taylor, P. (2007). *UNESCO and IUAV EGM on cosmopolitan urbanism: Urban policies for the social and spatial integration of international migrants*. Retrieved from http://www.unescochair-iuav.it/wp-content/uploads/2007/09/sarah-toner_paul-taylor.pdf

Thackeray, R., & Hunter, M. (2010). Empowering youth: Use of technology in advocacy to affect social change. *Journal of Computer-Mediated Communication, 15*(4), 575–591. doi:10.1111/j.1083-6101.2009.01503.x

Therborn, G. (2007). *Final report the expert group meeting on creating an inclusive society: Practical strategies to promote social integration*. Paris, France: DESA.

Thomas, C. (2004). Developing the social relational in the social model of disability: A theoretical agenda. In M. Corker & T. Shakespeare (Eds.), *Implementing the social model of disability: Theory and research* (pp. 32–47). London: Continuum.

Thomas, D. M. (2009). Culture and disability: A Cape Verdean perspective. *Journal of Cultural Diversity, 16*(4), 178–186. PMID:20069806

Thomas, R. M. (2003). *Blending qualitative and quantitative research methods in theses and dissertations*. London, UK: SAGE Publications. doi:10.4135/9781412983525

Tregaskis, C. (2004). *Constructions of disability: Researching the interface between disabled and non-disabled people*. London, UK: Routledge. doi:10.4324/9780203299517

United Nations Department of Economic and Social Affairs (UNDESA). (1995). *Report of the world summit for social development*. New York, NY: UNDESA.

United Nations Department of Economic and Social Affairs (UNDESA). (2000). *Millennium declaration*. Retrieved from http://www.un.org/millennium/declaration/ares552e.pdf

United Nations Department of Economic and Social Affairs (UNDESA). (2009). *Creating an inclusive society: Practical strategies to promote social integration*. New York, NY: UNDESA.

United Nations Department of Economic and Social Affairs (UNDESA). (2010). *Analysing and measuring social inclusion in a global context*. New York, NY: UNDESA.

United Nations Department of Economic and Social Affairs (UNDESA). (2016). *Leaving no one behind: The imperative of inclusive development (Report on the world social situation 2016)*. New York, NY: UNDESA.

Vernon-Feagans, L., Pancsofar, N., Willoughby, M., Odom, E., Quade, A., & Cox, M. (2008). Predictors of maternal language to infants during a picture book task in the home: Family SES, child characteristics and the parenting environment. *Journal of Applied Developmental Psychology, 29*(3), 213–226. doi:10.1016/j.appdev.2008.02.007 PMID:18618023

Wakelin, M. M. (2008). Challenging disparities in special education: Moving parents from disempowered team members to ardent advocates. *Northwestern Journal of Law and Social Policy, 3*(2), 263–288.

Wang, M., Mannan, H., Poston, D., Turnbull, A. P., & Summers, J. A. (2004). Parents' perceptions of advocacy activities and their impact on family quality of life. *Research and Practice for Persons with Severe Disabilities, 29*(2), 144–155. doi:10.2511/rpsd.29.2.144

Weatherby, A. M. (2006). Understanding and measuring social communication in children with autism spectrum disorders. In T. Charman & W. Stone (Eds.), *Social and communication development in autism spectrum disorders: Early identification, diagnosis, and intervention* (pp. 3–34). New York: Guilford Press.

Webster, A., Cumming, J., & Rowland, S. (2016). *Empowering parents of children with autism spectrum disorder: Critical decision-making for quality outcomes*. Singapore: Springer.

Wegner, J. R., Grosche, K., & Edmister, E. (2003). Students with speech and language disorders. In F. E. Obiakor, C. A. R. Utley, & A. F. Rotari (Eds.), *Effective education for learners with exceptionalities* (Vol. 15, pp. 181–193). Oxford, UK: Elsevier Sciences. doi:10.1016/S0270-4013(03)80039-9

Wellington, J., & Szczerbinski, M. (2007). *Research methods for the social sciences*. London: Continuum.

Westwood, P., & Graham, L. (2000). How many children with special needs in regular classes? Official predictions vs teachers' perceptions in South Australia and New South Wales. *Australian Journal of Learning Disabilities*, *5*(3), 24–35. doi:10.1080/19404150009546632

Wickremesooriya, S. F. (2012). *Talking is fun: Enhancing oral language development of students with learning difficulties, in a hard-to-reach area of Sri Lanka* (Unpublished doctoral dissertation). University of Sheffield, Sheffield, UK.

Williams, S. (2001). *Emotion and Social Theory*. London: Sage.

Wong, K. L., Ong, S. F., & Kuek, T. Y. (2012). Constructing a survey questionnaire to collect data on service quality of business academics. *European Journal of Soil Science*, *29*, 209–221.

Woodgate, R. L., Ateah, C., & Secco, L. (2008). Living in a world of our own: The experience of parents who have children with autism. *Qualitative Health Research*, *18*(8), 1075–1083. doi:10.1177/1049732308320112 PMID:18650563

World Health Organization (WHO). (2007). *The world health report 2007 - A safer future: Global public health security in the 21st century*. Geneva, Switzerland: World Health Organization.

Wright, A. C., & Taylor, S. (2014). Advocacy by parents of young children with special needs: Activities, processes, and perceived effectiveness. *Journal of Social Service Research*, *40*(5), 591–605. doi:10.1080/01488376.2014.896850

Wright, K. B. (2005). Researching internet-based populations: Advantages and disadvantages of online survey research, online questionnaire authoring software packages, and web survey services. *Journal of Computer-Mediated Communication*, *10*(3). Retrieved from http://onlinelibrary.wiley.com/doi/10.1111/j.1083-6101.2005.tb00259.x/full

Yun, G. W., & Trumbo, C. W. (2000). Comparative response to a survey executed by post, e-mail, and web form. *Journal of Computer-Mediated Communication*, *6*(1). Retrieved from http://onlinelibrary.wiley.com/doi/10.1111/j.1083-6101.2000.tb00112.x/full

Zikmund, W. G. (2003). *Business Research Methods* (7th ed.). Thompson/South-Western.

KEY TERMS AND DEFINITIONS

Advocacy: The act of speaking up for others.

Communication Disorders: A condition that is characterized by the inability to use a communication medium to successfully convey thoughts, feelings, beliefs, etc. to others.

Mixed Methods Approach: A method of data analysis that enables viewing information from quantitative and qualitative perspectives.

Online Surveys: A low-cost data collection mode that can be utilized when considering dispersed populations.

Self-Advocacy: Speaking up for one's self.

Social Exclusion: Excluding persons due to a range of reasons determined and influenced by culture, communities, attitudes, etc.

Social Inclusion: Including all persons regardless of any dividing factors to the social fabric of life. There are various types of inclusion: full, partial, and mainstreaming. It is a process that requires deliberate actions.

Social Model of Disability: First introduced in 1976, the model seeks to place responsibility on society to enable inclusion and to actively engage in eradicating barriers that subscribe to exclusion of people with disabilities.

APPENDIX: ONLINE SURVEY QUESTIONNAIRE

Mothers' Beliefs

1. "Every child has a right to social inclusion".
    a. Agree
    b. Somewhat Agree
    c. Neutral
    d. Disagree
    e. Somewhat Disagree
2. "Social Inclusion improves my child's well-being and self-esteem."
    a. Agree
    b. Somewhat agree
    c. Neutral
    d. Disagree
    e. Somewhat Disagree
3. "Social Inclusion helps my child to build friendships and be part of a community."
    a. Agree
    b. Somewhat agree
    c. Neutral
    d. Disagree
    e. Somewhat Disagree
4. "Social inclusion fosters understanding and acceptance of differences among communities."
    a. Agree
    b. Somewhat Agree
    c. Neutral
    d. Disagree
    e. Somewhat disagree
5. "Social Inclusion nurtures tolerance and patience among all members in a community."
    a. Agree
    b. Somewhat Agree
    c. Neutral
    d. Disagree
    e. Somewhat Disagree

Write as Many Relevant Details as Possible. Also, Include Examples.

6. "People react to my attempts to enable social inclusion of my child in different ways. They ..." __
    ____

Choose All Relevant Answers for Questions 7 to 10. Provide an Example or an Explanation for the Answers Chosen in the Space Provided.

7. "We encounter social exclusion when we attempt to mingle ..."
    a. With extended family ________________________
    b. With neighbors ________________________
    c. With members of our religious community ________________________
    d. With members of social groups ________________________
    e. Persons at recreational facilities e.g. playground ____________________
    f. With the school community ________________________
    g. At public spaces, e.g. shopping malls ________________________
    h. Whilst using public transit ________________________
    i. Other (please specify) ____________________________________
8. "My child is socially included by..."
    a. Family members ________________________
    b. Neighbors ________________________
    c. Friends ________________________
    d. Strangers ________________________
    e. Teachers and Peers ________________________
        j. Other (please specify) ____________________________________

Write as Many Relevant Details as Possible. Also, Include Examples.

9. "I have engaged in these strategies to enable social inclusion."

____

10. "I currently live in…"

    a. Australia
    b. New Zealand
    c. East Asia
    d. South Asia
    e. Central Asia
    f. Europe and UK
    g. Middle East
    h. African Continent
    i. Canada
    j. USA
    k. South America
        k. Name your country ____________________________________

Chapter 8
Stress and Anxiety Among Parents of Children With Communication Disorders

Kadambari Naniwadekar
All India Institute of Speech and Hearing, India

ABSTRACT

Parenting is a wonderful and rewarding experience, but in the case of parents of children with communication disorder, this experience is often accompanied with high levels of stress, due to difficulties, frustrations, and challenges that these parents face in everyday life. This chapter was carried out to find the status of stress in parents of children with communication disorder and also to find the levels of stress among mothers as well as fathers, and the level of support system available. The results revealed that most of the parents experience stress and anxiety in bringing up their child with communication disorder, although the stress being more in the mothers. Gender of the child also played a crucial role in determining the levels of stress. The results highlighted the fact that parents of children with autism spectrum disorder have a higher level of stress followed by parents of children with intellectual disability, multiple disability, and hearing impairment.

INTRODUCTION

The most valued relationships are found within the family. Family act as foundation for the child's holistic development, socialization and formation of his/her beliefs. Parenting is a wonderful and rewarding experience, although mostly accompanied by high levels of stress because of the difficulties and challenges that the parents face in everyday life, this stress being even more in the case of parents of children with communication disorders (Hodapp, Ricci, Ly, & Fidler, 2003). How the parents react to stress depends on a variety of factors like individual, family and environmental factors. Some families may view this as intimidating, while some may emerge stronger in this process. When the parent feels inundated by the stress associated with bringing up a child with communication disorder, there will be negative implications on the child, the parents and the family as a whole. For instance, increased

DOI: 10.4018/978-1-5225-4955-0.ch008

parental stress is associated with coercive parent-child interactions (Moes & Frea, 2000; Bor, Sanders, & Markie-Dadds, 2002), predicts drop-out from parent training interventions (Andra & Thomas 1998; Sanders, Markie-Dadds, Tully, & Bor, 2000; Schreibman 2000), and is linked with parental depression (Gray 2002; Vitaliano, Zhang, & Scanlan, 2003). In addition to that, heightened levels of stress can negatively influence a parent's interaction with other family members and thereby increase the risk of family maladjustment (Turnbull & Ruef, 1996).

Parents can never fully brace themselves for the news that their child is different (Pueschel, Bernier, & Weidenman, 1988). Whether the diagnosis of a disability is known after birth or in the later years, family dreams and expectations change unexpectedly. Although there are no universal reactions to the stress of raising a child with disability, several researchers have noted that there are some similar patterns or stages that the parents face emotionally (Miller, 1994). In the Indian context, disability is still viewed in terms of a misfortune. The cultural beliefs present in the society about disability plays an imperative role in influencing the way in which the family perceives the condition of the child and the kind of measures it takes for prevention, treatment and rehabilitation (Sen,1988). Dalal and Pande (1999) in their research explored the cultural beliefs and attitudes of a rural Indian community towards physical disability. The results revealed fatalistic approaches and external dependence in families with disabled children. In the same study, the respondents also felt that the disabled member cannot do anything and just needed help and sympathy.

Various studies reveal that negative attitudes will affect the parents negatively and they often experience harmful psychological effects. Such extreme levels of stress lead to heightened negative health outcomes like depression and marital dissatisfaction. Parents of children with communication disorders are found to be emotionally unstable, experience constant grief, and psychological ill health. They are also prone to be at a higher risk for marital disputes and social seclusion. Most of the mothers of children with communication disorders also experience extreme moodiness and are more prone to illness. They are found to be intensely affected by the way their child is accepted or rejected by the society. Mothers have also described themselves as unable to pursue their personal goals and as having little free time (Holroyd,1974), and concurrently report ambivalence and grief over the amount of time devoted to the disabled child at their own expense along with that of the family.

All parents of children with communication disorders deal with the similar tasks and demands that almost all of the parents face; however, one persistent point reported among these parents is the amount and degree of stress that they experience and the increased demands that is made by caring for the child with communication disorder. The everyday tasks of feeding, travelling, training their child is much more physically and emotionally demanding for the parents who have children with communication disorder (Ambert, 1992; Featherstone, 1980).

Having talked about stress in parents of children with communication disorders, we need to understand what stress actually means. Stress actually is a normal part of life and everyone experiences it in different degrees at various stages in life. According to the Merriam-Webster Dictionary (n.d.), one definition of stress is "a constraining force or influence such as physical, chemical, or emotional factor that causes bodily or mental tension and may be a factor for disease causation." Stress in anybody's life can be due to wide-range of reasons like change in person's life style, job pressures, financial problems, family problems, personal loss or negative emotions (Callanan 1990; Khalsa, Azok, & Leutenberg, 1994). Stress caused by any of these factors often leads to various physical, emotional and behavioral symptoms. The most common of them seen in parents of children with communication disorders being, frequent headaches, heart palpitations, weight loss or gain, constant tiredness, mood swings, crying, lack of concentration, feeling of helplessness etc.

As mentioned above one of the foremost causes of stress is change. Addition of a new member to an existing family is one of the changes that alter the family's social system. This stress can be even more traumatic if the child has any form of disability. Families of children with communication disorders are most likely to experience altered daily routines, roles, and expectations of their child, in addition to the regular stress of parenting. Parents of children with communication disorders are frequently bombarded with questions and concerns regarding their child's condition, along with dealing with the society's negative attitude. Although society's attitude and treatment of people with disabilities have changed considerably, there are still some people who may feel uncomfortable around their child. In the case of Autism, the contrast between the child's appearance, which shows no sign of disability, and his/her behavior, which is thought of as abnormal and "Strange" often puts parents in very unpleasant situations (Gray, 2002b; Portway & Johnson, 2005). Featherstone (1980) reports a sense of isolation and loneliness that many of these parents may experience. Social non-acceptance of the child's behavior often leads to stigmatization, experience of humiliation and the exclusion of these parents from normal social activities (Farrugia, 2009). The family's social and recreational patterns may also be altered due to the added care required by their child (Seligman, 1983). Having said this, it may also be taken into consideration that not all families of Children with Communication Disorder experience stress alike.

In the Indian context, as in the context of any other countries, parental stress might also be related to the attempts to trace appropriate services and education for their child (Bishop, Richler, Cain, & Lord, 2007). In the beginning, the parents generally lack information regarding their child's diagnosis and its management, thereby depending on the rehabilitation professionals for solutions. Along with the problem of finding appropriate services for their child, the medical expenses are greater for a child with communication disorder as compared to other children. Along with the daily expenses that comes for caring for any child, parents who have Children with Communication Disorder have an added burden of finding special clothing, adaptive equipment and making modifications at home (Thompson, 2000). One of the hardest things parents of children with communication disorders face is making a balance between the demands of other children and the family's normal life against the demands of the child with disability (Featherstone, 1980).

When there is an incongruity between expectations of a parent regarding their child's development by parenting, as opposed to what actually takes place, a crisis may occur. Depending upon the level of severity of the disability, many Children with Communication Disorder might master fewer skills of the normal developmental tasks faced in childhood (Bailey & Simeonsson, 1988). This impediment in the attainment of milestones becomes a major source of increased stress for parents (Hastings & Johnson, 2001; Hoffman, Sweeney, & Lopez-Wagner, 2008).

Each child and his or her disability is unique. Reactions of parents and the amount of stress they experience are subject to the child's behavior and personality characteristics (Bailey & Simeonsson, 1988; Bishop et al., 2007; Estes et al., 2009; Herring et al., 2006; Tomanik, Harris, & Hawkins, 2004; Walenski, Tager-Flusberg, & Ullman, 2006). Beckman (1983) in her studies, she examined the relationship between the child's characteristics and stress in the families of infants with a disability. She focused on five characteristics: rate of child's progress, responsiveness, temperament, repetitive behaviors and the presence of any additional or unusual demands. All of the child characteristics, except rate of child's progress were specifically related to the amount of stress reported by the mothers.

Interactions between the parent and their child with disability is another factor which influences the extent to which the family experiences stress. Parents may have to adjust their interaction styles depending on the child's ability to interact and communicate with them to meet the needs of the child (Pueschel et al., 1988). Children with developmental disabilities typically face difficulties in establishing eye contact, interacting with parents and communicating their needs and feelings. Parents who do not obtain cues or feedback from their child experience stress (Laborde & Seligman, 1983).

From the above studies, it can be understood that parents of children with communication disorders undergo stress and depression in their day to day lives. This stress, in turn, leads to various emotional problems, one of such is anxiety. Nanda and Shukla (1978) in their study found that diagnosis of a child with disability leads to severe emotional brunt on the parents of these children. It is beyond the understanding of the individual that has never thought of it or experienced it. The parents of these children start experiencing anxiety and have a feeling of enmity or rejection towards the child.

In another study by Lenhard, Breitenbach, Ebert, Schindelhaues-Deutscher, and Henn (2005) on psychological benefit for diagnostic certainty for the mother of children with disabilities, it was found that mothers of children with down's syndrome scored higher level of anxiety, feeling of guilt and emotional burden. Other family members also showed heightened level of anxiety. Hasting and Brown (2002) examined parental anxiety, depression, parental self-efficacy, and mental health and behavior problems in children with autism. Results of the study revealed that self-efficacy mediated the effect of child behavior problems on mothers' anxiety and depression.

Looking at the available literature, it can be said that there was an immense need to study the nature and degree of positive and negative impact of any disability on the parents and the families of children with communication disorders. While stress, factors leading to stress, coping mechanisms have been studied in various developed countries, very few studies have been conducted in India to find out the same. Keeping this in mind, this study was initiated to find out the level of stress and anxiety among caregivers/ parents of Children with Communication Disorder, to compare and contrast the levels of stress across four major disabilities (Hearing Impairment, Intellectual Disability, Autism Spectrum Disorder and Multiple/Physical Disabilities).

AIMS AND OBJECTIVES

1. To find out the factors leading to stress in parents of Children with Communication Disorder.
2. To find out the difference between the levels of stress and coping mechanisms of mothers and fathers.
3. To find out about the various support systems available.
4. To check which disability leads to higher levels of stress.

METHOD

With the above aim in mind, a survey type of research was conducted at the Department of Special Education, All India Institute of Speech and Hearing, Mysuru; hypothesising that presence of disabilities will adversely affect the psychological wellbeing among primary caregivers.

Participants

The participants of the study were selected through convenience sampling and the sample consisted of 73 parents of children with communication disorders out of which 20 parents had children who were diagnosed as having Autism Spectrum Disorder, 20 with Intellectual Disability, 20 with Hearing Impairment and remaining 13 were diagnosed as having multiple disability. The parents selected for this study were the ones whose children were attending one of the special educational services at the department of special education, AIISH, Mysuru.

Tools

A stress index scale was prepared as a part of the study taking inputs from various available inventories both in India and abroad (Parenting Stress Index, WHOQOL). Based on the references, a three-point rating scale viz. yes, sometimes no, comprising of 30 statements was prepared which covered domains like parental self-criticism, education, knowledge and pre-requisite skills of training their child, availability of various services, social and family support, financial stability, marital life, and general psychological well-being. The scale was translated to Kannada and then was sent for validation to experts in the field of special needs education. The suggestions hence received were incorporated in the scale and moved on to administration of the scale.

RESULTS AND DISCUSSION

After one to one administration of the scale on the parents of Children with Communication Disorder, the data was analysed to find out the level of stress the parents undergo and under which domain. The results are hence discussed under 6 heads.

Do the Parents of Children With Communication Disorders Experience Stress?

After careful analysis of data it was found that all the parents experienced stress in one or the other domain while bringing up their child with special need, irrespective of their child's disability (Eisenhower, Baker, & Blacher, 2005; Hodapp et al., 2003; Phetrasuwan & Miles, 2009; Tomanik et al., 2004). In a study by Gallagher, Beckman, and Cross (1983) and Kazak and Marvin (1984) were found similar results wherein, parents having children with disabilities stated to have higher amounts of physical, emotional, psychological, and financial demands; however the magnitude of stress depended upon a number of variables. One of the variables being the type of disability of their child (Gupta, 2007).

Comparison of Stress Level Across Disabilities

Once it was clear that all the parents experienced stress irrespective of their child's condition, the data was further analyzed to find out and compare the levels of stress among various disabilities. The results revealed that parents of children with autism spectrum disorder experienced the maximal stress with the highest mean (30.35), followed by parents of children with Intellectual Disability (29.25), children with hearing impairment (26.2) and multiple disability (26) respectively (refer Figure-1). The results found here are in concurrence with many similar studies (Deater-Deckard, Pinkerton, & Scarr, 1996; Abbeduto et al., 2004; Weiss, 2002). In a study by Mash and Johnston (1983), it was reported that mothers of children with attention deficits and hyperactivity disorders were more depressed, socially detached, and confined in their parental roles than mothers of children with normal behavior. The mothers of children with Autism are more concerned about their child's reliance on the care of others. In a study by Pisula (2007), the results indicated that mothers of children with autism in comparison to others of children with down syndrome had many difficulties in understanding their child's developmental problem and thereupon coped less effectively with these problems. While many studies have explored the relation between parenting stress and diagnoses, parenting stress depends upon the severity, visibility, unpredictability, and overall type of disability-behavioral, developmental or medical – rather than the medical diagnosis (Breslau, Staruch, & Mortimer, 1982; Bromley, Hare, Davison, & Emerson, 2004; Hastings & Johnson, 2001). Using the latter approach, Gupta (2007) reported that behavioral and developmental disability was associated with higher parenting stress than medical disability.

Comparison of Stress Under Different Domains

As mentioned before, the stress index scale was prepared covering domains like:

1. Self-Criticism
2. Early Intervention
3. Parental education and skills
4. Marital Life
5. Parental Health
6. Financial Condition
7. Social and Family support
8. General psychological wellbeing

Figure 1. Level of stress in parents across disabilities

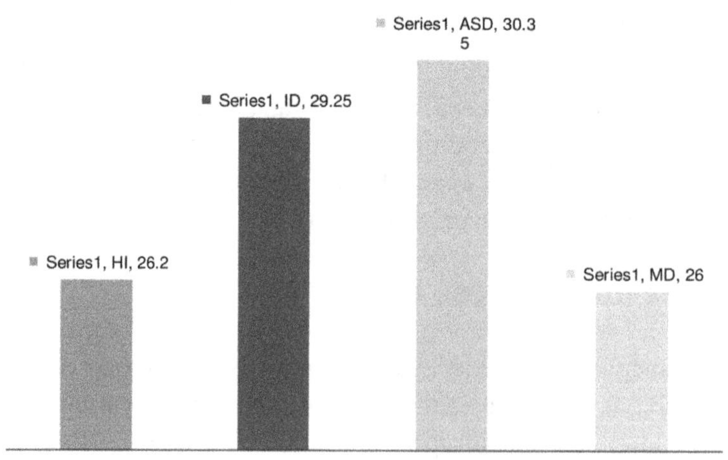

After analysis of the obtained data, it was found that the parents were more stressed in the items related to the domain of early identification followed by items under lack of education, knowledge and skills, spending excessive time with their disabled child, gender of their child and availability of services (refer Figure 2).

The parents were of the view that if their child's problem was identified at an early age (42% of the total participants), and services similar to AIISH would have been available at their native (29.2%), their child would have had a better prognosis. Another area of concern for parents was their knowledge and skills in handling their child (35%). In many studies (Barlow, Cullen-Powell, & Cheshire, 2006; Donovan, Leavitt, & Walsh, 1990; Florian & Fidler, 2001; Raikes & Thompson, 2005), it was found that parents with higher self-efficacy (more knowledge of the condition, and education) were found to have less stress as compared to parents who had lower self-efficacy. The primary caregiver in the Indian context is the mother, most of who have either low education or less exposure to the outside world were reported to feel more stressed as they were unable to meet the needs of their child and hence felt a gap in their relationship.

The next major concern of the parents especially the mothers was that they felt that they were giving up most of their time and energy in bringing up their children with communication disorder while ignoring their other children and family.

Figure 2. Level of stress across domains

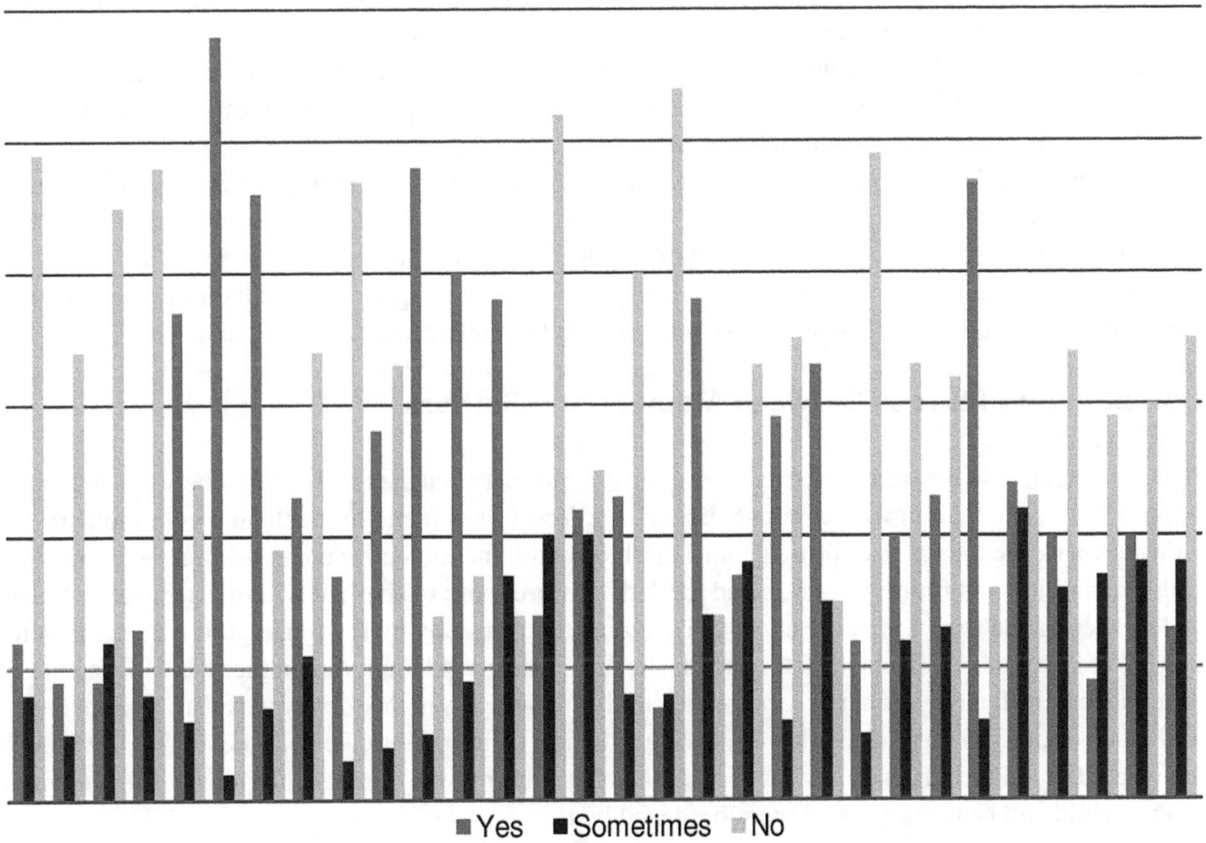

The mothers felt more guilty for the reason that their child is not getting appropriate care and love which he/she deserves. Also, this factor is strengthening the stress level in mothers, as their major concern is finishing therapy programs and getting back to their places.

As in most published reports, the parents of a girl child with disability are more stressed than those having a male child. This is more common in the Indian context as the gender of the child plays an important role in balancing the family relationships more so in the case of Children with Communication Disorder. Padencheri, Swamidhas, and Russell (2011) also found the similar results in his study. The results of the present study too revealed that the parents of girl child were more stressed as compared to those having a male child. Although the level of stress in parents of male children was also quite high. The parents of girl child, were concerned about the future of their daughters with respect to her marriage and security in the later years, whereas the parents of male child were disheartened to think of the future, as they felt that their child will not be able to earn for sustaining his family and also will not be able to take care of the parents in their old age.

While the data was being analyzed to check for the domains that were more stressful for the parents, it was seen that there were certain domains, in which parents were the least or not stressed at all. It was found that they were least stressed about their social life, i.e., going out with their children for various family functions followed by the support they receive from their family. The reason for being least stressed about social life might be that they have accepted the fact that their child has a problem, and thus they are not supposed to have a social life. Also, as most of the participants in the study are not residents of Mysore, they do not have a chance to attend family functions and hence the least stressed about. Another key factor being the social disapproval of their child's disability which often leads to stigmatization, experience of shame and thus exclusion from the social activities (Farrugia, 2009)

Taking about the other area where the parents have shown the least stress is in the domain of family support. It was found from the results that most of the participants/parents were satisfied with the support they received from the family and said that it would not have been possible to come for treatment to AIISH if they didn't have their family's support. In this regard, Taanila, Syrja, Kokkonen, and Ja¨rvelin (2002) found that families with better level of functioning explored for information about the disability, its treatment, worked towards maintaining family cohesion by sharing problems and seeking emotional support among family members, sought social support, looked for a space to be on their own and practice their hobbies, thereby having higher self-confidence and self-efficacy.

Comparison of Stress Between Mothers and Fathers

Another objective of the study was to compare and contrast between the level of stress between the mothers and fathers of children with communication disorders. It was found that although both mothers and fathers experience the stress of bringing up a disabled child, the mothers were more stressed about their child's condition and future prospects and the fathers were more concerned with the societal criticism and financial situations. Similar results were documented in a study by Hastings (2005). The reason for this difference can be attributed to the Indian societal structure wherein the mother has to take care of the child and the father goes out to earn for the family and mingles in the society. It can also be attributed to the role adopted by women within the caring situation (Pimm, 1996; Pelchat, Levert, & Bourgeois-Gue´rin, 2009). The fathers in our context are the ones who have to manage the finances for treatment of their child and hence might feel more burdened by this.

Effect of Stress on the Psychological Well-Being of the Parents

From the above results, it can be seen that most of the parents experience stress in one or the other form while raising their child with the communication disorder. A further probe was also conducted to find out how this stress affected these parents. From the results, it was found that out of the total participants 72% of them felt that they are giving up more of their life in raising this child and almost 63% of the population felt that this lead to the development of negative feeling and depression most of the times. This result reiterates the results of similar studies by Veisson (1999) and Keller & Honig (2004), who also reported that parents of children with disabilities experience heightened levels of stress leading to anxiety and depression. It was also seen that around 50% of the total participants often got suicidal thoughts. More than half of the participants reported that they remain unwell these days and this hinders their ability to work with their child, which in-turn makes them feel guilty and stressed. These results are in accordance with those found in other studies by Hamzat and Mordi, 2007; Kaya et al., 2010; Bella, Garcia, and Spadari-Bratfisch, 2011.

Positive Impact of Their Child's Condition

So far only the negative aspects of having a child with communication disorder were discussed. But an attempt was made to find out if there was any positive impact of the child's disability on the parents. It was found that most of the parents reported having a positive impact on their child, this being in congruence with results of the study by Scorgie, Wilgosh, and McDonald, 1998. Most of the mothers reported that they have become more self-sufficient, independent and have developed a lot of new skills and patience while working with their child. The mothers, in general, felt that they were able to come out of their cocoon and bring out their hidden talents while working with their child. Many mothers also reported that they learnt to read and write, which they didn't do during their growing up years. Indla, Indla, and Singh (2008) also found that 55.38% of parents felt their children with Intellectual Disability had positively impacted the family. Parents stated they had developed patience, tolerance, empathy, sensitivity, and experienced better spousal relations. In contrast, only 25.26% of respondents stated a negative impact of having a child with an Intellectual Disability. Mahoney (1958) found several positive effects of having a child with an Intellectual Disability on a family. These effects included the child having an integrative effect on the family by concentrating the family's energy in a positive manner. In another study by Scorgie and Sobsey (2000), it was found that some parents have focused on acquiring new traits like becoming more compassionate and less self-focused, learning they could achieve rather than remain powerless, developing endurance or greater personal strength in the midst of their feelings of weakness, progressing from depression to being able to view life as worthwhile and of value, and facing life with new boldness rather than capitulating to fear.

Hence, it can be seen that having a child with special needs does not necessarily lead to problems but also helps the parent grow as an individual too. To sum up, the following points can be highlighted based on the results:

1. All parents irrespective of their gender, age and qualifications experience stress while raising their child with communication disorders.
2. Parents of children with autism experience greater stress followed by parents of children with intellectual disability, hearing impairment and multiple disability.

3. Mothers experience more stress as compared to the fathers
4. Major stressors for parents of children with communication disorders being early identification and intervention, parents' level of knowledge and skills and the gender of their child.
5. It can also be highlighted that the parents reported enough family support in raising their child with special needs.

FUTURE RESEARCH DIRECTIONS

Through interactions on the sidelines of the research, it was further noticed that most of the families provided most advantageous support to the upbringing and rehabilitation of the children with the ultimately endeavouring to help them to develop optimally, irrespective of the stress and other adverse reactions to the presence of disability in the family. The progressive trend of acceptance of differential abilities and positive support both from the family as well as the society as a whole, extended to special needs in children assures a promising future. Provision of adequate caregiver support and guidance services may further enhance the constructive and comprehensive rehabilitation process.

CONCLUSION

The study was undertaken with an aim to find out the levels of stress and anxiety in the parents of children with communication disorders. In sum, the results of the study demonstrate that all the parents of children with communication disorders irrespective of their gender, age and qualifications undergo stress about the management and future of their child. Although, the level of stress was found to be a notch higher than others in the case of parents of children with autism spectrum disorder, which may be due to the discrepancy between the external appearance of the child versus the behavioral challenges that they face. This was followed by parents of children with intellectual disability, hearing impairment and then multiple disability, which was quite surprising. This can be attributed to the fact that parents of children with multiple disabilities have accepted the severity of their child's condition, as it is externally visible and there is no disparity in their appearance and activities.

The results also threw light on the much-studied fact that mothers of children with communication disorders experience more stress as compared to fathers. Although it should be noted that both parents do experience a certain level of stress. The study was also able to enlist the stressors which act as key factors in increasing or decreasing the level of stress in the parents. Some of the common stressors reported by most of the parents were lack of early identification and intervention services, level of their knowledge and skills in the management of their child's condition and the gender of the disabled child. With all these problems listed above, it was heartening to find that parents of children with communication disorders reported having enough support from their families. Taking all the aforementioned points into consideration, this study can be considered as a base for creating a better environment for children with communication disorders with the special focus on early intervention and parental guidance and counselling.

ACKNOWLEDGMENT

The author seeks to place on record the gratitude and credits due to participants in the study, Dr. M. Pushpavathi, Head-Department of Special Education for her guidance and Director, AIISH, Mysore, for the permission granted. A special reference and thanks to Ms. Shobha B N, and Dr. G. Malar for their continual support.

REFERENCES

Abbeduto, L., Seltzer, M. M., Shattuck, P., Krauss, M. W., Orsmond, G., & Murphy, M. M. (2004). Psychological well-being and coping in mothers of youths with autism, Down syndrome, or fragile X syndrome. *American Journal of Mental Retardation, 109*(3), 237–254. doi: PMID:15072518

Ambert, A. (1992). *The effect of children on parents*. New York: Haworth Press.

Andra, M. L., & Thomas, A. M. (1998). The influence of parenting stress and socioeconomic disadvantage on therapy attendance among parents and their behaviour disordered preschool children. *Education & Treatment of Children, 27*, 195–208.

Bailey, D. B., & Simeonsson, R. J. (1988). *Family assessment in early intervention.* Merrill Publishing Company.

Barlow, J. H., Cullen-Powell, L. A., & Cheshire, A. (2006). Psychological well-being among mothers of children with cerebral palsy. *Early Child Development and Care, 176*(3-4), 421–428. doi:10.1080/0300443042000313403

Beckman, P. A. (1983). Influence of selected child characteristics on stress in families of handicapped infants. *American Journal of Mental Deficiency, 88*(2), 150–156. PMID:6227240

Bella, G. P., Garcia, M. C., & Spadari-Bratfisch, R. C. (2011). Salivary cortisol, stress, and health in primary caregivers (mothers) of children with cerebral palsy. *Psychoneuroendocrinology, 36*(6), 834–842. doi:10.1016/j.psyneuen.2010.11.005 PMID:21146316

Bishop, S. L., Richler, J., Cain, A. C., & Lord, C. (2007). Predictors of perceived negative impact in mothers of children with autism spectrum disorder. *American Journal of Mental Retardation, 112*(6), 450–461. doi:10.1352/0895-8017(2007)112[450:POPNII]2.0.CO;2 PMID:17963436

Bor, W., Sanders, M. R., & Markie-Dadds, C. (2002). The effects of Triple P-Positive Parenting Program on preschool children with co-occurring disruptive behaviour and attentional/hyperactive difficulties. *Journal of Abnormal Child Psychology, 30*(6), 571–587. doi:10.1023/A:1020807613155 PMID:12481972

Breslau, N., Staruch, K. S., & Mortimer, E. A. (1982). Psychological distress in mothers of disabled children. *American Journal of Diseases of Children, 136*, 682–686. PMID:6213143

Bromley, J., Hare, D. J., Davison, K., & Emerson, E. (2004). Mothers supporting children with autistic spectrum disorders: Social support, mental health status and satisfaction with services. *Autism, 8*(4), 409–423. doi:10.1177/1362361304047224 PMID:15556959

Callanan, C. R. (1990). *Since owen*. Baltimore, MD: Johns Hopkins University Press.

Dalal, A. K., & Pandey, N. (1999). Cultural Beliefs and Family Care of the Children with Disability. *Psychology and Developing Societies*, *11*(1), 55–75. doi:10.1177/097133369901100103

Deater-Deckard, K., Pinkerton, R., & Scarr, S. (1996). Child care quality and children's behavioral adjustment: A four-year longitudinal study. *Journal of Child Psychology and Psychiatry, and Allied Disciplines*, *37*(8), 937–948. doi:10.1111/j.1469-7610.1996.tb01491.x PMID:9119941

Donovan, W. L., Leavitt, L. A., & Walsh, R. O. (1990). Maternal self-efficacy: Illusory control and its effect on susceptibility to learned helplessness. *Child Development*, *61*(5), 1638–1647. doi:10.2307/1130771 PMID:2245753

Eisenhower, A. S., Baker, B. L., & Blacher, J. (2005). Preschool children with intellectual disability: Syndrome specificity, behaviour problems, and maternal well-being. *Journal of Intellectual Disability Research*, *49*(9), 657–671. doi:10.1111/j.1365-2788.2005.00699.x PMID:16108983

Estes, A., Munson, J., Dawson, G., Koehler, E., Zhou, X.-H., & Abbott, R. (2009). Parenting stress and psychological functioning among mothers of preschool children with autism and developmental delay. *Autism*, *13*(4), 375–387. doi:10.1177/1362361309105658 PMID:19535467

Farrugia, D. (2009). Exploring stigma: Medical knowledge and the stigmatisation of parents of children diagnosed with autism spectrum disorder. *Sociology of Health & Illness*, *31*(7), 1011–1027. doi:10.1111/j.1467-9566.2009.01174.x PMID:19659737

Featherstone, H. (1980). *A difference in the family: Living with a disabled child*. New York, NY: Penguin Books.

Florian, V., & Findler, L. (2001). Mental health and marital adaptation among mothers of children with cerebral palsy. *The American Journal of Orthopsychiatry*, *71*(3), 358–367. doi:10.1037/0002-9432.71.3.358 PMID:11495338

Gallagher, J. J., Beckman, P., & Cross, A. H. (1983). Families of handicapped children: Sources of stress and its amelioration. *Exceptional Children*, *50*(1), 10–19. doi:10.1177/001440298305000102 PMID:6226529

Gray, D. E. (2002). 'Everybody just freezes. Everybody is just embarrassed': Felt and enacted stigma among parents of children with high functioning autism. *Sociology of Health & Illness*, *24*(6), 734–749. doi:10.1111/1467-9566.00316

Gupta, V. B. (2007). Comparison of parenting stress in different developmental disabilities. *Journal of Developmental and Physical Disabilities*, *19*(4), 417–425. doi:10.100710882-007-9060-x

Hamzat, T. K., & Mordi, E. L. (2007). Impact of caring for children with cerebral palsy on the general health of their caregivers in an African community. *International Journal of Rehabilitation Research. Internationale Zeitschrift fur Rehabilitationsforschung. Revue Internationale de Recherches de Readaptation*, *30*(3), 191–194. doi:10.1097/MRR.0b013e3281e5af46 PMID:17762763

Hastings, R. P. (2005). Child behaviour problems and partner mental health as correlates of stress in mothers and fathers of children with autism. *Journal of Intellectual Disability Research, 47*(4-5), 231–237. doi:10.1046/j.1365-2788.2003.00485.x PMID:12787155

Hastings, R. P., & Brown, T. (2002). Behavior problems of children with autism, parental self-efficacy, and mental health. *American Journal of Mental Retardation, 107*(3), 222–232. doi: PMID:11966335

Hastings, R. P., & Johnson, E. (2001). Stress in UK families conducting intensive home-based behavioral intervention for their young child with autism. *Journal of Autism and Developmental Disorders, 31*(3), 327–336. doi:10.1023/A:1010799320795 PMID:11518485

Herring, S., Gray, K., Taffe, J., Tonge, B., Seeney, D., & Einfeld, S. (2006). Behaviour and emotional problems in toddlers with pervasive developmental disorders and developmental delay: Associations with parental mental health and family functioning. *Journal of Intellectual Disability Research, 50*(12), 874–882. doi:10.1111/j.1365-2788.2006.00904.x PMID:17100948

Hodapp, R. M., Ricci, L. A., Ly, T. M., & Fidler, D. J. (2003). The effects of the child with Down syndrome on maternal stress. *British Journal of Developmental Psychology, 21*(1), 137–151. doi:10.1348/026151003321164672

Hoffman, Ch. D., Sweeney, D. P., Lopez-Wagner, M. C., Hodge, D., Nam, C. Y., & Botts, B. H. (2008). Children with autism: Sleep problems and mothers' stress. *Focus on Autism and Other Developmental Disabilities, 23*(3), 155–165. doi:10.1177/1088357608316271

Holroyd, J. (1974). The questionnaire on resources and stress: An instrument to measure family response to a handicapped family member. *Journal of Community Psychology, 2*(1), 92–94. doi:

Indla, R., Indla, V., & Singh, T. (2008). Impact of disability of mentally retarded persons on their parents. *Indian Journal of Psychological Medicine, 30*(2), 98–104. doi:10.4103/0253-7176.48482

Kaya, K., Unsal-Delialioglu, S., Ordu-Gokkaya, N. K., Ozisler, Z., Ergun, N., Ozel, S., & Ucan, H. (2010). Musculo-skeletal pain, quality of life and depression in mothers of children with cerebral palsy. *Disability and Rehabilitation, 32*(20), 1666–1672. doi:10.3109/09638281003649912 PMID:20170278

Kazak, E., & Marvin, R. S. (1984). Differences, difficulties and adaptation: Stress and social networks in families with a handicapped child. *Family Relations, 33*(1), 67–77. doi:10.2307/584591

Keller, D., & Honig, A. S. (2004). Maternal and paternal stress in families with school-aged children with disabilities. *The American Journal of Orthopsychiatry, 74*(3), 337–348. doi:10.1037/0002-9432.74.3.337 PMID:15291710

Khalsa, K. L., Azok, S. D., & Leutenberg, E. A. (1994). *Life management skills III.* Wellness Reproductions, Inc.

Laborde, P. R., & Seligman, M. (1983). Individual counselling with parents of handicapped children: Rationale and strategies. In M. Seligman (Ed.), *The family with a handicapped child: Understanding and treatment* (pp. 261–284). New York, NY: Grune & Stratton, Inc.

Lenhard, W., Breitenbach, E., Ebert, H., Schindelhaues-Deutscher, H. J., & Henn, W. (2005). Psychological benefit of diagnostic certainty for mothers of children with disabilities: Lessons from Down's syndrome. *American Journal of Medical Genetics. Part A, 133*(2), 170–175. doi:10.1002/ajmg.a.30571 PMID:15666306

Mahoney, S. C. (1958). Observations concerning counselling with parents of mentally retarded children. *American Journal of Mental Deficiency, 63*(1), 81–86. PMID:13559295

Mash, E. J., & Johnston, C. (1983). Parental perceptions of child behaviour problems, parenting self esteem, and mother's reported stress in younger and older hyperactive and normal children. *Journal of Consulting and Clinical Psychology, 51*(1), 86–99. doi:10.1037/0022-006X.51.1.86 PMID:6826870

Miller, N. B. (1994). *Nobody's perfect*. Baltimore, MD: Paul H. Brooks Publishing Co.

Moes, D. R., & Frea, W. D. (2000). Using family context to inform prevention planning for the treatment of a child with autism. *Journal of Positive Behavior Interventions, 2*(1), 40–46. doi:10.1177/109830070000200106

Nanda, J. L., & Sukla, G. D. (1978). Some probable factors causing mental retardation. *Child Psychiatry Quarterly, 10*, 4–106.

Padencheri, S., Swamidhas, P., & Russell, S. (2011). The role of gender of children with intellectual disability and their parents in marital intimacy in southern India. *Journal of Intellectual Disabilities, 15*, 241–251. PMID:22158461

Pelchat, D., Levert, M. J., & Bourgeois-Gue'rin, V. (2009). How do mothers and fathers who have a child with a disability describe their adaptation/ transformation process? *Journal of Child Health Care, 13*(3), 239–259. doi:10.1177/1367493509336684 PMID:19713407

Phetrasuwan, S., & Miles, M. S. (2009). Parenting stress in mothers of children with autism spectrum disorders. *Journal for Specialists in Pediatric Nursing, 188*(3), 157–165. doi:10.1111/j.1744-6155.2009.00188.x PMID:19614824

Pimm, P. L. (1996). Some of the implications of caring for a child or adult with cerebral palsy. *British Journal of Occupational Therapy, 59*(7), 335–341. doi:10.1177/030802269605900714

Pisula, E. (2007). A comparative study of stress profiles in mothers of children with autism and those of children with Down's syndrome. *Journal of Applied Research in Intellectual Disabilities, 20*(3), 274–278. doi:10.1111/j.1468-3148.2006.00342.x

Portway, S. M., & Johnson, B. (2005). Do you know I have Asperger Syndrome? Risks of a non-obvious disability. *Health Risk & Society, 7*(1), 73–83. doi:10.1080/09500830500042086

Pueschel, S. M., Bernier, J. C., & Weidenman, L. E. (1988). *The special child*. Baltimore, MD: Paul H. Brooks Publishing, Co.

Raikes, H. A., & Thompson, R. A. (2005). Efficacy and social support as predictors of parenting stress among families in poverty. *Infant Mental Health Journal, 26*(3), 177–190. doi:10.1002/imhj.20044 PMID:28682501

Sanders, M. R., Markie-Dadds, C., Tully, L. A., & Bor, W. (2000). The Triple P-Positive Parenting Program: A comparison of enhanced, standard, and self-directed behavioral family intervention for parents of children with early onset conduct problems. *Journal of Consulting and Clinical Psychology*, *68*(4), 624–640. doi:10.1037/0022-006X.68.4.624 PMID:10965638

Schreibman, L. (2000). Intensive behavioural/educational treatments for autism: Research needs and future directions. *Journal of Autism and Developmental Disorders*, *30*(5), 373–378. doi:10.1023/A:1005535120023 PMID:11098871

Scorgie, K., & Sobsey, D. (2000). Transformational outcomes associated with parenting children who have disabilities. *Mental Retardation*, *38*(3), 195–206. doi: PMID:10900927

Scorgie, K., Wilgosh, L., & McDonald, L. (1998). Parent's experiences managing life when a child has a disability. *International Journal of Special Education*, *13*, 102–110.

Seligman, M. (1983). Siblings of handicapped persons. In M. Seligman (Ed.), *The family with a handicapped child: Understanding and treatment* (pp. 147–174). New York: Grune & Stratton Inc.

Sen, A. (1988). *Psychosocial Integration of the Handicapped*. New Delhi: Mittal Publications.

Stress [Def.1]. (n.d.). In *Merriam-Webster*. Retrieved from https://www.merriam-webster.com/dictionary/stress

Taanila, A., Syrjala, L., Kokkonen, J., & Jarvelin, M.-R. (2002). Coping of parents with physically and/or intellectually disabled children. *Child: Care, Health and Development*, *28*(1), 73–86. doi:10.1046/j.1365-2214.2002.00244.x PMID:11856190

Thompson, C. E. (2000). *Raising a handicapped child*. New York: Oxford University Press Inc.

Tomanik, S., Harris, G. E., & Hawkins, J. (2004). The relationship between behaviors exhibited by children with autism and maternal stress. *Journal of Intellectual & Developmental Disability*, *29*(1), 16–26. doi:10.1080/13668250410001662892

Turnbull, A. P., & Ruef, M. (1996). Family perspectives on problem behavior. *Mental Retardation*, *34*, 280–293. PMID:8908993

Veisson, M. (1999). Depression symptoms and emotional states in parents of disabled and non-disabled children. *Social Behavior and Personality*, *27*(1), 87–98. doi:10.2224bp.1999.27.1.87

Vitaliano, P. P., Zhang, J., & Scanlan, J. M. (2003). Is caregiving hazardous to one's physical health? A meta-analysis. *Psychological Bulletin*, *129*(6), 946–972. doi:10.1037/0033-2909.129.6.946 PMID:14599289

Walenski, M., Tager-Flusberg, H., & Ullman, M. T. (2006). Language in autism. In S. O. Moldin & J. L. Rubenstein (Eds.), *Understanding autism: From basic neuroscience to treatment* (pp. 175–203). Florida: CRC Press.

Weiss, M. J. (2002). Hardiness and social support as predictors of stress in mothers of typical children, children with autism and children with mental retardation. *Autism*, *6*(1), 115–130. doi:10.1177/1362361302006001009 PMID:11918107

KEY TERMS AND DEFINITIONS

Anxiety: A mental health disorder characterized by feelings of worry or fear that is strong enough to interfere with one's daily activities.

Communication Disorders: Any disorder that affects an individual's ability to comprehend, perceive, or use language and speech to engage in conversation effectively with others.

Depression: A mental health disorder characterized by constantly depressed mood or loss of interest in activities, leading to significant impairment in daily life.

Disability: An impairment that may be cognitive, developmental, intellectual, mental, physical, sensory, or some combination of these and which affects the activities of daily living in one or the other way.

Family Support: The support of families to a member with a disability, which may include a child, an adult, or even the parent in the family.

Gender: The state of being male or female that is typically used with reference to social and cultural differences rather than biological ones.

Social Isolation: A state of complete or near-complete lack of contact between an individual and the society.

Stress: A feeling of strain and pressure or any unpleasant emotion and feeling.

Section 3

Communication Disorders:
Characteristics and Assessment

Chapter 9
Dysphagia in Persons With Communication Disorders

Gayathri Krishnan
All India Institute of Speech and Hearing, India

S. P. Goswami
All India Institute of Speech and Hearing, India

ABSTRACT

Dysphagia (swallowing disorders) is any difficulty in swallowing that interferes with safe and adequate intake of nutrition and hydration requirements in an individual. It may present itself as a symptom of another underlying medical condition or as a consequence of surgical and pharmacological treatment. While in few, dysphagia resolves itself as a transient phase; in the rest, dysphagia demands immediate treatment. It may be seen as an associated dysfunction in persons with communication disorders (PsWCD) as speech and swallowing functions share many neuro-musculo-skeletal structures at the oral, pharyngeal, and laryngeal level along with their central control processes. This chapter aims at introducing the readers to the signs and symptoms of dysphagia in PsWCD. This is expected to guide the team of professionals working with PsWCDin identification and making appropriate referrals to the concerned professional for effective intervention. This further can accelerate the progress and prognosis of PsWCD towards improved health, development, and quality of life.

INTRODUCTION

Dysphagia is defined as problems involving the oral cavity, pharynx, esophagus, or gastro esophageal junction because of which an individual fails in taking adequate hydration and/or nutrition essential for healthy survival. Any congenital or acquired condition that affects the central neural control of structures involved in swallow (For example: Stroke, Cerebral palsy, Amyotrophic Lateral Sclerosis etc.) or any impairment in the peripheral neuro-musculo-skeletal function of oro-pharyngo-laryngo-esophageal structures (For example, head and neck cancer, Gastro-esophageal reflux disorders, dental malformations etc) can result in difficulties during eating or drinking. An individual with dysphagia may or may not be aware of its presence and often seeks medical treatment when the condition worsens considerably leading

DOI: 10.4018/978-1-5225-4955-0.ch009

to deteriorated health and poor quality of life. Persons with communication disorders (PsWCD) often fall into this category of the neglected population with dysphagia because of the wide range and degree of symptoms presented. Issues with feeding and swallowing may range from mild to severe depending on the underlying cause of dysphagia. For example, in a child with cleft lip and palate (CLP), the initial focus of treatment is to ensure safe and adequate nutrition rather than cosmetic considerations. But the prime focus in the treatment of an individual diagnosed with oral carcinoma will be to improve life expectancy rather than feeding issues. In these individuals, dysphagia is neglected initially till it becomes a cause of distress in the individual and their family members, though prophylactic management is recently gaining appreciation across the world. It is often forgotten that basic nutrition and hydration will only accelerate recovery, development, and progress in all domains of life in a PsWCD (Ekberg, Hamdy, Woisard, Wuttge-Hannig, and Ortega, 2002; Farri, Accornero, and Burdese, 2007). This can immensely improve the overall quality of life (QoL) of the individual and add value to the treatment, management or rehabilitation services provided. A Speech-Language Pathologist (SLP) is trained to identify, assess and establish rehabilitation goals for these individuals' through varied approaches such as behavioral and motor skill training. Through graded sensory-motor stimulation and exercise based regimes combined with carefully selected dietary and environmental modifications, a qualified SLP can bring a marked difference in mealtime performance of PsWCD. A complete description of various strategies is beyond the scope of this chapter and readers are directed to reading elsewhere (Logemann and Logemann, 1983).

The aim of this chapter is to introduce the readers to various signs and symptoms of dysphagia that are commonly observed in PsWCD across the lifespan. By being observant and vigilant towards the possibility of the existence of this associated condition in their client group, the practicing rehabilitation professionals can identify and make appropriate referrals for the early and effective intervention of the individual for improving one of the basic functions and thereby accelerating betterment of overall health and wellbeing.

BACKGROUND

The term dysphagia is derived from the Greek words 'dys' meaning 'disordered' and 'phage' meaning 'eat'. Thus, dysphagia is disordered eating and hence this condition is often used alternatively with terms such as swallowing disorders, feeding disorders or deglutition disorders. Technically, all these terms (swallowing, feeding, eating and deglutition) refer to different dimensions of the same function. To elaborate, 'feeding' is the process of giving an edible substance to another individual for ingestion. The process of feeding thus involves at least two individuals, a mother and her newborn for example. Feeding disorders must then comprise of conditions that deviate from norms in the procedure of giving and taking the material to be ingested, whereas eating is a multi-dimensional self-performed act of ingestion of food. It involves the psychological readiness to eat such as interest and appeal of food, physical readiness such as hunger, motoric abilities to take the food from plate to the mouth for manipulation, and also the sensory-motoric integration of characteristics of the food and motoric activities that result in the quick and complete transfer of the manipulated food material to stomach. Thus eating disorders comprise of a whole lot of conditions resulting from deviations in any dimension of eating. For example, an extremely picky toddler or an individual under extreme psychological distress can have an eating disorder without feeding issues. The term 'swallowing' is more a medical term that denotes a series of actions that is initiated at the lips and that ends in the lower end of esophagus or stomach resulting in the transfer of food material from mouth to the stomach. The act of swallowing is referred to as deglutition. Thus, the term 'swallowing disorders' and 'deglutition disorders' may be used interchangeably by medical professionals and broadly refer to any impairment in the transfer of nutrition from lips to stomach (Leonard and Kendall, 1997).

From the above delineation of terms associated with dysphagia, it is clear that 'swallowing disorders' and/or 'deglutition disorders' are more physical in nature and come more in the practice purview of medical professionals for correction and with Speech-Language Pathologists for management. The group of 'eating disorders' and 'feeding disorders' are more behavioral in nature and requires team intervention from medical and allied professionals such as SLPs, Psychologists, Physio/Occupational therapists, Nutritionists, Dieticians, and many others. Therefore, treatment and management of dysphagia are essentially a multi-disciplinary and exact identification of the root cause of disordered function is central to this process. American Speech and Hearing Association (ASHA) emphasize on the inclusion of a number of medical and non-medical professionals in assessment and management of dysphagia in children and adults. The protocol followed for identification, assessment, treatment and rehabilitation vary across set up. Nevertheless, the focus of a dysphagia team is almost always to ensure adequate nutrition to the individual without encumbering the QoL and with minimal restrictions from normalcy at meal time. These decisions on the plan of action frequently cross borders of the individual profession and require deliberation and team consultations that are usually led and coordinated by an SLP. Depending on the setup, the dysphagia team takes joint decisions on treatment or rehabilitation plan or else serve as consultants.

Speech and swallowing share the common neuro-muscular-skeletal system starting from lips till the laryngeal structures. For this reason, any deviation in the structure or function of the lip to the laryngeal area can lead to deviations in both speech and swallow. While structural corrections are performed through surgical methods by qualified medical professionals, functional deficits are worked upon by rehabilitation professionals. This makes dysphagia a commonly associated dysfunction in PsWCD. Speech-Language Pathologists often face issues related to dysphagia in their routine practice. Their interest in holistic rehabilitation of their client has made dysphagia rehabilitation a special interest division of this profession but they are not the only professionals who deal with PsWCD (Figure 1).

Brain regions that integrate sensory-motor information for speech functions are known to participate in a similar function for deglutition also. The subcortical centers that relay afferent information to the frontal and parietal lobes for speech perform the same role for readiness and decision on performance during meal time. Other rehabilitation professionals such as psychologists, physio/occupational therapists, and special educators should play an equally important role in the identification of the earliest symptoms of dysphagia. They can ensure appropriate referrals to a qualified SLP for early and effective intervention before the individual develops complications such as malnutrition or aspiration pneumonia. The present chapter is prepared with the objective of briefly introducing the prominent symptoms of dysphagia in the most common group of communication disorders seen by psychologists and other allied health professionals in their daily practice.

Figure 1. The dysphagia team

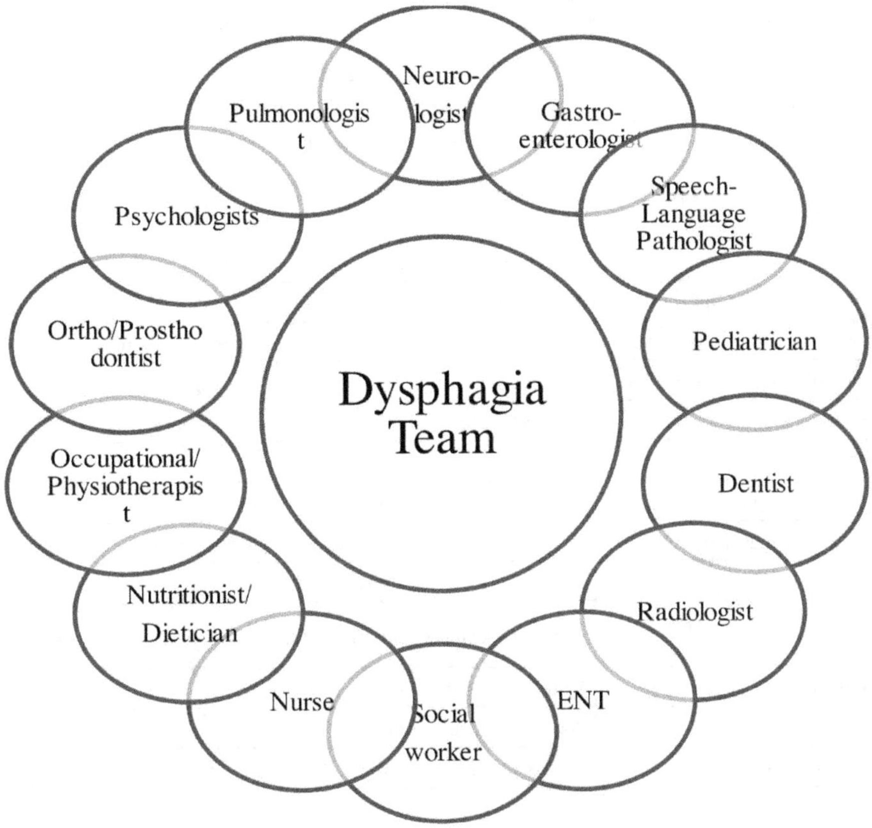

GENERAL SIGNS AND SYMPTOMS OF DYSPHAGIA IN PERSONS WITH COMMUNICATION DISORDERS

Symptoms are indications of deviant function that are experienced and reported by the affected persons themselves. These are individual's perception of their difficulties and indicate the immediate concerns of the individual and their family members. Signs are more objective in nature and are observed or derived by another individual and not the person complaining about dysfunction. In the context of dysphagia in PsWCD, Table 1 summarizes the most common symptoms reported by the individual/caretaker/ family members and the possible signs observed by the professionals. These symptoms may or may not be associated with aspiration or penetration which needs to be evaluated using detailed objective methods.

Recent reports suggest that 74% of children with developmental disabilities show some kind of feeding disorder (Burklow, Phelps, Schultz, McConnell, and Rudolph, 1998; Field, Garland, and Williams, 2003). The signs and symptoms of dysphagia in PsWCD depend on the type, locus, severity and complexity of underlying cause. When associated with isolated structural deficits, a correction of the structure may restore the overall efficiency of eating and swallowing. Functional and neural deficits at the peripheral structures usually show a wider range of impairments due to the typical complexity of swallow function. Neurogenic dysphagia is commonly due to impaired sensory-motor integration at the oral, pharyngo-laryngeal or esophageal stage of the swallow.

Table 1. Common signs and symptoms of dysphagia in PsWCD

Sl. No.	Symptom	Signs
1.	Pain during swallow	Inflammation, Infections, Ulcers
2.	Unexplained weight loss	Reduced quantity of food nutrient intake
3.	Loss of interest in eating	Effortful eating, Reduced quality of life
4.	Preferences to specific foods	Sensory issues, Oro-motor issues
5.	Long meal times	Poor oro-motor function
6.	Dry mouth	Thickened saliva, reduced amount of saliva and moisture in the oral cavity
7.	Leakage of food between lips	Lip and/or buccal weakness
8.	Repeated number of swallows	Poor lingual function, delayed initiation of swallow reflex
9.	Gagging of food placed in the mouth	Hypersensitivity, pre-mature posterior spillage
10.	Nasal regurgitation of food	Poor velar function
11.	Difficulty in swallowing	Delayed initiation of reflex
12.	Coughing or chocking on food	Pre-mature posterior spillage, aspiration/ penetration before, during or after swallow.
13.	Need to clear the throat frequently	Pharyngeal residue, regurgitated esophageal residue
14.	Sensation of food sticking in the throat	Poor pharyngeal or esophageal clearance
15.	Change in speech or voice over a period of time	Neuro-musculo-skeletal changes at the oral, pharyngeal or oro-pharyngeal passage
16.	Gastric complaints	Esophageal/ gastric dysfunction
17.	Frequent respiratory infections	Aspiration/ Penetration
18.	Burning sensation in the throat	Reflux gastric secretions

SIGNS AND SYMPTOMS OF DYSPHAGIA IN SPECIFIC COMMUNICATION DISORDERS

Developmental Delays (DD)

A delay in achieving typical age-appropriate milestones of thinking, language and motor activities are called developmental delays. The reasons for these delays can be many, most common being genetic factors, heredity, pre-natal complications and pre-mature birth. Pre-mature birth (< 37 weeks of gestation) is often associated with early feeding difficulties due to immature neuro-muscular system that is not yet ready to receive process or digest oral feeds. These infants gets short of their otherwise 40 weeks in-utero development of oral and swallowing reflexes before the introduction of oral feeding methods. Maintaining the rate of in utero weight gain in the post-natal period is a major challenge to the dealing medical professional during the pre-discharge period. The growth rate is necessarily monitored and maintained to avoid any delay in normal development of the pre-mature infant. It is normal for both term as well as pre-mature born infants to lose weight in the first days and then gradually catch up in the coming weeks with adequate nutrition. The already immature feeding system of a pre-term infant faces greater nutritional demands to catch up with the typical developmental rate. Many at times, they fail to compensate for their initial nutritional deficiency and continue to lag behind in average weight, length and developmental growth chart through early childhood (Su, 2014). Poor nutritional intake further causes delay in the physical, cognitive, emotional, and behavioral development of pre-term children (Cheong et al., 2017; de Kieviet, Piek, Aarnoudse-Moens, and Oosterlaan, 2009; Granuau et al., 2009; Hutton, Pharoah, Cooke, and Stevenson, 1997; Hornman, de Winter, Kerstjens, Bos, and Reijneveld, 2016).

Developmental delays are evident in feeding skills as well and a major concern for health professionals as well as caregivers for its role in growth and development. Though the sequence of feeding milestones remain similar, pre-term infants take more time to achieve and stabilize on these stages. The degree of delay is often associated with gestational age of the infant (Cooke, Ford, Werkman, Conner, and Watson, 1993; Ehrenkranz, Younes, and Lemons, 1999). An infant with poorly developed neuromuscular system and oral reflexes will face problems in sucking nutrition from the human or bottle nipples. Their immature brain often fails to integrate the suck-swallow-breathe pattern for safe, adequate and continued feeding sessions. This interferes with safe nutritional intake and places the infant at risk for serious medical complications secondary to aspiration during feeding (Ayuse et al., 2010; Bamford, Taciak, and Gewolb, 1992; Bu'Lock, Woolridge, and Baum, 1990; Gewolb, Vice, Schwietzer-Kenney, Taciak, and Bosma, 2001; Lau, 2006; Lau, Smith, and Schanler, 2003; Mizuno and Ueda, 2003; Nixon, Charbonneau, Kermack, Brouillette, and McFarland, 2008; Qureshi, Vice, Taciak, Bosma, and Gewolb, 2002; Sakalidis et al., 2013; Selley, Ellis, Flack, and Brooks, 1990). Decisions on introducing intravenous or tube feedings are made by professionals to ensure adequate growth and health until they are ready for oral feeding. Though the oro-pharyngeal inefficiency is bypassed with these non-oral feeding methods, digestion and adequate nutrient absorption through immature gastro-intestinal system remain as a barrier in normal development. Pre-mature babies are prone to gastro-intestinal reflux disorders, necrotizing enterocolitis and allergic reactions when external feeds are introduced to their immature gut. Further decisions on introducing normal oral feeding methods are indicated by the infant's development.

Infants with inefficient respiratory-swallow coordination indicate their discomfort with frowned eyebrows, irritability, crying, pulling back from nutrition source, coughing, wet eyes, increased breathing effort, discoloration of lips and face, loss of liquid from corners of the mouth and sometimes reduced heart rate. These indicate a feeding or swallowing difficulty that calls for professional intervention. Tube feeding and digestive disorders expose the infant to unpleasant experiences related to feeding. This can have long-term impact on meal times during early childhood and make feeding sessions a struggle or sometimes war. Long-term use of tube feeding leads to delayed development of oro-motor skills. Hence, the early intervention aimed at weaning tube feeding and introducing natural feeding methods are necessary to prevent development of long-term issues.

The best measure of feeding efficiency is the rate of weight gain in infants. Most pre-mature babies have lesser weight gain compared to term born babies at the time of discharge from hospital (Poindexter and Ehrenkranz, 2015). Though adequate and safe nutrition is essentially ensured at discharge, many young infants continue to show signs of distress at feeding time. Premature infants usually have more feeding issues and demand higher calorie for growth which is most frequently not met in the initial days. Consequently, longer duration of hospital stay for medical observation and general health stabilization is necessary. This is a period of great financial and emotional stress for the family and may also interfere with the mother-child bonding experience (Grunau et al., 2009).

As these children grow older, few issues are solved but new issues evolve. A report by Chatoor (2009) on oral feeding habits of children mention that food aversions and feeding difficulties are more common in pre-term more than term born children. Vomiting, gagging, strong food aversions, allergies, nausea, refusal to eat, irritability and crying are common in these children when complimentary feeds are introduced. These behaviors may continue to early childhood affecting their normal weight gain and growth. Most premature children remain small in stature compared to their age-matched term born peers throughout their childhood due to these feeding and nutritional issues.

Intellectual Disabilities (ID)

Feeding and eating are complex functions that involve complex relationships between cognitive, psychological, motor, sensory as well as para-sympathetic functions. In persons with intellectual disabilities, this function is deviant secondary to impaired cognitive functions. Prevalence of feeding issues is reported to be proportional to the severity of ID (Matson, Gardner, Coe, and Sovner, 1991; Rezaei, Rashedi, Gharib, and Lotfi, 2011). Around 80% of individuals with severe or profound intellectual disability were found to have mealtime issues (Perske, Clifton, McClean, and Stein, 1977). However, no reports have systematically described the characteristics of feeding issues in persons with ID. It may only be inferred that the lack of effective communication regarding the exact difficulties inhibits clear understanding of the underlying cause of inappropriate mealtime behavior. Feeding issues in ID are thought to be more behavioral than neuro-physiological. It has only been three decades since the first report on mealtime behavior of children with ID made its appearance in the literature (Linscheid, 1983). According to Sisson and Van Hasselt (1989), feeding difficulties in this population can be described under four main categories.

1. **Lack of Independent Skills:** Most children with ID depend on their caregivers for their routine activities, including feeding. They remain as 'feeders' for a longer time compared to their typical peers. Lack of self-feeding skill impairs their ability to take independent decisions on various aspects of feeding such as the quantity, method, positioning and manipulation of food taken into the mouth before swallow. Feeding dependency deprives the child with ID of a variety of oro-motor-sensory experiences that is an important aspect of feeding development. This further delay the development of chewing, sucking and swallowing function in these children.
2. **Disruptive Behaviors:** The cognitive deficits in ID lead to a number of behavioral issues in their day to day life and meal times are no exception. Parents often complain of irrepressible tantrums during meal times with the triggering factors varying from child to child and from time to time. These children develop peculiar eating habits secondary to cognitive and sensory deficits. Linscheid (1983) reported that children with ID fail to recognize edible and non-edible materials and unknowingly ingest harmful materials. This condition, called *'pica'*, cause serious damage to their overall health and may turn fatal if undetected (Matson, and Bamburg, 1999; Matson, Fodstad, and Boisjoli, 2008). Few children with ID bring up their swallowed food beyond their airway to the mouth, an act called rumination (Fredericks, Carr, and Williams, 1998). Long time chewing on ruminated food can cause oral infections and a reduction in overall nutrient intake. Continued rumination can also cause fatal consequences with aspiration pneumonia (Konarski, Favell, and Favell, 1992). Food refusal is common in young children and is more prevalent in young and older children with ID.
3. **Eating Too Much or Too Little:** Feeding dependency force the caregivers to make decisions on the quantity of food taken by the child irrespective of their hunger or metabolic state. This, along with communication difficulties, may lead to overeating behavior due to lack of expression of their state of fullness or hunger. The behavioral issues that interfere with successful feeding add on to the reduction in overall food intake leading to malnutrition and inadequate growth.
4. **Selectivity by Type or Texture:** While feeding, sensory processing issues make the child selective and picky about a particular type and texture of food. These children may show strong preferences to particular consistency (e.g.: pureed foods only), texture (e.g.: Crispy foods only), or sometimes

the temperature (e.g.: Room temperature only) or color of food (e.g.: Red colored vegetables only). These strong preferences make the child develop dislikes towards many other food items making nutritional adequacy a challenge to parents and professionals (Johnston, 1993; Matson and Kuhn, 2001; Riordan, Iwata, Finney, Wohl, and Stanley, 1984).

The profile of feeding issues in persons with ID is incomplete. Considering the background research of role of cognition in feeding behavior, it can only be supposed that feeding behaviors are significantly impaired in young and older children with ID. The existing reports in this direction suggest that feeding issues are more behavioral than developmental in nature.

Autism Spectrum Disorders (ASD)

Though eating is known to be disordered in children diagnosed within the Autistic Spectrum, not many objective researches have conducted towards this direction. However, it is very common that parents of children with ASD complain of mealtime melt downs (Cornish, 1998). Most often complaints of feeding difficulties are not reported during routine evaluations unless explicitly probed by the professionals. Untreated feeding issues and long-term deprivation of essential nutrients affect the normal growth patterns resulting in delayed development and maturation. Feeding difficulties are often severe when they are reported because of the negligence of minor indications in the early stages. Prevalence of feeding disorders ranges from 25% to 100% depending on the type of eating difficulty being probed (Cornish, 1998; Ledford and Gast, 2006; Patel and Piazza, 2001).

Feeding difficulties in children with ASD originates from extreme food selectivity (Ahearn, Castine, Nault, and Green, 2001; Collins et al., 2003; Cornish, 2002) leading to severe restriction in the range of diet (Bowers, 2002; Collins et al., 2003; Cornish, 1998). Other eating disorders reported by parents included obsessive eating (Collins et al., 2003) and nutritional deficits (Cornish, 1998; Cornish, 2002).

Eating disorders in ASD can be categorized into two types: Behavior based and Sensitivity based. Both these categories are usually not backed by any major medical condition. Among the 69% of children in the spectrum exhibiting feeding issues, 49% of them have behavioral based issues associated with eating (Williams, Dalrymple, and Neal, 2000). Children with ASD typically are impulsive in response, obsessive about their routines and repetitive in activities by nature. Minor changes from their preferences (including food) may elicit strong responses. This makes them very particular about the time, place, feeder, utensils, seating, food and many other characteristics associated with meal times. Changes can result in aggressive behaviors such as gagging, throwing, vomiting, and food refusal during meal times (Collins et al., 2003; Schreck, Williams, and Smith, 2004). Parental reactions to food refusal episodes and aggressive melt downs can further reinforce the unwanted behavior. The child who learns that refusal of specific foods can yield food items of their preference will only indulge in more refusals. Other reactions such as forced feeding make the child associate unpleasant experiences with mealtime and complicate the issue further.

Eating is a function that involves multiple sensory analyses and its integration. It involves visual, olfactory, gustatory, proprioceptive and tactile stimulation from the food presented. Eating becomes a pleasurable and comforting experience when these stimulations are accepted and appreciated. But, children with ASD are known to have issues in sensory processing (Kientz and Dunn, 1997) that leads to problem behaviors in communication and feeding sessions. Certain food characteristics such as color, taste, smell, texture, consistency, and temperature can trigger sensitivity issues and force children to exclude the whole category of food from their routine diet (Ahearn et al., 2001; Collins et al., 2003). Sensitivity issues can trigger aversive responses such as gagging or vomiting foods. Children learn to associate these unpleasant experiences with meal time and learn food refusal as a strategy. Children with hyposensitivity indulge in overeating by ingesting large portions of food into the mouth and also prefer extremely warm or cold foods. These children may refuse blunt tastes or soft cooked foods and prefer carbonated and crunchy foods, again limiting the range of food accepted. Chewing difficulties may be present and interfere from identifying items that require more effortful chewing and those that do not. The visual presentation of the food may also be a triggering factor for mealtime misbehaviors in children with ASD.

Among the many picky eaters and over-eaters in ASD, there are children who fail to understand differences between edible and non-edible items (Volkert and Vaz, 2010; Schreck, Williams, and Smith, 2004). Children with ASD may also present with *pica* and can turn into a very dangerous and fatal situation, if left untreated. This raises the risk of infections of the digestive system because of uncontrolled exposure to pathogens and ingestions of dangerous toxins. Immediate professional help is inevitable for management. Factors such as age, maturation and development of sensory-motor, cognition and communication skills are detrimental in understanding these feeding behaviors. Communication difficulties forbid children with ASD from indicating their difficulties and preferences making them indulge in inappropriate behaviors. Incidence of undetected food allergies may also be higher in this population.

Cerebral Palsy (Developmental Dysarthria)

Cerebral palsy (CP) is a condition that is congenital and interferes with the normal development of the brain from infancy. Epidemiological reports suggest that up to 75% of children with CP have issues with feeding (Rempel, Colwell, and Nelson, 1988). These issues may be in the oral preparatory, oropharyngeal or esophageal stages of swallow. The characteristics of feeding issues in this population depend on the severity and type of CP. For example, spastic CP caused by lesion in the cortico-bulbar and cortico-spinal tracts can have difficulty with the execution of voluntary movements of structures of the oral cavity. The severity of CP is a factor in understanding the extent of impairment in an individual. Mild impairments exhibit compensated growth patterns while severe growth retardation is common in children with severe CP. Mothers often find feeding problems as the first indication of the presence of abnormality in their babies (Reilly, Skuse, and Poblete, 1996).

Difficulty in feeding in newborns with inadequate neuro-motor system is usually seen as weak, interrupted sucking and inability to continue the feeding session for adequate nutritional intake. These oral phase difficulties inconsistently associated with inadequate apnea and bradycardia. Presence of rattling sounds, skin discoloration, cough, and gag are indicators of underlying pharyngeal phase difficulty. Children with mild impairments of the neuro-motor systemmay continue to grow within the developmental pattern if they are provided with longer and/or more frequent feeding. Some infants may benefit with low density supplements and energy boost diets to compensate and outgrow nutritional deficiency secondary to feeding difficulties (Lobstein, 1991). However, issues get more prominent with the introduction of solid foods as their masticatory inefficiency gets revealed. Most children prefer semi solids over solid foods. This adds on to nutritional deprivation and further growth deviations. Children with CP are commonly short by stature and hence their body mass index remains adequate though their weight gain remains lesser than expected. More than exception, these children are assessed and intervened much later, often after the first year of their life, when they become 'failure to thrive' (FTT) because of feeding issues.

Children with moderate and severe CP show similar but strong difficulties. Severe degree of CP is often associated with significant oro-motor sensory weakness and studies have revealed a direct association between degree of CP and feeding issues (Ruby and Matheny, 1962; Mosier, Grossman, and Dingman, 1965; Culley and Middleton, 1969; Tobis, Saturen, Larios, and Posnaik, 1961; Krick and Van Duyn 1984; Shapiro, Green, Krick, Allen, and Capute, 1986). Lack of adequate lip seal, drooling, tongue thrust, hyper/hyposensitivity, bite reflexes, difficulty controlling liquid bolus, preference to soft semisolids, nutritional deficiency, inappropriate weight and growth retardation are characteristic of this population. Detailed video-fluoroscopic studies revealed anterior leakage of saliva/bolus, inefficient management of secretions, masticatory inefficiency, lack of lingual control for bolus hold, inability to make a cohesive bolus, and pre-initiation posterior spillage of the bolus in the oral phase of swallow (Benfer, Weir, and Boyd, 2012a; Casas, Kenny, and McPherson, 1994; Couriel, Bisset, Miller, Thomas, and Clarke, 1993; Del Giudice et al., 1999; Erkin, Culha, Ozel, and Kirbiyik, 2010; Kim et al., 2013; van den Engel-Hoek et al., 2013). At the pharyngeal level, delay in initiation of swallow (van den Engel-Hoek et al., 2013), nasal regurgitation (Erkin et al., 2010; Kim et al., 2013; van den Engel-Hoek et al., 2013), reduced hyolaryngeal elevation, incomplete laryngeal vestibular closure and pooling may be visible leading to penetration or aspiration of pharyngeal residue into the airway (Bader and Niemann, 2010; Clancy and Hustad, 2011; Kim et al., 2013; van den Engel-Hoek et al., 2013; Weir et al., 2007a).This can elicit immediate protective reflexes such as cough, choking, tearing from eyes, gag, and clearing of throat. On long run, these symptoms may lead to bronchitis, pneumonia, and atelectasis. Unfortunately, aspiration may remain silent in this population (Kim et al., 2013) indicating the need for early and detailed evaluation for feeding and swallowing difficulties in this group. Many of them may also have associated esophageal symptoms.

Adding on to these physiological impairments, communication difficulties and other social factors hinder expression of their difficulties and experiences during meal times. For example, children with severe CP may fail to express their hunger or their food preferences. Many of these individuals depend on their caretaker for obtaining and maintaining feeding position and also the type, amount, rate and taste of their food (Rogers, Arvedson, Buck, Smart, and Msall, 1994). Inspite of this dependence, many caregivers report long feeding time in their wards with CP (Johnson and Deitz, 1985; Gisel and Patrick, 1988) secondary to impaired oral stage of swallow.

Such nutritional deprivation and inadequate weight gain in the early stages of development interferes with cognitive development of the child (Skuse, Pickles, Wolke, and Reilly, 1992) and reduces life expectancy. Inadequate growth of the child puts the mother under extreme psychological stress and probably is a cause of maternal depression (Hirst, 1985). Further, depression interferes with the mother's ability to nurture their young ones further completing a vicious circle of unpleasant events ultimately affecting the quality of life of the entire family. The quality of intervention depends on accurate diagnosis of the underlying impairments with detailed evaluations and tests by qualified professionals.

Structural and Oro-Facial Anomalies

Summarizing the presentation characteristics of feeding issues in this group is an enormous task as there are multiple permutations in the position, type, causes and associated deficits in this group of PsWCD. The feeding and swallowing issues in each individual with an oro-facial anomaly varies with the structural and functional abnormality. The characteristics also vary if the structural abnormality is associated with a cranial abnormality or a syndromic condition. If the oro-facial anomaly (OFA) is associated with cranio-facial syndromes, then feeding and swallowing issues emerge as a major concern from birth. The deviations in feeding secondary to structural abnormalities can be viewed under two categories: (1) Isolated cleft lip and/or cleft palate without associated conditions or sequel (CLP-I) (2) Cleft lip and/or cleft palate with associated conditions or sequel (CLP-AS).

Isolated Cleft Lip and/or Cleft Palate Without Associated Conditions or Sequel (CLP-I)

This category of individuals has a structural abnormality of lip and/or palate without any associated cognitive, neural, sensory or physiological malformations. The contribution of CLP-I towards feeding issues range from mild to moderate, depending on the extent of the abnormality. Their oral feeding deficits stem from the inability to suck nutrition effectively from the nipple source. Sucking deficits are secondary to their inability to attain or maintain lip seal or due to lack of a stable plate against which tongue can stroke the nipple source to eject milk. The presentation of feeding issues in CLP-I depends on side, extent and number of structures involved. Generally, an infant with cleft lip (CL) alone will eventually adapt the latch such that the breast tissue seals off the cleft while sucking. Mothers can also help them achieve this latching position. But an infant with cleft palate (CP) usually presents with more serious consequences in feeding activity. Incomplete palate provides an empty space against which the infant attempts to stabilize the nipple during sucking. The CP also couples the oral and nasal airway leading to nasal regurgitation of oral feeds leading to irritability and unpleasantness during the feeding sessions. Infants learn to cover posterior clefts with the back of their tongue to effectively stabilize and create the negative sucking pressure during feeding. Combined CL and CP is expected to have more serious impact on a child's feeding compared to CLP-I. A wide cleft makes feeding more troublesome compared to narrow cleft. Similarly, unilateral clefts are compensated easier compared to bilateral clefts.

CLP-I commonly lead to oral phase deficits with intact pharyngeal phase functioning. Loss of liquid from mouth through the cleft, inadequate lip seal, nasal regurgitation, low oral intake, inadequate weight gain, and irritability during feeding sessions are common. Feeding sessions need to last longer than typical, making it tiresome for the child as well as the mother. Careful observation may reveal short bursts of sucking episodes during which the infant attempts fast sucking on the nipple. Higher suck-swallow ratios and generation of a positive pressure during sucking motions are observed during feeding sessions (Masarei et al., 2007). Children with CLP tend to swallow a lot of air during feeding making them gassy (Wolf and Glass, 1992; Reid, Reilly, and Kilpatrick, 2007; Arvedson and Brodsky, 2002). These children need frequent and longer burping and comforting time compared to their typical peers. Pharyngeal and respiratory-swallow coordination remains intact in these children and are not at risk for aspiration. Adequate positioning and selection of appropriate feeding aids along with compensatory strategies identified by skilled SLP can create successful feeding sessions till the malformations are surgically repaired.

Cleft Lip and/or Cleft Palate With Associated Conditions or Sequel (CLP-AS)

When cleft lip and/ or palate are associated with CFA, its impact on feeding is more severe compared to CLP-I. These conditions present with a myriad of structural deformations at the oral, pharyngeal as well as esophageal structures and significantly impair its effective functioning. Many CFA place the individual at high risk for aspiration due to compromised aero-digestive pathway (Caron et al., 2015;

Dobbelsteyn, Peacocke, Blake, Crist, and Rashid, 2008; Khansa et al., 2016; Paes et al., 2017). Careful observation, detailed assessment and early intervention are necessary before oral feedings are initiated in CLP-AS. In most of these cases, feeding issues arise from difficulty in movement of oral structures such as lips, tongue and jaw. These structures are crucial in attaining effective and efficient feeding in newborns as well as in older children.

Many CFA present with hypoplasia of maxilla, mandible or midface along with multiple cranial nerve impairment. Structural abnormalities of nose, maxilla, mandible, pharynx and/ or larynx are also common. These abnormalities directly impair feeding and compromise the airway. Hypoplasia of maxillary and mandibular structures interferes with food or source positioning in the oral cavity and its preparation for swallow. In infants, this adversely affects the positioning of the nipples for nutrition sucking. Midface hypoplasia with high palate vault interferes with making adequate tongue-palate contact for generating negative sucking pressure. Certain conditions involve cleft of velum and velar insufficiency that causes coupling of nasal passage to oro-pharyngeal cavity during swallow. The food/liquid swallowed may then regurgitate to the nasal passage during the process. Inadequate velar functioning may also influence timely initiation of swallowing reflex as the afferent sensory information regarding the position of food at the anterior faucial pillars is thought to trigger swallowing reflex. Cleft of laryngeal or tracheal structures are serious considerations and quick decisions on mode of feeding is to be made after careful evaluation. Laryngeal clefts pose serious risks of aspiration that can be a threat to the life of the individual on long run. Careful and detailed instrumental and/ or radiological evaluations are warranted in these children. A brief description of various syndromes and sequences that are associated with CLP-AS along with their symptoms of feeding difficulties are presented in Table 2.

Repeated attempts to oral feed without understanding the physiological impairments underlying the structural malformations can make oral feeding fatal with continuous aspirations of swallowed food into the airway. Symptoms such as repeated respiratory infections, pneumonia and lung disorders should direct and warn the professionals towards undetected or untreated abnormalities at the aero-digestive level. Repeated hospitalization and long-term intervention for successful feeding induces great emotional, financial and social stress and also makes the infant-parent bonding an extremely taxing process.

Apraxia

The inability to volitionally initiate or execute a learned movement is termed as apraxia (Geschwind, 1975). Ongoing debates on its existence with unique characteristics and diagnosis criteria continue till date. Some researchers have gone forward to describing variants of apraxia based on its neurophysiological or behavioral attributes. For example, limb apraxia, bucco-facial apraxia, and apraxia of speech. Few available reports suggest that apraxia of swallow co-occur with some of the existing variants of apraxia.

It was in 1941 that the use of the term 'apraxia of swallow' (AOS) first appeared in the literature (Tuch and Nielson, 1941). Initial reports identified delay in initiating oral transfer on volitional swallow in spite of adequate oro-motor-sensory function, as the major symptom of AOS. Consequent reports described incoordination of tongue, mandible, buccal muscles and palate during deglutition (seen as groping movements) as symptoms of this condition (Daniels, 2000; Logemann, 1998). This incoordination between structures involved can ultimately lead to increased oral transit time. Delay in initiating the swallow reflex may be seen on radiological studies. Considering the definition of apraxia, learned or skilled movements are affected on volitional attempts. Swallow presents a unique scenario wherein the movements change from volitional to automatic (Kennedy and Kent, 1988). Hence AOS, if exists, should not alter the reflexive functions in the pharyngeal phase of swallow.

Table 2. Symptoms of feeding difficulties in various CLP-AS

Sl. No.	Syndrome Associated With CFA	Presenting Features	Remarks
Oral Phase Dysphagia			
1.	Van der Woude	CL/ CP Lip and salivary gland abnormalities Hypodontia	Loss of liquids from mouth through cleft, Nasal regurgitation, Inefficient sucking
2.	Oro-facio-digital syndrome Type II/ Mohr Syndrome	CL Poly lobed tongue Hypodontia Polydactyly Facial anomalies Digital anomalies	Poor sucking, poor lingual control over food, oral residue after swallow, poor reflex initiation for swallow, chewing difficulties.
3.	Hemifacial microsomia	Ear malformations Maxillary and mandibular hypoplasia CL/CP Facial nerve weakness	Loss of liquids from mouth through cleft, Nasal regurgitation, Excessive air intake during sucking, Poor of lingual control over the bolus, Poor sucking, oral residue after swallow, chewing difficulties.
4.	Fetal alcohol syndrome	Brain and cranial nerve damage, smooth philtrum, thin vermillion, small palpebral fissures, CL/CP, microcephaly, bone and joint deformities, heart defects	Poor oro-motor and sensory function, cleft and neurological impairment-oral motor and sensory dysfunction.
5.	Saethre-Chotzen syndrome	Craniosynostosis, facial asymmetry, midface hypoplasia, hypertelorism, ear malformations, Syndactyly, CP	Loss of liquids from mouth through cleft, Nasal regurgitation, Excessive air intake during sucking, poor oro-motor sensory function, loss of lingual control over bolus, poor oral transfer, residue after swallow.
6.	Crouzon syndrome	Craniosynostosis Hypertelorism Shallow eye sockets Stabismus Beaked nose Maxillary hypoplasia Dental problems Ear malformations CL/CP	Loss of liquids from mouth through cleft, Nasal regurgitation, Excessive air intake during sucking, poor oro-motor sensory function, and chewing difficulties.
7.	Beckwith-Wiedemann syndrome	Macrosomia Hemihyperplasia Abdominal wall defects Macroglossia Metabolic abnormalities	Limited range and movement of tongue, macroglossia may obstruct airway leading to breathing difficulties during swallowing.
Oro-Pharyngeal Dysphagia			
1.	Trisomy 13	Congenital heart defects Brain or Spinal cord abnormalities Microphthalmia Polydactyly Microcephaly Micrognathia CL/CP Hypotonia	Loss of liquids from mouth through cleft, Nasal regurgitation, Inefficient sucking, Airway compromise due to lung disorders, Reflux disorders, poor coordination of suck-swallow-breathe pattern. Severe feeding difficulties and FTT.
2.	Wolf-Hirschhorn syndrome	'Greek Warrior Helmet'appearance Hypertelorism Short philtrum Micrognathia Outer ear malformations Microcephaly Hypotonia Scoliosis and kyphosis Hypodontia CL/CP Abnormalities of eyes, heart, genitourinary tract and brain.	Loss of liquids from mouth through cleft, Nasal regurgitation, Inefficient sucking, Excessive air intake during sucking, Poor suck-swallow-breathe integration. Delayed growth and FTT.
3.	CHARGE association	Microphthalmia Coloboma Choanal stenosis Cranial nerve abnormalities Facial paralysis Hyposmia Hearing loss Heart defects CL/CP Genital abnormalities Tracheo-esophageal fistula	Loss of liquids from mouth through cleft, Nasal regurgitation, Excessive air intake during sucking, respiratory issues, oro-motor difficulties, airway compromise, choking/aspiration.

continued on following page

Table 2. Continued

Sl. No.	Syndrome Associated With CFA	Presenting Features	Remarks
4.	Pierre-Robin Syndrome	CP, retrognathia, micrognathia, glossoptosis	Loss of liquids from mouth through cleft, Nasal regurgitation, Excessive air intake during sucking, respiratory issues, airway obstruction.
5.	Stickler syndrome	Flattened facial appearance, midface hypoplasia, CP, Glossoptosis, micrognathia, vision difficulties, hearing loss	Loss of liquids from mouth through cleft, Nasal regurgitation, Excessive air intake during sucking, respiratory issues, airway obstruction.
6.	Velocardiofacial syndrome	Long face with prominent maxilla Flattened cheeks Mandibular hypoplasia Bluish pigmentation below the eyes Prominent nose with narrow nasal passage Long. Thin upper lip and down slanting mouth CP/ Sub mucous cleft Heart defects	Variable degrees of feeding difficulty. May have oro-motor dysfunction, difficulty in sequencing feeding movements, issues associated with cleft, and respiratory issues.
7.	Moebius syndrome	Palsy/paresis of multiple cranial nerves, eye abnormalities, microglossia, micrognathia, CP, ear malformations, dental abnormalities, skeletal malformations	Loss of liquids from mouth through cleft, Nasal regurgitation, Excessive air intake during sucking, poor oro-motor sensory function, loss of lingual control over bolus, poor oral transfer, residue after swallow, chewing difficulties, choking/aspiration secondary to cranial nerve involvement
8.	Apert syndrome	Craniosynostosis Syndactyly/ polydactyly Sunken appearance in the midface Hypertelorism Beaked nose Maxillary hypoplasia CL/CP Dental abnormalities Brain abnormalities	Loss of liquids from mouth through cleft, Nasal regurgitation, Excessive air intake during sucking, impaired oral mechanics, breathing difficulties during feeding.
9.	Pfeiffer syndrome	Craniosynostosis Hypertelorism Maxillary hypoplasia Beaked nose Ear malformations Dental problems Brachydactyly/syndactyly Narrow respiratory passage Brain abnormalities Cranial nerve involvement	Loss of liquids from mouth through cleft, Nasal regurgitation, Excessive air intake during sucking, impaired oral mechanics, chewing difficulties, breathing difficulties during feeding.
10.	Treachercollins	Micrognathia CP Narrow respiratory passage Eye malformations Eyelid Coloboma Ear malformations	Loss of liquids from mouth through cleft, Nasal regurgitation, Excessive air intake during sucking, respiratory issues, airway obstruction.
Oral Pharyngeal and Esophageal Dysphagia			
1.	Opitz/ BBB syndrome	Hypertelorism Defects of larynx, trachea and esophagus Hypospadias CL/CP Heart defects Imperforate anus Brain defects Facial dysmorphism	Loss of liquids from mouth through cleft, Nasal regurgitation, Inefficient sucking Airway compromise, Esophageal dysmotility and reflux, high risk of aspiration.

CFA= Cranio-Facial Anomalies; CP= Cleft Palate, CL= Cleft Lip; FTT= Failure to Thrive; CHARGE= Coloboma, Heart defects, Atresia Chonae, Retardation, Genital abnormalities, Ear abnormalities.

It is worth emphasizing that the abnormal movements of swallow can be observed only on cued swallows and not in spontaneous swallows, a feature that distinguishes this category of impairment from other disorders of swallow. Hence, it may be hypothesized that secretion management may be less impaired that mealtime swallows. However, symptoms of AOS may or may not overlap with symptoms of other associated problems. This further complicates clear diagnosis and management. Further research is needed to identify the specific symptoms of swallowing difficulties in persons with apraxia.

Aphasia

Stroke or cerebrovascular accidents leave a massive impact on cortical, subcortical or brainstem structures involved in speech and/or swallowing function. It is the most common cause of dysphagia and about 90% of individuals experience feeding and swallowing issues in the post-stroke period. The incidence of dysphagia ranges from 38-70% in the acute phase of stroke (Daniels et al., 1998; Horner and Massey, 1988; Horner, Massey, Riski, Lathrop, and Chase, 1988; Linden and Siebens, 1983). While most of the issues are temporary and resolve over time, some refuse to recover and leaves an impact on the quality of life of the stroke survivors (Ortiz and Marinelli, 2013). Because feeding and eating are not only a biological need but also a social activity, the impact of feeding issues after stroke turns into a family concern. The rate of post-stroke recovery depends on various internal and external factors, adequate nutrition and hydration being one among them. Post-stroke dysphagia presents with a wide range of symptoms depending on factors associated with stroke. The swallowing functions that are impaired vary with the extent, location, type, and hemisphere of stroke as well as age, associated problems and initial treatments provided at hospital admission. Repeated screening may be required in all individuals post-stroke to ensure earliest identification and intervention of dysphagia.

Brainstem infarcts increase the risk of persistent and severe dysphagia for this it has the central coordination structures of swallowing and also consists of several cranial nerve nuclei that are essential for initiating and performing the act of swallowing. Dysphagia post brainstem strokes go through minimal spontaneous recovery and results in long-lasting feeding handicap. Impairment in timely triggering of the swallowing reflex and sensory integration into the reflexive stages of swallowing is common. This is seen as a deficiency in processing the sensory information regarding bolus characteristics for the timed and coordinated airway decoupling. These individuals often are at high risk of silent aspiration as brainstem strokes suppress the protective cough reflex that is normally associated with laryngeal penetration or aspiration.

Cerebral hemispheric strokes are more common compared to brainstem strokes but fortunately, show milder residual impact because of the spontaneous recovery and neuronal reorganization in the post stroke period. The symptoms of dysphagia in cerebral hemispheric stroke depend on site, type and extent of infarct. Commonly, these strokes interfere with intent, planning, programming, sequencing and efficient execution of sensory-motoric commands for eating and swallowing. Strokes of sensory-motor cortex impair the oral and pharyngeal movements on the contralateral side of the body. Stroke in the frontal cortex affects cognitive involvement in eating such as concentrating on the feeding activity, extreme distractibility during meal times etc.

The characteristics also depend on the brain hemisphere involved in stroke. Published evidence suggest that left-sided lesions impair oral stages of swallowing while pharyngeal stages are impaired predominantly in right-sided lesions (Logemann et al.,1993; Teasell, Bach, and McRae, 1994). Hemorrhagic strokes are more devastating compared to ischemic strokes but are less common compared to ischemic strokes. Strokes that involve the subcortical structures and basal ganglia can result in bilateral impairment while unilateral hemispheric strokes affect the contralateral side only. Bilateral strokes are associated more frequently with dysphagia compared to unilateral strokes.

Early signs of dysphagia include difficulty managing oral secretions resulting in drooling or pooling, dysphonia, wet/gurgly voice before or after swallow, and abnormal gag reflex. The severity of symptoms may be influenced by the cognitive state of the individual, level of consciousness and also the orientation. Presence of symptoms of dysphagia indicates that the person may not be ready to re-start oral feeding. Also, individuals with posterior circulation strokes show signs of cough, abnormal gag reflex and dysphonia as symptoms of aspiration. Lateral medullary syndrome (Wallenburg syndrome) that results from thrombosis of the posteroinferior cerebellar artery differs from other strokes with increased tongue force for oral clearance.

Careful evaluation using clinical and instrumental procedures is necessary for various reasons. First, the most appropriate feeding method can be installed in place at the earliest. Second, adequate nutrition and hydration promote recovery. Third, mode of emergency medical supply can be decided. Early identification and management of dysphagia is expected to improve the overall treatment outcome by reducing further complications such as pulmonary infections and reducing the duration of hospital stay and related expenditures. Swallowing rehabilitation is especially crucial because stroke is common in the elderly and elderly individuals lose their ability to compensate for age related changes in the musculoskeletal structures post stroke.

COGNITIVE COMMUNICATION DISORDER (CCD/DEMENTIA)

The country is going through massive changes in the population dynamics and the relevance of understanding dysphagia in persons with dementia needs no further emphasis. It is estimated that the oldest range of Indian population (80 plus) will grow at a rate of 500% and will constitute the majority of population by 2050 (Helpage India, 2015) and hence, the incidence of CCD can also be projected to increase. As per the current reports, at least 50% of individuals with dementia experience dysphagia of varying degrees and is likely to increase in another two decades. It is important that the professionals prepare for confronting this enlarging client group.

Disorders of brain and nervous system such as Parkinson's disease (PD), Alzheimer' s disease (AD), Dementia of Lewy Bodies (DLB), Primary Progressive Dementia (PPD), and Fronto-temporal dementia (FTD) show symptoms of swallowing disorders at various stages of the condition. The appearance of initial symptoms of swallowing disorders and its characteristic presentation varies with the underlying medical condition that causes altered cognition and behavior. Dysphagia appears in the initial phases of AD while it may mark the transition to final stages of PD. While sensory processing issues contribute to dysphagia symptoms in AD, the same in PD is motoric in nature. In DLB, dysphagia is mostly cognitive in nature. Presence and progression of dysphagia in individuals with dementia complicate the course of illness and management decisions. Nevertheless, dysphagia makes its entry with all types of degenerative CCD but to varying degree (Affoo, Foley, Rosenbek, Shoemaker, and Martin, 2013; Alagiakrishnan, Bhanji, and Kurian, 2013; Easterling, and Robbins, 2008; Kalia, 2003; Leopold, and Kagel, 1996; Suh, Kim, and Na, 2009).

Symptoms of swallowing disorders appear as pocketing of food, difficulties in chewing and choking or coughing before, during or after swallow of thin or thick bolus. These individuals require frequent reminders about food that is placed inside the mouth and its clearance. Most individuals with dementia fail to identify their state of hunger or food items. Some may also have sensory processing deficits that impair the person's ability to appreciate the sight, smell, texture, consistency or temperature of the food presented. These individuals involved in overeating, compulsive and rapid eating by ingesting large boluses which may result in choking. This may turn fatal when they do not process the bolus flow through the pharynx that is necessary for initiating respiratory decoupling. Silent aspiration should be suspected in individuals with dementia with sensory processing deficits.

Swallowing difficulties in dementia with gradually declining motor movements start off as oral phase deficits. Liquids swallows are commonly the first to face difficulty followed by anterior leakage of liquids through lips and posterior spillage leading to cough or choking. Gradually the symptoms worsen with severely restricted oral movement dynamics that significantly increase the oral transit time. As the stages of illness progress, pharyngeal movements gets restricted with inadequate posterior retraction of tongue base to initiate the swallow and diminished pharyngeal responses to initiated swallow reflex. Restricted hyo-laryngeal elevation and weakened activity of cricopharyngeus muscles lead to severe pharyngeal dysphagia. Individuals with severe oro-pharyngeal dysphagia should be carefully evaluated for aspiration episodes using instrumental techniques. Along with cognitive decline, many also have associated apraxia of limbs or oro-facial structures. This restricts self-feeding skills and also impairs the oral stage of swallow with erroneous motor sequences. Consequences of unmanaged dysphagia are extreme weight loss, dehydration, and malnutrition (Easterling and Robbins, 2008; Hudson, Daubert, and Mills, 2000; Mendez, Friedman, and Castell, 1991; Mion, McDowell, and Heaney, 1994) that challenges the overall health and rehabilitation. Aspiration pneumonia remains as the most common cause of death in individuals with dementia.

CONCLUSION

Dysphagia or difficulty in swallowing is very common in PsWCD and affects all age groups irrespective of being a new born or a geriatric. The characteristic symptoms that may be present in each group of communication disorders vary. In some, dysphagia is behavioral while in others it is purely neurophysiological. Professionals engaged in rehabilitation of these individuals should be aware, alert and appreciate the slightest of indication of this devastating condition. This prevents further complications in the long run by reducing the risk of serious health issues such as lung infections. Identification and making appropriate referrals is important for early intervention and rehabilitation. Assessment and management of swallowing require team inputs and combined efforts of multiple disciplines. Treatments are led by medical professionals while training and rehabilitation are led by SLPs. Most importantly, cooperation and participation of the client and their caregivers decide the success of the management program. This makes a long way into ensuring adequate development or peaceful end-of-life.

FUNDING

This research received no specific grant from any funding agency in the public, commercial, or not-for-profit sectors.

REFERENCES

Affoo, R. H., Foley, N., Rosenbek, J., Shoemaker, K. J., & Martin, R. E. (2013). Swallowing dysfunction and autonomic nervous system dysfunction in Alzheimer's disease: A scoping review of the evidence. *Journal of the American Geriatrics Society*, *61*(12), 2203–2213. doi:10.1111/jgs.12553 PMID:24329892

Ahearn, W. H., Castine, T., Nault, K., & Green, G. (2001). An assessment of food acceptance in children with autism or pervasive developmental disorder-not otherwise specified. *Journal of Autism and Developmental Disorders*, *31*(5), 505–511. doi:10.1023/A:1012221026124 PMID:11794415

Alagiakrishnan, K., Bhanji, R. A., & Kurian, M. (2013). Evaluation and management of oropharyngeal dysphagia in different types of dementia: A systematic review. *Archives of Gerontology and Geriatrics*, *56*(1), 1–9. doi:10.1016/j.archger.2012.04.011 PMID:22608838

Arvedson, J., & Brodsky, L. (2002). *Pediatric Swallowing and Feeding*. New York, NY: Singular.

Ayuse, T., Ishitobi, S., Yoshida, H., Nogami, T., Kurata, S., Hoshino, Y., & Oi, K. (2010). The mandible advancement may alter the coordination between breathing and the non-nutritive swallowing reflex. *Journal of Oral Rehabilitation*, *37*(5), 336–345. doi:10.1111/j.1365-2842.2010.02067.x PMID:20337868

Bader, C. A., & Niemann, G. (2010). Dysphagia in children with cerebral palsy-fiber optic-endoscopic findings. *Laryngo- Rhino- Otologie*, *89*(2), 90–94. doi:10.1055-0029-1237348 PMID:19728257

Bamford, O., Taciak, V., & Gewolb, I. H. (1992). The relationship between rhythmic swallowing and breathing during suckle feeding in term neonates. *Pediatric Research*, *31*(6), 619–624. doi:10.1203/00006450-199206000-00016 PMID:1635825

Benfer, K. A., Weir, K. A., & Boyd, R. N. (2012). Clinimetrics of measures of oropharyngeal dysphagia for preschool children with cerebral palsy and neurodevelopmental disabilities: A systematic review. *Developmental Medicine and Child Neurology*, *54*(9), 784–795. doi:10.1111/j.1469-8749.2012.04302.x PMID:22582745

Bowers, L. (2002). An audit of referrals of children with autistic spectrum disorder to the dietetic service. *Journal of Human Nutrition and Dietetics*, *15*(2), 141–144. doi:10.1046/j.1365-277X.2002.00345.x PMID:11972743

Bu'Lock, F., Woolridge, M. W., & Baum, J. D. (1990). Development of co-ordination of sucking, swallowing and breathing: Ultrasound study of term and preterm infants. *Developmental Medicine and Child Neurology*, *32*(8), 669–678. doi:10.1111/j.1469-8749.1990.tb08427.x PMID:2210082

Burklow, K. A., Phelps, A. N., Schultz, J. R., McConnell, K., & Rudolph, C. (1998). Classifying complex pediatric feeding disorders. *Journal of Pediatric Gastroenterology and Nutrition*, *27*(2), 143–147. doi:10.1097/00005176-199808000-00003 PMID:9702643

Caron, C. J. J. M., Pluijmers, B. I., Joosten, K. F. M., Mathijssen, I. M. J., Van Der Schroeff, M. P., Dunaway, D. J., ... Koudstaal, M. J. (2015). Feeding difficulties in craniofacial microsomia: A systematic review. *International Journal of Oral and Maxillofacial Surgery*, *44*(6), 732–737. doi:10.1016/j.ijom.2015.02.014 PMID:25771070

Casas, M. J., Kenny, D. J., & McPherson, K. A. (1994). Swallowing/ventilation interactions during oral swallow in normal children and children with cerebral palsy. *Dysphagia*, *9*(1), 40–46. doi:10.1007/BF00262758 PMID:8131424

Chatoor, I. (2009). Sensory food aversions in infant and toddlers. *Journal of Zero to Three*, *29*(3), 43–49.

Cheong, J. L., Doyle, L. W., Burnett, A. C., Lee, K. J., Walsh, J. M., Potter, C. R., ... Spittle, A. J. (2017). Association between moderate and late preterm birth and neurodevelopment and social-emotional development at age 2 years. *JAMA Pediatrics*, *171*(4), e164805–e164805. doi:10.1001/jamapediatrics.2016.4805 PMID:28152144

Clancy, K. J., & Hustad, K. C. (2011). Longitudinal changes in feeding among children with cerebral palsy between the ages of 4 and 7 years. *Developmental Neurorehabilitation*, *14*(4), 191–198. doi:10.3109/17518423.2011.568467 PMID:21732803

Collins, M. S., Kyle, R., Smith, S., Laverty, A., & Roberts, S., and Eaton- Evans, J. (. (2003). Coping with the unusual family diet: Eating behavior and food choices of children with Down's syndrome, autistic spectrum disorders or cri du chat syndrome and comparison groups of siblings. *Journal of Learning Disabilities*, *7*, 137–155. doi:10.1177/1469004703007002004

Cooke, R. J., Ford, A., Werkman, S., Conner, C., & Watson, D. (1993). Postnatal growth in infants born between 700 and 1,500g. *Journal of Pediatric Gastroenterology and Nutrition*, *16*(2), 130–135. doi:10.1097/00005176-199302000-00006 PMID:8450378

Cornish, E. (1998). A balanced approach towards healthy eating in autism. *Journal of Human Nutrition and Dietetics*, *11*(6), 501–509. doi:10.1046/j.1365-277X.1998.00132.x

Cornish, E. (2002). Gluten and casein free diets in autism: A study of the effects on food choice and nutrition. *Journal of Human Nutrition and Dietetics*, *15*(4), 261–269. doi:10.1046/j.1365-277X.2002.00372.x PMID:12153499

Couriel, J. M., Bisset, R., Miller, R., Thomas, A., & Clarke, M. (1993). Assessment of feeding problems in neurodevelopmental handicap: A team approach. *Archives of Disease in Childhood*, *69*(5), 609–613. doi:10.1136/adc.69.5.609 PMID:7504911

Culley, W. J., & Middleton, T. O. (1969). Caloric requirements of mentally retarded children with and without motor dysfunction. *The Journal of Pediatrics*, *75*(3), 380–384. doi:10.1016/S0022-3476(69)80262-3 PMID:5804183

Daniels, S. K. (2000). Swallowing apraxia: A disorder of the Praxis system? *Dysphagia*, *15*(3), 159–166. doi:10.1007004550010019 PMID:10839830

Daniels, S. K., Brailey, K., Priestly, D. H., Herrington, L. R., Weisberg, L. A., & Foundas, A. L. (1998). Aspiration in patients with acute stroke. *Archives of Physical Medicine and Rehabilitation*, *79*(1), 14–19. doi:10.1016/S0003-9993(98)90200-3 PMID:9440410 de Kieviet, J. F., Piek, J. P., Aarnoudse-Moens, C. S., & Oosterlaan, J. (2009). Motor development in very preterm and very low-birth-weight children from birth to adolescence: A meta-analysis. *Journal of the American Medical Association*, *302*(20), 2235–2242. doi:10.1001/jama.2009.1708 PMID:19934425

Del Giudice, E., Staiano, A., Capano, G., Romano, A., Florimonte, L., Miele, E., ... Crisanti, A. F. (1999). Gastrointestinal manifestations in children with cerebral palsy. *Brain & Development*, *21*(5), 307–311. doi:10.1016/S0387-7604(99)00025-X PMID:10413017

Dobbelsteyn, C., Peacocke, S. D., Blake, K., Crist, W., & Rashid, M. (2008). Feeding difficulties in children with CHARGE syndrome: Prevalence, risk factors, and prognosis. *Dysphagia*, *23*(2), 127–135. doi:10.100700455-007-9111-6 PMID:18027028

Easterling, C. S., & Robbins, E. (2008). Dementia and dysphagia. *Geriatric Nursing*, *29*(4), 275–285. doi:10.1016/j.gerinurse.2007.10.015 PMID:18694703

Ehrenkranz, R. A., Younes, N., Lemons, J. A., Fanaroff, A. A., Donovan, E. F., Wright, L. L., ... Papile, L.-A. (1999). Longitudinal growth of hospitalized very low birth weight infants. *Pediatrics*, *104*(2), 280–289. doi:10.1542/peds.104.2.280 PMID:10429008

Ekberg, O., Hamdy, S., Woisard, V., Wuttge–Hannig, A., & Ortega, P. (2002). Social and psychological burden of dysphagia: Its impact on diagnosis and treatment. *Dysphagia*, *17*(2), 139–146. doi:10.100700455-001-0113-5 PMID:11956839

Erkin, G., Culha, C., Ozel, S., & Kirbiyik, E. G. (2010). Feeding and gastrointestinal problems in children with cerebral palsy. *International Journal of Rehabilitation Research. Internationale Zeitschrift fur Rehabilitationsforschung. Revue Internationale de Recherches de Readaptation*, *33*(3), 218–224. doi:10.1097/MRR.0b013e3283375e10 PMID:20216224

Farri, A., Accornero, A., & Burdese, C. (2007). The social importance of Dysphagia: Its impact on diagnosis and therapy. *Acta Otorhinolaryngologica Italica*, *27*(2), 83–86. PMID:17608136

Field, D., Garland, M., & Williams, K. (2003). Correlates of specific childhood feeding problems. *Journal of Paediatrics and Child Health*, *39*(4), 299–304. doi:10.1046/j.1440-1754.2003.00151.x PMID:12755939

Fredericks, D. W., Carr, J. E., & Williams, W. L. (1998). Overview of the treatment of rumination disorder for adults in a residential setting. *Journal of Behavior Therapy and Experimental Psychiatry*, *29*(1), 31–40. doi:10.1016/S0005-7916(98)00002-0 PMID:9627823

Geschwind, N. (1975). The apraxias: Neural mechanisms of disorders of learned movement: The anatomical organization of the language areas and motor systems of the human brain clarifies apraxic disorders and throws new light on cerebral dominance. *American Scientist*, *63*(2), 188–195. PMID:1115438

Gewolb, I. H., Vice, F. L., Schweitzer-Kenney, E. L., Taciak, V. L., & Bosma, J. F. (2001). Developmental patterns of rhythmic suck and swallow in preterm infants. *Developmental Medicine and Child Neurology*, *43*(1), 22–27. doi:10.1017/S0012162201000044 PMID:11201418

Gisel, E. G., & Patrick, J. (1988). Identification of children with cerebral palsy unable to maintain a normal nutritional state. *Lancet*, *1*(8580), 283–286. doi:10.1016/S0140-6736(88)90360-1 PMID:2893092

Grunau, R. E., Whitfield, M. F., Petrie-Thomas, J., Synnes, A. R., Cepeda, I. L., Keidar, A., ... Johannesen, D. (2009). Neonatal pain, parenting stress and interaction, in relation to cognitive and motor development at 8 and 18 months in preterm infants. *Pain*, *143*(1), 138–146. doi:10.1016/j.pain.2009.02.014 PMID:19307058

Hirst, M. (1985). Young adults with disabilities: Health, employment and financial costs for family carers. *Child: Care, Health and Development*, *11*(5), 291–307. doi:10.1111/j.1365-2214.1985.tb00471.x PMID:2934179

Horner, J., & Massey, E. W. (1988). Silent aspiration following stroke. *Neurology*, *38*(2), 317–319. doi:10.1212/WNL.38.2.317 PMID:3340301

Horner, J., Massey, E. W., Riski, J. E., Lathrop, D. L., & Chase, K. N. (1988). Aspiration following stroke: Clinical correlates and outcome. *Neurology*, *38*(9), 1359–1362. doi:10.1212/WNL.38.9.1359 PMID:3412582

Hornman, J., de Winter, A. F., Kerstjens, J. M., Bos, A. F., & Reijneveld, S. A. (2016). Emotional and behavioral problems of preterm and full-term children at school entry. *Pediatrics*, *137*(5), e20152255. doi:10.1542/peds.2015-2255 PMID:27244786

Hudson, H. M., Daubert, C. R., & Mills, R. H. (2000). The interdependency of protein-energy malnutrition, aging and dysphagia. *Dysphagia*, *15*(1), 31–38. doi:10.1007004559910007 PMID:10594256

Hutton, J. L., Pharoah, P. O., Cooke, R. W., & Stevenson, R. C. (1997). Differential effects of preterm birth and small gestational age on cognitive and motor development. *Archives of Disease in Childhood. Fetal and Neonatal Edition*, *76*(2), F75–F81. doi:10.1136/fn.76.2.F75 PMID:9135284

Johnson, C. B., & Deitz, J. C. (1985). Time use of mothers with pre-school children: A pilot study. *The American Journal of Occupational Therapy*, *39*(9), 578–583. doi:10.5014/ajot.39.9.578 PMID:2931990

Johnston, J. M. (1993). Phenomenology and treatment of rumination. *Eating and Growth Disorders*, *2*, 93–107.

Kalia, M. (2003). Dysphagia and aspiration pneumonia in patients with Alzheimer's disease. *Metabolism: Clinical and Experimental*, *52*, 36–38. doi:10.1016/S0026-0495(03)00300-7 PMID:14577062

Kennedy, J. G. III, & Kent, R. D. (1988). Physiological substrates of normal deglutition. *Dysphagia*, *3*(1), 24–37. doi:10.1007/BF02406277 PMID:3073916

Khansa, I., Hall, C., Madhoun, L., Splaingard, M., Baylis, A., Kirschner, R., & Pearson, G. (2016). Prospective evaluation of airway and feeding outcomes of mandibular distraction, tongue-lip adhesion and conservative management in Pierre-robin sequence. *The Cleft Palate-Craniofacial Journal*, *53*(4), E148.

Kientz, M. A., & Dunn, W. (1997). A comparison of the performance of children with and without autism on the sensory profile. *The American Journal of Occupational Therapy*, *51*(7), 530–537. doi:10.5014/ajot.51.7.530 PMID:9242859

Kim, J. S., Han, Z. A., Song, D. H., Oh, H. M., & Chung, M. E. (2013). Characteristics of dysphagia in children with cerebral palsy, related to gross motor dysfunction. *American Journal of Physical Medicine & Rehabilitation*, *92*(10), 912–919. doi:10.1097/PHM.0b013e318296dd99 PMID:23739271

Konarski, E. A., Favell, J. E., & Favell, J. E. (1992). *Manual for the assessment and treatment of the behavior disorders of people with mental retardation*. Western Carolina Center Foundation.

Krick, J., & Van Duyn, M. A. (1984). The relationship between oral-motor involvement and growth: A pilot study in a pediatric population with cerebral palsy. *Journal of the American Dietetic Association*, *84*(5), 555–559. PMID:6715752

Lau, C. (2006). Oral feeding in the preterm infant. *NeoReviews*, *7*(1), e19–e27. doi:10.1542/neo.7-1-e19

Lau, C., Smith, E. O., & Schanler, R. J. (2003). Coordination of suck-swallow and swallow respiration in preterm infants. *Acta Paediatrica (Oslo, Norway)*, *92*(6), 721–727. doi:10.1111/j.1651-2227.2003.tb00607.x PMID:12856985

Ledford, J. R., & Gast, D. L. (2006). Feeding problems in children with autism spectrum disorders: A review. *Focus on Autism and Other Developmental Disabilities*, *21*(3), 153–166. doi:10.1177/10883576060210030401

Leonard, R., & Kendall, K. (1997). Dysphagia Assessment and Treatment Planning: A Team Approach. San Diego, CA: Singular Publishing Group, Inc.

Leopold, N. A., & Kagel, M. C. (1996). Prepharyngeal dysphagia in Parkinson's disease. *Dysphagia*, *11*(1), 14–22. doi:10.1007/BF00385794 PMID:8556872

Linden, P., & Siebens, A. A. (1983). Dysphagia: Predicting laryngeal penetration. *Archives of Physical Medicine and Rehabilitation*, *64*(6), 281–284. PMID:6860100

Linscheid, T. R. (1983). Eating problems in children. In C. E. Walker & M. C. Roberts (Eds.), *Handbook of Clinical Child Psychology* (pp. 616–639). New York: Wiley.

Lobstein, T. (1991). *The Nutrition of Women on Low Income*. London: Food Commission.

Logemann, J., Shanahan, T., Rademaker, A., Kahrilas, P., Lazar, R., & Halper, A. (1993). Oropharyngeal swallowing after stroke in the left basal ganglion/internal capsule. *Dysphagia*, *8*(3), 230–234. doi:10.1007/BF01354543 PMID:8359043

Logemann, J. A. (1998). The evaluation and treatment of swallowing disorders. *Current Opinion in Otolaryngology & Head & Neck Surgery*, *6*(6), 395–400. doi:10.1097/00020840-199812000-00008

Logemann, J. A., & Logemann, J. A. (1983). *Evaluation and Treatment of Swallowing Disorders. National Student Speech Hearing Language Association*. NSSHLA.

Masarei, A. G., Sell, D., Habel, A., Mars, M., Sommerlad, B. C., & Wade, A. (2007). The nature of feeding in infants with unrepaired cleft lip and/or palate compared with healthy noncleft infants. *The Cleft Palate-Craniofacial Journal*, *44*(3), 321–328. doi:10.1597/05-185 PMID:17477749

Matson, J. L., & Bamburg, J. W. (1999). A descriptive study of pica behavior in persons with mental retardation. *Journal of Developmental and Physical Disabilities*, *11*(4), 353–361. doi:10.1023/A:1021870925227

Matson, J. L., Fodstad, J. C., & Boisjoli, J. A. (2008). Cutoff scores, norms and patterns of feeding problems for the Screening Tool of feeding Problems (STEP) for adults with intellectual disabilities. *Research in Developmental Disabilities*, *29*(4), 363–372. doi:10.1016/j.ridd.2007.06.001 PMID:17662575

Matson, J. L., Gardner, W. I., Coe, D. A., & Sovner, R. (1991). A scale for evaluating emotional disorders in severely and profoundly mentally retarded persons. Development of the Diagnostic Assessment for the Severely Handicapped (DASH) Scale. *The British Journal of Psychiatry*, *159*(03), 404–409. doi:10.1192/bjp.159.3.404 PMID:1958951

Matson, J. L., & Kuhn, D. E. (2001). Identifying feeding problems in mentally retarded persons: Development and reliability of the screening tool of feeding problems (STEP). *Research in Developmental Disabilities*, *22*(2), 165–172. doi:10.1016/S0891-4222(01)00065-8 PMID:11325163

Mendez, L., Friedman, L., & Castell, L. (1991). Swallowing disorders in the elderly. *Clinics in Geriatric Medicine*, *7*, 215–230. PMID:1855155

Mion, L. C., McDowell, J. A., & Heaney, L. K. (1994). Nutritional assessment of the elderly in the ambulatory care setting. *Nurse Practitioner Forum*, *5*(1), 46–51. PMID:8148658

Mizuno, K., & Ueda, A. (2003). The maturation and coordination of sucking, swallowing, and respiration in preterm infants. *The Journal of Pediatrics*, *142*(1), 36–40. doi:10.1067/mpd.2003.mpd0312 PMID:12520252

Mosier, H. D., Grossman, H. J., & Dingman, H. F. (1965). Physical growth in mental defectives. *Pediatrics*, *36*(3), 465–519. PMID:5825691

Nixon, G. M., Charbonneau, I., Kermack, A. S., Brouillette, R. T., & McFarland, D. H. (2008). Respiratory-swallowing interactions during sleep in premature infants at term. *Respiratory Physiology & Neurobiology*, *160*(1), 76–82. doi:10.1016/j.resp.2007.08.010 PMID:17942377

Ortiz, K. Z., & Marinelli, M. R. (2013). Investigation on the complaint of dysphagia in aphasic patients. *Revista CEFAC*, *15*(6), 1503–1511. doi:10.1590/S1516-18462013005000043

Paes, E. C., de Vries, I. A., Penris, W. M., Hanny, K. H., Lavrijsen, S. W., van Leerdam, E. K., ... Breugem, C. C. (2017). Growth and prevalence of feeding difficulties in children with Robin sequence: A retrospective cohort study. *Clinical Oral Investigations*, *21*(6), 2063–2076. doi:10.100700784-016-1996-8 PMID:27868158

Patel, M. R., & Piazza, C. C. (2001). Your finicky eater: A guide for parents. *Exceptional Parent*, *31*(6), 82–84.

Perske, R., Clifton, A., McClean, B. M., & Stein, J. I. (1977). *Meal Times for Severely and Profoundly Handicapped Persons: New Concepts and Attitudes*. Baltimore, MD: University Park Press.

Poindexter, B. B., & Ehrenkranz, R. A. (2015). Nutrient requirements and provision of nutritional support in the premature neonate. In R. J. Martin, A. A. Fanaroff, & M. C. Walsh (Eds.), *Neonatal-Perinatal Medicine* (10th ed.). Philadelphia, PA: Elsevier.

Qureshi, M. A., Vice, F. L., Taciak, V. L., Bosma, J. F., & Gewolb, I. H. (2002). Changes in rhythmic suckle feeding patterns in term infants in the first month of life. *Developmental Medicine and Child Neurology*, *44*(1), 34–39. doi:10.1017/S0012162201001621 PMID:11811648

Reid, J., Reilly, S., & Kilpatrick, N. (2007). Sucking performance of babies with cleft conditions. *The Cleft Palate-Craniofacial Journal*, *44*(3), 312–320. doi:10.1597/05-173 PMID:17477747

Reilly, S., Skuse, D., & Poblete, X. (1996). Prevalence of feeding problems and oral motor dysfunction in children with cerebral palsy: A community survey. *The Journal of Pediatrics*, *129*(6), 877–882. doi:10.1016/S0022-3476(96)70032-X PMID:8969730

Rempel, G. R., Colwell, S. O., & Nelson, R. P. (1988). Growth in children with cerebral palsy fed via gastrostomy. *Pediatrics*, *82*, 857–863. PMID:3186375

Rezaei, M., Rashedi, V., Gharib, M., & Lotfi, G. (2011). Prevalence of feeding problems in children with intellectual disability. *Iranian Rehabilitation Journal*, *9*, 56–59.

Riordan, M. M., Iwata, B. A., Finney, J. W., Wohl, M. K., & Stanley, A. E. (1984). Behavioral assessment and treatment of chronic food refusal in handicapped children. *Journal of Applied Behavior Analysis*, *17*(3), 327–341. doi:10.1901/jaba.1984.17-327 PMID:6239853

Rogers, B., Arvedson, J., Buck, G., Smart, P., & Msall, M. (1994). Characteristics of dysphagia in children with cerebral palsy. *Dysphagia*, *9*(1), 69–73. doi:10.1007/BF00262762 PMID:8131428

Ruby, D. O., & Matheny, W. D. (1962). Comments on growth of cerebral palsied children. *Journal of the American Dietetic Association*, *40*, 525–527. PMID:14494972

Sakalidis, V. S., Kent, J. C., Garbin, C. P., Hepworth, A. R., Hartmann, P. E., & Geddes, D. T. (2013). Longitudinal changes in suck-swallow-breathe, oxygen saturation, and heart rate patterns in term breastfeeding infants. *Journal of Human Lactation*, *29*(2), 236–245. doi:10.1177/0890334412474864 PMID:23492760

Schreck, K. A., Williams, K., & Smith, A. F. (2004). A comparison of eating behaviors between children with and without autism. *Journal of Autism and Developmental Disorders*, *34*(4), 433–438. doi:10.1023/B:JADD.0000037419.78531.86 PMID:15449518

Selley, W. G., Ellis, R. E., Flack, F. C., & Brooks, W. A. (1990). Coordination of sucking, swallowing and breathing in the newborn: Its relationship to infant feeding and normal development. *International Journal of Language & Communication Disorders*, *25*(3), 311–327. doi:10.3109/13682829009011980 PMID:2095838

Shapiro, B. K., Green, P., Krick, J., Allen, D., & Capute, A. J. (1986). Growth of severely impaired children: Neurological versus nutritional factors. *Developmental Medicine and Child Neurology*, *28*(6), 729–733. doi:10.1111/j.1469-8749.1986.tb03924.x PMID:3817311

Sisson, L. A., & Van Hasselt, V. B. (1989). Feeding Disorders. In J. K. Luiselli (Ed.), *Behavioral Medicine and Developmental Disabilities. Disorders of Human Learning, Behavior, and Communication* (pp. 45–73). New York, NY: Springer. doi:10.1007/978-1-4613-8844-9_3

Skuse, D., Pickles, A., Wolke, D., & Reilly, S. (1994). Postnatal growth and mental development: Evidence for a "sensitive period". *Journal of Child Psychology and Psychiatry, and Allied Disciplines, 35*(3), 521–545. doi:10.1111/j.1469-7610.1994.tb01738.x PMID:7515070

Su, B. H. (2014). Optimizing nutrition in preterm infants. *Pediatrics and Neonatology, 55*(1), 5–13. doi:10.1016/j.pedneo.2013.07.003 PMID:24050843

Suh, M. K., Kim, H., & Na, D. L. (2009). Dysphagia in patients with dementia: Alzheimer versus vascular. *Alzheimer Disease and Associated Disorders, 23*(2), 178–184. doi:10.1097/WAD.0b013e318192a539 PMID:19474573

Teasell, R. W., Bach, D., & McRae, M. (1994). Prevalence and recovery of aspiration post stroke: A retrospective analysis. *Dysphagia, 9*(1), 35–39. doi:10.1007/BF00262757 PMID:8131423

Tobis, J. S., Saturen, P., Larios, G., & Posnaik, A. O. (1961). Study of growth patterns in cerebral palsy. *Archives of Physical Medicine and Rehabilitation, 42*, 475–481. PMID:13777130

Tuch, B. E., & Nielson, J. M. (1941). Apraxia of swallowing. *Bulletin of the Los Angeles Neurological Society, 6*, 52–54.

van den Engel-Hoek, L., Erasmus, C. E., Hendriks, J. C., Geurts, A. C., Klein, W. M., Pillen, S., ... de Groot, I. J. (2013). Oral muscles are progressively affected in Duchenne muscular dystrophy: Implications for dysphagia treatment. *Journal of Neurology, 260*(5), 1295–1303. doi:10.100700415-012-6793-y PMID:23263593

Volkert, V. M., & Vaz, P. (2010). Recent studies on feeding problems in children with autism. *Journal of Applied Behavior Analysis, 43*(1), 155–159. doi:10.1901/jaba.2010.43-155 PMID:20808508

Weir, K., McMahon, S., Barry, L., Ware, R., Masters, I. B., & Chang, A. B. (2007). Oropharyngeal aspiration and pneumonia in children. *Pediatric Pulmonology, 42*(11), 1024–1031. doi:10.1002/ppul.20687 PMID:17893917

Williams, P. G., Dalrymple, N., & Neal, J. (2000). Eating habits of children with autism. *Pediatric Nursing, 26*(3), 259–264. PMID:12026389

Wolf, L., & Glass, R. (1992). *Feeding and Swallowing Disorders in Infancy: Assessment and Management*. Tucson, AZ: Therapy Skill Builders.

KEY TERMS AND DEFINITIONS

Aspiration: Entry of swallowed food or liquid into the region below vocal folds.

Aspiration Pneumonia: An infection of lungs caused by continued breathing in and accumulation of food/liquid into the airway.

Bradycardia: Slowing down of heart rate.

Communication Disorders: Any condition that hinders a person from expressing their needs and ideas due to difficulties in understanding and formulating language or execution of speech.

Failure to Thrive: Children who do not gain weight or are gaining weight inappropriately leading to survival difficulties.

Hypoplasia: Underdevelopment or incomplete development of a structure.

Mastication: The process of chewing to break down food particles so that it can be swallowed safely.

Non-Oral Feeding: The process of ingesting nutrition/hydration through methods other than the mouth. For example, tube feeding.

Penetration: Entry of swallowed food or liquid into the airway region above vocal folds.

Quality of Life: All parameters that can measure the general physical, personal, and social wellbeing of an individual.

Respiratory Apnea: A period of absence of breathing. In swallowing, apnea is the output of airway decoupling that is important in ensuring a safe swallow.

Sensory Processing: A function that receives information from peripheral senses and processes it to a motor or behavioral response.

Video-Fluroscopy: A radiological imaging procedure.

Chapter 10
Subjective Fatigue in Children and Adults:
Evidence From the Research on Speech Perception and Cognitive Abilities

Saransh Jain
JSS Institute of Speech and Hearing, India

Suma Raju
JSS Institute of Speech and Hearing, India

ABSTRACT

Fatigue is a common yet poorly understood topic. The psychological, physiological, social, emotional, and cognitive wellbeing of a person may be affected due to fatigue. Despite a century of research in understanding the effect of fatigue on human systems, there is no concrete explanation as how fatigue affects the perception of speech. Fatigue impairs auditory cognition and the reduced cognitive abilities further increase mental and physical fatigue. Since cognition is markedly affected in individuals experiencing mental fatigue, its consequences are widespread. According to the top-down approach of auditory processing, there is a direct link between cognition and speech perception. Thus, in the present chapter, the influence of fatigue on perception is reviewed. It is noted that the impact of fatigue on cognition and quality of life is different for children and adults. Training in music, meditation, and exposure to more than one language are some of the measures that help to reduce the effect of fatigue and improve cognitive abilities in both children as well as in adults.

INTRODUCTION

Our fatigue is often caused not by work, but by worry, frustration and resentment. Dale Carnegie (1888-1955)

Fatigue is a complex construct which can be defined in many ways. There is no universal definition of fatigue. The definition may vary with reference to the focus of the study and the person defining it. For

DOI: 10.4018/978-1-5225-4955-0.ch010

e.g. for a layman, fatigue is the feeling of tiredness after coming back from work place, and it fades off after sufficient rest; but for a clinical psychologist/psychiatrist, fatigue is a pathology which is often secondary to many neuro-psychological conditions, and require appropriate medical/rehabilitative attention. In general, fatigue is a subjective feeling of tiredness which is gradual in nature (Hawley and Reilly, 1997). It is a common symptom of almost every medical and psychiatric health condition as well as in non-pathological physical and psychological strain and stress (Radovic and Malmgren, 1998). Fatigue is not a disorder by itself, however, its existence may indicate multiple physical, physiological, psychological, cognitive and related disorders. Fatigue can be classified as being physical or mental in origin. Physical fatigue refers to the transient inability of the body muscles to maintain optimal physical performances (Gandevia, 2012), whereas mental fatigue may cause a temporary or permanent reduction in the cognitive abilities due to prolonged mental activities (Marcora, Staiano, and Manning, 2009).

Fatigue influences daily life and it is experienced by all human beings at many points throughout their lifespan. It is the most common complaint heard in primary healthcare settings (Wessely, Hotopf, and Sharpe, 1999). Yet, fatigue is seldom being studied and is poorly understood. Researchers do not really know much about fatigue despite more than 100 years of research. Still there is no mature theory of its origin or function (Hockey, 2013). The impact of fatigue is widespread and varies with children or adults. Thus, it is essential to understand the physiology behind fatigue and the effect of fatigue on speech perception and auditory cognition of the human beings. In the meantime, it is also important to discuss certain evidence-based measures to reduce the effect of fatigue and to improve the quality of life. In the present chapter, the authors tried to review some of the studies showing the effect of fatigue on cognitive abilities in children and adults, while high lighting the interconnections between cognition and speech perception, and possible measures to reduce the negative impact of fatigue.

CLASSIFICATION OF FATIGUE

Fatigue can be caused because of physical and/or mental exertion. Physical fatigue is the temporary inability of a muscle to perform optimally, and is usually reversible, i.e. the fatigue disappears after taking sufficient rest. It is usually due to excessive physical exertion, sleep deprivation, and may be because of poor overall health. This results in the lack of energy in the muscles, and the overall reduction in the control of the central nervous system over the peripheral body organs (Gandevia, 2001). Mental fatigue, on the other hand, is defined as temporary or permanent inability of the human brain to maintain optimal cognitive performances. Mental fatigue has also shown to be increased after excessive physical exercise(Marcora et al., 2009). But, unlike physical fatigue, mental fatigue results in more rigorous neuro-physiological changes.

Physical and mental fatigue is governed by different underlying processes. They are separate biological functions, but they may co-exist. For e.g. If one is physically exhausted, he/she may have difficulty in running, lifting, or playing, but their alertness and concentration will remain intact. On the other hand, when a person is mentally exhausted, his/her alertness will suffer but physical performance will be preserved. However, in certain circumstances, when a person is physically exhausted, his/her mental performance is affected, and vice versa. Experimental evidences suggested that mental fatigue limits the exercise tolerance in human beings and results in reduced threshold of physical fatigue (Marcora et al., 2009). The researchers attributed the co-morbidity of physical and mental fatigue as a consequence of neuro-physiological changes regulating fatigue in the human brain.

A series of physiological changes in the nervous system has been reported secondary to mental fatigue. Fan, Zhou, Liu and Zie (2015) did an electroencephalographic assessment of individuals suffering from mental fatigue. They reported increased alpha activity in the frontal, central, posterior temporal, parietal, and occipital lobes; and a dip in the beta activity in the pre-frontal, inferior frontal, posterior temporal and occipital lobes. The findings of many other research studies were also in the similar lines (Lal and Craig, 2001; Makeig and Jung, 1995; Okogbaa, Shell, and Filipusic, 1994; Wijesuriya, Tran, Thuraisingham, Nguyen, and Craig, 2008). Supporting evidences of reduction in frontal lobe potential amplitude for mentally fatiguing tasks are also available (Lorist, Boksem, and Ridderinkhof, 2005). fMRI studies of long duration psychomotor vigilance test task have also shown the evidence of reduced frontal-parietal activity with fatigue (Lim et al., 2010). Activity in the fronto-parietal network was lower during post fatigue condition compared to pre fatigue condition. The cerebral blood flow also decreased in this region in a manner correlated with a decline in task performance. Theta signal activity was reduced in the frontal executive network. This was in congruence with the increased alpha activity signals in the parietal regions (Murta, Leite, Carmichael, Figueiredo, and Lemieux, 2015). Researchers agreed with the notion that growing mental fatigue produces a shift away from executive function andattention and is accompanied by a shift in alpha frequency to the lower alpha band. Although electrophysiological evidence showing the effect of mental fatigue is limited, there are abundant behavioral manifestations.

Another classification of fatigue is based on the duration. On the basis of duration of symptoms, fatigue can be classified as recent (lasting from less than one month), prolonged (symptoms lasting from more than one month up to six months) and chronic fatigue (lasting from more than six months) (Griffith and Zarrouf, 2008). Studies have shown that the cognitive and perceptual symptoms of fatigue are visible mostly in the chronic stage (Jason, Boulton, Porter, Jessen, and Njoku, 2010). Thus, there is a direct relation between the duration of fatigue and its behavior manifestation. Some authors have also attempted to classify fatigue on the basis of its origin, as central (brain-derived) or peripheral (neuromuscular)(Jason et al., 2010). However, this classification is similar as mental (brain-derived) and physical (neuromuscular) fatigue.

EFFECT OF FATIGUE ON COGNITIVE ABILITIES

There is a close relationship between fatigue and cognitive abilities. On one hand, some researchers have reported that mild physical exercise improves individuals cognitive functioning (Hancock and McNaughton, 1986), whereas others have reported a marked reduction in cognitive abilities secondary to mental fatigue (Cian et al., 2000; Cian, Barraud, Melin, and Raphel, 2001). In the present chapter, the authors have restricted their review to the effect of mental fatigue on the cognitive performances. Further, the relationship between cognition and speech perception is reviewed, in the quest to establish an indirect liaising between fatigue and speech perception. The effect of mental fatigue on the cognitive performances can be seen in children as well as in adults. Consequently, the impact of subjective mental fatigue on the performance is also different for children and adults.

Ishii, Tanaka and Watanabe (2014) proposed a "dual regulation system model" to maintain cognitive task performances in mental fatigue. This model works on the dual performance of mental facilitation and inhibition. The mental workload activates the mental facilitation system to maintain cognitive performance. The mental facilitation increases the motivation activation, which in turn improves cognitive task performances. Contrarily, mental workload also activates mental inhibition. Mental inhibition impairs the cognitive performances. The tradeoff between mental facilitation and mental inhibition determines whether cognitive abilities are improved, maintained or reduced. When the fatigue activates mental inhibition more than mental facilitation, cognitive performance reduces. Thus, fatigue and cognitive abilities are related to each other. Below, some of the research findings examining this relationship are discussed.

EFFECT OF MENTAL FATIGUE ON COGNITIVE PERFORMANCE

In Children

Fatigue is a common complaint of children in a range of medical and psychological health conditions. Viner and Christie (2005) stated that around 33% of the young children experience fatigue at least 3-4 times a week. It is often associated with sleep deprivation, lethargy, poor general physical health and associated symptoms. Headaches and muscle aches, chronicity lasting for more than three months, stomach ache and back ache, and chronic pain are common symptoms associated with fatigue (Viner and Christie, 2005). It is also associated with a variety of negative social and psycho-educational problems in children (Eddy and Cruz, 2007; Garralda and Rangel, 2002).

Researchers have indicated that fatigue is associated with significant impairment of cognitive performances in children. Hanasoge, Ahmed, and Jain (2017) have reported that those children who are poor in their academic skills also have increased the subjective perception of fatigue. These findings were in congruence with their auditory cognitive skills. Verbal working memory, as assessed using forward and backward digit span test and verbal-visual working memory, as measured using operation span test, scores were below the normal range for children who were poor academic achievers. A structured equation model comparing subjective fatigue, academic performance and working memory abilities revealed an association between the three measures. These findings were in agreement with the earlier reports (Kahol et al., 2008; Shanks, Jason, Evans, and Brown, 2013; Tanaka et al., 2012). Cognitive dysfunction in children with fatigue was measured using a cross-sectional study on 120 adolescents (Sulheim et al., 2015). A complete neurocognitive test battery approach was used to measure processing speed, working memory, cognitive inhibition, cognitive flexibility, verbal learning and verbal memory. The results revealed that adolescents with fatigue have impaired cognitive functioning, and working memory and processing speed maximally represents the core cognitive difficulties.

Like working memory, other cognitive domains are also affected in children who experience mental fatigue. Cognitive processing and motor speed were reduced in children as a consequence of fatigue (Neu et al., 2011). Fatigue and sleeplessness were also related with reduced in intelligence quotient and other neuro psychological test scores in children (Mayes, Calhoun, Bixler, and Vgontzas, 2008). Liu et al. (2012) attempted to establish a relationship between fatigue and cognitive performance in Chinese kindergarten children within the age range of 4-6 years. The researchers found that the children, who reported to have fatigue, scored 3-6 points lower in IQ scale, than children who reported no fatigue. Memory and attention problem in 20 children who experienced subjective fatigue was also reported (Haig-Ferguson, Tucker, Eaton, Hunt, and Crawley, 2009). Using four item semi-structured questioner and neuropsychological test battery with 10 psychometric subtests, the researchers reported that attention and verbal memory was markedly affected in children experiencing subjective fatigue.

Deficits in attention and depression were noted in 49 children who were experiencing fatigue (Parrish, Weinstock-Guttman, Smerbeck, Benedict, and Yeh, 2013). All the children were assessed using pediatric quality of life-multidimensional fatigue scale (PedsQL-MFS) and the behavioral assessment of children (BAC, 2nded.). PedsQL-MFS scores fatigue in cognitive, sleep/rest and general domain. The scores on all the three domains were markedly reduced in children experience mental fatigue, as compared to their non-fatiguing counterparts. In another prospective cohort study on 142 elementary and junior high school students, the effect of fatigue on visual information processing and attention was measured (Mizuno et al., 2011). The participants completed paper and pencil based behavioral and computerized cognitive tasks. The testing was done at two time points, first, at the day of the admission to the schools and second, after attending the school for one year. The fatigue was measured using the Japanese version of Chalder fatigue scale. Among 142 students, 40 students confirmed as having fatigue after one year. The multivariate logistic regression analysis for the responses of these 40 students revealed that fatigue caused reduction in the visual information processing speed and attention abilities. The researchers also reported that both visual processing and attention are independent predictors of fatigue in elementary and junior high school students.

Later, in another study (Mizuno, Tanaka, Fukuda, Imai-Matsumura, and Watanabe, 2013), the researchers reported that divided attention of adolescents is related to lifestyle, academic and family conditions and fatigue decreases the ability to divide attention and also causes low academic performance. Betts, McKay, Maruff and Anderson (2006) assessed the effect of mental fatigue by increasing task load on certain measures of sustained and divided attention. The test of everyday attention for children was used to measure the attention abilities of 57 children within the age range of 5-12 years. The findings suggested that, as the task complexity increased, the performance generally reduced irrespective of the child's age.

Another related factor as a consequence of fatigue is sleep deprivation, which has marked impact on cognitive abilities. A series of scholarly papers have reported that sleeplessness is the most common and prevalent outcome of mental fatigue (Armstrong and Gilbert, 2012; Chorney, Detweiler, Morris, and Kuhn, 2008; Findlay, 2008; Stores and Stores, 2013). The association between sleep deprivation and fatigue is so close that some researchers have even used the term interchangeably (Myles, 1985). Cognitive dysfunctions are related to sleep deprivations and fatigue in children. Beebe (2011) found that inadequate sleep in children causes increased mental fatigue and decreases their cognitive abilities. Sleep deprived children tend to be less attentive during the day. Increased mental fatigue further increases sleeplessness, and the attention is further affected (Fallone, Acebo, Arnedt, Seifer, and Carskadon, 2001).

As true for all the domains of cognition, the auditory processing is also affected as a consequence of fatigue. In a recent report (Key, Gustafson, Rentmeester, Hornsby, and Bess, 2017), the researchers suggested that attention and processing resources are effective markers of fatigue in children. Young children who spend the majority of their school days in listening to the classroom instructions and who reported greater subjective fatigue were selected. Increases lapses of attention and longer reaction time were measured as a consequence of listening fatigue. Johnson, DeLuca, Diamond, and Natelson (1996) observed that individuals with fatigue have selective impairment of auditory processing. The researchers also reported that in comparison to visual processing, auditory processing is more affected in fatiguing situations.

Apart from the children with normal hearing sensitivity, subjective fatigue is also a potential problem affecting cognitive abilities in children with hearing loss. Fatigue is a complaint of children with a range of pathological health conditions (Eddy and Cruz, 2007). Researchers have suggested that children with sensorineural hearing loss are at greater risk for fatigue and its negative effects (Bess, Dodd-Murphy, and Parker, 1998; Hick and Tharpe, 2002). Hick and Tharpe (2002) stated that children with hearing loss exert more effort and hence the occurrence of fatigue is high in such children. The problem is more evident in adverse listening situations. For children, classroom environment itself is potential enough to cause fatigue. Classrooms always exceed maximum permissible noise limits, even when unoccupied (Knecht, Nelson, Whitelaw, and Feth, 2002; Shield and Dockrell, 2003). High levels of background noise are especially challenging for children with sensori-neural hearing loss, and are known to increase stress and fatigue (Walinder, Gunnarsson, Runeson, and Smedje, 2007).

Bess and Hornsby (2014) proposed a computational model to link the hearing loss in noise and fatigue with a decline in the cognitive processes and ultimately decline in the scholastic performances. Children nowadays have different mental workload, and they are required to complete many tasks simultaneously or in close succession to one another. Above all, the parental/caregiver expectations further increase the mental workload on children. The quest to perform similarly as normal hearing children do causes excessive mental exertion for the children with hearing impairment. This leads to fatigue. Excessive fatigue reduces the attention and concentration abilities of the children, and ultimately decline their cognitive abilities. The working memory capacity also simultaneously decline as a consequence of excessive fatigue. This follows a sequence of disengagement and compromise in learning skills. Finally, the academic/scholastic performance drops.

The perception of speech is also reported to be affected due to fatigue. Jain, Usha, and Jain (2017) found that speech perception in noise abilities were affected because of physical and mental fatigue. It has been observed that greater effort is required to perceive speech in presence of noise (Lewis et al., 2016). The cognitive resources required to understand speech (a.k.a. listening effort) increases (Gosselin and Gagné, 2010). Since, the cognition is already affected as a consequence of fatigue, the listening effort might not be appropriate, which indirectly influences the speech perception.

Thus, it may be observed form the literature review that subjective fatigue not only affects the day to day performance in children, but also causes a significant decline in their cognitive abilities. In the present day world, with such high competition and race to be the first/best, the subtle cognitive decline can also lead to a marked decrement in the child's performance at the later stages of life. This may further lead to emotional, social, psychological, physiological and related impairments. Furthermore, since fatigue is a hidden symptom, it is difficult to identify it in the regular situations. Hence it is very important for the parents/caregivers/teachers/educators to understand the adverse consequences of fatigue on the well-being and quality of life of children. It is also important for them to identify the fatigue in children at the earliest and employ appropriate measures to eliminate it or to reduce its impact. In the later section of this chapter, the authors have discussed some widely accepted measures to reduce the subjective perception of fatigue in children and adults.

In Adults

The effects of mental fatigue on cognitive abilities in adults are different from that of children. Where, for children, the effect is limited to academic/scholastic performances and psycho-social well-being, for adults the effect of fatigue is extensive. Fatigue affects social, psychological, emotional, neurological, physiological, and cognitive, well-being of the adults. The adults with fatigue frequently complaint of irritability, sleeplessness, restlessness, and anxiety. Due to the relevance of the topic, in the present section, the authors are restricting their review only to the effect of fatigue on cognition, and its association with speech perception abilities in adults.

Cognitive skills are affected in all fatiguing conditions (Abd-Elfattah, Abdelazeim, and Elshennawy, 2015) and prolonged fatigue may result in irritability, depression, mood swings, panic attacks, anxiety, impairment in concentration and memory loss ("CDC - Diagnosis - Chronic Fatigue Syndrome (CFS)," n.d.). Some of these symptoms improve over time after the cessation of the fatiguing conditions, but others such as memory loss leaves a permanent imprint on the sufferer life. The fatigue is associated with significant impairment of cognitive functioning (Cian et al., 2001; Neu et al., 2011). In a magneto encephalographic study, an association of increased mental fatigue with cognitive impairment was established, and the researchers reported that selected cognitive processing is more vulnerable to mental fatigue (Tanaka, 2015).

Researchers have reported that fatigue and sleepiness associated conditions can result in significant impairment in cognitive functioning and psychomotor performances in adults (Neu et al., 2011). Kahol et al. (2008) had also reported that fatigue and sleepiness causes significant deterioration in the cognitive skills. The cognitive skills were measured in terms of memory, attention and intermodal coordination using virtual reality simulation technique. Holtzer, Shuman, Mahoney, Lipton, and Verghese (2010) examined the effect of subjective fatigue on attention network test. A significant fatiguing effect was observed on executive attention. Van der Linden, Frese, and Meijman (2003) have also reported reduced executive attention function after two hours of the cognitive demanding task in normal adults.

Sustained attention, i.e. the ability to maintain attention with changing conditions, is also reported to be impaired as a consequence of mental fatigue. Dorrain, Roach, Fletcher, and Dawson (2007) measured the effect of fatigue on cognitive disengagement in 20 train drivers. The researchers investigated low, moderate, and high levels of fatigue on psychomotor vigilance, self-rated performance, and subjective alertness. They reported that as the level of fatigue increases, the ability to sustain the attention decreases. In another study, Langner, Steinborn, Chatterjee, Sturm, and Willmes (2010) assessed the effect of mental fatigue and temporal preparation in simple reaction time performance. The results revealed that mental fatigue generally reduces cognitive efficiency, but temporal preparation time certainly remains unaffected.

In an event-related potential study, the effect of mental fatigue on attention was studied (Boksem, Meijman, and Lorist, 2005). The fatigue was induced by asking the participants to perform a three-hour visual attention task, without rest. The subjective perception of fatigue was correlated with the EEG recordings. The results indicated dissociation in the effect of mental fatigue on top down and bottom up processing. Mental fatigue results in a reduction in the top down processing in the form of decreased goal-directed attention ability. Van der Linden and Eling (2006) had assessed the differential effect of mental processing on local and global processing. The results of their study showed that in comparison to non-fatigued participants, fatigued participants particularly showed compromised local processing. These findings indicated that divided attention abilities are also affected as a consequence of fatigue.

Kato, Endo, and Kizuka (2009) examined the effect of mental fatigue on cognitive resources and associated response-related processes. The researchers reported that the mental fatigue apparently slows down the time course of response inhibition and impairs the intensity of response execution. Planning and mental preparation ability were also assessed using task switching paradigm (Lorist et al., 2000). The researchers found that mental planning reduces after excessive mental fatigue. Later and Lorist (2008) assessed the impact of top-down control during mental fatigue. He reported that the information processing ability diminishes with increasing mental fatigue.

The effect of mental fatigue on verbal working memory was examined by Jain, Usha and Jain (2017). The working memory was assessed using forward and backward digit span test and operation span test. Subjective fatigue contributes to 62.7% of the variance in the working memory skills. Using the partial least square regression model, the weight of each test of working memory i.e., digit span and operation span was also measured to observe that which test maximally predicts the decline in working memory due to fatigue. The results revealed that general (86.6%) and cognitive fatigue (86.0%) both contribute maximally to reduced working memory skills. Among the working memory tests, operation span most reliably predicts the decline in working memory skills (93.8%). Even the digit span test reasonably predicts the decline in the working memory (89%).

Dobbs, Dobbs, and Kiss (2001) stated that cognitive impairment in terms of decline in the working memory is one of the most common symptoms of mental fatigue. In an experiment, the researchers assessed the working memory ability using digit span testing and found that the central executive function is a deficit in individuals having mental fatigue. Other researchers have also reported deficits in working memory secondary to mental fatigue (DeLuca, Johnson, Ellis, and Natelson, 1997; Krupp, Sliwinski, Masur, Friedberg, and Coyle, 1994; Taillefer, Kirmayer, Robbins, and Lasry, 2002, 2003).

The decline in the cognitive abilities was more evident in individuals with hearing loss. Qualitative research data indicated that individuals with hearing loss often have difficulty in understanding speech and other environmental sounds. As a consequence, they increase their attention, concentration and effort at the workplace. This leads to increase in fatigue and stress. This fatigue is sometimes so much that individuals are unable to perform their daily activities without feeling tired (Hetu, Riverin, Lalande, Getty, and St-Cyr, 1988).

Kramer, Kapteyn, and Houtgast (2006) assessed the occupational difficulty faced by workers with and without hearing loss. The workers reported excessive effort during work time because of their hearing loss, in comparison to normal hearing peers at the same work place. The researchers also reported that a number of sick leaves availed by the workers with hearing loss due to fatigue, strain or burnout, were four times more than those without hearing loss.

The relationship between hearing ability and work efficiency was assessed by Nachtegaal and his colleagues in a couple of studies (Nachtegaal et al., 2009; Nachtegaal, Festen, and Kramer, 2012). The researchers reported that the reduced hearing ability was significantly associated with the lower self-reported absolute productivity and increased need for recovery. The employees attributed the reduction in work performance to excessive mental fatigue at the work place due to hearing loss.

Likewise, Hornsby, and Kipp (2016) found reduced vigor in adults with hearing loss than age-matched normal. The researchers also found that individuals with hearing loss were more likely to experience severe vigor deficits (32%) in comparison to normal peers (7%). This difference was also seen on the fatigue scale. Individuals with hearing loss reported 8% more fatigue than normal hearing individuals. Thus, it was clear that hearing loss is related to fatigue and vigor deficits.

As evident from the above research review, subjective perception of fatigue affects individual's cognitive abilities. Such effect is seen in both normal hearing and individuals with hearing impairment. Cognitive decline due to fatigue affects individuals work performance and personal well-being. Ultimately, their social, emotional, and psychological life is affected. Hence, fatigue is an important lifestyle related issue which should be addressed at the earliest. It may also be noted that this effect of fatigue on cognitive abilities, indirectly affects the speech perception skills. According to the Broadbent's limited resource capacity model (Broadbent, 1969), human brain has limited capacity to attend to the sensory input. The capacity of brain is directly related to the subjective fatigue. Increase fatigue reduces the brain capacity to process any information (Mizuno et al., 2011, 2013; Tanaka et al., 2012). Thus, the top-down processing, which is important for speech perception is affected as a consequence of fatigue. Different management options are proposed in the literature to address fatigue and reduce its impact on daily living and quality of life. Some of these measures are discussed below.

MANAGEMENT OF FATIGUE

In the present day world, academic achievement surmounts all other non-academic skills in children. The 'quest for the best' has forced parents and teachers to pressurize their children for excellence. Such situations increase the fatiguing experienced by children. A study to measure the 'effect of subjective fatigue on the academic performance of children and its relation with working memory' (Hanasoge, Ahmed and Jain, 2017) revealed that good academic achievers reported less subjective fatigue than poor academic achievers. Verbal working memory abilities were also better for children with good academic performances. In a subsequent study (Kothari, Rohit, and Jain, 2017), speech perception and cognitive abilities were correlated in specific learning disabled children (SLD) and the authors found a good positive correlation between two variables. It was also observed that SLD children experience increased subjective perception of fatigue, and have poor speech perception abilities. The impact of excessive physical and mental fatigue on the work performances and its relation with cognitive skills and speech perception in noise in adults were also measured. Jain et al. (2017) reported that working memory was significantly affected by fatiguing conditions, and cognitive and general fatigue contributed maximally to impaired professional outcomes in adults. The speech perception in noise abilities were also found to be affected as a consequence of fatigue in adults.

These findings reveal that individuals with subjective experiences of fatigue more often encounter cognitive deficits and speech perception problems. The relationships between these variables are mutual. The fatiguing experiences reduce the cognitive processing, the affected cognitive processes impact the academic/work performances negatively, and the poor academic/work performances increase the subjective perception of fatigue. Since cognition and speech perception are also associated to each other, the top-down cognitive processing affects the perception of speech. Thus, appropriate measures to break the interlinkage between subjective perception of fatigue and cognition, and indirectly on speech perception, should be adapted.

Measures can be employed to improve cognitive abilities and reduce the subjective perception of fatigue. Some scientifically proven measures which helped in improving cognitive performance are discussed. One such measure is musical training which proved to be effective in improving perceptual processing and cognitive abilities in human beings (Divyashree, Divyashree, Sudha, and Jain, 2014; Jain, Kashyap, and Vinutha, 2016; Jain et al., 2016; Krupanidhi, Urs, Prateeksha, and Jain, 2016; Ranjini, Natesh, and Jain, 2017). Divyashree et al. (2014) assessed the categorical perception ability for voiced and voiceless sounds between musicians and non-musicians. The findings showed that the categorical boundary is sharper, i.e. significantly reduced region of ambiguity, for musicians. Their results indicated that auditory processing of the speech stimuli, which is often monitored by the top-down cognition, is better for musicians. Similarly Jain, Kashyap, and Vinutha (2016) assessed the effect of training in music on the perception of temporal fine structure cues in children. The researchers reported significantly enhanced temporal fine structure cue perception by children undergoing training in music in comparison to non-trained peers. Since temporal fine structure sensitivity and cognitive abilities are related (Neher, Lunner, Hopkins, and Moore, 2012), it was hypothesized that working on temporal processing may improve cognitive ability and speech perception in children.

Ranjini et al. (2017) measured auditory stream segregation, verbal working memory and speech perception in noise abilities in musicians and the scores were compared with age and gender matched non-musicians. The previous literature review indicated that musicians have better auditory processing and cognitive abilities than non-musicians, but such measure with respect to auditory stream segregation had seldom being investigated. Stream segregation was measured using inter-aural time and level difference, and working memory skills were evaluated using forward andbackward digit span test. The results revealed better performance of musicians for all the measures of auditory and cognitive processing in comparison to non-musicians. Multiple linear regression results revealed a good positive association between measures of auditory stream segregation and verbal working memory. Working memory is a good predictor of stream segregation, and hence the measures of improving auditory stream segregation can be employed as a therapeutic tool for management of children and adults for whom, the cognitive abilities are otherwise compromised. In the same study, the association of auditory stream segregation, verbal working memory and speech perception in noise was also measured. The speech perception in noise abilities were found to be better in musicians, and a close association between stream segregation, working memory and speech perception abilities was observed. Further, in consonance with the available literature, that study also supported the notion of improving auditory and cognitive processing through training in music.

Clark et al. (2006) used preferred music as a tool to reduce emotional stress and fatigue in individuals undergoing radiation therapy for the treatment of cancer. They reported that although the music had no effect on symptoms, patients reported a marked reduction in emotional and mental stress and fatigue after listening to music. Fredenburg and Silverman (2014) assessed the effect of cognitive-behavioral music therapy on fatigue. The qualitative data obtained from the patients hospitalized for blood and bone marrow transplantation showed that therapy reduces cognitive fatigue by increasing motivation and self-efficiency, and by promoting relaxation and restful states. The researchers concluded that cognitive-behavioral music therapy is an effective intervention tool for plummeting the effect of fatigue.

The behavioral and electrophysiological evidence of music on mental fatigue was given by Guo, Ren, Wang, and Zhu (2015). The researchers selected 36 university undergraduate students and randomly divided them into two groups. All the participants did one hour of continuous performance task, to induce mental fatigue. Music group participants listened to relaxing music along with the task, whereas participants of control group performed the task without listening to any music. Reaction time and error rate were measured as behavioral variables and N2-P3 late latency endogenous potentials were recorded electro physiologically. The results revealed that the music group demonstrated significantly reduced mental fatigue than the control group. The reaction time and error rate were significantly more for the participants of the control group. Finally, larger amplitude of P3 wave was also detected in the electro physiological responses of the participants of music group. These result combined with anecdotal research findings suggested that music training is a potential tool to reduce mental fatigue in children and adults.

The review of potential research studies along with some experimental evidences suggested that music training may be used as a potential tool for reducing the effect of fatigue and improving cognitive and speech perception abilities. In children, music influences brain plasticity (Barrett, Ashley, Strait, and Kraus, 2013; Herholz and Zatorre, 2012; Moreno and Bidelman, 2014). Luo et al. (2012) had reported increased functional connectivity between motor and multi-sensory areas in the fMRI scan of the cerebellum for children undergoing training in music. Other studies have also shown greater plastic changes in the brain of children under going training in music (Hensch, 2004; Knudsen, 2004; Weinberger, 2004). In adults also, music ability improves listening abilities for second/ non-native language learning (Milovanov, Huotilainen, Välimäki, Esquef, and Tervaniemi, 2008). These empirical research studies show that music training can be used as a potential tool to reduce the effect of fatigue and improve cognitive and speech perception abilities in both children and adults.

Apart from training in music, meditation has also proved to be an effective measure to reduce mental fatigue and improve speech perception and cognitive abilities. Studies have reported a significant reduction in fatigue, anxiety, and increased mindfulness following brief meditation training (Zeidan, Johnson, Diamond, David, and Goolkasian, 2010). Kaplan (2001) also reported that traditional eastern meditation is a useful and successful measure to reduce the effect of mental fatigue. Other researchers have also reported that mindfulness meditation helps in improving the cognitive abilities and reduce mental fatigue (Germer, Siegel, and Fulton, 2005).

Johansson, Bjuhr, and Ronnback (2012) have assessed the effect of mindfulness based stress reduction training on long-term mental fatigue after the stroke and traumatic brain injury. 18 patients with stroke and 11 patients with traumatic brain injury were included in the study. Mental fatigue was assessed using self-assessment scale and neuropsychological tests. The training was given for eight weeks. The testing was done at the baseline (before training) and the scores were compared with that obtained after training. The results revealed a significant improvement in self-assessment of mental fatigue and digit symbol coding and trail making neuropsychological test scores. The authors concluded that mindfulness based meditation technique is a promising non-pharmacological tool for mental fatigue.

Prasad, Varreyand, and Sisti (2016) measured the effect of meditation on the reduction of stress and fatigue and the sense of wellbeing among medical students. A prospective case control study was carried out from first to third year. The stress and fatigue were measured using standardized scales and self-assessment. After six weeks of meditation program, the researchers reported significant improvement in feeling of peace, focus, personal satisfaction and self-confidence. The patience and fatigue were found to be markedly improved. Other researchers have also reported marked improvement in subjective mental fatigue after short or long term meditation training (Fjorback, 2012; Hevezi, 2016; Kasai et al., 2017; Moss et al., 2012; Scherz, 2015; Tang et al., 2007). Thus, meditation can also be used as a therapeutic tool to reduce mental fatigue.

Marchand (2014) reviewed some of the neuro-imaging studies which showed evidences of neural changes due to meditation. The reviewers found compelling evidences of functional changes in the medial cortex (Zeidan et al., 2010) and associated default mode network, in insula (Lutz, McFarlin, Perlman, Salomons, and Davidson, 2013), amygdala and hippocampus (Zeidan et al., 2011), as well as in the lateral frontal region (Zeidan, Martucci, Kraft, McHaffie, and Coghill, 2014) and basal ganglion (Baerentsen et al., 2010), secondary to mindfulness and meditation training. In light of such structural and functional changes in the brain, it is likely that meditation not only reduces the perception of fatigue but also improves cognitive and speech perception abilities.

Another such measure is linguistic competence. Studies have shown that cognitive performances are superior for children having bi/multi-lingual brain than mono-lingual brain. Raju and Nataraja (2016a) found that verbal and visuospatial working memory skills are better in bilinguals and multi-linguals. The speech perception in noise skill was also reported to be better in bilingual and multilingual children (Mendel and Widner, 2016; Tabri, AbouChacra, and Pring, 2011). Thus, such measures can be employed to reduce subjective experiences of fatigue by children and their cognitive performances can be improved at least to a reasonable extent. Research with older children and adults has also shown that bilinguals outperform monolinguals in different tasks involving executive function (Bialystok, 1999; Bialystok, Craik, and Luk, 2008; Costa, Hernández, and Sebastián-Gallés, 2008)

Bialystok (2009) reported that the exercise of speaking two or more languages on a daily basis may produce changes in cognitive performance of the bilingual speakers. Research evidence have supported the viewpoint that in bilingual speakers, two languages are active in mind to some extent during both comprehension and production of language. Hence, the cognitive changes are considered to be contributed by the mechanisms using which bilinguals monitor attention to the target language in the context of joint activation of the other language when there is activation of two languages in bilingual mind during language execution (Blumenfeld and Marian, 2007; Francis, 1999; Kroll, Bobb, and Wodniecka, 2006; Marian, Spivey, and Hirsch, 2003; Rodriguez-Fornells, Rotte, Heinze, Nösselt, and Münte, 2002).

Bialystok (2001) reviewed studies of the effects of bilingualism on cognitive processes of children and stated that ''the most consistent empirical finding of the cognition of bilingual children is their advantage in selective attention and inhibition''. A study by Suarez et al.(2014) reported an advantage in inhibitory control among bilinguals. A similar finding was reported in a study by Bialystok and Viswanathan (2009) which examined the differences in inhibitory control between monolingual and bilingual children, belonged to one of three groups: monolinguals in Canada, bilinguals in Canada, and bilinguals in India. It was found that the bilingual children in both settings were faster than monolinguals in conditions based on inhibitory control.

Raju and Nataraja (2016b) also investigated inhibitory control skills in monolingual and bilingual children. Children in the age range of 8 to 10 years belonging to monolingual and bilingual groups participated in the study. Two subtasks namely verbal inhibition and nonverbal motor inhibition was used to examine the inhibitory control skills in all the participants. Response accuracy and reaction times were measured in each task. The results of the study revealed that in both subtasks of inhibition, bilinguals were fast in inhibiting the verbal and nonverbal responses. Authors concluded that enhanced inhibitory control skills are noted in bilinguals.

Feng, Diamond, and Bialystok (2007) assessed working memory in children using tasks that varied in their demands for executive control. It was reported that bilinguals maintained their performance level better than the monolinguals and outperformed monolinguals on tasks where the executive control demands increased. Raju and Nataraja (2016) investigated the executive loaded working memory skills in Kannada-English bilingual children. The study compared verbal and visuo-spatial working memory skills between mono and bilinguals of two different age groups. A total of 120 monolingual and 120 bilingual children participated in the study. Results of the study revealed that bilinguals performed better than monolinguals on two different working memory tasks. Thus, it was hypothesized that bilingual children may exhibit an advantage in working memory that is evident when the task demanded additional executive function.

The central aspect of the bilingual experience that may be responsible for generalized effects on cognitive performance comes from the well-documented observation that for fluent bilinguals who use both languages regularly, both languages are active and available when one of them is being used (Chee, 2006; Crinion et al., 2006; Dijkstra, Grainger, and van Heuven, 1999; Kaushanskaya and Marian, 2007; Kroll et al., 2006; Marian et al., 2003; Rodriguez-Fornells et al., 2005; Sumiya and Healy, 2004). This situation creates a problem of attentional control that is unique to bilinguals that are not only the need to correctly select a form that meets all the linguistic criteria for form and meaning, but is also part of the target language and not the competing system.

Some studies on the cognitive development of bilingual children focused on metalinguistic abilities of children. Metalinguistic awareness refers to "the ability to make language forms opaque and attend to them in and for themselves" (Cazden, 1974). Research studies have shown metalinguistic awareness to be an important element in intellectual development, including the development of reading skills (Barac and Bialystok, 2011). A study investigating metalinguistic awareness in bilinguals was conducted by Ben-Zeev (1977). The researcher reported that bilinguals outperformed monolinguals on tasks involving 'symbol substitution', e.g., constructing grammatically-violated sentences according to the experimenter's direction. Such tasks are designed to measure children's awareness of language features as well as the ability to control the automatic production of correct sentences. Bilingual children were shown to have greater capacities to evaluate tautological and contradictory statements than their monolingual peers (Cummins, 1978).

Bilingual children acquire two phonological systems and thus, receives additional 'practice' manipulating the sounds of language. Importantly, studies reliably showed that phonological awareness skills in bilingual children easily transfer from one language to another. This has been shown for English-Spanish bilinguals (Lindsey, Manis, and Bailey, 2003), English-French bilinguals (Comeau, Cormier, Grandmaison, and Lacroix, 1999), and English-Chinese bilinguals (Luk and Bialystok, 2008). Overall, the literature provides the fact that bilingualism positively affects the cognitive abilities of children as well as adults. These cognitive benefits of bilingualism are more prominent in individuals who use two languages equally in day to day basis. Studies in this regard may be useful to consider bilingualism as a condition fostering better cognitive development and detain cognitive decline.

The above review on bi/multi lingual brain indicates that being proficient in more than one language significantly improve the cognitive abilities. There are no direct study to support the view that being bilingual reduces fatigue and related symptoms, but improvement in cognitive ability indicated that the learning two or more languages, that too early in life may help in reducing the distress caused due to fatigue in the later stages of life. However, a direct relationship between the two is yet to be investigated. Other than these three measures, other techniques and strategies to overcome fatigue is also suggested in literature. Cognitive behavior therapy have also shown to reduce the impact of fatigue and improve cognitive well-being in individuals suffering from cognitive fatigue syndrome (Heins, Knoop, Burk, andBleijenberg, 2013; O'Dowd, Gladwell, Rogers, Hollinghurst, and Gregory, 2006). Other techniques to reduce the effect of fatigue as reported in literature include aquatic therapy (Andreasen, Stenager, and Dalgas, 2011; Kargarfard, Etemadifar, Baker, Mehrabi, and Hayatbakhsh, 2012), massage (Chunco, 2011; Mori et al., 2004), baleno therapy (Rapolien, Razbadauskas, Salyga, and Martinkenas, 2016) and other individual based fatigue management programs (Mulligan et al., 2016). However, the research support for these techniques is limited and there are numerous therapist based variations. Hence, it is difficult to report a common protocol for these programs/ techniques. Future research is required to justify the utility of these programs in the management of fatigue.

CONCLUSION

Fatigue is a subjective perception of being tired or loss of energy and vigor. It can affect the physiological, psychological, social, emotional, academic, professional, etc. wellbeing of an individual. Cognitive decline and difficulty in speech perception are most important characteristics of mental fatigue. Research studies have shown that almost all aspects of cognition and speech perception are affected in children and adults experiencing fatigue. Thus, measures such as music training, meditation and exposure to more than one language (bilingualism) may be adapted to reduce the impact of fatigue and to improve the quality of life.

REFERENCES

Abd-Elfattah, H. M., Abdelazeim, F. H., & Elshennawy, S. (2015). Physical and cognitive consequences of fatigue: A review. *Journal of Advanced Research*, *6*(3), 351–358. doi:10.1016/j.jare.2015.01.011 PMID:26257932

Andreasen, A., Stenager, E., & Dalgas, U. (2011). The effect of exercise therapy on fatigue in multiple sclerosis. *Multiple Sclerosis Journal*, *17*(9), 1041–1054. doi:10.1177/1352458511401120 PMID:21467189

Armstrong, T. S., & Gilbert, M. R. (2012). Practical strategies for management of fatigue and sleep disorders in people with brain tumors. *Neuro-Oncology*, *14*(suppl 4), 65–72. doi:10.1093/neuonc/nos210 PMID:23095832

Baerentsen, K. B., Stødkilde-Jørgensen, H., Sommerlund, B., Hartmann, T., Damsgaard-Madsen, J., Fosnaes, M., & Green, A. C. (2010). An investigation of brain processes supporting meditation. *Cognitive Processing*, *11*(1), 57–84. doi:10.100710339-009-0342-3 PMID:19876663

Barac, R., & Bialystok, E. (2011). Cognitive development of bilingual children. *Language Teaching*, *44*(01), 36–54. doi:10.1017/S0261444810000339

Barrett, K. C., Ashley, R., Strait, D. L., & Kraus, N. (2013). Art and science: How musical training shapes the brain. *Frontiers in Psychology*, *4*. doi:10.3389/fpsyg.2013.00713 PMID:24137142

Beebe, D. W. (2011). Cognitive, behavioral, and functional consequences of inadequate sleep in children and adolescents. *Pediatric Clinics of North America*, *58*(3), 649–665. doi:10.1016/j.pcl.2011.03.002 PMID:21600347

Ben-Zeev, S. (1977). The influence of bilingualism on cognitive strategy and cognitive development. *Child Development*, *48*(3), 1009–1018. doi:10.2307/1128353

Bess, F. H., Dodd-Murphy, J., & Parker, R. A. (1998). Children with minimal sensorineural hearing loss: Prevalence, educational performance, and functional status. *Ear and Hearing*, *19*(5), 339–354. doi:10.1097/00003446-199810000-00001 PMID:9796643

Bess, F. H., & Hornsby, B. W. Y. (2014). The complexities of fatigue in children with hearing loss. *Perspectives on Hearing and Hearing Disorders in Childhood*, *24*(2), 25. doi:10.1044/hhdc24.2.25

Betts, J., Mckay, J., Maruff, P., & Anderson, V. (2006). The development of sustained attention in children: The effect of age and task load. *Child Neuropsychology*, *12*(3), 205–221. doi:10.1080/09297040500488522 PMID:16837396

Bialystok, E. (1999). Cognitive complexity and attentional control in the bilingual mind. *Child Development*, *70*(3), 636–644. doi:10.1111/1467-8624.00046

Bialystok, E. (2001). *Bilingualism in development: Language, literacy, and cognition*. Cambridge, UK: Cambridge University Press. doi:10.1017/CBO9780511605963

Bialystok, E. (2009). Claiming evidence from non-evidence: A reply to Morton and Harper. *Developmental Science*, *12*(4), 499–501. doi:10.1111/j.1467-7687.2009.00868.x PMID:19635076

Bialystok, E., Craik, F., & Luk, G. (2008). Cognitive control and lexical access in younger and older bilinguals. *Journal of Experimental Psychology. Learning, Memory, and Cognition*, *34*(4), 859–873. doi:10.1037/0278-7393.34.4.859 PMID:18605874

Bialystok, E., & Viswanathan, M. (2009). Components of executive control with advantages for bilingual children in two cultures. *Cognition*, *112*(3), 494–500. doi:10.1016/j.cognition.2009.06.014 PMID:19615674

Blumenfeld, H. K., & Marian, V. (2007). Constraints on parallel activation in bilingual spoken language processing: Examining proficiency and lexical status using eye-tracking. *Language and Cognitive Processes*, *22*(5), 633–660. doi:10.1080/01690960601000746

Boksem, M. A. S., Meijman, T. F., & Lorist, M. M. (2005). Effects of mental fatigue on attention: An ERP study. *Brain Research. Cognitive Brain Research*, *25*(1), 107–116. doi:10.1016/j.cogbrainres.2005.04.011 PMID:15913965

Broadbent, D. E. (1969). *Perception and communication*. Oxford, UK: Pergamon Press.

Cazden, C. B. (1974). Play and metalinguistic awareness: One dimension of language experience. *The Urban Review*, *7*(1), 28–39. doi:10.1007/BF02223202

CDC - Diagnosis - Chronic Fatigue Syndrome (CFS). (n.d.). Retrieved September 15, 2016, from http://www.cdc.gov/cfs/diagnosis/index.html

Chee, M. W. L. (2006). Dissociating language and word meaning in the bilingual brain. *Trends in Cognitive Sciences*, *10*(12), 527–529. doi:10.1016/j.tics.2006.09.009 PMID:17049907

Chorney, D. B., Detweiler, M. F., Morris, T. L., & Kuhn, B. R. (2008). The interplay of sleep disturbance, anxiety, and depression in children. *Journal of Pediatric Psychology*, *33*(4), 339–348. doi:10.1093/jpepsy/jsm105 PMID:17991689

Chunco, R. (2011). The effects of massage on pain, stiffness, and fatigue levels associated with ankylosing spondylitis: A case study. *International Journal of Therapeutic Massage & Bodywork*, *4*, 12–17. PMID:21589691

Cian, C., Barraud, P. A., Melin, B., & Raphel, C. (2001). Effects of fluid ingestion on cognitive function after heat stress or exercise-induced dehydration. *International Journal of Psychophysiology*, *42*(3), 243–251. doi:10.1016/S0167-8760(01)00142-8 PMID:11812391

Cian, C., Koulmann, N. A. P., Raphel, C., Jimenez, C., & Melin, B. (2000). Influences of variations in body hydration on cognitive function: Effect of hyperhydration, heat stress, and exercise-induced dehydration. *Journal of Psychophysiology*, *14*, 29–36. doi:10.1027//0269-8803.14.1.29

Clark, M., Isaacks-Downton, G., Wells, N., Redlin-Frazier, S., Eck, C., Hepworth, J. T., & Chakravarthy, B. (2006). Use of preferred music to reduce emotional distress and symptom activity during radiation therapy. *Journal of Music Therapy*, *43*(3), 247–265. doi:10.1093/jmt/43.3.247 PMID:17037953

Comeau, L., Cormier, P., Grandmaison, E., & Lacroix, D. (1999). A longitudinal study of phonological processing skills in children learning to read in a second language. *Journal of Educational Psychology*, *91*(1), 29–43. doi:10.1037/0022-0663.91.1.29

Costa, A., Hernández, M., & Sebastián-Gallés, N. (2008). Bilingualism aids conflict resolution: Evidence from the ANT task. *Cognition, 106*(1), 59–86. doi:10.1016/j.cognition.2006.12.013 PMID:17275801

Crinion, J., Turner, R., Grogan, A., Hanakawa, T., Noppeney, U., Devlin, J. T., ... Price, C. J. (2006). Language Control in the Bilingual Brain. *Science, 312*(5779), 1537–1540. doi:10.1126cience.1127761 PMID:16763154

Cummins, J. (1978). Bilingualism and the development of metalinguistic awareness. *Journal of Cross-Cultural Psychology, 9*(2), 131–149. doi:10.1177/002202217892001

DeLuca, J., Johnson, S. K., Ellis, S. P., & Natelson, B. H. (1997). Cognitive functioning is impaired in patients with chronic fatigue syndrome devoid of psychiatric disease. *Journal of Neurology, Neurosurgery, and Psychiatry, 62*(2), 151–155. doi:10.1136/jnnp.62.2.151 PMID:9048715

Dijkstra, T., Grainger, J., & van Heuven, W. J. B. (1999). Recognition of cognates and interlingual homographs: The neglected role of phonology. *Journal of Memory and Language, 41*(4), 496–518. doi:10.1006/jmla.1999.2654

Divyashree, M. S., Divyashree, G., Sudha, P. N., & Jain, S. (2014). Categorical perception in musicians and non musicians. *Proceedings of International Symposium on Frontiers of Research on Speech and Music.*

Dobbs, B. M., Dobbs, A. R., & Kiss, I. (2001). Working memory deficits associated with chronic fatigue syndrome. *Journal of the International Neuropsychological Society, 7*(3), 285–293. doi:10.1017/S1355617701733024 PMID:11311029

Dorrian, J., Roach, G. D., Fletcher, A., & Dawson, D. (2007). Simulated train driving: Fatigue, self-awareness and cognitive disengagement. *Applied Ergonomics, 38*(2), 155–166. doi:10.1016/j.apergo.2006.03.006 PMID:16854365

Eddy, L., & Cruz, M. (2007). The relationship between fatigue and quality of life in children with chronic health problems: A systematic review. *Journal for Specialists in Pediatric Nursing, 12*(2), 105–114. doi:10.1111/j.1744-6155.2007.00099.x PMID:17371554

Fallone, G., Acebo, C., Arnedt, J. T., Seifer, R., & Carskadon, M. A. (2001). Effects of acute sleep restriction on behavior, sustained attention, and response inhibition in children. *Perceptual and Motor Skills, 93*(1), 213–229. doi:10.2466/pms.2001.93.1.213 PMID:11693688

Fan, X., Zhou, Q., Liu, Z., & Xie, F. (2015). Electroencephalogram assessment of mental fatigue in visual search. *Bio-Medical Materials and Engineering, 26*(s1), S1455–S1463. doi:10.3233/BME-151444 PMID:26405908

Feng, X., Diamond, A., & Bialystok, E. (2007). Manipulating information in working memory: An advantage for bilinguals. *Proceedings of Biennial meeting of the Society for Research in Child Development.*

Findlay, S. M. (2008). The tired teen: A review of the assessment and management of the adolescent with sleepiness and fatigue. *Paediatrics & Child Health, 13*(1), 37–42. doi:10.1093/pch/13.1.37 PMID:19119351

Fjorback, L. O. (2012). Mindfulness and bodily distress. *Danish Medical Journal, 59*, B4547. PMID:23171754

Francis, W. S. (1999). Analogical transfer of problem solutions within and between languages in Spanish–English bilinguals. *Journal of Memory and Language*, *40*(3), 301–329. doi:10.1006/jmla.1998.2610

Fredenburg, H. A., & Silverman, M. J. (2014). Effects of cognitive-behavioral music therapy on fatigue in patients in a blood and marrow transplantation unit: A mixed-method pilot study. *The Arts in Psychotherapy*, *41*(5), 433–444. doi:10.1016/j.aip.2014.09.002

Gandevia, S. C. (2001). Spinal and supraspinal factors in human muscle fatigue. *Physiological Reviews*, *81*(4), 1725–1789. doi:10.1152/physrev.2001.81.4.1725 PMID:11581501

Gandevia, S. C. (2012). Some central and peripheral factors affecting human motoneuronal output in neuromuscular fatigue. *Sports Medicine (Auckland, N.Z.)*, *13*(2), 93–98. doi:10.2165/00007256-199213020-00004 PMID:1561512

Garralda, M. E., & Rangel, L. (2002). Annotation: Chronic Fatigue Syndrome in children and adolescents. *Journal of Child Psychology and Psychiatry, and Allied Disciplines*, *43*(2), 169–176. doi:10.1111/1469-7610.00010 PMID:11902596

Germer, C. K., Siegel, R. D., & Fulton, P. R. (Eds.). (2005). *Mindfulness and psychotherapy*. New York: Guilford Press.

Gosselin, P. A., & Gagné, J. P. (2010). Use of dual-task paradigm to measure listening effort. *Canadian Journal of Speech-Language Pathology and Audiology*, *34*, 43–51.

Griffith, J. P., & Zarrouf, F. A. (2008). A systematic review of chronic fatigue syndrome: Don't assume it's depression. *Primary Care Companion to the Journal of Clinical Psychiatry*, *10*(02), 120–128. doi:10.4088/PCC.v10n0206 PMID:18458765

Guo, W., Ren, J., Wang, B., & Zhu, Q. (2015). Effects of relaxing music on mental fatigue induced by a continuous performance task: Behavioral and ERPs evidence. *PLoS One*, *10*(8), e0136446. doi:10.1371/journal.pone.0136446 PMID:26305353

Haig-Ferguson, A., Tucker, P., Eaton, N., Hunt, L., & Crawley, E. (2009). Memory and attention problems in children with chronic fatigue syndrome or myalgic encephalopathy. *Archives of Disease in Childhood*, *94*(10), 757–762. doi:10.1136/adc.2008.143032 PMID:19001478

Hanasoge, S., Ahmed, A., & Jain, S. (2017). Effect of subjective fatigue on the academic performance of children and its relation with working memory. *Proceedings of Indian Speech and Hearing Association Conference*.

Hancock, S., & McNaughton, L. (1986). Effects of fatigue on ability to process visual information by experienced orienteers. *Perceptual and Motor Skills*, *62*(2), 491–498. doi:10.2466/pms.1986.62.2.491 PMID:3503256

Hawley, J. A., & Reilly, T. (1997). Fatigue revisited. *Journal of Sports Sciences*, *15*, 245–246. PMID:9232549

Heins, M. J., Knoop, H., Burk, W. J., & Bleijenberg, G. (2013). The process of cognitive behaviour therapy for chronic fatigue syndrome: Which changes in perpetuating cognitions and behaviour are related to a reduction in fatigue? *Journal of Psychosomatic Research*, *75*(3), 235–241. doi:10.1016/j.jpsychores.2013.06.034 PMID:23972412

Hensch, T. K. (2004). Critical period regulation. *Annual Review of Neuroscience*, *27*(1), 549–579. doi:10.1146/annurev.neuro.27.070203.144327 PMID:15217343

Herholz, S. C., & Zatorre, R. J. (2012). Musical training as a framework for brain plasticity: Behavior, function, and structure. *Neuron*, *76*(3), 486–502. doi:10.1016/j.neuron.2012.10.011 PMID:23141061

Hetu, R., Riverin, L., Lalande, N., Getty, L., & St-Cyr, C. (1988). Qualitative analysis of the handicap associated with occupational hearing loss. *British Journal of Audiology*, *22*(4), 251–264. doi:10.3109/03005368809076462 PMID:3242715

Hevezi, J. A. (2016). Evaluation of a meditation intervention to reduce the effects of stressors associated with compassion fatigue among nurses. *Journal of Holistic Nursing*, *34*(4), 343–350. doi:10.1177/0898010115615981 PMID:26598000

Hick, C. B., & Tharpe, A. M. (2002). Listening effort and fatigue in school-age children with and without hearing loss. *Journal of Speech, Language, and Hearing Research: JSLHR*, *45*(3), 573–584. doi:10.1044/1092-4388(2002/046) PMID:12069009

Hockey, R. (2013). *The psychology of fatigue: Work, effort and control.* Cambridge, UK: Cambridge University Press. doi:10.1017/CBO9781139015394

Holtzer, R., Shuman, M., Mahoney, J. R., Lipton, R., & Verghese, J. (2010). Cognitive fatigue defined in the context of attention networks. *Neuropsychology, Development, and Cognition. Section B, Aging, Neuropsychology and Cognition*, *18*(1), 108–128. doi:10.1080/13825585.2010.517826 PMID:21128132

Hornsby, B. W. Y., & Kipp, A. M. (2016). Subjective ratings of fatigue and vigor in adults with hearing loss are driven by perceived hearing difficulties not degree of hearing loss. *Ear and Hearing*, *37*(1), e1–e10. doi:10.1097/AUD.0000000000000203 PMID:26295606

Ishii, A., Tanaka, M., & Watanabe, Y. (2014). Neural mechanisms of mental fatigue. *Reviews in the Neurosciences*, *25*, 469–479. PMID:24926625

Jain, H., Usha, M. N., & Jain, S. (2017). Effect of physical and mental fatigue on working memory skills and speech perception in noise. Proceedings of Indian Speech and Hearing Association, 2017.

Jain, S., Kashyap, S., & Vinutha, M. M. (2016). Effect of musical training on perception of temporal fine structure cues in children. *Proceedings of International Symposium on Frontiers of Research on Speech and Music*.

Jason, L. A., Boulton, A., Porter, N. S., Jessen, T., Njoku, M. G., & Friedberg, F. (2010). Classification of myalgic encephalomyelitis/chronic fatigue syndrome by types of fatigue. *Behavioral Medicine (Washington, D.C.)*, *36*(1), 24–31. doi:10.1080/08964280903521370 PMID:20185398

Johansson, B., Bjuhr, H., & Rönnbäck, L. (2012). Mindfulness-based stress reduction (MBSR) improves long-term mental fatigue after stroke or traumatic brain injury. *Brain Injury: [BI]*, *26*(13-14), 1621–1628. doi:10.3109/02699052.2012.700082 PMID:22794665

Johnson, S. K., DeLuca, J., Diamond, B. J., & Natelson, B. H. (1996). Selective impairment of auditory processing in chronic fatigue syndrome: A comparison with multiple sclerosis and healthy controls. *Perceptual and Motor Skills*, *83*(1), 51–62. doi:10.2466/pms.1996.83.1.51 PMID:8873173

Kahol, K., Leyba, M. J., Deka, M., Deka, V., Mayes, S., Smith, M., ... Panchanathan, S. (2008). Effect of fatigue on psychomotor and cognitive skills. *American Journal of Surgery*, *195*(2), 195–204. doi:10.1016/j.amjsurg.2007.10.004 PMID:18194679

Kaplan, S. (2001). Meditation, restoration, and the management of mental fatigue. *Environment and Behavior*, *33*(4), 480–506. doi:10.1177/00139160121973106

Kargarfard, M., Etemadifar, M., Baker, P., Mehrabi, M., & Hayatbakhsh, R. (2012). Effect of aquatic exercise training on fatigue and health-related quality of life in patients with multiple sclerosis. *Archives of Physical Medicine and Rehabilitation*, *93*(10), 1701–1708. doi:10.1016/j.apmr.2012.05.006 PMID:22609300

Kasai, Y., Sakakibara, T., Kyaw, T. A., Soe, Z. W., Han, Z. M., & Htwe, M. M. (2017). Psychological effects of meditation at a Buddhist monastery in Myanmar. *Journal of Mental Health (Abingdon, England)*, *26*(1), 4–7. doi:10.3109/09638237.2015.1124405 PMID:26698922

Kato, Y., Endo, H., & Kizuka, T. (2009). Mental fatigue and impaired response processes: Event-related brain potentials in a Go/NoGo task. *International Journal of Psychophysiology*, *72*(2), 204–211. doi:10.1016/j.ijpsycho.2008.12.008 PMID:19135100

Kaushanskaya, M., & Marian, V. (2007). Bilingual language processing and interference in bilinguals: Evidence from eye tracking and picture naming. *Language Learning*, *57*(1), 119–163. doi:10.1111/j.1467-9922.2007.00401.x

Key, A. P., Gustafson, S. J., Rentmeester, L., Hornsby, B. W. Y., & Bess, F. H. (2017). Speech processing fatigue in children: Auditory event-related potential and behavioral measures. *Journal of Speech, Language, and Hearing Research: JSLHR*, 1–15. PMID:28595261

Knecht, H. A., Nelson, P. B., Whitelaw, G. M., & Feth, L. L. (2002). Background noise levels and reverberation times in unoccupied classrooms: Predictions and measurements. *American Journal of Audiology*, *11*(2), 65–71. doi:10.1044/1059-0889(2002/009) PMID:12691216

Knudsen, E. I. (2004). Sensitive periods in the development of the brain and behavior. *Journal of Cognitive Neuroscience*, *16*(8), 1412–1425. doi:10.1162/0898929042304796 PMID:15509387

Kothari, S., Rohit, V. S., & Jain, S. (2017). Effect of Specific Leaning Disability on Auditory Stream Segregation, Auditory Working Memory and Speech Perception in Noise Abilities in Children. *Proceedings of Indian Speech and Hearing Association Conference*.

Kramer, S. E., Kapteyn, T. S., & Houtgast, T. (2006). Occupational performance: Comparing normally-hearing and hearing-impaired employees using the Amsterdam Checklist for Hearing and Work. *International Journal of Audiology*, *45*(9), 503–512. doi:10.1080/14992020600754583 PMID:17005493

Kroll, J. F., Bobb, S. C., & Wodniecka, Z. (2006). Language selectivity is the exception, not the rule: Arguments against a fixed locus of language selection in bilingual speech. *Bilingualism: Language and Cognition*, *9*(02), 119–135. doi:10.1017/S1366728906002483

Krupanidhi, P., Urs, B., Prateeksha, K., & Jain, S. (2016). Effect of musical training on the perception of instrumental music. Proceedings of Indian Speech and Hearing Association, 2016.

Krupp, L. B., Sliwinski, M., Masur, D. M., Friedberg, F., & Coyle, P. K. (1994). Cognitive functioning and depression in patients with chronic fatigue syndrome and multiple sclerosis. *Archives of Neurology*, *51*(7), 705–710. doi:10.1001/archneur.1994.00540190089021 PMID:8018045

Lal, S. K., & Craig, A. (2001). A critical review of the psychophysiology of driver fatigue. *Biological Psychology*, *55*(3), 173–194. doi:10.1016/S0301-0511(00)00085-5 PMID:11240213

Langner, R., Steinborn, M. B., Chatterjee, A., Sturm, W., & Willmes, K. (2010). Mental fatigue and temporal preparation in simple reaction-time performance. *Acta Psychologica*, *133*(1), 64–72. doi:10.1016/j.actpsy.2009.10.001 PMID:19878913

Lewis, D., Schmid, K., O'Leary, S., Spalding, J., Heinrichs-Graham, E., & High, R. (2016). Effects of noise on speech recognition and listening effort in children with normal hearing and children with mild bilateral or unilateral hearing loss. *Journal of Speech, Language, and Hearing Research: JSLHR*, *59*(5), 1218–1232. doi:10.1044/2016_JSLHR-H-15-0207 PMID:27784030

Lim, J., Wu, W., Wang, J., Detre, J. A., Dinges, D. F., & Rao, H. (2010). Imaging brain fatigue from sustained mental workload: An ASL perfusion study of the time-on-task effect. *NeuroImage*, *49*(4), 3426–3435. doi:10.1016/j.neuroimage.2009.11.020 PMID:19925871

Lindsey, K. A., Manis, F. R., & Bailey, C. E. (2003). Prediction of first-grade reading in Spanish-speaking English-language learners. *Journal of Educational Psychology*, *95*(3), 482–494. doi:10.1037/0022-0663.95.3.482

Liu, J., Zhou, G., Wang, Y., Ai, Y., Pinto-Martin, J., & Liu, X. (2012). Sleep problems, fatigue, and cognitive performance in Chinese kindergarten children. *The Journal of Pediatrics*, *161*(3), 520–525.e2. doi:10.1016/j.jpeds.2012.03.018 PMID:22521112

Lorist, M. M. (2008). Impact of top-down control during mental fatigue. *Brain Research*, *1232*, 113–123. doi:10.1016/j.brainres.2008.07.053 PMID:18687317

Lorist, M. M., Boksem, M. A. S., & Ridderinkhof, K. R. (2005). Impaired cognitive control and reduced cingulate activity during mental fatigue. *Brain Research. Cognitive Brain Research*, *24*(2), 199–205. doi:10.1016/j.cogbrainres.2005.01.018 PMID:15993758

Lorist, M. M., Klein, M., Nieuwenhuis, S., De Jong, R., Mulder, G., & Meijman, T. F. (2000). Mental fatigue and task control: Planning and preparation. *Psychophysiology*, *37*(5), 614–625. doi:10.1111/1469-8986.3750614 PMID:11037038

Luk, G., & Bialystok, E. (2008). Common and distinct cognitive bases for reading in English–Cantonese bilinguals. *Applied Psycholinguistics*, *29*(02), 269–289. doi:10.1017/S0142716407080125

Luo, C., Guo, Z., Lai, Y., Liao, W., Liu, Q., Kendrick, K. M., ... Li, H. (2012). Musical training induces functional plasticity in perceptual and motor networks: Insights from resting-state fMRI. *PLoS One*, *7*(5), e36568. doi:10.1371/journal.pone.0036568 PMID:22586478

Lutz, A., McFarlin, D. R., Perlman, D. M., Salomons, T. V., & Davidson, R. J. (2013). Altered anterior insula activation during anticipation and experience of painful stimuli in expert meditators. *NeuroImage*, *64*, 538–546. doi:10.1016/j.neuroimage.2012.09.030 PMID:23000783

Makeig, S., & Jung, T. P. (1995). Changes in alertness are a principal component of variance in the EEG spectrum. *Neuroreport*, *7*(1), 213–216. doi:10.1097/00001756-199512000-00051 PMID:8742454

Marchand, W. R. (2014). Neural mechanisms of mindfulness and meditation: Evidence from neuroimaging studies. *World Journal of Radiology*, *6*(7), 471–479. doi:10.4329/wjr.v6.i7.471 PMID:25071887

Marcora, S. M., Staiano, W., & Manning, V. (2009). Mental fatigue impairs physical performance in humans. *Journal of Applied Physiology*, *106*(3), 857–864. doi:10.1152/japplphysiol.91324.2008 PMID:19131473

Marian, V., Spivey, M., & Hirsch, J. (2003). Shared and separate systems in bilingual language processing: Converging evidence from eye tracking and brain imaging. *Brain and Language*, *86*(1), 70–82. doi:10.1016/S0093-934X(02)00535-7 PMID:12821416

Mayes, S. D., Calhoun, S. L., Bixler, E. O., & Vgontzas, A. N. (2008). Nonsignificance of sleep relative to IQ and neuropsychological scores in predicting academic achievement. *Journal of Developmental and Behavioral Pediatrics*, *29*(3), 206–212. doi:10.1097/DBP.0b013e31816d924f PMID:18480734

Mendel, L. L., & Widner, H. (2016). Speech perception in noise for bilingual listeners with normal hearing. *International Journal of Audiology*, *55*(2), 126–134. doi:10.3109/14992027.2015.1061710 PMID:26189557

Milovanov, R., Huotilainen, M., Välimäki, V., Esquef, P. A. A., & Tervaniemi, M. (2008). Musical aptitude and second language pronunciation skills in school-aged children: Neural and behavioral evidence. *Brain Research*, *1194*, 81–89. doi:10.1016/j.brainres.2007.11.042 PMID:18182165

Mizuno, K., Tanaka, M., Fukuda, S., Imai-Matsumura, K., & Watanabe, Y. (2013). Divided attention of adolescents related to lifestyles and academic and family conditions. *Brain & Development*, *35*(5), 435–440. doi:10.1016/j.braindev.2012.07.007 PMID:22877835

Mizuno, K., Tanaka, M., Fukuda, S., Yamano, E., Shigihara, Y., Imai-Matsumura, K., & Watanabe, Y. (2011). Low visual information-processing speed and attention are predictors of fatigue in elementary and junior high school students. *Behavioral and Brain Functions*, *7*(1), 20. doi:10.1186/1744-9081-7-20 PMID:21672212

Moreno, S., & Bidelman, G. M. (2014). Examining neural plasticity and cognitive benefit through the unique lens of musical training. *Hearing Research*, *308*, 84–97. doi:10.1016/j.heares.2013.09.012 PMID:24079993

Mori, H., Ohsawa, H., Tanaka, T. H., Taniwaki, E., Leisman, G., & Nishijo, K. (2004). Effect of massage on blood flow and muscle fatigue following isometric lumbar exercise. *Medical Science Monitor*, *10*, CR173–CR178. PMID:15114265

Moss, A. S., Wintering, N., Roggenkamp, H., Khalsa, D. S., Waldman, M. R., Monti, D., & Newberg, A. B. (2012). Effects of an 8-week meditation program on mood and anxiety in patients with memory loss. *Journal of Alternative and Complementary Medicine (New York, N.Y.)*, *18*(1), 48–53. doi:10.1089/acm.2011.0051 PMID:22268968

Mulligan, H., Wilkinson, A., Barclay, A., Whiting, H., Heynike, C., & Snowdon, J. (2016). Evaluation of a fatigue self-management program for people with multiple sclerosis. *International Journal of MS Care, 18*(3), 116–121. doi:10.7224/1537-2073.2015-019 PMID:27252598

Murta, T., Leite, M., Carmichael, D. W., Figueiredo, P., & Lemieux, L. (2015). Electrophysiological correlates of the BOLD signal for EEG-informed fMRI. *Human Brain Mapping, 36*(1), 391–414. doi:10.1002/hbm.22623 PMID:25277370

Myles, W. S. (1985). Sleep deprivation, physical fatigue, and the perception of exercise intensity. *Medicine and Science in Sports and Exercise, 17*(5), 580–584. doi:10.1249/00005768-198510000-00011 PMID:4068965

Nachtegaal, J., Festen, J. M., & Kramer, S. E. (2012). Hearing ability in working life and its relationship with sick leave and self-reported work productivity. *Ear and Hearing, 33*(1), 94–103. doi:10.1097/AUD.0b013e318228033e PMID:21826005

Nachtegaal, J., Kuik, D. J., Anema, J. R., Goverts, S. T., Festen, J. M., & Kramer, S. E. (2009). Hearing status, need for recovery after work, and psychosocial work characteristics: Results from an internet-based national survey on hearing. *International Journal of Audiology, 48*(10), 684–691. doi:10.1080/14992020902962421 PMID:19863354

Neher, T., Lunner, T., Hopkins, K., & Moore, B. C. J. (2012). Binaural temporal fine structure sensitivity, cognitive function, and spatial speech recognition of hearing-impaired listeners (L). *The Journal of the Acoustical Society of America, 131*(4), 2561–2564. doi:10.1121/1.3689850 PMID:22501036

Neu, D., Kajosch, H., Peigneux, P., Verbanck, P., Linkowski, P., & Le Bon, O. (2011). Cognitive impairment in fatigue and sleepiness associated conditions. *Psychiatry Research, 189*(1), 128–134. doi:10.1016/j.psychres.2010.12.005 PMID:21196050

O'dowd, H., Gladwell, P., Rogers, C. A., Hollinghurst, S., and Gregory, A. (2006). Cognitive behavioural therapy in chronic fatigue syndrome: A randomised controlled trial of an outpatient group programme. *Health Technology Assessment-Southampton, 10*(37).

Okogbaa, O. G., Shell, R. L., & Filipusic, D. (1994). On the investigation of the neurophysiological correlates of knowledge worker mental fatigue using the EEG signal. *Applied Ergonomics, 25*(6), 355–365. doi:10.1016/0003-6870(94)90054-X PMID:15676987

Parrish, J. B., Weinstock-Guttman, B., Smerbeck, A., Benedict, R. H. B., & Yeh, E. A. (2013). Fatigue and depression in children with demyelinating disorders. *Journal of Child Neurology, 28*(6), 713–718. doi:10.1177/0883073812450750 PMID:22805247

Prasad, L., Varrey, A., & Sisti, G. (2016). Medical students' stress levels and sense of well being after six weeks of yoga and meditation. *Evidence-Based Complementary and Alternative Medicine, 2016*, 1–7. doi:10.1155/2016/9251849 PMID:28053644

Radovic, S., & Malmgren, H. (1998). Fatigue and Fatiguability- semantic and etiologic perspectives. *Proceedings of Neural Correlates of Consciousness: Empirical and conceptual issues*. Retrieved from http://www.phil.gu.se/posters/fatigue.html

Raju, S., & Nataraja, N. P. (2016a). Assessment of working memory in bilingual children. *Indian Journal of Positive Psychology*, *7*, 159.

Raju, S., & Nataraja, N. P. (2016b). Lexical-semantic production and inhibitory control skills in monolingual (Kannada) and bilingual (Kannada-English) children. *Journal of All India Institute of Speech and Hearing*, *34*, 90–100.

Ranjini, A., Natesh, G., & Jain, S. (2017). Auditory stream segregation abilities in musicians and its association with verbal working memory and speech perception in noise. Proceedings of Indian Speech and Hearing Association.

Rapolienė, L., Razbadauskas, A., Sąlyga, J., & Martinkėnas, A. (2016). Stress and fatigue management using balneotherapy in a short-time randomized controlled trial. *Evidence-Based Complementary and Alternative Medicine*, *2016*, 1–10. doi:10.1155/2016/9631684 PMID:27051455

Rodriguez-Fornells, A., Rotte, M., Heinze, H.-J., Nösselt, T., & Münte, T. F. (2002). Brain potential and functional MRI evidence for how to handle two languages with one brain. *Nature*, *415*(6875), 1026–1029. doi:10.1038/4151026a PMID:11875570

Rodriguez-Fornells, A., van der Lugt, A., Rotte, M., Britti, B., Heinze, H.-J., & Münte, T. F. (2005). Second language interferes with word production in fluent bilinguals: Brain potential and functional imaging evidence. *Journal of Cognitive Neuroscience*, *17*(3), 422–433. doi:10.1162/0898929053279559 PMID:15814002

Scherz, N. (2015). Mindfulness meditation improves sleep quality in the elderly. *Praxis (Bern)*, *104*, 591–592. doi:10.1024/1661-8157/a002018 PMID:26098158

Shanks, L., Jason, L. A., Evans, M., & Brown, A. (2013). Cognitive impairments associated with CFS and POTS. *Frontiers in Physiology*, *4*. doi:10.3389/fphys.2013.00113 PMID:23720636

Shield, B., & Dockrell, J. (2003). The effects of noise on children at school: A review. *Building Acoustics*, *10*(2), 97–116. doi:10.1260/135101003768965960

Stores, G., & Stores, R. (2013). Sleep disorders in children with traumatic brain injury: A case of serious neglect. *Developmental Medicine and Child Neurology*, *55*(9), 797–805. doi:10.1111/dmcn.12163 PMID:23662906

Suarez, P. A., Gollan, T. H., Heaton, R., Grant, I., & Cherner, M. (2014). Second-language fluency predicts native language stroop effects: Evidence from Spanish-English bilinguals. *Journal of the International Neuropsychological Society*, *20*(03), 342–348. doi:10.1017/S1355617714000058 PMID:24622502

Sulheim, D., Fagermoen, E., Sivertsen, Ø. S., Winger, A., Wyller, V. B., & Øie, M. G. (2015). Cognitive dysfunction in adolescents with chronic fatigue: A cross-sectional study. *Archives of Disease in Childhood*, *100*(9), 838–844. doi:10.1136/archdischild-2014-306764 PMID:25791841

Sumiya, H., & Healy, A. F. (2004). Phonology in the bilingual Stroop effect. *Memory & Cognition*, *32*(5), 752–758. doi:10.3758/BF03195865 PMID:15552352

Tabri, D., Chacra, A., Smith, K. M., & Pring, T. (2011). Speech perception in noise by monolingual, bilingual and trilingual listeners. *International Journal of Language & Communication Disorders*, *46*, 411–422. PMID:21771217

Taillefer, S. S., Kirmayer, L. J., Robbins, J. M., & Lasry, J. C. (2002). Psychological correlates of functional status in chronic fatigue syndrome. *Journal of Psychosomatic Research*, *53*(6), 1097–1106. doi:10.1016/S0022-3999(02)00566-4 PMID:12479992

Taillefer, S. S., Kirmayer, L. J., Robbins, J. M., & Lasry, J. C. (2003). Correlates of illness worry in chronic fatigue syndrome. *Journal of Psychosomatic Research*, *54*(4), 331–337. doi:10.1016/S0022-3999(02)00332-X PMID:12670610

Tanaka, M. (2015). Effects of mental fatigue on brain activity and cognitive performance: A magnetoencephalography study. *Anatomy & Physiology*, *s4*. doi:10.4172/2161-0940.S4-002

Tanaka, M., Shigihara, Y., Ishii, A., Funakura, M., Kanai, E., & Watanabe, Y. (2012). Effect of mental fatigue on the central nervous system: An electroencephalography study. *Behavioral and Brain Functions*, *8*(1), 48. doi:10.1186/1744-9081-8-48 PMID:22954020

Tang, Y.-Y., Ma, Y., Wang, J., Fan, Y., Feng, S., Lu, Q., ... Posner, M. I. (2007). Short-term meditation training improves attention and self-regulation. *Proceedings of the National Academy of Sciences of the United States of America*, *104*(43), 17152–17156. doi:10.1073/pnas.0707678104 PMID:17940025

van der Linden, D., & Eling, P. (2006). Mental fatigue disturbs local processing more than global processing. *Psychological Research*, *70*(5), 395–402. doi:10.100700426-005-0228-7 PMID:15968553

van der Linden, D., Frese, M., & Meijman, T. F. (2003). Mental fatigue and the control of cognitive processes: Effects on perseveration and planning. *Acta Psychologica*, *113*(1), 45–65. doi:10.1016/S0001-6918(02)00150-6 PMID:12679043

Viner, R., & Christie, D. (2005). Fatigue and somatic symptoms. *British Medical Journal*, *330*(7498), 1012–1015. doi:10.1136/bmj.330.7498.1012 PMID:15860829

Walinder, R., Gunnarsson, K., Runeson, R., & Smedje, G. (2007). Physiological and psychological stress reactions in relation to classroom noise. *Scandinavian Journal of Work, Environment & Health*, *33*(4), 260–266. doi:10.5271jweh.1141 PMID:17717617

Weinberger, N. M. (2004). Specific long-term memory traces in primary auditory cortex. *Nature Reviews. Neuroscience*, *5*(4), 279–290. doi:10.1038/nrn1366 PMID:15034553

Wessely, S., Hotopf, M., & Sharpe, M. (1999). *Chronic fatigue and its syndromes (Repr)*. Oxford, UK: Oxford University Press.

Wijesuriya, N., Tran, Y., Thuraisingham, R. A., Nguyen, H. T., & Craig, A. (2008). Effects of mental fatigue on 8-13Hz brain activity in people with spinal cord injury. *Conference Proceedings: ... Annual International Conference of the IEEE Engineering in Medicine and Biology Society. IEEE Engineering in Medicine and Biology Society. Annual Conference*, *2008*, 5716–5719.

Zeidan, F., Johnson, S. K., Diamond, B. J., David, Z., & Goolkasian, P. (2010). Mindfulness meditation improves cognition: Evidence of brief mental training. *Consciousness and Cognition*, *19*(2), 597–605. doi:10.1016/j.concog.2010.03.014 PMID:20363650

Zeidan, F., Martucci, K. T., Kraft, R. A., Gordon, N. S., McHaffie, J. G., & Coghill, R. C. (2011). Brain mechanisms supporting the modulation of pain by mindfulness meditation. *The Journal of Neuroscience*, *31*(14), 5540–5548. doi:10.1523/JNEUROSCI.5791-10.2011 PMID:21471390

Zeidan, F., Martucci, K. T., Kraft, R. A., McHaffie, J. G., & Coghill, R. C. (2014). Neural correlates of mindfulness meditation-related anxiety relief. *Social Cognitive and Affective Neuroscience*, *9*(6), 751–759. doi:10.1093can/nst041 PMID:23615765

KEY TERMS AND DEFINITIONS

Auditory Processing: The way in which speech/sound signals are processed by the human hearing and associated nervous system.

Bilingual/Multilingual: A person who is proficient in speaking and/or writing two or more languages.

Cognition: Individual's mental ability to understand, reason, enquire, and learn.

Communication Disorders: A condition that is characterized by the inability to use a communication medium to successfully convey thoughts, feelings, beliefs, etc. to others.

Fatigue: A feeling of extreme tiredness.

Music Training: A formal structured training in instrumental music and/or singing.

Neurophysiology: The function of the nervous system.

Psychoacoustics: A study from the psychological perspectives of speech/sound perception.

Review Studies: A compilation of many peer-reviewed research studies.

Chapter 11
Behavioral Approach to Speech, Language, Hearing, and Communication Disorders

Srinivasan Venkatesan
All India Institute of Speech and Hearing, India

ABSTRACT

This chapter seeks to outline the overarching scenario of behavioral approaches to developmental and childhood speech, language, hearing, and communication disorders. By adopting the dichotomy of skill and problem behaviors, the steps or sequence, procedures, and practices of behavioral assessment and interventions are explained. While doing so, the uniquely Indian cultural underpinnings are highlighted with evidence-based empirical supports for the optimal benefits of the affected individuals. Additionally, two separate segments are focused on guidelines for skill training and problem behavior management along with case illustration on the format for their mapping procedures. The concluding section covers a critique of this approach which continues to hold promise for some more explorations in the contemporary circumstances for the optimum habilitation of these affected individuals.

INTRODUCTION

It is not the load that breaks you down, it is the way you carry it. – Lou Holtz

There are varied approaches to understanding speech, language, hearing, and communication disorders (Figure 1). This chapter attempts to explain behavioral approach.

BEHAVIORAL APPROACH

The behavioral approach focuses on *here-and-now, observable and measurable actions.* Behaviors are typically analyzed or understood as their *antecedents and consequences* within a given learning environment. Such observations must be precise, accurate, objective and unbiased. For example, the statement

DOI: 10.4018/978-1-5225-4955-0.ch011

Figure 1. Approaches to understanding speech, language, hearing, and communication disorders

Longitudinal or Life Span Approach takes into account the context of human aging and the regular transformations that occur with time to explain disorders in communication (Owens, 2017; Oller, Oller, and Badon, 2010).

Normative or Psychometric Approach involves comparative evaluation of individual typical behaviors against those of a large collectively representative sample of the general population known as norm or reference group. It helps in screening, identification, diagnostic labelling of individuals for given psychological variables on standard scores (Hegde, 2007; McCauley, 2001).

Systems Approach view communication as an integral part of an organized entity made up of inter-related and inter-dependent parts with well-defined checks or balances, barriers or boundaries. For example, an individual is viewed as a family which is a social unit comprising all members in an inter-connected dynamic system (Purves and Phinney, 2012).

Neuropsychological Ipsative or Idiometric Approach views communication disorders as outcome of deficit cognitive functions whose identification becomes the basis for their remediation (Ferguson and Armstrong, 2009; p. 86).

Sociolinguistic Approach argue against use of a 'de-contextualized' scheme of viewing language and cognition in isolation without taking into account the everyday social settings during communication (Kovarsky, 2014; Ball, 2005).

Psychoanalytic or Psychodynamic Approach is concerned with the relation of conscious and unconscious in dictating current behavior that is determined by past experiences. Manifest disturbances are caused by repressed trauma from latent or hidden unresolved issues during development periods (Gedo, 1988; Glauber, 1982).

Rights-Based Approach is gaining momentum after the advent of International Classification of Functioning, Disability and Health (ICF-CY; WHO, 2007), This approach uses a 'person-in-environment' social perspective (Fougeyrollas and Beauregard, 2001) to argue that human disabilities, including communication disorders, are the consequences of several intended or unintended barriers imposed by the larger social system on the affected individual (Ormerod, 2005).

Medical, Clinical or Disease Approach explain the taxonomy and aetiology of communication disorders as based on organic, bodily or biological basis before prescribing cures or solutions thereof (Miller, Vandome, and McBrewster, 2010);

The Magical-Religious or Laypersons Approach understands causes and treatments of disability-disorder conditions as mediated by curses or blessings of supernatural elements (Venkatesan, 2015a).

that a child 'hits others' is preferred expression rather than 'naughty' or 'mischievous', which would be dubbed as a subjective description (Miltenberger, 2012). The role of historical elements, organic causes, biology and heredity as causative factors to explain behavior is discounted. Any or *all behaviors are presumed to be learned and they can also be unlearned.* More than labeling or diagnosis, this approach underscores a *functional-utilitarian relationship* between the person and their behavior. As agents of behavior change, professionals in the area of communication disorders are involved in creating, strengthening, sustaining or increasing speech, or language skills. They are also concerned with decreasing undesirable behaviors that interfere with therapy. *Experimental backup* derived from animal or human subjects is the basis for all behavioral assertions. Behaviourally based interventions are action therapies contrasting verbal therapies like psychoanalysis or client-centered therapy (Spiegler, 2016).

PRINCIPLES AND APPLICATIONS

Known by several names, depending on their applications and alternatives, such as, Behavior Therapy, Behavior Modification, Applied Behavior Analysis, Clinical Behavior Analysis, Functional Behavior Analysis, Behavior Management Program, Behavioral Economics, Behavior Finance, Behavioral Medicine, Behavioral Geriatrics, Early Intensive Behavioral Intervention and others; all of them share common assumptions for understanding the underlying process through which people learn to behave the way they do. Based on principles of classical and operant conditioning, the role of rewards or reinforcements to increase behaviors and punishments to decrease them is underscored as the cardinal principle of behaviorism (Martin and Pear, 2016). Irrespective of the area of application, nomenclature or variants, behavioral practices are targeted toward developing new behavior, strengthening already achieved behavior, maintaining an established behavior, and for decreasing, stopping or eliminating inappropriate behaviors (Jena, 2008). They follow a characteristically systematic step-wise algorithm. It begins with designating a therapeutic agent, followed by identifying or listing of skill deficits or problem behaviors, prioritizing, selection of target behaviors for intervention, selection, and preparation of rewards, baseline, selection or implementation of treatment techniques, terminal evaluation, review and generalization (Spiegler, 2015; p. 60).

There are many behavioural techniques for skill training and problem behavior management. Some of them are based on classical techniques like flooding, systematic desensitization, and aversion therapy. Others based on operant conditioning principles are: token economy, prompting, cueing, shaping, chaining, modelling, behavioural rehearsal, extinction, self-instructional training, response costs, activity scheduling, shadowing, masking, reinforcement training, contingency contracting, over-correction, time out, negative practice, and others (Lewis, 2010; Lee and Axelrod, 2005). These techniques have been successfully used on a variety of clinical conditions including speech, language, hearing and communication disorders, such as, stuttering (Menzies, Onslow, Packman, and O'Brian, 2009; Menzies et al., 2008), autism (Hewitt, 2014; MacDonald, Parry-Cruwys, Dupere, and Ahearn, 2014; Vismara and Rogers, 2010), aphasia (Goldfarb, 2006), traumatic brain injury (Ylvisaker, Turkstra, and Coelho, 2005), voice disorders (Hackworth, 2007), and others. In recent times, new formats of behavioural approaches are being floated, such as Dialectical Behavior Therapy (DBT), Functional Analytic Psychotherapy (FAP) and Acceptance and Commitment Therapy (ACT), whose application in the field of communication disorders is still open to the investigation (Haynes et al., 2004).

BEHAVIOR ASSESSMENT

Behavioural interventions are preceded by behavior assessment. The purpose of behavior assessment is not so much to diagnose or label conditions. It is not meant to classify or compare people behaviors against one another or on a normative standard. Its process and procedure seek to list, gather and organize information systematically about what an individual can do (assets), cannot do (deficits), never had the opportunity to do (missed chances), and does not want to do (problem behavior). Behaviors are classified as skill-problem behaviors, adaptive-maladaptive behaviors, asset-deficit-excess behaviors, positive-negative behaviors, overt-covert behaviors, and verbal-non verbal behaviors. Behavior assessment is carried out by using techniques like observation, self-report data, interviews, and by using checklists developed for such purpose (Kazdin, 2013; Haynes, O'Brien, and Kaholokula, 2011; Hersen, 2006;

Venkatesan, 1994). At the easiest informal level, behavior assessments typically profile observable-measurable actions, focus on the circumstances under which they occur, elicit details on when, where, how much (intensity), how many times (frequency), or how long (duration) they occur, what happens just before (antecedents) or immediately after occurrence (consequence) of the behavior (Kazdin, 2013; Hegde and Freed, 2011).

Some well known behavior assessment tools relevant for children, adolescents or adults with communication related problems developed in India are: Madras Developmental Programming System (MDPS; Jeyachandran, Vimala, and Kumar, 1992), Behavior Assessment Scales for Indian Children with Mental Retardation (BASIC-MR; Peshawaria and Venkatesan, 1992), Assessment Scale for Speech and Language (Rao, 1992), Upanayan Early Intervention Program (UEIP; Krishnaswamy, 1992), Functional Assessment Checklist for Programming (DSE, 1994), NIMH Vocational Assessment and Programming System (NIMH-VAPS; Thressiakutty, 1998), Behavior Assessment Scales for Adult Living with Mental Retardation (BASAL-MR; Peshawaria et al. 2000), Portage Guide to Early Child Education (PGECE; Rao, 2002; Venkatesan, 2010a), Activity Checklist for Preschool Children with Developmental Disabilities (ACPC-DD; Venkatesan, 2004), Functional Assessment Checklist for Programming of Students with Profound Mental Retardation (FACP-PMR; Myreddi et al., 2004), Communication DEALL Developmental Checklist (Com-DEALL; Karanth, 2007), and others. Venkatesan (2004) compiled a list of 15 behavior assessment tools available for different age groups of clinical populations. It was noted that most of them were specific institution-based arm-chair preparations lacking details of standardization or needed manual, reliability, validity or sensitivity indices. While the tools listed above address the clinical population of developmental and intellectual disabilities, there are some instruments developed or standardized for other conditions too. For example, in recent times, despite the peril of pseudo-diagnosis (Venkatesan, 2015b), professional and parent interests have shifted upon autism resulting in the production of assessment tools, such as, Indian Scale for Assessment of Autism (ISAA; Mukherjee et al., 2015; Patra and Arun, 2011; MSJE, 2009), and Autism Behavior Checklist for Disability Estimation (A2E; Venkatesan and Ravindran, 2015). There are clinical conditions, such as attention-deficit/hyperactivity disorder and dysexecutive syndrome, for which such exclusive scales are still unavailable. Another weakness is that most of these behavior assessment tools address only skill behavior components and ignore the problem behavior dimension of the targeted population. Ideally, as in BASIC-MR and FACP-PMR, they must cover both sides of behavior. Otherwise, another problem behavior tool like Problem Behavior Survey Schedule (PBSS; Venkatesan, 2013; 2015c) is additionally used.

BEHAVIOR THERAPY IN INDIA

H. Narayan Murthy (1924-2011) is credited with introducing the concept of behavior therapy during the 1970s in Indian settings at National Institute of Mental Health and Neurosciences in Bangalore. Earlier called as 'Behavior Therapy and Biofeedback Unit' in Department of Clinical Psychology of the institute, the nomenclature was later changed as 'Behavior Medicine Unit' with three-fold aim of providing behavior therapy services, training postgraduates and conducting research in the field (Veeraraghavan, 1998; Veeraraghavan and Malik, 1994). In 1983, a state-of-the-art soundproofed air-conditioned room with one-way viewing mirror and another miniature 20-seater auditorium with stage lighting and acoustics for undertaking psychodrama sessions for patients with stuttering were designed with the help of structural engineers in Department of Clinical Psychology, All India Institute of Speech and Hearing (AIISH), Mysore, Karnataka.

Emphasis on cognitive behavior therapy services, training, and research for a wide range of psychological and physical problems including mood, anxiety, personality disorders, eating disorders, substance abuse, psychotic symptoms and lifestyle disorders has become a contemporary area of interest in the unit. A variety of behavioral strategies such as relaxation training, graded exposure and response prevention, anger management, assertiveness, social skills training, biofeedback, stress management and cognitive strategies are used to identify and handle faulty or dysfunctional thought patterns that underlie such problems. Mindfulness-based cognitive behavior therapies as a third wave of new generation CBT with its roots in ancient Buddhist tradition is used (Bhattacharya, Chaudari, Saldanha, and Menon, 2013; Mishra, 1998; De Silva, 1984; Mikulas, 1981). Another early contribution was the publication of a book titled '*Behaviour Therapy and Speech Disorders*' by AIISH, Mysore (Rathna, 1968). Recently, a multipurpose behavior therapy room was set up in Post Graduate Institute of Medical Education and Research, Chandigarh (Sharma et al. 2017). While there are exclusive journals on behavior therapy or modification in the west, there are no such exclusive journals in India. A few professional bodies dedicated to behavior therapy or modification in the country are: Association for Behavior Analysis-India (ABA-I) affiliated to Association of Behavior Analysts International, USA, which publishes its ABA-India Newsletter; the Indian Association of Cognitive Behavior Therapy (IACBT), Applied Behavior Analysis-India (www.aba-india.org), Behavior Medicine Society of India (BMSI), Alpha Behavior Therapy and Counseling, Chevayur, Kerala. Other online based get-well clinics merchandize behavior counseling, relaxation therapy, behavior rectification, psychobehavioral therapy, cognitive behavior therapy and dialectical behavior therapy (www.dir.indiamart.com; www.whatclinic.com; www.drnehamalhotra.com; www.docgautham.com). Although no systematic clinical trials of such supplies have been attempted, there is scope for innovation in the application of behavioral technology or management techniques in Indian settings.

Wherein speech, language, hearing (listening) and communication are viewed as skills, the role of behavioral approaches in their acquisition, maintenance, or enhancement becomes a needed application in routine clinical practice. In this context, it would be worthwhile to raise the question as to how much behavioral training components are incorporated in the formal graduate or post-graduate programs for audiologists and speech-language professionals. While some online, as well as institutional credits based add-on refresher programs degrees or diplomas, are available on applied behavior analysis, behavioral psychology, behavioral sciences, or cognitive-behavior therapy for such professionals at few places in abroad, there is no such formal courses made available anywhere in India. A perusal of the prescribed syllabus for 4-year UG programs in Audiology and Speech-Language Pathology and the 2-year PG Programs in Audiology/Speech-Language Pathology (RCI, 2009a; 2009b) show that there are no inputs at all about behavior therapy/modification. There is a semblance of an optional soft core subject paper on 'Clinical Behavior Analysis' offered for PG students at AIISH, Mysore. There are less than five hours of theoretical orientation on 'behavior therapy' in one of the units under the paper titled 'psychology' for students pursuing Diploma Course in Hearing, Language and Speech (DHLS; RCI, 2009c).

A turning point in application of behavior modification techniques for persons with intellectual disabilities in the country was the initiation of an UNICEF-funded 'BM Project titled: Application of Behavioral Technology with Mentally Handicapped Children in School Settings' (1989-1992) at National Institute for Empowerment of Persons with Intellectual Disabilities (formerly National Institute for the Mentally Handicapped). This initiative led to streamlining the issue of 'what to target or teach' such affected school-aged children in Indian settings. There was then a paradigm shift in the field from reliance upon western tools to an entirely indigenous device called 'Behavioral Assessment Scales for Indian Children with Mentally Retardation' (BASIC-MR; Peshawaria and Venkatesan, 1992) along with its accompanying manual for teachers titled 'Behavioral Approaches in Teaching Mentally Handicapped Children' (Peshawaria and Venkatesan, 1992) in English and Hindi. Apart from being included in the official curriculum for compulsory study in various RCI recognized professional courses, these tools have revolutionized skill training and problem behavior management programs for such affected children across special schools in the country. It has impacted publication of several research articles on the theme (Ganale, 2014; Lakhan, 2014; Lakhan and Singh, 2014; Ghosh, Shah, Dhir, and Merchant, 2008; Kishore and Nagar, 2008; Upadhyaya and Havalappanavar, 2008; Jain and Passi, 2005). A lower extension of BASIC-MR is now available as 'Activity Checklist for Preschool Children with Developmental Disabilities' (ACPC-DD; Venkatesan, 2004) just as another upward expansion is 'Behavior Assessment Scales for Adult Living with Mental Retardation (BASAL-MR; Peshawaria et al. 2000)

COMMUNICATION DISORDERS

Communication is a complex behavior seeking exchange of messages between two or more individuals. It is defined as 'ability to receive or convey a message, regardless of the mode, to communicate effectively and independently in a given environment' (ASHA, 2008). Communication disorder is impairment in the ability to receive, send, process and comprehend concepts or verbal, nonverbal, and graphic symbol systems. It becomes evident in the process of hearing, language and speech. It may range in severity from mild to profound. It may be developmental or acquired. Individuals may show one or any combination of communication disorders. It may result in a primary disability to it may be secondary to other disabilities (Owens, 2017). One classification system differentiates communication disorder, a hearing disorder, speech disorder, processing disorder. Another classification lists developmental speech disorders, language disorders, communication disorders of mental illness, acquired speech disorders, acquired language disorders, disorders of voice, disorders of fluency, and hearing disorders (Cummings, 2014).

It covers speech disorders of articulation (articulation disorders, phonological disorders, and motor speech disorders), fluency (stuttering and cluttering), resonance (hyper-nasality and hypo-nasality), cognitive (developmental or acquired), literacy (reading and writing disorders) or voice (aphonia or dysphonia). As disorders of language, it may be characterized by impaired comprehension (receptive language disorder) and use of spoken, written and other symbol systems (expressive language disorder). It may affect the form (phonology, morphology or syntax), content (semantics) or function (pragmatics) of the language in any combinations. A hearing disorder is the result of impaired auditory sensitivity as conductive, sensorineural, and mixed losses. Individuals with hearing impairment may be described as deaf or hard of hearing. Further, communication disorders may also result in central auditory processing disorders (Schindler, Ruoppolo, and Barillari, 2010). Sometimes, distinctions are also made between psychogenic/functional, developmental, and neurogenic communication disorders. Although swallowing disorder is not technically a communication disorder, it is a major area of concern for speech-language pathologists (Fogle, 2017). Telling communication disorders from mere problems, difficulties or interference in communication as something that is unexpectedly long lasting, persistent or recurring hindrance with normal, successful communication is important. Only those conditions wherein speech therapy might be appropriate or indicated could be labeled as communication disorders (Gunter and Koenig, 2011).

EVIDENCE-BASED BEHAVIORAL RESEARCH IN COMMUNICATION DISORDERS

A review of 42 research papers published on behavior therapy appearing in *Indian Journal of Psychiatry* beginning 1952 till 2009 showed 10 of them were case reports. None followed A-B-A-B design to prove or disprove its efficacy (Kuruvilla, 2010). Classical conditioning, rather than operant approaches were predominantly used or reported in these studies. Aversion therapy and relaxation technique was frequently mentioned. Behavior therapy was reported as used by Indian researchers on clinical conditions like sexual dysfunctions, obsessive-compulsive disorders, writer's cramp, anxiety neurosis, tension headache, hysteria, trichotillomania, alcoholism, and depression. There is no report on behavior therapy directed towards communication disorders. While formal training modules for practice of cognitive-behavior therapy is still unavailable, albeit, in a modified Guru-Chela paradigm, it has been reported to be more suitable for Indian culture (Beck, Virudhagirinathan, Santosham, and Begum, 2014; Neki, 1976).

Condition-specific application of behavioral techniques in the treatment of various speech-hearing, language, and communication disorders have been sporadically attempted by different investigators of Indian origin. Addressing the problem of stuttering with or without anxiety, for example, case studies have reported the usefulness of cognitive behavior therapy (Gupta, 2016; Ansari, Gorji, and Shafie, 2013; Reddy, Sharma, and Shivashankar, 2010). A solitary study has attempted operant training for children with language delays (Hegde and Gierut, 1979). Another pair of studies has focussed on the issue of skill enhancement and simultaneous reduction or elimination of problem behaviors in children with autism using customised behavioral intervention program (Kadambari and Venkatesan, 2014; Naniwadekar and Venkatesan, 2014). Most studies using behavior modification in the country are case studies on skill training of individual or groups of children with intellectual and developmental disabilities (Aniah, Kumaraiah, and Mishra, 1991; Abraham, 1990; Abraham, Mishra, and Kumaraiah, 1989; Rao, Barnabas, and Gopinath, 1989; Prasad and Sitholey, 1988; Das, 1973). Others have attempted to ascertain the effect of orienting parents and teachers on behavior techniques to train their children (Kaushik, 1984; Mehta and Ochaney, 1984; Singh and Kaushik, 1982; Kaushik, 1981).

A series of studies have targeted problem behaviors in children with developmental communication disorders (Singh, 1973). Beginning with an early analysis of parent demands for greater professional help to tackle behavioural issues in their children (Peshawaria, Venkatesan, and Menon, 1988; Singh and Dagar, 1982) and the empirical observation that matters related to management of problem behaviors are ranked second in presenting complaints after speech or language difficulties in children with intellectual disabilities (Peshawaria, Venkatesan, and Menon, 1990), the need for active collaboration between speech therapists and clinical psychologists has been repeatedly stressed. It has been noted that there is a differential between parents and teachers in the perception of problem behaviors for the same population of children (Peshawaria, Venkatesan, Mohapatra, and Menon, 1990), as well as in the perception of its causes and use of management strategies (Venkatesan and Vepuri, 1993). For instance, most parents attribute the 'cause' of problem behaviors to the primary condition in their children rather than owing to anomalies in their own parenting and/or environmental issues. Further, they were found to vacillate between extremes of either over appeasement or excessive of physical coercion often punctuated in between with a state of indecision, helplessness or ignorance about how to handle them. A similar trend is reported with regard to reward preferences, parents erroneously assuming that only expensive or primary and material rewards will work in their children. They did not seem to realize the potential of easily available and inexpensive acts like praise, hugs, pats or allied social rewards in changing behaviors of children (Venkatesan, Peshawaria, and Anuradha, 1996).

These differential perceptions of problem behaviors between parents, teachers, and therapists were further confirmed as the biggest hurdle in the effective management of children (Venkatesan and Lokesh, 2016). When child handlers differ in the key aspects of identification, listing, prioritizing, and recording or reporting the frequency, duration, intensity or extensity of problem behavior for the same child or group of children, there is enough ground to endanger the behavior correction program. Wherein a treatment program between the child-parent-teacher-therapist quartets begins without consensus on a single problem, chances are high that such intervention will fail (Hawley and Welsz, 2003).

SKILL TRAINING

The application of behavior-based approaches while handling children with communication disorders carry two aspects: (a) skill training; and, (b) problem behavior management. Actually, both these dimensions need to be addressed and worked on individual or groups, for such cases. Inherent in the behavioral approach is a systematized, objective, individualized, tailor-made, ecology-based, functional, pragmatic, and target-specific skill behavior training or problem behavior correction program that has been shown to be effective even in child clinical population (Eyberg, 2008). There are many excellent texts that explain the systematic step-wise sequence for implementation of skill training and problem behavior remediation programs (Spiegler, 2015; Kazdin, 2013; Marr, 2010; Venkatesan, 2004; Peshawaria and Venkatesan, 1992).

Ideally, the problem behavior management program must precede a skill training program. When a child has problem behaviors it becomes difficult to extract compliance for skill training activities. Many times, children with communication disorders may not be as yet ready for the skill training. At the simplest level, they may not be able to follow commands or even single step instructions with or without associated gestures. Their receptive vocabulary may be minimal if not absent. It might appear that they are following some commands. But, it may be actually that the caregiver imagines it to be so or that, unwittingly, they are just automatic situation-based responses. Many times, the caregivers themselves unknowingly give away many cues and then believe that the child is communicating with them. An example is when the mother thinks he is reaching out for toilet or indicating thirst when he routinely goes to the designated place to fulfill them. When the place, person or time is changed, it will be seen that the child is unable to make the person understand.

Many trainers are unable to distinguish between skill behavior deficit and problem behavior. For example, chewing at the ends of footwear might be because the child makes no distinction between edible and non-edible. It can also be because the child is seeking negative attention in the scolding or reprimand of the parent for the misbehavior. In the former instance, the child requires a skill training program to help differentiate edibles from non-edibles. In the later occasion, a problem behavior program involving the use of ignoring or extinction techniques may be needed.

Skill training proceeds along a clearly identified course in accordance with systematic steps. By abandoning layperson descriptions of behavior, such as lazy, mischievous, inattentive, dull, naughty, careless, hasty, unruly, or other adjectives, the identified therapeutic agent must commence by making a comprehensive list of the assets, desirable, adaptive or positive skill behaviors in a given child. One can take recourse to use the readymade or available behavior assessment tools already mentioned in an earlier section. A developmental perspective is crucial for effective implementation of skill behavior training programs. Take the example of contemporary skew of young children being overly exposed to adult-child dyadic interactions in preference for minimal child-child contacts. The result is that children with communication disorders particularly are bereft of social-language skills required for kindergarten level peer-mediated activities. It typically ends up with issues like a short span of attention-concentration, poor turn taking, waiting, indulgence in solitary gadget-based play, the absence of cooperative rule-based play, and deficient sharing behaviors. Within the adult-child interaction, the adults are likely to give way to the child's behaviors which may not happen without friction when such children move on into child-child peer interactions.

Going by the same developmental viewpoint, the area or domains of skills to be assessed and targeted for skill training can vary according to the age or stage of the child. For example, during *preschool years*, the areas like sensory, fine-gross motor, receptive-expressive language skills, social and self-care activities may be important. In *primary school years*, apart from sharpening or whetting sensory-motor skills their speech, dexterity, and control need to be enhanced. Further usage or practice of language skills, presentation of social skills and attainment of independence in self-care is to be achieved by the end of this stage. During *middle school years,* along with the above, effective communication, social-interpersonal relationships, community living, safety, leisure and hobby skills need to be cultivated. The basics of life skills including decision making, coping with stress or emotions, problem-solving, creative and critical thinking require being given priority. The essence of all this saying is that the specific behavioral objectives or teaching targets to be subsumed under a skilled behavior training program for a given child with communication disorder will have to be tailor-made according to age, gender, health condition, and other socio-demographic correlates (Reddy, Kumari, and Kusuma, 2004).

Goal setting best fit behavioral objectives is a daunting task for the success of skill training program. The chosen objective is something the child has to achieve at the end of a therapeutic module. It must be clearly stated by including four components: (a) a clearly observable-measurable behavior activity; (b) situations or conditions under which the said behavioural activity is to be performed; (c) amount or level of performance that is expected; and, (d) the date or deadline that has been set for achieving it. Ideally, such skill training objectives for children with communication disorders must be activity based, functional, child-initiated, developmentally appropriate, interactive, inclusive, and play based rather than concept driven, book based, and trainer initiated (Venkatesan, 2015d). Empirical observations carried out based on 'w' question matrix on what objectives are set, who plans them, where, when and/or how they are earmarked for children with developmental disabilities has shown that bulk of the training reportedly happens at home than in schools. The onus of the training appears to fall on mothers. The chosen training objectives are overly skewed (>40%) towards skill activities involving pre-academic, academic and communication skills (20%). Low priority is accorded for targeting play, sensory stimulation, and self-help skills. As many as 9.13 goals were set per child which is on the higher side of caregiver expectations from these children. It was also reported that observation of other children or informal discussions with fellow parents, rather than professional advice or guidance was the basis for their setting behavioral objectives. Gap analysis has shown teacher-caregiver skewed prioritizing, an imposed agenda setting, over expectancy error and demand overload resulting in the child's achievement deficit and perceived pendency, non-compliance or failed habilitation (Venkatesan, 2015e; Venkatesan, Yashodharakumar, Gupta, and Vasudha, 2015).

Prioritizing is a crucial element in setting few behavior objectives that are easy to handle and quick to achieve. This must be done after a baseline frequency or duration recording for those behaviors. This is followed by selection and preparation of rewards for use during the implementation of the behavior modification program. There are specific varieties of rewards and there are rules about them for implementation as when, where, how much, amounts as rewards, which must be dispensed. Implementation of the behavior change techniques must be carried out consistently, constantly, clearly and effectively. It must be noted that great efforts might be dispensed in planning skill training or problem behavior change programs which bring unsuccess due to their poor implementation in school, home or the environmental settings. There may not be the needed resources or cooperation from everyone involved with the program, or there may be apprehensions whether the program implementation will really work. It might be that the tempo is sustained across stakeholders continually over a period of time or it might be simply a matter of poor motivation and will to implement the program (Ostergren, 2014).

PROBLEM BEHAVIOR MANAGEMENT

Skill or adaptive behavior contrasts maladaptive, dysfunctional, and non-productive problem behaviors. Problem behaviors are considered as negative, maladaptive, unproductive, undesirable, or challenging. By definition, such behaviors are deemed as not being age or situation appropriate, interfering in the learning of new behaviors, harmful to self or others, occurring in a magnitude sufficient to cause stress on others (Venkatesan, 2004). Such behaviors may be seen extended over a period of time and across persons, situations to such a marked degree and by nature that it could adversely affect the acquisition or performance of their positive, skill or asset behaviors. Typical categories of such behaviors vary according to different authors perceptions. A specific example of problem behaviors are hits others, screams, falls on the floor, etc. Contrast this with skill behavior examples like buttons, greets others, eats on own, names colors, etc.

A distinction is to be made between behavior problems of non-clinical nature from those which is part of full-fledged clinical diagnostic conditions like Opposition Defiant Disorder, Attention Deficit/Hyperactivity Disorder, or Conduct Disorder (APA, 2013; WHO, 2013). A developmental, socio-economic and cultural perspective is vital for identification or definition of behavioral abnormalities in children (Venkatesan, 2010b). Bed-wetting, avoidance of strangers or fear of darkness, for example, in a particular age is typical and beyond a developmental stage, they are viewed as the problem behavior. More than being a passing age-related phenomenon, persisting behavior problems are shown to have a long-term negative outcome for affected children, their family, and society (Sroufe and Rutter, 1984).

The value or role of identifying antecedents and consequences for given problem behaviors in a child is critical. An antecedent is something that happens 'before' just as a consequence happen 'after' behavior. Antecedent triggered behavior problems need techniques like environmental manipulation, cue recognition, use of Premack's principle, self-control techniques, they form a verbal/graphic portrayal or description of those variables that are hypothesized to contribute to the initiation and maintenance of a given problem behavior. It is done by specifying the functional relationships among one another. It is a kind of path analysis or causal modeling diagram developed for a given instance for particular problem behaviors (Cosco, Moore, and Islam, 2010). It was recently found that the taxonomy, structure, content, and characteristics of consequence maps depicting events or happenings following problem behaviors are found to vary by setting, gender, diagnosis, and parent variables. Further, it was found that there were multiple, ambiguous, inconsistent, self-contradictory, ad hoc and arbitrary consequences for specific problem behaviors which mediated and only aggravated its occurrence (Venkatesan and Lokesh, 2017). Thus, based on Antecedent-Behaviour-Consequence (A-B-C Model) of understanding problem behaviors; in the Indian context, consequences appear to play a more powerful role in the acquisition, mediating, and maintenance of such behaviors in children.

Functional-utilitarian models of behavior analysis recognize that problem behaviors in children are mediated by five important functions: (a) attention; (b) self-stimulation; (c) skill deficits; (d) escape; and, (e) tangible rewards. Negative behaviors in children owing to attention-seeking factors are easily identified by instances when their occurrence increases whenever attention is paid. In such instances, the apt management technique would be to use extinction or withdrawing the attention being given as means of reinforcement for the child. Rather increased attention must be paid to the non-occurrence of such maladaptive behaviors. Children with sensory impairments, severe hearing loss, and intellectual disabilities are likely to show problem behaviors mediated by self-stimulation. Since they are left with nothing much to do or lack social skills and opportunities, they may end up indulging in stereotyped, stimming or self-stimulation behaviors like repetitive or monotonous motor actions, repetitive speech utterances, body rocking, etc. Such behaviors indulges must be managed through activity scheduling by providing meaningful activities that reinforce the child. Behavior problems occurring as means of escape or avoidance in a child can be handled through the use of behavior techniques like compliance training, contingency reinforcement, and over correction. Lastly, misbehaviors learned by faulty use of reward techniques, such as a crying child being given a candy as a pacifier, must be corrected by the withdrawal of such rewards. All behavior change programs for skill training or problem behavior management must conclude with a terminal evaluation on whether or not the implemented program has been indeed effective.

A simplistic *format of problem behavior mapping* is depicted (Figure 2) for illustrative purpose only by drawing reports from different stakeholders involved with the same given child. Note the stark differences between the various caregiver reports on all aspects of problem behavior identification, listing, recognition of antecedents and consequences, as well as their use of techniques to manage them. Many times, such disparities themselves unknowingly become the basis for the origins and maintenance of problem behaviors in children. Some *golden rules in the management of problem behaviors* are also listed (Figure 3) for quick reference.

CRITIQUE

The strength of behavior modification is that it provides the practitioners with many concrete things to do. It offers a number of tools and techniques for use in behavior change programs. It offers means to appropriately deal with stress, anxiety, negative thoughts and maladaptive behaviors. One learns to act in the world rather than being passive towards it. Behavior therapy is often a relatively short-term and cost-effective. The treatment lasts anywhere between 6-10 sessions unless multiple problems are to be addressed. In some cases, as in the management of children's behavior problems, there is a temporary increase of symptoms followed by a lowering in due course of time. There is a phenomenon called 'testing of limits' when a child attempts to retain its problem behaviors or even up-scales it in anticipation of the earlier benefits. However, it will gradually disappear if the changed strategies are consistently

Figure 2. Problem behavior mapping

Name of Child: Mukund   Age: 6 years   Class: UKG

A. Listing of Problem Behaviors

(a) Father's Report

- Does not follow a schedule
- Does not share things

(b) Mother's Report

- Does not obey commands
- Does not write neatly
- Demands for things

(c) Grandparent's Report

- Cries (or the parents make him to cry)
- Does not sit in a place
- Disturbs other children
- Demands to go for toilet frequently

No problem behaviors are noted or reported from school

B. Techniques Used to Handle Problem Behaviors

(a) Father's Report

- Advise
- Scold
- Make a timetable
- Raise voice

(b) Mother's Report

- Instruct him repeatedly
- Hit him
- Yield to demands
- Become silent
- Pacify
- Scold
- Compel him to comply
- Leave him to his wishes

(c) Grandparent's Report

- Give him candy secretly
- Plead or beg to behave well

C. Analysis of Situations (WHEN, WHERE, HOW and WHY REPORTS)

- When denied something
- When cannot verbalize
- When hungry
- When sleepy
- In public places
- In front of guests at home

implemented. Behavior therapy offers a wide range of techniques as options in combinations to select. In stressing 'doing', its techniques can be extended to more areas of human functioning than any other therapeutic approach. The whole scheme and system of behavioral treatment are backed up by evidence-based research (Goldfried and Cstonguay, 1993).

Figure 3. Some golden rules in management of problem behaviors

Some Do's...

- Make a clear distinction between a deficit skill behavior and excess problem behavior
- All stakeholders must unanimously agree on the list of skill deficits and/or problem behaviors for a given child
- Prefer use of rewards to punishment
- Always reward in small quantities to maintain the motivation value or interest of the child on the incentive
- Follow the rules of consistency, constancy, clarity and immediacy when dispensing rewards
- Catch them doing good than wait for a wrong doing to say 'NO' or punish children
- Although well intended, avoid comparison with others. It will only communicate negative reactions
- Rewarding the non-occurrence of a problem behavior is preferable to punishment of is occurrence
- Remember that you are NOT against the child. You are only against their negative behaviours
- Keep in mind that no two children are the same
- Understand, respect and accept individual differences between children
- Note that rearing or caring for children or disciplining them is serious time consuming hard work
- Realise that there are no quick fixes to behaviour issues like a tonic, medicine, or surgery
- Desist from Helicoptering. This is to do with keeping a round-the-clock vigil on all the activities of the child
- Training in 3 Rs (reading, writing and arithmetic) is NOT the only skills to be targeted for teaching children
- Develop the habit of keeping a simple daily record of the home-based behavior program being undertaken
- Develop short-term and long-term goals for skill training to review them periodically
- Plan skill training activities for a child based on their developmental age rather than chronological age
- Note that every skill training objective has a prerequisite which unless identified and trained cannot help achieve the next target
- Understand that children learn better or faster from same developmentally aged peers than from older ones
- Children minimally exposed to other kids may require more time for warm-up to get used to larger groups
- Prepare a 24-hour activity log for the child with equitable distribution of engagements throughout the day
- For skill training proceed from easy to difficult, familiar to unfamiliar, concrete to abstract, and general to specific
- For very young children, prefer one-to-one brief physical or play based gross motor activities than group-based activities requiring high levels of attention and sustained concentration
- For older children make small written or oral contracts of 'If-then' clause and implement them accordingly
- Combine the use of social rewards like 'good' or 'well done' along with other rewards
- Learn to fade the use of primary rewards like edibles gradually
- Specify the rules for dispensing rewards and follow them scrupulously
- Learn to ignore behaviors that increase when you pay attention
- Always praise in public and use punishment in private
- Be brief while giving instructions

Some Don'ts...

- Never debate/discuss strategies for managing problem behaviors in front of the child
- Never reward a problem behavior either knowingly or unknowingly
- Never beg or bargain with the child to behave or not to behave in certain ways
- Never use spanking, hitting, or physical punishment
- Do not bother or worry about what others will think or say when using some behaviour techniques
- Never make false promises and refuse them later
- Never give long lectures, multiple instructions
- Use positive instructions like 'Do this!' than negative instructions like 'Don't do this!'
- Never give instructions that you yourself are unable or not prepared to enforce
- Never give prophecy-fulfilling instruction. "I know, you are like your father who gets angry at the very sight of this dish... Now, you don't get angry!" This statement invites the child to get angry and fulfil the expected role model of an angry father.

However, some of the potential disadvantages of behavior therapy are it ignores the role of thoughts, feelings and unconscious processes in human behavior. It is argued that behavior therapy may change behavior but it does not change feelings. The symptoms are treated rather than causes. It does not provide insight to the client. When it comes to the application of behavioral techniques through parents or care-givers as therapeutic agents it poses an additional challenge of demystifying its techniques/technology in simple formats. The commitment in terms of time and involvement is demanding. There are added concerns regarding generalization of the therapeutic gains to natural settings of what happened within the clinical settings. Invulnerable populations with communication disorders, while establishment and maintenance of self-help skills for daily living have been successfully taught using techniques of behavior modification, their use even to teach rudimentary levels of useful communication to them has proved relatively unrewarding. Useful communication means spontaneous, self-initiated and discursive communication rather than simply labeling, or question answering through parroting repeatedly paired talk or conversation. Therefore, response generalization is a huge challenge especially in improving deficit communication behaviors (Bentley, 1987; Morrow and Gochros, 1970).

A share of criticism has been directed towards the use of aversion techniques and flooding or implosion as unethical or against basic respect for human rights. The use of pinpricks or electric shocks, lemon peel squirting or water dousing for problem behaviors, application of bitter castor/neem oil for thumb sucking, using physical restraint by draping in blankets, and administration of nausea-inducing drugs, are some of the frequently reported aversion techniques that are no longer approved by contemporary behaviour therapists. Ethical considerations are raised against the use of such techniques that cause physical or psychological pain.

SUMMARY

In sum, this chapter has sketched an overall picture of behavioral approaches to developmental and childhood speech, language, hearing and communication disorders. In doing so, no attempt is made either to discount the contributions of other approaches nor is claims made to demonstrate the superiority of this approach alone. Ideally, it is recommended that the helping professionals in the field must draw from all the sources and tailor make interventions to suit the individual or small groups of such affected persons. Although an arbitrary distinction is made between skill and problem behaviors for the convenience of understanding or explanation, they must not be viewed as separate compartments. Undoubtedly, they are interrelated. A lowered level of skills can inversely increase the occurrence of challenging behaviors. There is also an exclusively Indian twist for understanding and handling children with or without com-

Figure 4. Common misconceptions about behavioral treatments

Common Misconceptions about Behavioral Treatments

- Rewards or reinforcements are nothing more than bribes
- It only changes peripheral symptoms and not the underlying cause of the problems
- When one symptom is eliminated it gets substituted or replaced by another in its place
- It can be applied to simple but not complex problems
- Its approaches are atomistic, dehumanizing, mechanical, and dictatorial
- Behavior therapists are cold, detached and non-empathetic professionals

munication disorders given the social-cultural settings. This is exemplified in concepts like behavioral or consequence mapping. This occasion and opportunity are used to invite mutual dialogue between behaviourally based therapist and speech, language and hearing professionals for ameliorating the optimum habilitation of individuals affected by communication disorders.

REFERENCES

Abraham, A. (1990). Behavior modification in institutionalized mentally retarded children: Case reports. *Journal of Personality and Clinical Studies*, *6*(1), 124–126.

Abraham, A., Mishra, H., & Kumaraiah, V. (1989). The effectiveness of behavior modification in institution-based mentally retarded children. *Journal of Personality and Clinical Studies*, *5*(3), 153–160.

American Psychiatric Association. (2013). *Diagnostic and Statistical Manual of Mental Disorders* (5th ed.). Washington, DC: Author.

American Speech Hearing Association. (2008). *Communication facts*. Rockville, MD: ASHA, Science and Research Department.

Aniah, U., Kumaraiah, V., & Mishra, H. (1991). Behavior modification in self-help skills of mentally retarded children. *Journal of Personality and Clinical Studies*, *7*(1), 15–19.

Ansari, P., Gorji, Y., & Shafie, B. (2013). An empirical study on the effect of speech therapy with cognitive behavior therapy on reducing the severity of stuttering and anxiety. *Management Science Letters*, *3*(12), 2957–2962. doi:10.5267/j.msl.2013.11.001

Ball, M. J. (2005). *Clinical Sociolinguistics*. Oxford, UK: Blackwell Publishing. doi:10.1002/9780470754856

Beck, A., Virudhagirinathan, B. S., Santosham, S., & Begum, F. J. (2014). Developing cognitive behavior therapy training in India: Using the Kolb learning cycle to address challenges in applying trans-cultural models of mental health and mental health training. *International Review of Psychiatry (Abingdon, England)*, *26*(5), 572–578. doi:10.3109/09540261.2014.918024 PMID:25343633

Bentley, K. J. (1987). Major legal and ethical issues in behavioral treatment: Focus on institutionalized mental patients. *Behavioral Sciences & the Law*, *5*(3), 359–372. doi:10.1002/bsl.2370050309

Bhattacharya, L., Chaudari, B., Saldanha, D., & Menon, P. (2013). Cognitive behavior therapy. *Medical Journal of DY Patil University*, *6*(2), 132–138. doi:10.4103/0975-2870.110294

Cosco, N., Moore, R., & Islam, M. (2010). Behaviour mapping: A method for linking preschool physical activity and outdoor design. *Medicine and Science in Sports and Exercise*, *42*(3), 513–519. doi:10.1249/MSS.0b013e3181cea27a PMID:20068497

Cummings, L. (2014). *The Communication Disorders Workbook*. Cambridge, UK: Cambridge University Press. doi:10.1017/CBO9781107295117

Das, J. P. (1973). How to teach retardates to control their behavior. *Indian Journal of Mental Retardation*, *6*(1), 5–20.

De Silva, P. (1984). Buddhism and behavior modification. *Behaviour Research and Therapy*, *22*(5), 661–678. doi:10.1016/0005-7967(84)90129-3 PMID:6517830

DSE. (1994). *Functional Assessment Checklist for Programming. Secunderabad.* Department of Special Education, National Institute for the Mentally Handicapped.

Eyberg, S. M., Nelson, M. M., & Boggs, S. R. (2008). Evidence-based psychosocial treatments for children and adolescents with disruptive behavior. *Journal of Child Clinical and Adolescent Psychology*, *37*(1), 215–257. doi:10.1080/15374410701820117 PMID:18444059

Ferguson, A., & Armstrong, E. (2009). *Researching communication disorders*. New York, NY: Palgrave Macmillan. doi:10.1057/9780230594340

Fogle, P. T. (2017). *Essentials of communication sciences and disorders*. Burlington, MA: Jones and Bartlett Learning.

Fougeyrollas, P., & Beauregard, L. (2001). Disability: An interactive person-environment social creation, Chapter 6 under part 1: The shaping of disability studies as a field. In G. L. Albrecht, K. D. Seelman, & M. Bury (Eds.), *Handbook of disability studies* (pp. 171-194). Sage Publications.

Ganale, S. A. (2014). A study on association among sleep pattern, sleep disturbance and problem behavior in persons with developmental disabilities. *International Journal of Behavioral Research and Psychology*, *2*(2), 18–26. doi:10.19070/2332-3000-140005

Gedo, J. E. (1988). Disorders of communication: Language, affects, and vegetative signs. In *The mind in disorder: Psychoanalytic models of pathology* (pp. 177–186). Lawrence Erlbaum Associates.

Ghosh, M., Shah, A. H., Dhir, K., & Merchant, K. F. (2008). Behavior in children with Down syndrome. *Indian Journal of Pediatrics*, *75*(7), 685–689. doi:10.100712098-008-0129-z PMID:18716736

Glauber, I. P. (1982). *Stuttering: A psychoanalytic understanding*. New York: Human Sciences Press.

Goldfarb, R. (2006). Operant conditioning and programmed instruction in aphasia rehabilitation. *The Journal of Speech and Language Pathology, Applied Behavior Analysis*, *1*(1), 56–65. doi:10.1037/h0100186

Goldfried, M. R., & Cstonguay, L. G. (1993). Behaviour therapy: Redefining strengths and limitations. *Behavior Therapy*, *24*(4), 505–526. doi:10.1016/S0005-7894(05)80315-6

Gunter, C. D., & Koenig, M. A. (2011). Communication development and disorders for partners in service. Oxfordshire, UK: Plural Publishing.

Gupta, S. K. (2016). The efficacy of cognitive behavior therapy in an adult who stutters. *Indian Journal of Psychiatry*, *58*(4), 477–778. doi:10.4103/0019-5545.196726 PMID:28197011

Hackworth, R. S. (2007). The effect of vocal hygiene and behavior modification instruction on the self-reported vocal health habits of public school music teachers. *International Journal of Music Education*, *25*(1), 20–28. doi:10.1177/0255761407074889

Hallowell, B. (2017). The WHO ICF and its relevance to acquired neurogenic communication disorders. In *Aphasia and other acquired neurogenic language disorders: A guide for clinical excellence* (pp. 69–65). San Diego, CA: Plural Publishing.

Hawley, K. M., & Welsz, J. R. (2003). Child, parent, and therapist (dis) agreement on target problems in outpatient therapy: The therapist's dilemma and its implications. *Journal of Consulting and Clinical Psychology*, *71*(1), 62–70. doi:10.1037/0022-006X.71.1.62 PMID:12602426

Haynes, S. C., Masuda, A., Bissett, R., Lucoma, J., & Guerrero, L. F. (2004). DBT, FAP, and ACT: How empirically oriented are the new behavior therapy technologies? *Behavior Therapy*, *35*(1), 35–54. doi:10.1016/S0005-7894(04)80003-0

Haynes, S. N., O'Brien, W. H., & Kaholokula, J. K. (2011). *Behavioral assessment and case formulation*. John Wiley and Sons.

Hegde, M. N. (2007). *Hegde's pocket guide to communication disorders*. Boston, MA: Thomson Delmar Learning.

Hegde, M. N., & Freed, D. (2011). Assessment of communication disorders in adults. Oxfordshire, UK: Plural Publishing.

Hegde, M. N., & Gierut, J. (1979). The operant training and generalization of pronouns and a verb form in a language delayed. *Journal of Communication Disorders*, *12*(1), 23–34. doi:10.1016/0021-9924(79)90018-2 PMID:422745

Hersen, M. (2006). *Handbook of behavioral assessment*. Boston: Academic Press.

Hewitt, L. (2014). Social anxiety and pragmatics in autism spectrum disorders: Cognitive behavioral therapy and its relation to speech-language pathology. *Perspectives on Language Learning and Education*, *21*(1), 5–12. doi:10.1044/lle21.1.5

Jain, M., & Passi, G. R. (2005). Assessment of a modified mini-mental scale for cognitive functions in children. *Indian Pediatrics*, *42*, 907–991. PMID:16208050

Jena, S. P. K. (2008). *Behavior therapy: Techniques, research, and applications*. New Delhi: Sage Publications.

Jeyachandran, P., Vimala, K., & Kumar, S. (1992). *Madras Developmental Programming System* (5th ed.). Madras: Vijay Human Services.

Kadambari, N., & Venkatesan, S. (2014). Concurrent use of customized behavioral interventions in skill enhancement and problem behavior reduction in children with autism. *Guru Journal of Behavioral and Social Sciences*, *2*(3), 270–283.

Kanfer, F. H., & Saslow, G. (1969). Behaviour diagnosis. In C. M. Franks (Ed.), *Behaviour therapy: Appraisal and status* (pp. 417–444). New York: McGraw Hill.

Karanth, P. (2007). *Communication DEALL Developmental Checklists*. Bangalore: Com DEALL Trust.

Kaushik, S. S. (1981). *Parents are teachers: A study in behavior modification of mental sub-normal*. New Delhi: Northern Book Center.

Kaushik, S. S. (1984). Behavior modification workshop for parents and teachers of mentally retarded: Program evaluation. *The Journal of Rehabilitation in Asia*, *25*(2), 47.

Kazdin, A. E. (2013). *Behavior modification in applied settings*. Long Grove, IL: Waveland Press.

Kishore, T. M., & Nagar, R. K. (2008). Mountaineering expedition by persons with intellectual disability. *Journal of Intellectual Disabilities*, *12*(3), 183–189. doi:10.1177/1744629508095322 PMID:18728141

Kovarsky, D. (2014). The ethnography of communication disorders revisited. In M. J. Ball, N. Muller, & R. L. Nelson (Eds.), *Handbook of Qualitative research in communication disorders* (pp. 55–78). New York, NY: Psychology Press.

Krishnaswamy, J. (1992). The Upanayana early intervention program (UEIP). *Indian Journal of Pediatrics*, *59*(8), 701–705. doi:10.1007/BF02859404 PMID:1340858

Kuruvilla, K. (2010). Indian contribution to behavior therapy. *Indian Journal of Psychiatry*, *52*(7S1), S371–S377. doi:10.4103/0019-5545.69271 PMID:21836708

Lakhan, R. (2014). Behavioral management in children with intellectual disabilities in a resource-poor setting in Barwani, India. *Indian Journal of Psychiatry*, *56*(1), 39–45. doi:10.4103/0019-5545.124712 PMID:24574557

Lakhan, R., & Singh, A. (2014). Early intervention tool for children with developmental delay: A pilot study. *The European Health Psychologist*, *16*(1), 18–25.

Lee, D. L., & Axelrod, S. (2005). *Behavior modification: Basic principles*. Austin, TX: Pro-Ed.

Lewis, D. J. (2010). *Foundations of behavioral therapy*. London: Transaction Publishers.

MacDonald, R., Parry-Cruwys, D., Dupere, S., & Aheam, W. (2014). Assessing progress and outcome of early intensive behavioral intervention for toddlers with autism. *Research in Developmental Disabilities*, *35*(12), 3632–3644. doi:10.1016/j.ridd.2014.08.036 PMID:25241118

Marr, J. N. (2010). *Manual of behavior modification: A guide for parents*. Bloomington, IN: Xlibris Corporation.

Martin, G., & Pear, J. J. (2016). *Behavior modification: What it is and how to do it*. New York: Routledge.

McCauley, R. J. (2001). *Assessment of language disorders in children*. New York: Psychology Press.

Mehta, M., & Ochaney, M. (1984). Training mental retardation: Involving mothers in the operant conditioning program. *Indian Journal of Clinical Psychology*, *11*, 45–49.

Menzies, R. G., O'Brian, S., Onslow, M., Packman, A., St. Clare, T., & Block, S. (2008). An experimental clinical trial of a cognitive-behavior therapy package for chronic stuttering. *Journal of Speech, Language, and Hearing Research: JSLHR*, *51*(6), 1451–1464. doi:10.1044/1092-4388(2008/07-0070) PMID:18664696

Menzies, R. G., Onslow, M., Packman, A., & O'Brian, S. (2009). Cognitive-behavior therapy for adults who stutter: A tutorial for the speech-language pathologist. *Journal of Fluency Disorders*, *34*(3), 187–200. doi:10.1016/j.jfludis.2009.09.002 PMID:19948272

Mikulas, W. L. (1981). Buddhism and behavior modification. *The Psychological Record*, *31*(3), 331–334. doi:10.1007/BF03394746

Miller, F. P., Vandome, A. F., & Mc Brewster, J. (2010). *The medical model of disability*. VDM Publishing.

Miltenberger, R. G. (2012). *Behavior modification: Principles and procedures*. Belmont, CA: Wadsworth Cengage Learning.

Mishra, H. (1998). Cognitive behavior therapy. *Behavior Medicine Journal*, *1*(1), 14–19.

Morrow, W. R., & Gochros, H. L. (1970). Misconceptions regarding behavior modification. *The Social Service Review*, *44*(3), 293–307. doi:10.1086/642579

MSJE. (2009). *Ministry of Social Justice and Empowerment. Scientific Report on Research Project for Development of Indian Scale for Assessment of Autism*. New Delhi: Government of India.

Mukherjee, S. B., Malhotra, M. K., Aneja, S., Chakraborty, S., & Deshpande, S. (2015). Diagnostic accuracy of Indian scale for assessment of autism (ISAA) in children aged 2-9 years. *Indian Pediatrics*, *52*(3), 212–216. doi:10.100713312-015-0608-z PMID:25848996

Myreddi, V., Narayan, J., Saleem, S., Sumalini, K., & Padma, V. (2004). *Functional assessment checklist for programming of students with profound mental retardation (FACP-PMR)*. National Institute for the Mentally Handicapped.

Naniwadekar, K., & Venkatesan, S. (2014). Impact of behavioral intervention on reduction of problem behaviors in children with autism. *Journal of Disability Management and Special Education*, *4*(2), 1–15.

Oller, J. W., Oller, S. D., & Badon, L. C. (2010). Cases: Introducing Communication Disorders across the lifespan. Oxfordshire, UK: Plural Publishing.

Ormerod, M. (2005). Understanding access audits and appraisals: An inclusive design approach. *Journal of Building Appraisal*, *1*(2), 140–152. doi:10.1057/palgrave.jba.2940013

Ostergren, J. A. (2014). *Speech-language pathology assistants: A resource manual*. San Diego, CA: Plural Publishing.

Owens, R. E. (2017). *Introduction to communication disorders: A lifespan evidence-based perspective*. Content Technologies.

Patra, S., & Arun, P. (2011). Use of Indian scale for assessment of autism in child guidance clinic: An experience. *Indian Journal of Psychological Medicine*, *33*(2), 217–219. doi:10.4103/0253-7176.92043 PMID:22345858

Peshawaria, R., Menon, D. K., Bailey, D., Skinner, D., Ganguly, R., & Rajshekar, C. (2000). *Behavior Assessment Scales for Adult Living with Mental Retardation (BASAL-MR)*. National Institute for the Mentally Handicapped.

Peshawaria, R., & Venkatesan, S. (1992a). *Behavioral Assessment Scales for Indian Children with Mentally Retardation (BASIC-MR)*. National Institute for the Mentally Handicapped.

Peshawaria, R., & Venkatesan, S. (1992b). *Behavioral Approaches to training mentally handicapped children: A manual for teachers*. National Institute for the Mentally Handicapped.

Peshawaria, R., Venkatesan, S., & Menon, D. K. (1988). Consumer demand for services by parents of mentally handicapped individuals. *Indian Journal of Disability and Rehabilitation*, *2*(2), 43–57.

Peshawaria, R., Venkatesan, S., & Menon, D. K. (1990). Behavior problems in mentally handicapped persons: An analysis of parent needs. *Indian Journal of Clinical Psychology*, *17*(2), 63–70.

Peshawaria, R., Venkatesan, S., Mohapatra, B., & Menon, D. K. (1990). Teachers' perception of problem behaviors among mentally handicapped persons in special school settings. *Indian Journal of Disability and Rehabilitation*, *4*(1), 23–30.

Prasad, M., & Sitholey, P. (1988). Behavior therapy in a retarded adolescent with conduct disorder: A case report. *Indian Journal of Clinical Psychology*, *15*(2), 74–76.

Purves, B. A., & Phinney, A. (2012). Family voices: A family systems approach to understanding communication in dementia. *Canadian Journal of Speech-Language Pathology and Audiology*, *36*(4), 284–300.

Rao, I. (2002). *Portage Guide to Early Child Education (PGECE)*. Bangalore: CBR Network. *South Asia*.

Rao, K., Barnabas, I., & Gopinath, P. S. (1989). Behavior modification in a rehabilitation setting. *Journal of Personality and Clinical Studies*, *5*(1), 23–27.

Rao, T. A. S. (1992). *Manual on developing communication skills in mentally retarded persons*. National Institute for the Mentally Handicapped.

Rathna, N. (Ed.). (1968). *Behaviour therapy and speech disorders*. Mysore: All India Institute of Speech and Hearing.

Reddy, G., Kumari, P. S., & Kusuma, A. (2004). *Language disorders and intervention strategies: A practical guide to the teachers*. New Delhi: Discovery Publishing House.

Reddy, R. P., Sharma, M. P., & Shivashankar, N. (2010). Cognitive behavior therapy for stuttering: A case series. *Indian Journal of Psychological Medicine*, *32*(1), 49–53. doi:10.4103/0253-7176.70533 PMID:21799560

Rehabilitation Council of India. (2009a). *Bachelor of Audiology and speech-language pathology (BASLP): Semester scheme regulations, norms, scheme of exam and curriculum*. New Delhi: Author.

Rehabilitation Council of India. (2009b). *Master of science in audiology/speech-language pathology: Semester scheme regulations, norms, scheme of exam and curriculum*. New Delhi: Author.

Rehabilitation Council of India. (2009c). *Diploma course in the hearing, language, and speech: Course curriculum*. New Delhi: Author.

Schindler, A., Ruoppolo, G., & Barillari, U. (2010). Communication and its disorders: Definition and taxonomy from a phoniatric perspective. *Audiological Medicine*, *8*(4), 163–170. doi:10.3109/1651386X.2010.530023

Sharma, R., Dhaliwal, L. K., Suri, V., Kaushal, P., Singhal, N., Rana, A. K., & Singh, A. (2017). Implementing a life cycle approach through the establishment of multipurpose behavior therapy room in PGIMER, Chandigarh for enhancing the fitness level of women. *Journal of Postgraduate Medicine Education, and Research*, *51*(3), 115–122.

Singh, A. N. (1973). Behavior problems of the mentally retarded deaf. *Social Welfare*, *19*, 4.

Singh, M. V., & Dagar, B. (1982). Sociological aspects of behavior problems in a community child guidance center. *Child Psychiatry Quarterly*, *15*(2), 43–49.

Singh, R., & Kaushik, S. S. (1982). Parent training techniques in acquisition and generalization of behavior modification skill to train the retarded. *Indian Journal of Clinical Psychology*, *9*(2), 193–201.

Spiegler, M. D. (2016). *Contemporary behavior therapy*. Boston, MA: Cengage Learning.

Sroufe, L. A., & Rutter, M. (1984). The domain of developmental psychopathology. *Child Development*, *55*(1), 17–29. doi:10.2307/1129832 PMID:6705619

Thressiakutty, A. T. (1998). *NIMH Vocational Assessment and Programming System (NIMH-VAPS)*. National Institute for the Mentally Handicapped.

Upadhyaya, G. R., & Havalappanavar, N. B. (2008). Stress in parents of the mentally challenged. *Journal of the Indian Academy of Applied Psychology*, *34*, 53–59.

Veeraraghavan, V. (1998). Behavior medicine: Its relevance to the 21st century. *Behavior Medicine Journal*, *1*(1), 1–9.

Veeraraghavan, V., & Malik, S. C. (Eds.). (1994). *Readings in behavior medicine*. New Delhi: Phoenix Publishing.

Venkatesan, S. (1994). Recent trends and issues in the behavioral assessment of individuals with mental handicap in India. *The Creative Psychologist*, *6*(1), 1–7.

Venkatesan, S. (2004). *Children with developmental disabilities: A training guide for parents, teachers and caregivers*. Thousand Oaks, CA: Sage Publications.

Venkatesan, S. (2010a). Book Review; Portage Guide to Early Childhood Education. *Journal of All India Institute of Speech and Hearing*, *29*(1), 128–130.

Venkatesan, S. (2010b). Cultural factors in clinical assessment: The Indian perspective. *Indian Journal of Clinical Psychology*, *37*(1), 75–85.

Venkatesan, S. (2013). Preliminary try out and validation of problem behavior survey schedule for children with developmental disabilities. *Journal of Disability Management and Special Education*, *3*(2), 9–22.

Venkatesan, S. (2015a). Socio-cultural dimensions of cleft lip and palate in India. *Global Journal of Interdisciplinary Social Sciences*, *4*(3), 72–77.

Venkatesan, S. (2015b). A growing trend in pseudo-diagnosis: A field study on children frequently mistaken for autism in India. *Psychological Studies*, *60*(1), 91–100. doi:10.100712646-015-0302-1

Venkatesan, S. (2015c). *Problem Behavior Survey Schedule*. Bangalore: Psychotronics.

Venkatesan, S. (2015d). Evaluation of teaching objectives earmarked for children with developmental disabilities. *Disabilities and Impairments*, *29*(2), 85–96.

Venkatesan, S. (2015e). Revisiting goal setting for children with developmental disabilities. *Journal of Disability Management and Special Education*, *5*(2), 19–27.

Venkatesan, S., & Lokesh, L. (2016). Differential perception of problem behaviors between parents, teachers, and therapists. *The International Journal of Indian Psychology*, *3*(4), 21–33.

Venkatesan, S., & Lokesh, L. (2017). Consequence mapping of problem behaviors in children with developmental delays. *Disabilities and Impairments*, *31*(3), 47–64.

Venkatesan, S., Peshawaria, R., & Anuradha, M. P. (1996). Reward preferences in parents/caregivers of children with mental handicaps. *Indian Journal of Applied Psychology*, *33*(1), 11–17.

Venkatesan, S., & Ravindran, N. (2015). Autism behavior checklist for disability estimation: A preliminary field tryout. *Psychological Studies*, *60*(2), 215–225. doi:10.100712646-015-0304-z

Venkatesan, S., & Vepuri, V. G. D. (1993). Parental perceptions of causes and management of problem behaviors in individuals with a mental handicap. *Disabilities and Impairments*, *7*(2), 29–37.

Venkatesan, S., Yashodharakumar, G. Y., Gupta, S. K., & Vasudha, H. H. (2015). Gap analysis for evaluation of individualized education programs for children with developmental disabilities. *International Journal of Psychology and Psychiatry*, *3*(2), 64–76. doi:10.5958/2320-6233.2015.00017.6

Vismara, L. A., & Rogers, S. L. (2010). Behavioral treatments for autism spectrum disorder: What do we know? *Annual Review of Clinical Psychology*, *6*(1), 447–468. doi:10.1146/annurev.clinpsy.121208.131151 PMID:20192785

World Health Organization. (2007). *International Classification of Functioning, Disability, and Health: Children and Youth Version*. Geneva: Author.

World Health Organization. (2013). *The ICD-10-CM codes and criteria*. Retrieved from http://www.icd10data.com/search?s=autism%20

Ylvisaker, M., Turkstra, L. S., & Coelho, C. (2005). Behavioral and social interventions for individuals with traumatic brain injury: A summary of the research with clinical implications. *Seminars in Speech and Language*, *26*(4), 256–267. doi:10.1055-2005-922104 PMID:16278797

KEY TERMS AND DEFINITIONS

Antecedent: A thing or event that existed before or logically precedes another.

Applied Behavior Analysis: A scientific discipline concerned with developing techniques of behavior change based on principles of behaviorism.

Attention Deficit/Hyperactivity Disorder: A childhood developmental disorder characterized by short attention span, impulsivity, and overactivity.

Autism: A childhood developmental disorder characterized by social-interaction difficulties, communication challenges, and a tendency to engage in repetitive behaviors.

Behavior Assessment: A method used to observe, describe, explain, predict, and correct behaviors based on the tenets proposed by behaviorism.

Behavior Therapy: A form of psychotherapy which follows the tenets espoused by behaviorism in the correction, change, remediation, or treatment of maladaptive behaviors.

Behavioral Mapping: A depiction of events or happenings related to observable and measurable actions in terms of their nature, setting, frequency or duration, before and after events.

Biofeedback: A training process of gaining awareness of the physiological functions using instruments that provide information on the activity of those systems with a goal of being able to manipulate them.

Chaining: An instructional procedure used by behaviorists that involves reinforcing individual responses occurring along a sequence of complex behavior.

Challenging Behavior: Any behavior that interferes with learning, is harmful to the learner or others in the environment.

Communication Disorders: Any disorder that affects an individual's ability to comprehend, detect, or apply language and speech to engage in interaction with others.

Compliance Training: A non-coercive procedure involving the teaching of certain behavioral responses for particular stimulus conditions.

Conduct Disorder: A condition presenting itself as repetitive and persistent pattern of behavior in which basic rights of others or age-appropriate norms are violated.

Consequence: The result or effect that is seen or occurs after a behavior.

Contingency Contracting: An agreement between the therapist-client which states the offering of particular rewards contingent upon performance of certain agreed upon behaviors.

Differential Rewards: A procedure of reinforcement of certain specified behaviors while abstaining from rewarding certain other kinds of other or alternate behaviors.

Extinction: The disappearance of previously learned behavior when the behavior is not reinforced anymore.

Functional Analysis: It is the application of the laws of operant and respondent conditioning to establish the relationships between stimulus and response.

Functional-Utilitarian Model: It refers to the assumption in behavioral approach that all human actions are learned or maintained as means of some benefit or utility they provide to the person exhibiting them.

Generalization: A tendency to respond in the same way to different but similar stimuli.

Human Rights Model: An approach in psychology that champions promotion of human rights, health, wellbeing, and dignity.

Intellectual Disability: A new term for mental retardation that reflects a condition of significant limitations in cognitive functioning and in adaptive behavior.

Life Span Approach: A perspective that accounts for human behavior across stages of development beginning from conception to death.

Normative Approach: A perspective which assumes that all behavioral phenomenon exists according to the normal distribution curve thereby signifying that a majority population lies in the center while the rest of them occupy less portions in the either extreme ends.

Operant Techniques: Also called instrumental techniques, it refers to methods of learning through rewards and punishments for behavior.

Opposition Defiant Disorder: A disorder in a child marked by defiant and disobedient behavior to authority figures.

Premack Principle: The reinforcement of preferred more probable behaviors for the non-preferred low probable behaviors.

Problem Behavior: A negative, unwanted, or maladaptive human action that causes stress on others, is either harmful to self or others, is age inappropriate and interferes in the learning or teaching of skill behaviors.

Prompting: An act of helping or teaching a behavior to occur.

Psychometric Approach: An approach that seeks to study individual differences while making measurements of various variables in psychology.

Punishment: A thing or event that occurs after a behavior and that which leads to reduction of that behavior.

Reward: A thing or event that occurs after a behavior and that which leads to increase in the occurrence of that behavior.

Shaping: A technique that involves differential reinforcement of successive approximations.

Situational Analysis: A framework for understanding behavior in the context, ambience, environment, or ecology of their occurrence.

Skill Behavior: A positive, wanted, or adaptive human action that is sought to be taught for the benefit of the learner.

Symptom Substitution: At the core of psychoanalytic approach, it refers to the development of new symptoms that replaces an old symptom when they have been already cleared after the treatment.

Testing of Limits: The use of behavioral counter-strategies by a subject by maintaining the same maladaptive behavior to see how far one can go in the enforcement of behavior modification strategies.

Token Economy: A system of contingency management based on systematic reinforcement, is target behavior using tokens that can be exchanged for other reinforcements.

Chapter 12
Discourse Elicitation in Aphasia: An Indian Framework

S. P. Goswami
All India Institute of Speech and Hearing, India

Brajesh Priyadarshi
All India Institute of Speech and Hearing, India

Sharon Mathews
All India Institute of Speech and Hearing, India

ABSTRACT

Persons with aphasia (PWA) face varying difficulties of communication breakdown through different stages of recovery. With speech-language therapy, significant recovery may be seen at unitary levels, but the ultimate success of therapy is evident when the PWA uses all of the units as a whole and is able to communicate optimally to sustain social identities. An individualized intervention program as the focus, a protocol is proposed with seven semi-structured interviews aimed at eliciting discourse incorporating the philosophies of the social model, LPAA, SCA, AphasiaBank Protocol, and Protocol to Measure Participation of Persons with Aphasia. The interviews with the PWA and their communication partners in individual and joint sessions can help the clinician answer questions regarding the PWA's physical abilities, dietary issues, functional independence, personal traits, relationships at home, different social roles played, and subsequently plan a treatment program, and track the holistic recovery of the PWA.

DISCOURSE IN COMMUNICATION

Successful social bonds form the foundations of human communication. Social networking is cemented with concrete conversational episodes whose primary purpose is information exchange. Each individual's innate desire to communicate brings about the multitude of language forms witnessed in the environment. Language is molded, modified, scaffolded and presented as discourse for sharing of ideas, thoughts and feelings. This transmission of information between individual units is indispensable for the existence of the unit as a whole. Language disorders hinder the smooth flow of information causing an imbalance in

DOI: 10.4018/978-1-5225-4955-0.ch012

the social unit. The presence of discourse elicitation works as an appendage buttressing the connections in this network.

Discourse is defined as the basic unit of human communication. Pragmatics-component of language-defines the contextual use of language. The mutual relationship of language and context determine "why a speaker says something, when the speaker says it; to whom the speaker says it and how it is said". Yet, words and sentences alone cannot completely describe how discourse is produced, given the variations in the linguistic structures based on the context. The cognitive and social aspects of language play exhibit a symbiotic reaction in discourse. Cognition and language are two interrelated domains working on the various aspects of information processing in the brain. The role of cognition in language dissemination is visible in the pragmatic ability of an individual. Discourse being the denouement of the interaction of cognition, language and context, deserves a multifaceted investigation (Cherney, Shadden, and Coelho, 1998). The pragmatic appropriateness of discourse revolves around three context: extra-linguistic, paralinguistic and linguistic contexts (Davis, 1986). The extra-linguistic context is inclusive of external-physical surroundings, time of the day and the number and location of the participants- and internal factors of participants. The paralinguistic context refers to the prosodic and suprasegmental component of an utterance. The linguistic context refers to the verbal output. Discourse is a series of connected sentences that convey a message. Although typically discourse is longer than a word, it has been argued that when a word alone expresses a message, it may be considered discourse. This is particularly relevant for persons with aphasia (PWA) in which the unit of analysis may be as short as a word.

Types of discourse entail descriptive, narrative, procedural, persuasive, expository and conversational. Discourse is classified based on the functions it serves. Analysis of discourse involves multilevel examination that (a) assesses PWAs' performance across discourse tasks that require different cognitive and discourse skills and (b) assesses different aspects of discourse performance within the same task. Microstructural analyses focus at the local level of the word. They are concerned with the small elements in a text and the relations between these small elements. Macrostructural analyses focus at the level of the entire text. Superstructural analysis overlies the text and includes the analysis of story grammar. PWA may show differential impairments at each level. Therefore, it is important to use a variety of discourse elicitation and analysis procedure to identify the specific discourse impairments of the PWA.

ASSESSMENT OF DISCOURSE

The proliferation of research on discourse analysis has occurred concomitantly with changes in health care that emphasizes the need for determining functional goals for communicatively impaired PWA and measuring functional outcomes in clinical practice. The environment determines the nature of communication; if the environment changes, the communication changes accordingly. Functional communication goals for a specific person can be determined only with respect to that persons' own social and physical setting and therefore can be defined only with respect to the individual (Hartley, 1995). Discourse analysis procedures provide the clinician with a set of evaluation tools that (a) describe the impairment in objective and measurable terms, (b) help identify the underlying cognitive or linguistic processes that contribute to the discourse impairment, (c) assist in treatment planning, and (d) are sensitive to changes over time. It is important to consider the discourse of PWA. However, the systematic application of discourse analysis procedures may not be warranted for all individuals, particularly, if the communication problem is severe and the output is limited. Therefore, for each PWA, clinicians must make decisions about when and what kind of discourse is to be sampled and how the discourse is to be analyzed.

For a keen assessment, the selection of tasks for eliciting a substantive sample for discourse should encompass a broad range of behaviors especially focusing on the individual strengths and deficits of a person. As the etiology and the ramifications of stroke vary with each individual, the method of assessment of discourse also follows a distinctive pattern. These specific decisions need to be made considering the variety of task-related variables. As for the stimulus used, the different modes of presentation can be simple to complex, auditory and/ or visual with a shared and/or absent reference between the PWA and clinician. The memory and sequential organization at the level of PWA can set the macro-structural level of discourse. Disruptions, like repetitions, revisions, excessive pausing in the task can be anticipated by the clinician, but not often, while setting the complexity of the stimulus. The testing instructions are solely at the disposal of the clinician and how s/he conveys them effectively. For example, instructions for a picture description task can vary from direct to elaborate as in, 'Describe this picture' to 'Connect the events in the picture to form a story' will influence the quality of the verbal performance. Similarly, a request to tell a story in their own words or follow the clinician would affect the elicited response. Personal relevance comes into play when the clinician intends to tap into the individual's emotional plane. Overall functioning can be assessed using a general topic of conversation, but with a topic of personal relevance, the PWA may not just give the details about the topic, but also state personal experiences that add to the content of discourse, and higher quality of performance. For instance, upon asking an older gentleman about smart phones, the quality of the description and information content would clearly be different from when the same topic is given to a teenager. The factor of personal style in discourse is also associated closely with the aspect of personal relevance, again left to the judgment of the clinician. Open-ended tasks generally allow the individual to exercise their personal style. Accounts of past events and general conversation gives a good opportunity for the person to exhibit their stylistic variations in discourse, than do constrained tasks such as story retelling or picture descriptions. Discourse analysis procedures, although vast, provide the clinician with an extensive understanding of the strengths and weaknesses of an individual. An attempt to include all the variability in a discourse elicitation task is analogous to pattern in chaos. A clinician's discretion even though aims at individualized analysis, may more often seem subjective, with the clinician choosing only tasks that are adept at assessing the overt needs of the PWA. Having a specified framework for discourse assessment, builds on the confidence of the clinician as s/he would not miss the minute details, simultaneously working on the initiation of rehabilitative services.

DISCOURSE ELICITATION IN PERSONS WITH APHASIA

The essence of discourse elicitation lies in the purpose of reintegration of the PWA in society. The scope of recovery is measured by the number of social roles the individual can carry off after the advent of stroke followed by aphasia. The current treatment models focusing on the narrow linguistic parameters assessed by standardized test batteries allow only as much improvement as can be achieved within the clinical setting and the recovery tends to remain incomplete. Termination of traditional language intervention programs reflects the sheer ignorance of the social aspect of recovery. Issues on lack or change in social identities of PWA remain disregarded when clearly the "ceiling effect" in their recovery is an effect of their social isolation. An understanding of this idea leads us to the social model applied to aphasia (Simmons-Mackie, 1998a; Gee, 1999). The social model looks at aphasic impairments from two different perspectives that are essentially two sides of the same coin! Societal and communicative perspective constitute the 'social model' with the former addressing issues of social barriers to communication and life participation and the latter focusing on the individualistic interactions of the PWA with his/her environment. This model projects the outlook that the treatment approach should follow a social holistic pattern wherein along with addressing the language impairment the PWA and his family comes forth as a thriving social unit.

Supported Conversation Analysis (SCA; Simmons-Mackie, 1998b; Kagan, 1999) as a technique embodies that a supportive environment assuages the conversational episodes of PWA; thereby improving one's opportunity for restoring social identities. SCA (Parr and Byng, 1998) helps in revealing the inner strength of person in conversational interactions which play a central role in life participation. This is achieved by training the caregiver to view PWA as a competent conversational partner by providing a communicative ramp. The philosophy of SCA is derived from the Life Participation Approach to aphasia (LPAA; Chapey et al., 2001). The LPAA is based on the premise that whatever be the strengths or weaknesses of the PWA, a supportive environment dampens the effect of disability on the individual's life. This approach advocates the need for intervention at three levels, classifying the different activities of a PWA, i.e., at the body level, individual level and the society level. Anomia or hemiparesis reflects problems at body level, and is differentiated from problems at the individual level that involve difficulties in taking bath or reading a book. The society level comprises of activities like practicing one's profession, being a part of a social gathering, or going to a movie. Targeting treatment at all three levels ensures quality services for the PWA and professional support for the PWA and family throughout the course of recovery. Keeping in mind the importance of life enhancement changes with its dependence on social model, clinician may also look into the environment in which activity or discourse is carried out. The conversation partner in the adjoining environment is the key to understanding how the situated meaning, grammar and social identities in conversation vary within discourse. Thus, the recovery of PWA involves a reorientation of the conversation partner to the communicative needs of the reformed person. The social integration of PWA falls within the purview of the International Classification of Functioning, Disability and Health (ICF) schematic (World Health Organization, 2001) which centralizes on the activity and is co-dependent on the health condition, body functions, contextual factors and participation levels of the PWA. The social perspective of treatment for PWAs focuses not only on the medical aspects of improving the body functions and structures, but also enhancing the participation levels by improving the life activities, wherein the environmental factors and personal factors act as either a barrier or a facilitator.

THE PROPOSED PROTOCOL FOR DISCOURSE ELICITATION IN PERSONS WITH APHASIA

The road to social recovery of a PWA begins with identification and assessment of the person and the family as a holistic unit (Joanette and Brownell, 1993). Assessment of aphasia entails precise and extensive tools each having their own advantages. The decision lies in the hands of the clinician on how to use these tools in a time effective manner. A discourse analysis incorporated in the assessment of aphasia helps to strike a balance between an extensive and precise assessment procedure, in order to accomplish an efficient assessment. It is a tedious job to approximate an appropriate discourse elicitation procedure without any specific guidelines. This study introduces a manual consisting of seven semi-structured interviews enabling to gather copious amounts of information right from the first session. These interviews, accommodating a range of tasks were designed keeping in view the problems in PWA, and to obtain information about the subtle changes in their discourse production. Whilst giving structure to what kind of data needs to be collected, it provides freedom to clinicians for organizing interviews in discrete sessions. This ensures that the assessment duration does not outgrow the duration of rehabilitative services provided.

The proposed protocol prepared for discourse elicitation is a result of the incorporation of philosophies of the social model, LPAA, SCA, AphasiaBank Protocol, Protocol to Measure Participation of Persons with Aphasia and an opinion of how a uniform protocol aimed at holistic recovery enables a person with aphasia. Priority should be given to the person as a whole and not the disability as discussed in these aforementioned concepts. The PWA's social identities and his life as an individual are valued and it is believed that every individual contributes to the society in the minutest and the biggest possible ways.

The present protocol is a booklet of questions that set the stage for elaborate discourse elicitation via semi-structured interviews with PWA and others who are a part of his social unit. A social unit in this study comprised of the PWA, the conversation partner, an employer or colleague. A conversation partner can be the spouse, parents or friends who is vital to the PWA's current communication episodes. In the proposed manual, specific demeanor of clinician in each interview and their attitude through which they can create maximum opportunities for detailed responses is outlined. The proposed interviews are divided into definite topics with a single open-ended question and a set of prompt questions for each topic. Each session is expected to be conducted in 45-60 minutes, wherein a single interview may extend for more than one session based on the discourse abilities of the PWA and the quality of discourses itself. Prior to beginning the interviews, informing the PWA and caregiver about the format of the interviews and the confidentiality of the information provided by them helps the clinician build a better rapport. It is also easier when the PWA is informed that he/she may take a break at any point during the interview, or even choose not to answer certain questions.

Interview 1

The first semi-structured interview is a joint interview involving the PWA and caregiver(s) and begins with questions that help build a rapport with the clinician. The first interview format is illustrated in Appendix 1. Beginning with a brief introduction and a casual exchange of information, this interview session kicks off the assessment by obtaining information about the PWA and caregivers, covering all facets of demographic detail, specifics of stroke and neurological, psychological, behavioral, motor, linguistic aftermath. Further, the details of any alternate therapies, allied and medical assessments and treatments to improve the overall quality of life are also inquired by the clinician. Having gathered these basic demographics of the individual, the clinician can now move to communication with the PWA at a discourse level. Discourse topics listed in the protocol such as relationships at home, dietary issues, physical abilities, social life, functional independence and personal traits include questions that will help direct the PWA-clinician conversation. This provides an opportunity for the clinician to understand the communicative level of the PWA in the presence of the caregivers and the extent and type of support received from the caregiver when there is a communication breakdown. The clinician can directly observe the communicative roles of the PWA and caregiver as being active or passive partners during this interview.

In addition to gathering information, the first joint interview session sets the way to establishing a professional trust between the social unit and the clinician. As the clinician and the social unit move further, the format of the interviews enable the clinician to build an understanding within this unit, and intervention goals can be focused on the unit as a whole and not PWA alone.

Interview 2

The AphasiaBank Protocol (http://aphasia.talkbank.org/protocol/) forms the second interview session with the PWA. The AphasiaBank Protocol which is freely available online was used with linguistic and ethno-cultural adaptations for Indian languages. The AphasiaBank protocol is a detailed procedure assessing all aspects of linguistic competence and has two major sections and various sub-sections. The first section is broken down into four subsections: conversation, picture description, story re-telling and procedural discourse. Each of these subsections has set of tasks and questions that elicit verbal discourse. The first subsection (illustrated in Appendix 2) involves the clinician inquiring about the stroke story, coping with the condition and an important event that molded the PWA's life. The second subsection is a picture description task that includes three stimuli: broken window, refused umbrella and cat rescue. The first two stimuli consisted of a four-panel and six-panel sequence. The clinician may simply present these stimuli and instruct the PWA to look at the pictures carefully and describe what they see. The PWA's may require prompts to help them connect the story sequence at the beginning of this subsection and the clinician is free to decide the type of prompts to be used with each of these picture description tasks.

Keeping in mind the cultural variations of the target population, certain adaptations and modifications are made to the subsections in the AphasiaBank Protocol as in the third subsection. Story re-telling requires the PWA to tell the 'Hare and Tortoise' story commonly known to the target population. This section can employ a different story based on the target population. When assessing PWA from varied ethno-cultural background, childhood fables specific to them should be assessed. For Indian population, the 'Hare and Tortoise' story is an appropriate option. The fourth subsection which elicits procedural discourse skills entails the step-by-step delineation of making tea. Making a peanut butter-jelly sandwich is a concept alien to the Indian population. However, tea is a common drink throughout the country and the procedure would be known to all individuals albeit with certain variations. This change in the procedural task is only made to make the evaluation relevant to the target population. The second section of the AphasiaBank Protocol involves administration of Western Aphasia Battery-Revised (Kertesz, 1982), Aphasia Bank Repetition Test and Verb Naming Test. The word and sentence repetition test and verb naming test are translated into Indian languages or appropriately adapted such that the stimuli has an ascending level of difficulty and are culturally appropriate. Observations and results from these tests will help the clinician specifically target the linguistic challenges faced by the PWA during language therapy. Administration and scoring of each test is explained systematically in the manual as is in the online AphasiaBank protocol.

The incorporation of internationally developed and recognized AphasiaBank protocol assists the clinician to establish a clear understanding of the PWA's linguistic abilities and deficits. Comprehensive knowledge of the PWA's shortcomings becomes the basis of the succeeding interviews with the clinician being the sole communication partner, finds it easier to carry out supported conversations.

Interview 3

The third interview (see Appendix 3) is an individual interview session with the PWA, investigating the personal feats, relations, work expertise, public relations, current responsibilities, financial status, quality of service delivery and further expectations. This session brings the focus on the PWA; the clinician is free to enquire about the individual's feelings and thus, gather an understanding of his/her fears, anxieties, and sorrows and how they are coping with these feelings over the continuum of recovery. The interview format for this session lists questions that are directed toward the individual and his experiences, helping the clinician drive the conversation into understanding the PWAs personality. The clinician can trace out the various changes in the individual's personality with respect to each of their social identities. Most individuals may put on a strong face in front of their dear ones and hide the deepest fears about their condition. In many situations, PWAs are dependent on their caregivers for activities of daily living, and the extent of help required depends on their communicative and motor difficulties. They often consider themselves as a burden on the family and thus, hide their worries and fears hoping not to cause any further problems to their caregivers. Difficulty accepting change in their social role could be another reason for not sharing their feelings with the caregiver, which could be sometimes expressed in terms of anger or frustration. For most PWAs, a space to talk about themselves in the absence of the caregiver gives them an opportunity to vent out suppressed feelings over the whole situation, something that they keep thinking about every minute of their life post-stroke. This gives them a chance to talk about their anxieties, fears, depression and hope for recovery from their own perspective. Clinicians may bear in mind that, although an individual interview is intended to gather subtle information about the PWA, it is the choice of the PWA to disclose any of the information. By establishing oneself as an ardent listener who is neither biased nor detached, the clinician is able to gain the trust of the PWA. This further emphasizes the role of the speech-language pathologist as a professional with a better understanding of the PWA's current situation.

With this interview session, the clinician discusses matters that are of the highest priority to the PWA, matters concerning the past, present and future. This way, the clinician can track the change within and across interviews, from feelings solely of anger and depression to more positive attitudes toward life changes.

Interview 4

The fourth interview session (see Appendix 4) is an individual session with the conversation partner or caregiver to explore the changes in the dynamics of their relationship after the onset of stroke and aphasia, extent of setback faced by this event and strength of the support system coming into play for coping up. It goes on to understand the scope of hope and good-will, factors responsible for improvement, people who have come forward to be a part of the PWA's recovery and the need for training of conversation partner. It also maps out the conversation partner's personal life and career plans and where PWA's recovery falls on this timeline. A strong support system is imperative for inclusion of PWA in his social circles post aphasia.

Interview 5

The fifth session lays out the administration of Protocol to Measure Participation of Persons with Aphasia for appraising the ability of PWA to participate in desired life situations, and was developed by Mathur and Goswami in 2010. This tool measures the effect of aphasia on a person's life in the horizon with the goals of ICF schematic (World Health Organization, 2001). It is a picture based rating measure wherein the PWA rates on a 5 point rating scale for an extensive set of questions broadly categorized under (a) understanding and expression, (b) general tasks and demands, (c) interpersonal interactions and relationships (d) facilitators and barriers. The clinician begins the session by explaining PWA about the questionnaire and how to rate each question using an illustration of the scale provided. The clinician continues by asking the questions and prompting the PWA to choose a number on the scale based on their experiences in the present and based on their perception of how easy or difficult an activity is. The questionnaire also includes certain questions wherein the PWA has to compare the pre-morbid abilities and skills to the present condition. This self-rating scale gives a vivid picture on how the PWA perceives his/her life with aphasia. Having meticulously observed PWA's discourse skills over the days, the clinician must now be able to decide if these ratings are in line with the actual difficulties faced by the individual. Moreover, PWA's self-perception is also an indication of their confidence in carrying out various communicative and daily life activities. The Protocol to Measure Participation of Persons with Aphasia tremendously helps in the early phase of assessment as the included illustrations supplement the verbal instructions and traditional quality of life measures.

Interview 6

The sixth session (see Appendix 5) draws attention to the work arena. Taking into consideration the ICF model and social model, the identities and activities of the PWA are not only restricted to family and home, but to the society and the workplace too. The session would be applicable if the PWAs were pre-morbidly employed or held an identity that was away from home and family members. The clinician interviews an employer or colleague for the new found expectations and consignment of duties to the individual who now has aphasia. This interview attempts to consider the demands of PWA's job and tries to make it clear to the employer/colleague that PWA still has the abilities to contribute though in an altered way. The session observes if the co-worker/ employer is willing to keep the PWA employed despite their communicative and/or physical difficulties. It gives an opportunity for the clinician, PWA and the co-worker/employer to discuss the modifications, accommodations and adjustments that can be made at workplace. As professionals, it gives a chance to counsel the employer that taking a PWA back at workplace will be a determiner of good prognosis.

Interview 7

The seventh session (see Appendix 6) is communicative counseling session that consolidates a profile description of PWA to the social unit. The employer, conversation partner/caregiver and PWAs are all privy to the results of the seven semi-structured interview sessions. These sessions will help in knowing the strengths, weaknesses, opportunities, threats, barriers and facilitators with respect to home, community and workplace, understanding and interpreting the findings to unearth to improve and maintain the role of PWA in house, work and community; thereby, improving the mental, physical, social well being of the PWA, conversation partner and the employer. Each session provides an opportunity to PWAs to clarify doubts, queries, suggestions, views they have regarding the assessment and treatment plan. This manual provides a conglomerate of multichannel communicative access between the PWA family, employer and clinician serving as confidence building measure for better recovery.

CONCLUSION

The present protocol for discourse elicitation in PWA is fundamentally a semi-structured questionnaire that enables the clinician to be feasible with the questions as per PWA's emotional state. It helps in building a strong foundation for intervention. Voicing out personal stories of PWA and caregiver establishes a bond between them and the clinician. By empathizing with the PWA whilst keeping a professional outlook, the clinician is able to build the rapport for future sessions. It enumerates life participation goals for PWA. In order for clinician to attend to life enhancement skills of PWA, it is important to establish the different activities of PWA pre and post-stroke. This manual with its vast range of discourse elicitation task gives a better picture of PWA's life at personal, individual and societal levels. It is instrumental in charting changes/ improvements in PWA. It evaluates the motivational level of PWA in terms of volubility and overall demeanor while coming for rehabilitative services. A set of seven sessions is important for PWA and clinician to accept and adjust to the new situation, forge new bonds, come to terms with new way of life. A week of discourse between the clinician, PWA and his social unit builds confidence, connects them on a personal level, co-ordinates the flow of service delivery, and improves communication amplifying the caliber of all involved.

Starting from first interview session, the current discourse manual becomes a rich source of information for carrying out clinical services and detailed research programs outlining the road to recovery. The number of sessions is flexible and can be selected based on what the situation demands. A clinician can pick and choose the topics to be elicited and manipulate the manual as per the needs of PWA and the environment. The current study describes a manual that paves the way for qualitative research as the quantity and quality of data gathered can be enormous. Further, it entails a discourse analysis incorporating the ideas of LPAA and ICF, providing a true insight about the feelings, coping mechanisms, expectations, failures and course of recovery.

ACKNOWLEDGMENT

This research was funded by the All India Institute of Speech and Hearing, Mysuru [grant number SH/CDN/ARF-19/2016-17].

REFERENCES

Chapey, R., Duchan, J. F., Elman, R. J., Garcia, L. J., Kagan, A., Lyon, J. G., & Simmons-Mackie, N. (2001). Life participation approach to aphasia: A statement of values for the future. In R. Chapey (Ed.), *Language intervention strategies in aphasia and related neurogenic communication disorders* (pp. 235–245). Baltimore, MD: Lippincott, Williams and Wilkins.

Cherney, L. R., Shadden, B. B., & Coelho, C. A. (1998). *Analyzing discourse in communicatively impaired adults*. Gaithersburg, MD: Aspen Publishers, Inc.

Davis, G. A. (1986). Pragmatics and treatment. In R. Chapey (Ed.), *Language intervention strategies in adult aphasia* (pp. 251–265). Baltimore, MD: Williams and Wilkins.

Gee, J. P. (1999). *An introduction to discourse analysis: Theory and practice*. London: Routledge.

Hartley, L. L. (1995). *Cognitive-communicative abilities following brain injury: A functional approach*. San Diego, CA: Singular Publishing Group.

Joanette, Y., & Brownell, H. H. (Eds.). (1993). *Narrative discourse in neurologically impaired and normal aging adults*. San Diego, CA: Singular Publishing Group.

Kagan, A. (1999). *Supported conversation for adults with aphasia: Methods and evaluation* (Published doctoral dissertation). Toronto: University of Toronto.

Kertesz, A. (1982). *Western Aphasia Battery*. New York: Grune and Stratton.

Mathur, R., & Goswami, S. P. (2010). *Protocol to Measure Participation of Persons with Aphasia* (Unpublished dissertation). University of Mysore.

Parr, S., & Byng, S. (1998). Breaking new ground in familiar territory: A response to 'Supported conversation for adults with aphasia' by Aura Kagan. *Aphasiology*, *12*(9), 839–844. doi:10.1080/02687039808249579

Simmons-Mackie, N. (1998a). A solution to the discharge dilemma in aphasia: Social approaches to aphasia management. *Aphasiology*, *12*(3), 231–239. doi:10.1080/02687039808249451

Simmons-Mackie, N. (1998b). In support of supported conversation for adults with aphasia. *Aphasiology*, *12*(9), 831–838. doi:10.1080/02687039808249576

World Health Organisation. (2001). *Classification of Functioning, Disability and Health. Retrieved from* http://www.who.int/classifications/icf/en/

KEY TERMS AND DEFINITIONS

Aphasia: It is the condition resulting from any kind of damage to the brain leading to impaired ability to comprehend speech or formulate language in terms of verbal or even written mode.

Cohesion: It is one of the integral parts of discourse which refers to the continuity in text or speech, within and between sentences giving lexical and semantic links in the discourse. The cohesiveness determines the connectivity and overall understanding of a discourse.

Communication: Communication is the act of exchanging one's ideas, thoughts, and opinions effectively with one or multiple participants. This transferring of information can be made using verbal or nonverbal modes.

Discourse: Discourse refers to the continuity and appropriateness of the use of words during conversation. It reflects the ability of an individual to retain the theme of conversation using varied linguistic components. In persons with aphasia, loss of language should not be viewed only from a linguistic perspective pertaining to phonology, syntax, and semantics but also from a holistic view including discourse in communication. Thus, discourse should be an integral component in the assessment and treatment of persons with aphasia.

Language: It is an arbitrary system of communication consisting of symbols like words, gestures, signs, and written text. It follows a set of rules to convey information and ideas in a group or within a community.

Life Participation Approach: This is a service delivery model in aphasia which is more individual-centered and advocates the activities which are focused to improve the activity and participation of an individual from a holistic perspective.

Recovery: Recovery in aphasia refers to the improvement in the condition post-stroke where the individual regains the lost skills and is able to gain independency thereby improving quality of life. The recovery is, however, dependent on various factors including severity of the stroke and the individual's ability.

Social Identity: The identity of a person in the society is the sense of understanding of the person's beliefs and opinions which builds a perception of their recognition in a particular social group.

APPENDIX 1

The following is an illustration of the first semi-structured interview in the proposed protocol for discourse elicitation in PWA. This interview is a joint session with the patient and family members

- **For the Researcher:** This session will record the relationship between the patient and the spouse/ communication partner. It will try to gauge the comfort levels between them, the level of dependency of the patient on the spouse/ communication partner and each of their contribution in successful communication during the meeting.
- **Note:** The researcher should follow the role of a conversation partner, be assertively involved in the conversation, should speak encouragingly to extend the conversation, speak in smaller sentences that help the patient put up a better discourse. The researcher should use the following questions to shape the interview into a conversation. The researchers should make sure all points are discussed, but feel free to change the ordering of the questions in order to follow conversational topics. The researcher should create opportunities for eliciting stories from the patient by being cooperative and not authoritative during the sessions.
- **For the Participant:** We intend to cement a strong bond amongst all of us for laying out your ideas, feelings and expectations which will help us in better understanding of the issues resulting in improved health, functioning and service delivery.

Introductory Conversation

Hello.

How are you feeling today?

Did you have your breakfast? Tell me about your favorite breakfast and how you prepare it? Do you get it in a restaurant and where is it?

Do you like the weather here? Which is your favorite season and why do you like it so much? What is the one thing that you like to do in that season?

Documenting Details

- **Demographic Details:** Name, Age/Gender, Education, Pre and post-morbid: vocation, socioeconomic status, languages known, handedness, family status, geographical location
- **Details of Stroke:** Site of lesion, Age, Medical Treatment
- **Results of Stroke:** Neurological, Psychological, Behavioral, Motor, Linguistic aftermath of stroke (Based on the available reports from PWA viz. hospital discharge reports, case files or any other sources available.)
- **Type of Services:** Medical, Physical, Occupational, Speech-Language, Psychotherapy and any other treatment (Eg: Ayurveda, Homeopathy etc.) and/or rehabilitation.

Framework

Clinician should use this framework but also use situational prompts and questions to encourage the patient in a discourse.

Family and Home

Tell me about your family.

Prompts from the clinician:

Oh, so all of them are living with you at your home?

How are the household chores divided?

Is this similar to before the accident/stroke?

Do both of you enjoy close-knit family activities?

Nutrition

Tell me about your favorite food and how you cook it?

Prompts

Has your diet changed since some days?

Any change in your feeding schedule?

Who helps you in cooking?

Does your spouse enjoy cooking?

What is your spouse's favorite meal?

Physical Status

Tell me about your health.

Prompts

You fancy a walk in the park?

How do you go to the market?

Does your family accompany you to the market?

Tell me about a day spend in the market/ park with your family members.

Social Life

Tell me about your friends.

Prompts

Where do you use to meet them? And where do you meet them now?

What is your favorite pastime? Tell me about a day you have done that recently.

What are your hobbies and interests?

Who is your best friend?

Tell me when you first met them/ tell me about your fondest memory with them.

Functional Independence

Tell me the directions to your hospital.

Prompts

How often do you meet your doctor?

What is your daily schedule?

Who takes care of you around the house?

Personality

Tell me what do you like best about yourself?

Prompts

Are people impressed with this attribute?

What do you like best about your spouse?

Do you feel there is a change in her/his behavior?

This brings us to the end of this session. If you have any queries now or later, we will oblige with pleasure. Hope you all had a good time. Thank you for your time. I really appreciate it. See you soon. Bye.

APPENDIX 2

Conversation: Stroke Story and Coping

1. "I'm going to be asking you to do some talking. How do you think you speak in English/Hindi, Kannada/Malayalam?" (Choose the dominant language spoken by the PWA pre-morbidly)
    a. If no response in approximately 10 seconds, prompt: "How's your talking/ability to tell a story?"
    b. Listen, encourage full response.
    c. If no response, ask, "Are you having trouble with your talking?"
2. "Do you speak any languages besides your mother tongue?" (ask to specify)
3. "Have you ever had a stroke or serious illness?"
    a. If yes, "Please tell me about it."
    b. If no, "Well how about anyone in your family or anyone you know? Can you tell me about that?"
    c. If no response in approximately 10 seconds prompt: "Try to tell me about the day you/they had your/their stroke/illness."
4. At a natural juncture add: "Tell me about your/their recovery. What kinds of things have you/they done to try to get better since your/their stroke/illness?"
    a. If no response in approximately 10 seconds, prompt: "Tell me about any changes you/they needed to make in your/their daily life."

Important Event

Thinking back, can you tell me a story about something important that happened to you in your life? It could be happy or sad or from any time -- from when you were a kid or more recently.

If no response in approximately 10 seconds, prompt:

For instance, you could tell me about a trip you took or something about your family or your work -- anything.

APPENDIX 3

Session 3: Individual Session With Patient

This session is aimed at understanding how you feel about yourself on a personal level and how you deem your future to be.

Leisure

Tell me the most fun time you have had.

Prompts

Pick on the activity that the patient explains and ask questions about it. In case of not understanding the question or no answer, ask these

Do you like shopping?

Do you like hanging out with friends?

Do you like adventure sports?

What are your hobbies?

What do you like to do for fun at home?

What does your family enjoy on holidays?

After stroke, tell me a time when you have done your favorite activity (whichever is mentioned by the patient) with your friends/family?

Work

Tell me what you were/are doing for a living.

Prompts

What do you hope to achieve in the next one year in office?

Are your colleagues helpful?

Has your work environment changed?

What are your employer/boss's expectations from you before and now?

How are you coping with the work in your present medical condition?

How do you go to your office?

Social Identities

Tell me the things that you have done in your neighborhood.

Prompts

Pick on the role that the patient speaks about and ask,

Why do you like it so much?

Is the recipient of your love and attention equally responsive?

Tell me about your wedding.

Tell me about your fondest memory with your child.

Tell me about a promotion/ successful moment at work?

Tell me about your biggest accomplishment.

Communication

Tell me how best you communicate.

Prompts

Do you write to communicate?

Are you able to understand the body language and express in the same way?

Do you use gestures for common everyday situations?

Have you learnt any sign language?

How do people react when you communicate?

Responsibilities

Tell me about your work and finances.

Prompts

Do you want to go back to work?

Who makes the budget of your house?

How has this budget planning with the medical expenditures?

Service Delivery

Tell me about all treatments you have received so far?

Prompts

Are you satisfied with them?

Do you want some changes in them?

How has your spouse helped you during the treatment?

This is the end of this session. Please ask if you have any queries, doubts or any suggestions for improving these meetings. Thank you for your time and participation. We will see you soon. Bye.

APPENDIX 4

Session 4: Individual Interview With Caregiver/Spouse

This meeting aims to understand the caregiver's idea of his future life in the company of a patient with aphasia and what are his individual hopes and dreams.

Change

Tell me what changes you see in the PWA since the stroke/ accident?

Prompts

In terms of his behavior, mobility, intellect, mood, attitude towards work and life?

Have both of your reactions changed towards each other?

How did you meet your spouse?

Was your wedding love/ arrange?

How has your life in terms of the emotional bond and physical relations with him/her before and post-stroke?

Are your children affected by his condition?

Do they still consider him an authoritative figure in the household?

How has your life changed since the stroke?

Do you feel there are added responsibilities?

Do you get enough rest?

Hope

Where do you see the PWA and yourself in the future?

Prompts

Which area has he improved in?

Are you hopeful of his improvement?

Do you hope for improvement over a period of time?

What do you think whether the PWA is hopeful or not?

Where do you wish to see yourself in the work arena 5 years from now?

How do you see your married life in the future?

Improvement

What is the improvement that you have seen in him post-stroke rehabilitation?

Prompts

What do you think are the main barriers and facilitators in his recovery?

Tell me how his recovery is improving your personal life.

Caregiver Training

Have you undergone any specific training to help his/ her condition and has it helped?

Prompts

Are you satisfied with the training?

Do you feel that PWA is able to perform better with your trained approach?

Are you able to cope with his/her condition?

People

Tell me about your friends and relatives and how they have helped.

Prompts

Are your relatives coming in to help?

Are your friends visiting and encouraging?

Are your work colleagues helping with your work schedule and his colleagues with his?

Do you hope to achieve a stable family life for all of you?

This is the end of this session. We will answer your doubts and queries with pleasure. Please give us any suggestions for improvement. Thank you for your help. We will see you soon. Bye

APPENDIX 5

Session 6: Individual Session With the Employer

This session is to explain his current and future recovery pattern at work.

Q. What are your expectations from PWA?
Q. How do you feel towards the PWA?
Q. Do you think the PWA is an asset/ liability to the workplace?
Q. Compare the pre-and post morbid role of PWA in workplace?
Q. Do you see a recovery pattern since the accident?
Q. How would you rate his current performance and expect the progress to be?
Q. What are the barriers and facilitators in his improvement?
Q. Are you planning to change his work duties?
Q. What changes can be made in the office to accommodate him?
Q. Do you have confidence in his work?
Q. Do you see an improvement in the near future?

This is the end of this session. What do you feel about your office decorum and its flexibility? We will answer your doubts and queries with pleasure. Please give us any suggestions for improvement. We will see you soon. Bye

APPENDIX 6

Session 7: Communicative Counseling Session

This is a concluding session to make the PWA and important people in his life understand about his health, his feelings, their mental state and contribution to his effective social functioning in the future.

- Results of the interview will be explained- weakness and strength, barriers and facilitators with respect to home, community and workplace, understand and interpret the finding to find a decent correlation
- Ways to improve and maintain the role of the PWA in house, work and community.
- Mental, physical, social well being of the PWA, communication partner, and employer

This is the end of this session. We are very thankful for all the help in this study and hope that these meetings have helped you realize the importance of each other and the relevance of personal ideas and identities for the effective functioning of the society and its members. Have a good day. All the best for your future. Bye

Chapter 13
Assessment of Significant Other's Burden and Their Communication Strategies to Enhance the Treatment Outcome in Aphasia

Pinki Singh
All India Institute of Medical Sciences-Bhopal, India

Apoorva Pauranik
MGM Medical College and Hospital, India

ABSTRACT

Post-stroke management of person with aphasia (PWA) needs the crucial involvement of significant others (SOs) or caregivers of PWA. The manners in which SOs perceive the burden and execute their supportive communication strategies (SCS) are highly variable and are influenced by many factors like their motivation, emotional attachment, constraints of time and economy, self-confidence, and the clinical and individualistic attributes of the PWA herself or himself. There are variations regarding motivation, supportive communication strategies (SCS), significance and burden of communication to PWA by SO. These variations lead to a prognosis of a PWA, which needs to be evaluated for a better understanding of the diversity of burden and SCS before incorporating tailor-made treatment planning. These aspects have a significant bearing on the prognosis of aphasia, hence must be evaluated prior to treatment planning.

INTRODUCTION

Aphasia is an acquired language disorder resulting from an injury to the brain, such as from a stroke or traumatic brain injury (TBI). Symptoms of aphasia include difficulty in finding words, using sentences, and communicating with others. All the treatment approaches related to aphasia focused on improvement of communication skills of the person with aphasia (PWA). In order to achieve this goal, significant others (SOs) of PWA follow and execute all the recommended communication facilitating activities in their natural settings.

DOI: 10.4018/978-1-5225-4955-0.ch013

In the literature, terms "carer" or "caregiver" are used more often to refer the individuals who are involved with the PWA and considered as equivalent to the term "family".In many studies, a narrower term i.e. Partner (spouse or cohabitant) of the PWA is also being used frequently. The use of the appropriate term is significant to understand the extent and intensity of its implied meaning. "Carer" or "caregiver" could be perceived to imply a nursing role that may not be present, and "family" might be taken as the too narrow term (Blom Johnsson, 2012). When a person suffers from a stroke and aphasia, life not only changes for him or her, but also for their significant others (Le Dorze and Brassard, 1995; Michallet, Tétreault, and Le Dorze, 2003). To acknowledge the significant involvement of family members, friends and other persons who are important to the PWA, they are termed as "Significant Others (SOs)" in this chapter. Post-stroke responsibilities of SOs towards PWA, their home and family increases suddenly. They need to plan their everyday life i.e. social and personal more carefully than before (Kitzmüller, Asplund, and Häggström, 2012).They also have to act as "interpreters" at social events as well as at formal encounters e.g. doctor visits (Michallet et al., 2003).

Irrespective of the aphasia treatment approaches i.e. functional, environmental, language-oriented, the involvement of significant others (SOs) of a PWA during therapy and rehabilitation are robust and crucial. In many severe cases with aphasia, it is found that family member tends to focus on only verbal output in initial years. Later, when they fail to get success in achieving a verbal output, then most of them ignore other modes of communication i.e. written, drawing and other innovative modes. SOs act as an active receiver of the message (assumed to be sent by PWA) i.e. SOs perceives and understand the need ofa PWA without any evident or specific indication given to them. They try to understand the need of PWA based primarily on environmental context or regular routine/time scheduled activity. Due to these communication gaps, incidences of frequent misunderstanding and feeling of the burden of SOs to interpret communication intention of PWA are quite evident.

Post-stroke physical and communicative deficits lead to the reduction in communication opportunities, communicative effectiveness, interactional competence, language, and communication-related activities. It generates frequent irritation and frustration to both i.e. PWA and SOs and gives rise to many interpersonal problems and communication burden on each other.

REVIEW OF THE LITERATURE

Conversations between two people who do not have communication impairment often follow a basic structure, to begin with a greeting, an act of introduction of the main topic, conversational turn-taking where each partner exchange message as needed and then a closing of a topic (Sacks, Schegloff, and Jefferson, 1974; Stokoe, 2013). When one partner experiences communication impairment such as aphasia, this exchange becomes difficult, yet the behaviors by both the PWA and their SO can influence the course of the conversation.

Several authors have discussed various conversational facilitators, defined as behaviors that move the conversation forward. Other authors discuss barriers or behaviors that tend to impede information exchange (Bauer and Kulke, 2004; Perkins, 2014; Simmons-Mackie and Kagan, 1999; Stokoe, 2013). When SOs encounters a breakdown in communication, they often attempt to engage in repairing strategy. Repairingstrategy such as starting the conversation again, repeating questions in a simplified manner or otherwise repeating the use of facilitating behaviors in order to repair the miscommunication.

Facilitating behaviors is a general term that covers a variety of behaviors that SOsuse to keep the conversation moving forward. Examples include the SOs and PWA using acknowledgement tokens such as *uh-hum, yeah right,* and *I see* to let the other person know that they are still listening, the SOs giving the PWA time to answer, and use of gestures and writing for alternate communication (Simmons-Mackie and Kagan, 1999; Kagan and Black, 2001).

Simmons-Mackie and Kagan (1999) highlighted the importance of facilitating behaviours by identifying a number of strategies demonstrated by SOs that separated successful communication exchanges from unsuccessful exchanges. They also accepted the use of alternate communication methods such as gestures, drawing, and writing, as opposed to remaining fixated on verbal communication (Simmons-Mackie and Kagan, 1999).

Another facilitation strategy that has been frequently used in repair sequences is the SOs use of multiple choices and yes/no question formats to clarify the PWA's intended message (Kagan and Black, 2001). Instead of allowing the miscommunication to continue, a SO's request for additional information is considered a repair behavior. Identification and use of these facilitating and repair behaviors may reduce the struggle and tension in communications between dyads and lead to more successful communication exchanges.

Barrier behaviors lead to unsuccessful communication and include behaviors such as language exercising, not acknowledging the contributions of the other person, or interrupting when the other person has the floor (Simmons-Mackie and Kagan, 1999; Bauer and Kulke, 2004; Simmons-Mackie, Kearns, and Potechin, 2005). Simmons-Mackie and Kagan (1999) found that unsuccessful SOs tended to talk over the PWA when the PWA was attempting to communicate and tended to remain fixated on the SO's agenda, rather than follow the natural flow of conversation as the PWA took it. Language exercising is the practicing of language at the expense of the intended communication.

Simmons-Mackie and Kagan (1999) found that when one partner had language impairment, the focus became on restoring the language ability, and the couple engaged in continual "practicing language" only. In these situations, the SOs became the teacher and the PWA the student, instead of partners in communication.

Hence, it is vital to incorporate assessment of severity and diversity of communication and other burden among SOs and Supportive Conversation Strategies (SCS) used by them for PWA. The inclusion of these domains in test battery would make treatment program efficient and tailor-made. It would help them to maintain and generalize the effect of treatment in the long-term.

MAIN FOCUS OF THE CHAPTER

Communication is not just dependent on one person; it is an interaction between two or more people. Treatment approach in aphasia therapy has to focus on the communication strategies used by the communication partner of the PWA (Cunningham and Ward, 2003; Kagan and Black, 2001). The goal of all intervention approaches is to try to help both the SOs and PWA in developing strategies for communicating with each other, rather than the burden of communication placed on the person with communication impairment or his/her communication partner.

To achieve this goal, it is required to understand and assess the type and extent of difficulties they are facing in daily situations. It is also mandatory to understand the perception of SOs towards PWA and pattern of SCS, they are using through all modalities i.e. spoken, comprehension, reading, writing, pictorial representations. It would be of great importance to evaluate and incorporate these findings as a part of comprehensive rehabilitation program of PWA. Along with this, the inclusion of SOs as an active participant might also reduce the risks of negative psychosocial consequences due to their diverse burden. In the present scenario, the assessment procedure is mostly focused on language domains of PWA only.

AIM

To incorporate assessment of Significant others (SOs) in a test battery for tailor-made or individualized treatment plan and better prognosis.

MATERIALS

Two types of questionnaires were incorporated; one, to understand the magnitude and diversity of burden faced by SOs of PWA in the different domain of communication and related activities; and second, Supportive Conversation Strategies (SCS) used by SOs for communication facilitation.

Details About Questionnaire to Be introduced in Test Battery

- The Questionnaire to assess magnitude and diversity of communication and language related burden of SOs. It was developed and standardized by cross- sectional survey (Pinki and Pauranik, 2013; Appendix-1).

It has following subheadings and details:

1. **Extent of Changes in Experience (Physical, Cognition) of SOs with PWA:** Consisting of the pre and post stroke changes.
    a. This section consists of 30 items.
    b. Purpose: To assess changes in experiences of SOs related to changes in communication and personal activity after stroke.
2. **Communication Effectiveness (CE):** Communication goals of a language user vary enormously from context to context; hence this part of questionnaire may not be straight forward. There are three aspects of communicative effectiveness i.e. ease of comprehension; stylishness of the language produced; and the perceived linguistic proficiency.
    a. This section consists of 8 items.
    b. **Purpose:** To estimate communication ability of PWA in different communicative situations (i.e., Basic needs, Social needs, life skills).
3. **Interaction Competence (IC):** It is a replacement for communicative competence because individuals don't acquire a general, practice independence competence; rather they acquire a practice specific interactional competence by participating with more experienced others in specific interactive practices (He and Young, 1998, p.7).
    a. This section consists of 7 items.
    b. **Purpose:** To assess the level participation of PWA in terms of communication with others.

4. **Language and Communication Related Activities (LCA):** It is consisting of both knowledge, or competence, and the capacity for implementing it, or executing that competence in appropriate, contextualized communicative language use (Bachman, 1990, p.84).
    a. This section consists of 11 items.
    b. **Purpose:** To assess language and communication-related activity of PWA.
5. **Significant Others (SOs) Oriented:** It includes perception of SOs towards post stroke changes of PWA as a burden.
    a. This section consists of 7 items
    b. **Purpose:** To investigate the mental status of SOs of PWA.
        2. **Questionnaire about Supportive Conversation Strategies (SCS)** (Singh and Pauranik, 2014; Appendix 2)

Additionally a 44-item specific language domain based questionnaire was developed for qualitative descriptive study. It contains polar questions to assess Supportive Conversation Strategies (SCS) used by SOs of PWA.

The use of communication strategies by SOs to reduce burden also needs to get assessed by questionnaire based on each language domain specific SCS e.g. auditory comprehension, spoken language, reading, writing and others. All sections were containing positive and negative polar questions in random order. In every section, 30%-47% negative statements were included (Singh and Pauranik, 2014).

Details About Supportive Conversation Strategies (SCS) Questionnaire

1. **Auditory Comprehension:** This section consists of total 10 items with three negative questions.
2. **Spoken Language:** This section consists of total 13 items with five negative questions.
3. **Reading:** This section consists of total 9 items with three negative questions.
4. **Writing:** This section consists of total 8 items with three negative questions.
5. **Other:** This section consists of total 4 items.

The focus of assessment should be to get information about SCS used by SOs and extent of the diverse burden they experience in everyday environments. These findings would facilitate tailor-made training to SOs and make them more confident in familiar and novel settings. Different ways of communications would enhance the overall communication effectiveness.

To understand the significant input by SOs of PWA, it is important to understand the diversity of their burden and SCS separately.

RESULTS

Assessment of diverse burden on SOs towards 56% PWA of age range 40-60 years with anterior aphasia has reflected the perception of the majority of the SOs as being less stimulating and enjoyable than conversation before stroke onset. It also increased the communicative responsibilities and burden of the SOs due to reduced language and communication-related activities (LCA), interaction competence (IC) and communication effectiveness (CE) of PWA.Reduced LCA, IC and CE of PWA are closely associated with education, aphasia type and its severity (Chi-square,$p< .001$). Border-line association ($p\leq$

0.046) has also been observed between type of family and their impact on competencies of PWA. As a contra indicatory response, denial or unawareness about the perception of communication burden was prominently evident in the nuclear family (Pinki and Pauranik, 2013).

On the other hand, SCS used by SOs to reduce the communication burden was studied by Singh and Pauranik (2014) for auditory comprehension, verbal expression, reading, writing, and others. It was found that 17.14% SOs do not consider factors like rate of speech, face to face communication, emphasis on keywords etc. during the conversation. 34.28% and 37.14% SOs tends to hinder the communication through frequent changing the topics and involving many people during the conversation. In terms of verbal language, 77.14% SOs have insisted on verbal mode only. In terms of reading and writing approach, 60% SOs have conceded that they do not provide any reading material to their relatives and 45.71% SOs do not direct any pattern to start writing. Even, 51.43% SOs do not facilitate simple gesture too. Hence, SCS oriented questionnaire might not show what actually occurs to the conversational situation but it would describe helpful and unhelpful strategies precisely.

DISCUSSION

Communication is a source for human beings to interact with the family member and society. Unlike physical limitation which is evident and visible, communication impairment is invisible in nature but has a larger impact on patients and their family member's social and functional life.

Due to the variation of type and severity of aphasia; PWAs are not only restricted in verbal output but also in their comprehension, reading, writing and other skills severely. Aphasic disorder might affect all pattern of communication mode (at input/output level) other than verbal one. To overcome these communication difficulties, some PWA participates in speech-language therapy but some do not. In both conditions, directly or indirectly SOs has to suffer a lot along with PWA which in turn creates a burden regarding physical, cognition, language, communication, interaction competence, communication effectiveness and mental status to SOs.

Pinki and Pauranik (2013), reported that 57.14% SOs tended to use many yes/no questions frequently took the form of information clarifications, which was consistent with Simmons-Mackie and Kagan (1999) who found that Communication Partners (CPs) often used a clarification questions during conversations. This tendency to use many yes/no questions could be a result of the SOs prior experiences that one question at a time and using the yes/no format assisted with communication with the PWA. While the SOs themselves seldom initiated the use of alternative communication (i.e., writing/drawing and gestures), they also rarely dismissed the PWA's attempts to use alternative communication when it was offered. This was in contrast to Simmons-Mackie and Kagan (1999) who wrote that some CPs in their study rejected the PWA attempts at alternate communication methods in favour of speech. It could be that the participants in this study were not averse to using alternate modalities, but that it was simply not in their habit to use them.

The experiences of using Supportive Conversation Strategies (SCS) vary considerably among the family member of PWA. Even acceptance towards use of new strategies or communicative means by PWA also differs in a wide range i.e. some try hard to make them understood through any mode to other who refuse any other mode except verbal. Simmons-Mackie and Kagan (1999) have found the low acceptance attitude of PWA and SOs towards strategies, communication aid devices which aim to facilitate communicative means other than spoken words in everyday life. This behaviour and perception of SOs and PWA might be based on their fear/anxiety about the interference of alternate modality on the restoration of their language and its unnaturalness appearance. The importance of the attitudes of the speech-language pathologist (SLP) and family member in using SCS could strongly influence the readiness of PWA. Initially, SOs might be hesitant to use total communication strategies or SCS due to barriers connected to the strategy or communication aid device itself. These barriers could be related to difficulties in its use, insufficient practice, their attitudes inclined towards only verbal mode, lack of awareness and motivation of the PWA and their SOs.

The families might take help of a specialized professional to reduce all kind of burden through organized treatment planning i.e. understanding of the diverse burden of SOs. The later could be analysed and quantified through standard test battery or planned interview by professional so that treatment goal may be planned in a better manner, thereby reducing the amount of burden of SOs. This kind of treatment goal will help in the facilitation of the functional communication of PWA, and consequentially it will provide motivation to both of them to work ahead.

Treatment could also be planned for whom follow-up would be a difficult whatever reasons with the means of recommended videos (as per planning or target goal), supportive conversation strategies or home training program (written or verbally explained). These measures would not be that effective as one to one treatment, but these guidelines (on the basis of type and severity of aphasia) could be planned or incorporated in a daily living environment of PWA in a such a manner that it would help in reducing the burden of SOs. It would result in enhancement of quality of life of the whole family member.

Eriksson, Hartelius, and Saldert (2016) have advocated for Interaction focused training to provide an individualized intervention to PWA. They have studied the effects on conversation partner's ability to support the PWA in conversation and on the PWAs' perception of their functional communication. It was found that two of the six participants had small improvements in the ability to support their partner with aphasia in conversation. Half the PWA and half the SOs reported improvements in perceived functional communication in the person with aphasia after the intervention.

Due to the large subjective variations among SOs, PWA, their relations, natural environment, experiences; their responses towards SCS would also vary largely. For some SCS might act as a hindrance or less beneficial but for other, it could be a boon. So, authors believed that custom-made treatment plan based on this assessment approach would help all i.e. SOs, PWA and clinician to great extent in terms of reduction in communication burden, more communication opportunity and future research concept respectively.

On the other hand, rating scales assessment of ability to support communication can be reliably applied but are susceptible to factors outside the actual assessment. Factors inherent in SOs seem to influence the ability of SOs to support disordered communication in conversation. To learn and use the SCS in natural everyday conversation with PWA might not be effective for everyone but may have an impact on the perceived functional communication of PWA.

LIMITATIONS

There are several limitations to this study that need to be addressed. First, the type and severity of aphasia were not controlled, to study the correlation between type, the severity of aphasia and SCS used by SOs. Though there was the small size of participants in each severity group to determine if aphasia severity played a role in the conversational behaviours of the SOs. Second, PWA with co-morbidities such as dementia was not excluded from this sample, because the primary concern of this study was focused on the behaviour changes (in terms of strategies and communication burden) of SOs.

The third limitation, the experience of SOs including the number of hours spent by them pre and post-stroke were taken in the account which might determine the rapport and quality of language inputs required for the better outcome. Fourth, the impact of relationships of SOs with PWA was not analyzed separately i.e. involvement of wife/husband, mother/father, sister/brother and others. Rather all significant communication partners were collectively taken as significant others (SOs) of PWA. Fifth, other socio-demographic variables like age, gender, education and its impact on diverse communication burden and SCS were not analysed separately. These factors could also obstruct the use of adequate amount and quality of communication strategies. But this sort of analysis would be significant only in a large sample and pre-post comparative study.

Additionally, this chapter sought to contribute to the literature by revealing some of the changes in communication effectiveness, language and communication-related activities and interactional competence as a communication burden along with the very often and rarely used SCS. But It is possible that with additional research and understanding into the attitudes of SOs and PWA, clinicians will be able to target and change behaviours more effectively.

FUTURE RESEARCH DIRECTIONS

Supportive Conversation Strategies (SCS) need to be implemented and monitored in custom-made approach due to the numerous variations among PWA and their SOs. In a broader sense, SCS monitoring in terms of the topic of conversation, its utility, frequency and length, number of communication breakdown and use of breakdown resolving strategies could be done in natural settings through video recorded clips. These clips would be beneficial for the clinician to analyse the pattern of SCS and to provide feedback to SOs. In addition, the environmental modification could also be considered in terms of noise, physical barriers and materials which are being used during practice tasks in terms of its lexical frequency and use.

CONCLUSION

Use of questionnaires for assessing the burdens being faced by SOs of PWA and also the SCS used by SOs routinely as a part of aphasia assessment protocol would be effective and helpful. It would help the clinician to understand the significance of these measures in the treatment plan of PWA; it would also make them understand that which strategies should be used in particular case. Along with this, it would direct the facilitation of coping strategies to be maintained through all modalities, i.e., spoken, comprehension, reading, writing, pictorial representation and others to reduce the communicative burden of SOs. It would also help in learning and planning family-oriented interventions programs i.e. communication partner training. On the basis of the feedback or experience of SOs, many effective, practical strategies could be extracted and generalised among other PWA to make them active in their social life.

REFERENCES

Bachman, L. F. (1990). *Fundamental consideration in language testing*. Oxford, UK: Oxford University Press.

Bauer, A., & Kulke, F. (2004). Language Exercises for dinner: Aspects of aphasia management in family settings. *Aphasiology*, *18*(12), 1135–1160. doi:10.1080/02687030444000570

Blom Johansson, M. (2012). *Aphasia and Communication in Everyday Life: Experience of persons with aphasia, significant others, and speech-language pathologists* (Doctoral Thesis). Uppsala: Acta Universitatis Uppsaliensis.

Cunningham, R., & Ward, C. D. (2003). Evaluation of training programme to facilitate conversation between people with aphasia and their partners. *Aphasiology*, *17*(8), 687–707. doi:10.1080/02687030344000184

Eriksson, K., Hartelius, L., & Saldert, C. (2016). On the diverse outcome of communication partner training of significant others of people with aphasia: An experimental study of six cases. *International Journal of Language & Communication Disorders*, *51*(4), 402–414. doi:10.1111/1460-6984.12216 PMID:26947265

He, A., & Young, R. (1998). Language proficiency interviews: A discourse approach. In R. Young & W. He (Eds.), *Talking and Testing: Discourse approaches to the assessment of oral proficiency* (pp. 1–24). Philadelphia: John Benjamins. doi:10.1075ibil.14.02he

Kagan, A., Black, S., Duchan, J. F., Simmons-Mackie, N., & Square, P. (2001). Training Volunteers as Conversation Partners Using "Supported Conversation for Adults with Aphasia" (SCA): A Controlled Trial. *Journal of Speech, Language, and Hearing Research: JSLHR*, *44*(3), 624–638. doi:10.1044/1092-4388(2001/051) PMID:11407567

Kitzmüller, G., Asplund, K., & Häggström, T. (2012). The long-term experience of family life after stroke. *The Journal of Neuroscience Nursing*, *44*(1), E1–E13. doi:10.1097/JNN.0b013e31823ae4a1 PMID:22210306

Le Dorze, G., & Brassard, C. (1995). A description of the consequences of aphasia on aphasic persons and their relatives and friends, based on the WHO model of chronic diseases. *Aphasiology*, *9*(3), 239–255. doi:10.1080/02687039508248198

Michallet, B., Tétreault, S., & Le Dorze, G. (2003). The consequences of severe aphasia on the spouses of aphasic people: A description of the adaptation process. *Aphasiology*, *17*(9), 835–859. doi:10.1080/02687030344000238

Perkins, M. (2014). Linguistic recycling in typical and atypical interactions. *Clinical Linguistics & Phonetics*, *28*(6-7), 590–601. doi:10.3109/02699206.2014.926995 PMID:25000380

Pinki & Pauranik, A. (2013). The diversity of burden for significant others of person with aphasia. *Journal of All India Institute of Speech and Hearing, 32,* 167-172.

Pound, C., Parr, S., Lindsay, J., & Woolf, C. (2000). *Beyond Aphasia: Therapies for Living with Communication Disability*. Bicester: Speechmark.

Purdy, M., & Hindenlang, J. (2005). Educating and training caregivers of persons with aphasia. *Aphasiology, 19*(3-5), 377–388. doi:10.1080/02687030444000822

Rautakoski, P. (2011). Partners' self-perceptions of the use of different communication strategies during total communication intervention. *Aphasiology, 25*(12), 1523–1542. doi:10.1080/02687038.2011.624164

Rautakoski, P. (2011). Training total communication. *Aphasiology, 25*(3), 344–365. doi:10.1080/02687038.2010.530671

Reis, A., & Petersson, K. M. (2003). Educational level, socioeconomic status and aphasia research: A comment on Connor et al. (2001)-effect of socioeconomic status on aphasia severity and recovery. *Brain and Language, 87*(3), 449–452. doi:10.1016/S0093-934X(03)00140-8 PMID:14642547

Sacks, H., Schegloff, E. A., & Jefferson, G. (1974). A simplest systematics for the organization of turn-taking for conversation. *Language, 50*(4), 696–735. doi:10.1353/lan.1974.0010

Simmons-Mackie, N., & Kagan, A. (1999). Communication strategies used by "good" versus "poor" speaking partners of individuals with aphasia. *Aphasiology, 13*(9-11), 807–820. doi:10.1080/026870399401894

Simmons-Mackie, N., Kearns, K., & Potechin, G. (2005). Treatment of aphasia through family member training. *Aphasiology, 19*(6), 583–593. doi:10.1080/02687030444000408

Singh, P., & Pauranik, A. (2014). Supportive conversational strategies for person with aphasia (PWA) and their significant others (SO). *Proceedings of 8th World Congress for Neuro Rehabilitation (WCNR).*

Stokoe, E. (2013). Overcoming barriers to mediation in intake calls to services: Research-based strategies for mediators. *Negotiation Journal, 29*(3), 289–314. doi:10.1111/nejo.12026

Young, R. (1999). Sociolinguistic approaches to SLA. *Annual Review of Applied Linguistics, 19*, 105–132. doi:10.1017/S0267190599190068

KEY TERMS AND DEFINITIONS

Alternate Modality: It refers to the unpopular modalities of communication other than the verbal mode. Use of alternate modality reduces the communication gap between society and PWA.

Comprehensive Rehabilitation Program: The program offering a wide variety of additional programs and services to support and make PWA able to participate in social communities.

Custom-Based Approach: This approach would suggest the designing of the treatment plan for the patient's diverse individual needs and desire.

Diverse: It is related to the different character or quality of persons/thoughts/feeling/burden which makes them distinct from one another.

Natural Settings: It refers to actual environment, where PWA actually resides and faces the communication difficulties. Communication assessment and management in natural setting facilitates authentic and functional communication.

Strategy: It is a planned process or actions used to facilitate and accelerate particular target performance.

Video Recorded Clips: It refers to short clips of video from a part of the longer video. It could be used for monitoring, analysis and feedback related to natural settings.

APPENDIX 1

Table 1. Extent of Changes in Experience (Physical, Cognition, Social) of Significant Others with Person with Aphasia (PWA)

पूर्णतः सहमत (SA) पूर्णतः असहमत (SD)

		SA SD
1	मेरे परिजन को कपड़े पहनाने में मेरी सहायता की जरूरत पड़ती है।	
2	मेरे परिजन को उनकी देख.रेख करने के लिए मेरी सहायता की जरूरत पड़ती है।	
3	स्ट्रोक के बाद से मेरे परिजन फोन का इस्तेमाल ठीक से नही कर पाते जैसे पहले कर पाते थे।	
4	मेरे परिजन सामाजिक कार्यक्रमों में शामिल होने में सक्षम हैं।	
5	मेरे परिजन स्ट्रोक से पहले सामाजिक रूप से सक्रिय थे ।	
6	मेरे परिजन यह उम्मीद करते है कि मैं हमेशा हर समय उनके साथ रहूं	
7	मेरे परिजन किसी भी चीजों में मजा आनन्द नहीं लेते।	
8	अब मेरे परिजन घर की चीजों के लिए पैसे का हिसाब नहीं रख पाते हैं।	
9	मेरे परिजन काम करने के बजाय बैठना पसंद करते हैं।	
10	मेरे परिजन को खाना खाने के लिए मेरी जरूरत पड़ती हैं।	
11	स्ट्रोक के बाद से मेरे परिजन जितना हो सके उतना सामाजिक रूप से सम्मिलित होने की कोशिश करते हैं।	
12	अब मेरे परिजन कभी कभी बच्चों की तरह व्यवहार करते है।	
13	स्ट्रोक से पहले मेरे परिजन पूरा समय फोन पर बने रहते थे।	
14	मेरे परिजन बड़े समूह से ज्यादा छोटे समूह में रहना पसंद करते हैं	
15	मेरे परिजन को उनकी देख-रेख के लिए मेरी सहायता लेना पसंद है।	
16	मेरे परिजन कुछ बोलने से ज्यादा लिखते है।	
17	मेरे परिजन को पार्टीयों में जाना घूमना ज्यादा पसंद है।	
18	मेरे परिजन को मेरी जरूरत हर समय होती है।	
19	मेरे परिजन पहले जैसे मनोरंजन वाली चीजों में आनन्द नहीं महसूस करते हैं।	
20	स्ट्रोक से पहले मेरे परिजन घर के खर्च के लिए रुपये का हिसाब रख लेते थे।	
21	स्ट्रोक से पहले मेरे परिजन मेरे समय के लिए बहुत इच्छा रहती थी।	
22	अब मेरे परिजन दूसरे से बात करने से कतराते/बचते है।	
23	मेरे परिजन ये सोचते है कि वो अब कुछ नहीं कर सकते।	
24	मेरे परिजन पड़ोसी के घर जाने से ज्यादा टी वी देखना पसद करते है।	
25	मेरे परिजन खाना खाने में मेरी मदद पसंद करते हैं।	
26	अब मेरे परिजन मुझे और मेरे समय को लेकर ज्यादा इच्छुक हो गए।	
27	मेरे परिजन वैसी सामाजिक गतिविधियों से बचते है जो वो नहीं कर सकते है।	
28	अब मेरे परिजन अपने बैंक खाते को उपयोग नहीं करते।	
29	मेरे परिजन के सिर्फ वहीं मित्र हैं जो कि उनकी तरह स्ट्रोक के कारण ग्रसित है।	
30	स्ट्रोक से पहले मेरे परिजन छुट्टियाँ लेना पसंद नहीं करते थे।	

Communication Effectiveness

५- लगभग हमेशा ४-अधकितर ३- कभी कभी २- बहुत कम १- कभी नहीं

1. क्या वो सामूहकि बातचीत में शामलि होना पसंद करते हैं?
2. क्या वो हाँ/न का सही उतर दे तेहैं?
3. क्या वो अपनी भावनाओ को बयक्त कर पाते हैं/या उन के बारे में बात कर पाते हैं?
4. क्या वो उस वयक्तकि नाम बता पात है, जो उसके सामने हो?
5. क्या वो अपनी शारीरक जरूरते (जैसे दर्द या चोट) को बता पाते हैं?
6. क्या वो कसिी वषिय पर बात या अपनी प्रतक्रियिा व्यक्त कर पातेहै ?(हाँ /न के सहति लेकनि बनिा शब्दों के प्रयोग कयि)
7. क्या वो लखिा हुआ समझ पाते हैं?
8. क्या वो अनजान लोगो के साथ बातचीत कर पाते हैं?

Interactional Competence

Table 2.

	1	2	3	4	5	6	7
१. आपके परजिन पारस्परकि वचिार वमिर्श में कतिना सम्मलति होते हैं?	बलि्कुल नहीं			कुछ- कुछ			बहुत
२. लगभग कतिने बार वक्ता "x" अपने सन्देश को समझा पाते हैं?	बलि्कुल नहीं			कुछ- कुछ			बहुत
३. लगभग कतिने बार वक्ता "x" पारस्परकि वचिार वमिर्श के दौरान प्रश्न पुछ कर, अनचाही टप्पिणी या अपनी वचिार वयक्त कर के सक्रयि भूमकिा नभिाते हैं?	बलि्कुल नहीं			कुछ- कुछ			बहुत
४. लगभग कतिने बार वक्ता "x" अपनी सन्देश को समझाने के लयि अन्य तरीकों का इस्तेमाल करते हैं (जैसे बोलना,लखिना, चत्रि बनाना एवं अन्य)?	बलि्कुल नहीं			कुछ- कुछ			बहुत
५. दुसरो द्वारा वक्ता "x" की बात नहीं समझ पाने पर वो अपनी बात समझाने के लयि कतिने लचीले एवं सामरकि हो जाते हैं ?	बलि्कुल नहीं			कुछ- कुछ			बहुत
६. बातचीत करते वक्त वक्ता "x" कतिनी चीजो (जैसे,प्रश्न पूछना, तर्क करना, सलाह देना, टप्पिणी देना, इशारा करना) का इस्तेमाल करते हैं?	बलि्कुल नहीं			कुछ- कुछ			बहुत
७. १ से ७ के मापांक पर आप वक्ता "x" को उनकी बातचीत के सक्षमता के अनुसार कतिना मूल्याङ्कन करोगे ?	बलि्कुल कम क्षमता			थोड़ी क्षमता			अच्छी क्षमता

Language and Communication Related Activities

५- लगभग हमेशा ४- अधकितर ३- कभी कभी २- बहुत कम १- कभी नहीं

1. क्या आपके परजिन इस बात पर ध्यान देते हैं की दुसरे क्या कह रहे हैं?
2. क्या आपके परजिन अपनी बात को बनिा कसिी की सहायता के कह पाते है?
3. क्या आपके परजिन अपने कसिी भी वचिारो पर खुलकर बात कर पाते हैं?
4. क्या आपके परजिन दुसरे व्यक्ति के वचिारो पर अपनी प्रतक्रियिा व्यक्त कर पाते हैं?
5. क्या वो अपने बात करने की क्षमता पर अपने वचिार व्यक्त कर पाते हैं?
6. क्या वो दुसरो की बातचीत के दौरान बीच में बोलते हैं?
7. अन्य लोगो की बातचीत न समझ में आने पर क्या वो दोहराने को बोलते हैं?
8. जब अन्य लोग आपके परजिन की बात न समझ पाने के कारण जब उन्हे दोहराने को बोलते है तो क्या वो अपनी बात को दुबारा समझा पाते हैं?
9. क्या आपके परजिन के शब्द अस्पष्ट और दुर्बोध होते हैं?
10. आपके परजिन बातचीत के दौरान सवाल पूछ्के, अपने वचिार व्यक्त करके कतिना सक्रयिाए भूमकिा नभिाते हैं ?
11. आपके परजिन दुसरो को अपनी बात समझाने में कतिने सक्षम हैं?

Significant Others (SOs) Oriented

५- लगभग हमेशा ४- अधकितर ३- कभी कभी २- बहुत कम १- कभी नहीं

१. क्या आप अपने परजिन से बात करते बक्त अपना धैर्य खो देते हैं?
२. जब आप अपनी परजिन द्वारा बोली बाते नहीं समझ पाते तो क्या आप दुखी हो जाते हैं?
३. बातचीत के दौरान क्या आप अक्सर अपनी परजिन द्वारा बोली बात को गलत समझते हो?
४. बातचीत के दौरान जब आपके परजिन अचानक से बातचीत के वषिय बदल देते हैं तो तो क्या आप नाराज़ होते हो ?
५. आपके परजिन के बीमारी के बाद आपकी आर्थकि स्थतिि ख़राब होने का कारण क्या आप उनको मानते हो?
६. दनिभर अपने परजिन की देखभाल करने के कारण क्या आप आराम या अपने लयि वक्त नहीं दे पाते?
७. अपने परजिन के लयि दैनकि दनिचर्या में सारे कार्य करना क्या अब बोझ मससूस होने लगा है?

APPENDIX 2

Supportive Conversation Strategies (SCS) Questionnaire

Auditory Comprehension

1. Do you maintain clear, slightly slow rate of speech than usual and emphasize on the key words in the sentence?
2. Do you always insist on face to face communication with attention of your relative's / family?
3. Do you mostly avoid talking with your relative/family in a busy, noisy and distracting environment?
4. Do you concentrate on single theme/subject at a time with usage of simple sentences during communication?

5. Do you write down the key words of related conversation to make/help/assist them to follow topic easily?
6. Do you talk normally to your relatives/family without considering rate and clarity of speech/information?
7. Do you use visual cues mostly during conversation to make them (relatives/family) understand better?
8. Do you use simple gesture during conversation?
9. Do you change topics rapidly during conversation?
10. Do many people take part/involve in conversation at same time?

Language Spoken

1. Do you provide opportunities to your relative/friend to involve conversation?
2. Do you usually choose/phrase question in manner that can only be answered in "yes" or "no".
3. Do you mostly provide alternatives of key words to your relative/friend to make them easy to choose among those e.g. do you want "rice", or "roti"?
4. Do you allow ample amount of time to your relatives/family member to communicate and then helps in selecting words during conversation, if required?
5. Do you always try to guess communicative intent of your relative/friend?
6. Do you use other ways (e.g. gestures, facial expressions and body language) also to facilitate communication?
7. Do you reveal it (that you don't understand what he/she is saying) to your relative/friend and try to find out alternative way to help you understand what your relative/friend is saying?
8. Do you adopt direct way of communication always?
9. Do you always insist for only verbal communication to your relatives/family member?
10. Do you avoid their (your relatives/ family member) involvement in most of the conversation due to their inability to speak?
11. Do you provide their (your relatives/ family member) all required stuff as per their need on time so, that they don't require to speak?
12. Do you quit conversation, if not understanding their (your relatives/ family member) conversation?
13. Do their (your relatives/ family member) proximity not essential during conversation?

Reading

1. Do you read aloud so that they (your relative/family) can understand?
2. Do you provide them reading material with their (your relative/family) interest oriented contents instead of children oriented?
3. Do you try to make them read and understand the headlines of newspaper through showing associated/related pictures?
4. Do you often use books, magazines that are printed in big letters?
5. Do you always use meaningful and useful material to increase reading potential of your family member?

6. Do you avoid providing any reading material to him/her, due to their (family member) inability to read?
7. He/ She does not know to read (illiterate).
8. Do you give anything to them (relatives/family member) to read e.g. children's poem, alphabet?
9. Due to their (relatives/family member) inability to read, do you avoid reading aloud in front of them or to make them try to speak?

Writing

1. During writing, do you dictate only words to them (relatives/family member) without any guidance of hands movement and its coordination?
2. Do you provide them (relatives/family member) only easy words and shapes e.g. cups, pens, alphabet, straight line to copy?
3. Do you try to make them (relatives/family member) write to dictation of simple words/sentences?
4. Do you avoid giving options (written/verbal) to assist/help them (relatives/family member) in completing their spoken/written sentences?
5. Do you make them write the name of objects/materials (which they need or want to speak) from memory?
6. Do you ask them to name objects/materials (of daily use) "what is this?" and then ask them to write its name?
7. Do you help them in writing by providing cues (written/spoken) of initial letter when they start?
8. Do you avoid making them describe pictures of newspaper and magazines by writing because they are unable to write?

Others

1. Do you ask them (your relative/family) to create imaginary images?
2. Do you ask them to use clear and simple gesture (if one side is paralyzed then do you ask to use only one hand)?
3. Do you use only those gestures/ signals which primarily reflects the same action/content (such as ' pen ' point for writing)?
4. Do you use facial gestures mostly to convey message and to make them understand and express their feelings/emotions through face?

Chapter 14
Assessment of Cognitive-Communicative Functions in Persons With Mild Cognitive Impairment and Dementia of Alzheimer's Type

Reuben Thomas Varghese
All India Institute of Speech and Hearing, India

S. P. Goswami
All India Institute of Speech and Hearing, India

ABSTRACT

According to world population prospects data report, older individuals, especially those aged 60 years and above, have increased substantially over the recent year, which is going to accelerate in the coming decades. The most common problems the aging population faces are dementia of the Alzheimer's type (DAT) and mild cognitive impairment (MCI). Assessment of cognitive-communicative markers is essential for persons with MCI and DAT. Furthermore, it can help in the differential diagnosis of DAT and MCI. Proper assessment by speech-language pathologists is warranted in this area as it will throw light on the differential diagnosis of MCI and DAT, the clinical description of the characteristics between the two clinical groups, the prognosis for improved outcomes, recommendations for intervention and support, and referral for other professionals for assessments or services.

INTRODUCTION

According to world population prospects data report (DESA, 2015), older individuals especially those aged who are 60 years and above have increased substantially over the recent year, which is going to accelerate in the coming decades. The number of people in the world aged sixty years or over is expected to increase by 56 percent between the years 2015 and 2030. The recent advancement in health care facilities and better living conditions has resulted in the longevity of human life. Due to this change, it is

DOI: 10.4018/978-1-5225-4955-0.ch014

indeed time to pay more focus to the problems that the aging population faces, one of the most common amongst them is dementia. Persons having Dementia of Alzheimer's type (DAT) is one of the fastest growing clinical populations. Prince et al. (2013) reported that by the year 2030, around 65.7 million people will be affected and 115.4 million will be affected by 2050 by Dementia. Speech-Language Pathologists (SLPs) form one of the core team members who are qualified to treat the cognitive-communicative disorders associated with dementia. Early identification of dementia along with Mild Cognitive Impairment-which constitutes the earliest manifestation of clinical symptoms of dementia, has become a matter of research recently.

MILD COGNITIVE IMPAIRMENT (MCI)

According to the Diagnostic and Statistical Manual of Mental Disorders- Fourth Edition (DSM-IV) American Psychiatric Association (1994), Mild Cognitive Impairment (MCI) is defined as an intermediary stage between the cognitive stages of normal elderly aging and the mild degree of dementia. Petersen et al. (2001a) reported that persons with MCI have more risk of progressing to clinically probable DAT.

Sub-Types of MCI

According to Petersen et al. (2001b), based on cognitive features MCI can be divided into

1. **Amnestic MCI:** These individuals have impairment predominantly in memory.
2. **Multiple Domain MCI:** These individuals have impairments noticed in more than one cognitive domain which can include memory.
3. **Single Domain Non-Amnestic MCI:** These individuals have impairment in any one cognitive domain apart from memory.

Dementia

Dementia describes a group of brain disorders which can progressively lead to brain damage, and subsequently lead to gradual deterioration of a person's functional capacity and socio-cultural relations. The term dementia is originally derived from Latin word 'de mens' meaning a decline in mental abilities. Cummings, Benson, and LoVerme (1980) reported that at least three out of the following five areas-memory, language, visuospatial skills, emotional skills, personality and cognition must be disrupted in persons with dementia. The definition according to Diagnostic and Statistical Manual of Mental Disorders- Fourth Edition (DSM-IV) (1994) states that the most prominent feature among dementia is the impairments in both short-term (STM) and long-term memories (LTM). These memory deficits may also be associated with one or more concomitant features like agnosia, aphasia, apraxia, impairment in abstract thinking, and personality changes. The salient features for diagnosis of dementia are

1. Impairment in both short term and long-term memory.
2. Impairment in abstract thinking and judgment.
3. Personality changes.
4. Specific organic factor.
5. The absence of a non-organic factor as a reason for the symptoms like depression.

DEMENTIA OF ALZHEIMER'S TYPE (DAT)

It is reported as the most common cause of DAT. The classic DAT symptoms involve initial memory deficits due to dysfunction of the medial temporal lobe structures -particularly the hippocampus and entorhinal cortex. However, as the disease progresses the person also exhibits deficits in the parietal and frontal regions, thus affecting language, executive functions, personality and visuospatial systems. Other than disturbances in cognitive abilities, there are often neuropsychiatric and behavioural symptoms which includes depression, anxiety, irritability, agitation, hallucinations, impulsivity, insensitivity and sleep problems. While the predominant presentation of DAT is an amnestic one (typical DAT) where the individual has poor recent memory and better remote memory events, there also exist non-amnestic DAT which exhibits language, visuospatial and executive dysfunction deficits. Thus, the above symptoms for persons with DAT can lead to problems in their quality of life, activities of daily living and self-care. As older persons tend to live well, beyond 70 years due to better healthcare advancements, the prevalence of DAT is anticipated to rise 2-3 fold in the coming decades. The major risk factors of developing DAT are older age (above 65 years); family history of DAT, vascular risk factors (diabetes, hypertension, dyslipidemia, stroke), repeated brain trauma and low cognitive reserve, Down's syndrome and genetic factors mainly apolipoprotein-E (APOE).

Diagnostic Criteria for MCI and DAT

According to McKhann et al. (2011), the four neurobehavioral criteria that define MCI are

1. **Concern Regarding Change in Cognitive Level Compared With Prior Level:** This can be elicited by the patient, caregiver, informant or clinician.
2. **Impairment in One or More Cognitive Skills:** It can be noticed that for persons with MCI, there will be impairment in one or more cognitive domains like attention, memory, language abilities, executive function and visuospatial skills that is much lower than the client's age and socio-economic background.
3. **Preservation of Independence in Performing Functional Abilities:** It can be noticed that although persons with MCI maintain their ability to manage their daily living activities, they are less efficient doing so and require more time for completion of the task.
4. **Not Demented:** In persons with MCI, the cognitive and behavioral changes are significantly mild to affect social and occupational functioning.

Procedure for Clinical Diagnosis of DAT

Diagnosing dementia and determining what type it is can be challenging. There is no single procedure to diagnose dementia; the professionals use a test battery to diagnose. First and foremost the clinician will obtain an accurate case history. The clinician may interview both the caregiver as well as the client to get a better picture. Along with cognitive impairments, depression is also screened as well as neuropsychiatric symptoms such as disinhibition, irritation, apathy etc. are also noted by the clinician. Physical examination by a physician is also done to identify co-morbid conditions such as atrial fibrillation, heart disease or pulmonary problems. Cognitive & Neuropsychological assessment is also carried. Neurological evaluation is carried out by a neurologist where cranial nerve examination, focal weakness and gait are assessed. Cerebro-spinal fluid (CSF) evaluation, as well as neuroimaging techniques like Computed Tomography scan (CT), magnetic resonance imaging (MRI) and Positron emission tomography (PET) etc. are useful in providing clinical diagnosis of dementia.

Cognitive Deficits in Persons With DAT

Numerous studies report that persons with DAT exhibit cognitive deficits which vary with the different subtypes (Brandt et al., 2009; Saunders & Summers, 2010; Bozoki, Giordani, Heidebrink, Berent, & Foster, 2001; Hodges, Erzinclioglu, & Patterson, 2006). Since various cognitive processes such as attention, memory, perception, speed of processing and various executive functions play an important role in language functions there exist a strong correlation between language and cognitive domains. Cognitive deficits in Persons with DAT are discussed.

Memory Deficits

Memory problems are exhibited as the major sign of cognitive decline in persons with dementia. Working memory (WM) deficits are seen in persons with dementia due to the poor executive control system. There are also studies that have reported reduced memory span and short-term memory (STM) capacities in persons with dementia (Morries, 1986). Belleville, Peretz and Malenfant (1996) investigated the verbal and attention components of working memory in patients with DAT, normal elderly, and healthy young adults. It was also noticed that Persons with DAT showed a reduced attention span but were sensitive to word length.

Deficits in Executive Function (EF)

Voss and Bullock (2004) explored the role of executive control function (ECF) within DAT and Vascular Dementia. The results indicated that DAT performed more poorly than Vascular Dementia on most of the cognitive tests.

Attention and Concentration Deficits

Perry and Hodges (1999) reported that Persons with DAT have more difficulty in performing complex tasks which require divided attention such as listening for the target word in a list. While simple tasks like selecting and sustaining are not typically impaired in early stages of dementia (Assal & Cummings, 2003).

Abstraction and Problem Solving Deficits

Cummings and Benson (1992) reported that impaired abstract thinking and problem-solving abilities are often prominent clinical features of dementia. These problems differ across the stages of dementia and are more prominent in the middle stage of the disease. Freedman and Oscar-Berman (1986) investigated the problem-solving impairment in persons with dementia using a tactile discrimination test. The impaired performance in these people was a result of the impaired cognitive flexibility that is required to alternate responses and shift mental set.

Linguistic Deficits in Dementia

The presence of memory impairment deficits in persons with dementia will also interfere with their linguistic abilities and will vary over the course of the illness. Early cognitive linguistic changes in discourse might be helpful for the preclinical identification of dementia.

Syntactic Comprehension Deficits

Bickel, Pantel, Eysenbach, and Schroder (2000) investigated the syntactic comprehension abilities of German speakers with dementia. The authors used semantically reversible sentences using a sentence-picture matching paradigm. Syntactic complexity was in the range from simple active voice sentences to complex sentences. Persons with dementia showed deficits in all the categories. However, syntactic comprehension is only mildly affected in the early stages of DAT.

Word Finding Difficulties

Ash et al. (2006) investigated the discourse abilities in persons with progressive non-fluent aphasia (PNFA), non-aphasic persons with a social disorder and persons with semantic dementia (SemD). The authors reported significant discourse impairments in all three groups of individuals. Persons with PNFA had the least verbal output, producing few narratives per minute. Persons with SemD had difficulty retrieving words while aphasics' persons with a disorder of social comportment and executive functioning had profound difficulty in organizing and expressing their narratives.

Discourse Abilities in Persons With Dementia

Impairment in discourse abilities of persons with dementia has become the area of recent research. Studies have reported that persons with mild to moderate dementia show relatively preserved phonologic, syntactic and lexical knowledge, while semantic and pragmatic knowledge is affected (Appell, Kertesz, & Fisman, 1982). Gracia and Joanette (1997) investigated the topic shifts in the spontaneous speaking abilities of persons with dementia of Alzheimer's type. Persons with dementia of Alzheimer's type demonstrated impaired topics shifts than healthy elderly which were due to failure to continue and repetition of ideas.

Cognitive-Linguistic Deficits in MCI

The cognitive –linguistic deficits in MCI are found to be similar to those found in DAT. These include deficits in category fluency and confrontation naming including Reaction time for language comprehension. Persons with MCI also tend to exhibit impairments in syntactic reasoning (Collie et al., 2002) and as well as naming rhyming words (Dwolatzky et al., 2003). Picture-description task, such as the Cookie Theft Picture, is less likely to reveal alterations in MCI or mild DAT (Bschor et al., 2001). Thus, it appears that linguistic impairments in MCI are most likely located at the semantic level which is exhibited in early DAT. It is reported that timed tests are especially sensitive to the declines seen in MCI. Massoud et al. (2002) reported that word-reading threshold may be useful in discriminating MCIs from DAT; Similarly lexical decision tasks (Taler & Jarema, 2006) and Event-related potentials (ERPs; Olichney et al., 2002) studies have shown to distinguish well between MCI and healthy controls and early DAT .

Neuroimaging Techniques in Dementia Assessment

Neuroimaging has become a vital fundamental part of a routine dementia assessment to find the causes of cognitive impairment, and also to support early, accurate dementia subtype diagnosis. Neuroimaging techniques used in the assessment of dementia can be mainly classified into three types-Structural, Functional, and Molecular.

Structural imaging basically includes computed tomography (CT) and magnetic resonance imaging (MRI). The images produced by these techniques allow one to visualize the anatomical 'structure' of cerebral tissue.

Functional imaging consists of Tc-HMPAO single positron emission CT scan (HMPAO-SPECT), F-FDG positron emission tomography (FDG-PET) and DaTscan, which uses radioactive tracer elements to give an indication of the functioning of the brain tissues. HMPAO-SPECT scan uses a lipophilic tracer element that crosses the blood-brain barrier and moves into brain tissue by diffusion technique, the resulting SPECT image shows the degree of cerebral blood perfusion. FDG-PET uses a glucose analogue to show the degree of cerebral glucose metabolism. Thus, in practice, these two imaging modalities give similar information and are used to identify impaired brain physiology prior to the onset of obvious atrophy. Finally, Molecular imaging use radioactive traces that helps to bind specific molecules of interest is an emerging field.

Team Approach in the Assessment of Dementia

The trans-disciplinary team approach is essential for the diagnosis of dementia. This inter-professional team consist of speech-language pathologists, neurologists, physicians, nurses, social workers, psychologists, health educators, other allied health professionals and support staff. An excellent trans-disciplinary approach allows shared commitment for better quality care and strong communication skills among team members.

Role of the Speech-Language Pathologist in the Assessment of MCI and DAT

According to American Speech Language Hearing Association (ASHA), the primary aim of a speech-language pathologist (SLP) is to evaluate cognitive-communication deficits in persons with dementia and to identify socio-cultural factors that delay functioning. During the evaluation, the SLP determines the appropriate assessment protocol to be used based on the severity of dementia as well as the client's communication needs. Furthermore, while selecting screening and other comprehensive tests, the speech pathologists must also consider the socio-economic factors. SLP's also play an important role while planning treatment, especially when working with persons with DAT; is to make sure that communication and cognitive goals are based on the client's skill. The primary focus of SLPs is working on the patient's strengths, rather than their weaknesses. In due course of time, as a patient's condition progresses, SLPs need to spot appropriate compensatory strategies and educate family members and caregivers to improve the quality of life in persons with DAT and MCI.

Factors to Consider Prior to Screening in Older Individuals

Before screening for cognitive-communication functions associated with dementia/MCI, it is essential to consider the impact of sensory issues, depression, and effect of current medications on cognitive skills.

Hearing Loss

Since hearing loss is prevalent in older adults it is mandatory to conduct an audiological evaluation prior to the screening of cognitive-communicative deficits. Traditional behavioral hearing tests like pure tone audiometry and speech audiometry are helpful in the initial stages of dementia/MCI with the help of certain modifications such as reiterating/paraphrasing instructions, slowing presentation of speech stimuli, using pulse tones and by providing constant reminders to the client to respond. During the later stages, more objective tests like Auditory Steady State response (ASSR) and Otoacoustic emissions can be used. If the Person with Dementia fails in the hearing screening, a referral has to be made to an audiologist for further evaluation. If the client is diagnosed as having hearing loss, it is necessary that the clinician make sure that client wears hearing aids during testing. If clients hearing status cannot be determined, the clinician can administer speech discrimination test present in the Arizona Battery of Communication Disorders of Dementia (ABCD).

Visual Impairment

Since visual acuity decreases with age, it is necessary to check the visual abilities of the client prior to cognitive-communication screening. If vision is corrected, eyeglasses have to be worn by the client while screening and adequate lighting must be present in the testing environment. The clinician can check for the presence of visual field deficits by administering a simple letter cancellation task present in Arizona Battery of Communication Disorders of Dementia (ABCD).

Depression

Depression is very common among older individuals and can be mistaken for dementia as it can significantly affect test scores. The cognitive changes associated with depression can be similar to the cognitive changes due to dementia which is referred as pseudo-dementia. If depression symptoms are present, the client should be referred to a clinical psychologist for further evaluation.

Effect of Medications

Older individuals take many medications like sedatives and antidepressants to manage diseases related to aging. Furthermore, these medications can exacerbate the cognitive-communicative functions due to drug interactions. Thus, before the screening, the clinician should consider the effects of drugs on cognitive-communicative functions.

Screening Tests for MCI and Dementia

Few of the screening tests for MCI and dementia are listed below.

1. **Mini-Mental State Examination (Folstein, Folstein, & McHugh, 1975):** The Mini-Mental State Examination (MMSE) is commonly used by SLPs and neuropsychologists. MMSE evaluates the client in terms of - orientation to place, person, time, memory, knowledge skills, communication and copying. The total score is 30, while scores less than 24 are indicative of dementia by most clinicians (Desmond, 2002). Bayles, Tomoeda, Montgomery, Cruz, and Azuma (2000) have reported that early dementia or MCI can be reported in clients having scores of 25 to 26. In another study by Monsch et al. (1995), the authors have reported that a score of less than 26 in MMSE is indicative of cognitive impairment.
2. **Montreal Cognitive Assessment (Rossetti, Lacriz, Cullum, & Weiner, 2011):** The Montreal Cognitive Assessment was designed as a quick screening tool for mild cognitive impairment to assess attention, concentration, executive functions, memory, language, visuospatial construction, conceptual thinking, calculation and orientation. The maximum score that person can get is 30, while scores of 26 and higher are considered normal; scores less than 25 indicating of cognitive impairment. Rossetti, Lacriz, Cullum, and Weiner (2011) have reported that MoCA was sensitive to detecting 90% of clients diagnosed with MCI, while MMSE was able to detect only 18% diagnosed with MCI.
3. **Mini-Cog (Borson, Scanlan, Brush, Vitaliano, & Dokmak, 2000):** This test was given by Mini-Cog uses a clock- drawing test with a simple un-cued three item word recall task. Clients are instructed to listen to and repeat three unrelated words, then draw a clock and finally recall the three previously presented words. The time taken to administer this test is four minutes. The cut-off score of less than three is indicative of dementia.
4. **Memory Impairment Screen (Buschke, Kuslansky, & Katz, 1999):** The Memory Impairment Screen (MIS) is a test that uses four item delayed free and cued recall tasks. The client is asked to read the word aloud (e.g., 'potato') and associate it with its semantic category cue (e.g. vegetable). The patient is engaged in a distractor task (counting from 1-20 forward and backward). After that the client is asked to freely recall the 4 items (free recall). Category cues are provided only if the item is not retrieved during the free recall (cued recall). MIS score is calculated as (2x [Free- recall]+(Cued -recall). The maximum score is eight. Scores of four or less are considered indicative of cognitive impairment.

Comprehensive Tests for Assessment of Dementia

Comprehensive evaluation of cognitive-communicative functions should provide information about the client's mental status, language comprehension and expression, memory, orientation and visuospatial skills.

Two of the most commonly used comprehensive tests for dementia are listed below:

1. **Arizona Battery for Communication Disorders of Dementia (Bayles & Tomoeda, 1993):** The ABCD consists of 14 subtests that evaluate mental status, verbal memory, language comprehension and expression and visuospatial memory. This test also contains four screening measures including speech discrimination, visual perception and literacy, visual field and visual agnosia. The subtests

of ABCD can be used individually or administered as a full battery. There are 5 constructs and 14 subtests. Language comprehension constructs consists of the following subtests (i) following commands (ii) comparative questions (iii) repetition (iv) reading comprehension. Language expression construct consists of the following subtests (i) object description (ii) generative naming (iii) confrontation naming (iv) concept definition. Verbal memory constructs consists of the following subtests (i) story retelling-immediate (ii) story retelling-delayed (iii) Word learning. Visuospatial skill construct consists of the following subtests (i) generative drawing (ii) figure copying. Mental status constructs consists of mental status subtest of ABCD. The full ABCD requires 90 minutes to complete. Total overall Score less than 18 is indicative of cognitive impairment.

2. **Functional Linguistic Communication Inventory (Bayles & Tomoeda, 1994):** FLCI evolved from longitudinal studies of individuals with DAT. FLCI tests the following skills Naming and greeting, Answering questions, Participation in a conversation, Comprehending signs and matching objects to pictures, Reading and comprehending words, Following commands, Reminiscing, Gesturing, Pantomiming, and writing. It takes approximately thirty minutes to administer this test. The advantage of FLCI is that it allows clinicians to compare the performance of the client with normative. The client's intact communication functions can be charted and predictions of communicative skills vulnerable to dementia can be charted. The test results are useful in the preparation of functional maintenance programs and caregiver counselling.

Indian Assessment Tests for Dementia

1. **Dementia Assessment Battery:** Sunil and Shyamala (2009) aimed at developing a diagnostic test battery in Kannada to assess persons with dementia. The test battery consists of four major domains such as memory, linguistic expression, linguistic comprehension, and visuospatial construction skills. The battery was administered on a control group (90 normal participants; 30 each into three groups). The groups consisted of young adults in the age range of 20-40 years; older adults in the age range of 40-60 years and geriatrics above 60 years. The experimental group consisted of 30 persons with dementia (10 in each severity group). The performance of persons with mild dementia was near normal in most of the subtests which included, spontaneous speech, reading comprehension, following commands, etc. Persons with moderate dementia exhibited difficulty in tasks related to memory – working memory, episodic memory, picture naming, generative naming, and generative drawing. Persons with severe dementia failed to elicit responses to any of the tasks due to the poor spontaneous speech output. The limitations of the study were less number of participants in the dementia group. The participants with dementia had different pathologies like Parkinsonism, Multi-infarct dementia, Alzheimer's etc.
2. **Comprehensive Cognitive Assessment Protocol for Persons with Dementia in Malayalam (CCAP-M; Malayalam):** Anjana and Shanbal (2010) aimed at developing a comprehensive cognitive Assessment Protocol in Malayalam (CCAP-M) for persons with Dementia to help Speech Language Pathologists to get in-depth knowledge of impairments. The other aim was to differentially diagnose Persons with Dementia from a normal elderly population. The test consisted of 6 domains mainly Memory, Linguistic comprehension, Linguistic expression, Visuospatial construction and Problem solving and Organization. Persons with Dementia performed poorly on the following tasks like generative naming, delayed recall, picture naming, categorization abilities, problem-solving etc. compared to other domains.

Role of Family in Dementia Care

Family can assist persons with dementia in dealing with the physical and psychological consequences of dementia. DAT impacts the client's ability to live independently and perform activities of daily living. Family members should provide emotional support, financial aid and personal care assistance to persons with DAT. Establishing a good working relationship with doctors and other team members helps in ensuring good care and ongoing support to persons with dementia. Many families provide care for a person with dementia at home. While this very rewarding experience, on the other hand, it can be stressful also. Caring for persons with dementia is more stressful than caring for someone with a physical impairment. It is also essential that caregivers take sometime to care for themselves both physically and emotionally so that caregiver burden can be avoided. It is necessary that family members take help from friends, other family members or community agencies so that they can continue to provide good care to persons with dementia without becoming exhausted, frustrated or simply burned out.

Assessment of Swallowing

A swallowing assessment should also be performed in persons with Dementia and MCI. However, assessment regarding swallowing issues is overlooked by SLPs. Studies have reported that forty-five percent of individuals with dementia who were residing in an institutional set up had dysphagia (Easterling & Robbins, 2008), which was more prevalent in patients with Dementia of Alzheimer's type (DAT) compared to normal elderly persons (Horner, Alberts, Dawson, & Cook, 1994).

Swallowing assessment with individuals with dementia involves evaluation of

1. The oro-motor examination
2. The client's ability to comprehend along with using compensatory strategies
3. The client's oral preparatory, oral, pharyngeal, and esophageal phases
4. The client's recognition of food and utensils;
5. Environmental factors like the appearance of the food, lighting, and distractions;
6. Food and liquid with a variation in textures, tastes etc
7. The effect of the persons prescribed medications on swallowing function;
8. The effect of cognitive factors on swallowing.

An instrumental evaluation is performed to determine safety as well as to identify effective treatment techniques. The instrumental evaluation may also give additional information about the oral and pharyngeal bolus transit time, airway protection reflux, the impact of bolus texture and size, and appropriate pacing (Easterling & Robbins, 2008).

CONCLUSION

Assessment of cognitive-communicative markers is essential for persons with MCI and DAT. Furthermore, it can help in the differential diagnosis of DAT and MCI. Proper assessment by SLPs is warranted in this area as it will throw light on the differential diagnosis of MCI and DAT, the clinical description of the characteristics between the two clinical groups, the prognosis for improved outcomes, recommendations for intervention and support; and referral for other professionals for assessments or services.

REFERENCES

American Psychiatric Association. (1994). *Diagnostic and statistical manual of mental disorders (DSM-IV)*. Washington, DC: American Psychiatric Association.

Anjana, A. V., & Shanbal, J. (2010). Cognitive communication assessment protocol for persons with dementia-Malayalam (Part B, VIII, pp. 12-28). Mysore: Students Research at All India Institute of Speech and Hearing.

Appell, J., Kertesz, A., & Fisman, M. (1982). A study of language functioning in Alzheimer patients. *Brain and Language*, *17*(1), 73–91. doi:10.1016/0093-934X(82)90006-2 PMID:7139272

Ash, S., Moore, P., Antani, S., McCawley, G., Work, M., & Grossman, M. (2006). Trying to tell a tale discourse impairments in progressive aphasia and frontotemporal dementia. *Neurology*, *66*(9), 1405–1413. doi:10.1212/01.wnl.0000210435.72614.38 PMID:16682675

Assal, F., & Cummings, J. L. (2003). Cortical and frontosubcortical dementias. *Dementia: Presentations, Differential Diagnosis, and Nosology*, 3-30.

Bayles, K. A., & Tomoeda, C. K. (1993). *Arizona battery for communication disorders of dementia*. Tucson, AZ: Canyonlands Publishing.

Bayles, K. A., & Tomoeda, C. K. (1994). *FLCI: Functional Linguistic Communication Inventory*. Canyonlands Publishing, Incorporated.

Bayles, K. A., Tomoeda, C. K., Montgomery, E. B., Cruz, R. F., & Azuma, T. (2000). The relation of mental status to performance on lexical-semantic tasks in Parkinson's disease. *Advances in Speech Language Pathology*, *2*(2), 67–75. doi:10.3109/14417040008996792

Belleville, S., Peretz, I., & Malenfant, D. (1996). Examination of the working memory components in normal aging and in dementia of the Alzheimer type. *Neuropsychologia*, *34*(3), 195–207. doi:10.1016/0028-3932(95)00097-6 PMID:8868277

Bickel, C., Pantel, J., Eysenbach, K., & Schröder, J. (2000). Syntactic comprehension deficits in Alzheimer's disease. *Brain and Language*, *71*(3), 432–448. doi:10.1006/brln.1999.2277 PMID:10716871

Borson, S., Scanlan, J., Brush, M., Vitaliano, P., & Dokmak, A. (2000). The Mini-Cog: A cognitive 'vital signs' measure for dementia screening in multi-lingual elderly. *International Journal of Geriatric Psychiatry*, *15*(11), 1021–1027. doi: PMID:11113982

Bozoki, A., Giordani, B., Heidebrink, J. L., Berent, S., & Foster, N. L. (2001). Mild cognitive impairments predict dementia in nondemented elderly patients with memory loss. *Archives of Neurology*, *58*(3), 411–416. doi:10.1001/archneur.58.3.411 PMID:11255444

Brandt, H. E., Deliens, L., Steen, J. T. V. D., Ooms, M. E., Ribbe, M. W., & Wal, G. V. (2005). The last days of life of nursing home patients with and without dementia assessed with the palliative care outcome scale. *Palliative Medicine*, *19*(4), 334–342. doi:10.1191/0269216305pm1018oa PMID:15984506

Bschor, T., Kühl, K. P., & Reischies, F. M. (2001). Spontaneous speech of patients with dementia of the Alzheimer type and mild cognitive impairment. *International Psychogeriatrics*, *13*(3), 289–298. doi:10.1017/S1041610201007682 PMID:11768376

Buschke, H., Kuslansky, G., Katz, M., Stewart, W. F., Sliwinski, M. J., Eckholdt, H. M., & Lipton, R. B. (1999). Screening for dementia with the memory impairment screen. *Neurology*, *52*(2), 231–231. doi:10.1212/WNL.52.2.231 PMID:9932936

Collie, A., Maruff, P., & Currie, J. (2002). Behavioral characterization of mild cognitive impairment. *Journal of Clinical and Experimental Neuropsychology*, *24*(6), 720–733. doi:10.1076/jcen.24.6.720.8397 PMID:12424647

Cummings, J. L., & Benson, D. F. (1992). *Dementia: A clinical approach*. Butterworth-Heinemann Medical.

Desa, U. (2015). World population prospects: The 2015 revision, key findings and advance tables. New York: United Nations.

Desmond, D. W., Moroney, J. T., Sano, M., & Stern, Y. (2002). Mortality in patients with dementia after ischemic stroke. *Neurology*, *59*(4), 537–543. doi:10.1212/WNL.59.4.537 PMID:12196645

Dwolatzky, T., Whitehead, V., Doniger, G. M., Simon, E. S., Schweiger, A., Jaffe, D., & Chertkow, H. (2003). Validity of a novel computerized cognitive battery for mild cognitive impairment. *BMC Geriatrics*, *3*(1), 4. doi:10.1186/1471-2318-3-4 PMID:14594456

Easterling, C. S., & Robbins, E. (2008). Dementia and dysphagia. *Geriatric Nursing*, *29*(4), 275–285. doi:10.1016/j.gerinurse.2007.10.015 PMID:18694703

Folstein, M. F., Folstein, S. E., & McHugh, P. R. (1975). “Mini-mental state”: A practical method for grading the cognitive state of patients for the clinician. *Journal of Psychiatric Research*, *12*(3), 189–198. doi:10.1016/0022-3956(75)90026-6 PMID:1202204

Freedman, M., & Oscar-Berman, M. (1986). Comparative neuropsychology of cortical and subcortical dementia. *The Canadian Journal of Neurological Sciences*, *13*(S4), 410–414. doi:10.1017/S0317167100037008 PMID:3791055

Garcia, L. J., & Joanette, Y. (1997). Analysis of conversational topic shifts: A multiple case study. *Brain and Language*, *58*(1), 92–114. doi:10.1006/brln.1997.1871 PMID:9184097

Hodges, J. R., Erzinçlioğlu, S., & Patterson, K. (2006). Evolution of cognitive deficits and conversion to dementia in patients with mild cognitive impairment: A very-long-term follow-up study. *Dementia and Geriatric Cognitive Disorders*, *21*(5-6), 380–391. doi:10.1159/000092534 PMID:16601329

Horner, J., Alberts, M. J., Dawson, D. V., & Cook, G. M. (1993). Swallowing in Alzheimer’s disease. *Alzheimer Disease and Associated Disorders*, *8*(3), 177–189. PMID:7986487

Massoud, F., Chertkow, H., Whitehead, V., Overbury, O., & Bergman, H. (2002). Word-reading thresholds in Alzheimer disease and mild memory loss: A pilot study. *Alzheimer Disease and Associated Disorders*, *16*(1), 31–39. doi:10.1097/00002093-200201000-00005 PMID:11882747

McKhann, G. M., Knopman, D. S., Chertkow, H., Hyman, B. T., Jack, C. R., Kawas, C. H., & Mohs, R. C. (2011). The diagnosis of dementia due to Alzheimer’s disease: Recommendations from the National Institute on Aging-Alzheimer’s Association workgroups on diagnostic guidelines for Alzheimer’s disease. *Alzheimer’s & Dementia*, *7*(3), 263–269. doi:10.1016/j.jalz.2011.03.005 PMID:21514250

Monsch, A. U., Foldi, N. S., Ermini-Fünfschillin, D. E., Berres, M., Taylor, K. I., Seifritz, E., & Spiegel, R. (1995). Improving the diagnostic accuracy of the Mini-Mental State Examination. *Acta Neurologica Scandinavica*, *92*(2), 145–150. doi:10.1111/j.1600-0404.1995.tb01029.x PMID:7484063

Morris, R. G. (1986). Short-term forgetting in senile dementia of the Alzheimer's type. *Cognitive Neuropsychology*, *3*(1), 77–97. doi:10.1080/02643298608252670

Olichney, J. M., Morris, S. K., Ochoa, C., Salmon, D. P., Thal, L. J., Kutas, M., & Iragui, V. J. (2002). Abnormal verbal event related potentials in mild cognitive impairment and incipient Alzheimer's disease. *Journal of Neurology, Neurosurgery, and Psychiatry*, *73*(4), 377–384. doi:10.1136/jnnp.73.4.377 PMID:12235303

Perry, R. J., & Hodges, J. R. (1999). Attention and executive deficits in Alzheimer's disease. *Brain*, *122*(3), 383–404. doi:10.1093/brain/122.3.383 PMID:10094249

Petersen, R. C., Doody, R., Kurz, A., Mohs, R. C., Morris, J. C., Rabins, P. V., ... Winblad, B. (2001a). Current concepts in mild cognitive impairment. *Archives of Neurology*, *58*(12), 1985–1992. doi:10.1001/archneur.58.12.1985 PMID:11735772

Petersen, R. C., Stevens, J. C., Ganguli, M., Tangalos, E. G., Cummings, J. L., & DeKosky, S. T. (2001b). Practice parameter: Early detection of dementia: Mild cognitive impairment (an evidence-based review) Report of the Quality Standards Subcommittee of the American Academy of Neurology. *Neurology*, *56*(9), 1133–1142. doi:10.1212/WNL.56.9.1133 PMID:11342677

Prince, M., Bryce, R., Albanese, E., Wimo, A., Ribeiro, W., & Ferri, C. P. (2013). The global prevalence of dementia: A systematic review and metaanalysis. *Alzheimer's & Dementia*, *9*(1), 63–75. doi:10.1016/j.jalz.2012.11.007 PMID:23305823

Rossetti, H. C., Lacritz, L. H., Cullum, C. M., & Weiner, M. F. (2011). Normative data for the Montreal Cognitive Assessment (MoCA) in a population-based sample. *Neurology*, *77*(13), 1272–1275. doi:10.1212/WNL.0b013e318230208a PMID:21917776

Saunders, N. L., & Summers, M. J. (2011). Longitudinal deficits to attention, executive, and working memory in subtypes of mild cognitive impairment. *Neuropsychology*, *25*(2), 237–248. doi:10.1037/a0021134 PMID:21381828

Sunil, R., & Shyamala, K. C. (2009). Dementia assessment battery (Part B, VII, pp. 262-275). Mysore: Students Research at All India Institute of Speech and Hearing.

Taler, V., & Jarema, G. (2006). On-line lexical processing in AD and MCI: An early measure of cognitive impairment? *Journal of Neurolinguistics*, *19*(1), 38–55. doi:10.1016/j.jneuroling.2005.07.002

Voss, S. E., & Bullock, R. A. (2004). Executive function: The core feature of dementia? *Dementia and Geriatric Cognitive Disorders*, *18*(2), 207–216. doi:10.1159/000079202 PMID:15211077

KEY TERMS AND DEFINITIONS

Communication: It is the act of the imparting or exchanging information by means of speaking, writing, or using some other medium.

Dementia of Alzheimer's Type (DAT): It is the most common cause of dementia, affecting memory, language, thinking, and behavior of an individual in middle or older age groups. The pathological conditions reveal plaque formations and tangles which progressively affects the individual's daily living activities.

Diagnosis: It is the identification of the nature and cause of a certain phenomenon.

Executive Function: It is a set of mental skills that help you get things done. These skills are controlled by an area of the brain called the frontal lobe.

Memory: It is defined as the power or process of reproducing or recalling what has been learned and retained especially through associative mechanisms.

Mild Cognitive Impairment (MCI): It is a condition characterized by significant cognitive impairment in the absence of dementia. It primarily affects memory, but it might cause changes in daily function in subtle ways. MCI is different from Alzheimer's disease or other dementias. It does not typically affect a person's ability to complete daily tasks or cause general confusion.

Section 4
Communication Disorders:
Rehabilitation and Intervention

Chapter 15
Changing Socio-Cultural Models and Policy Programs in Rehabilitation of Persons With Communication Disorders

Srinivasan Venkatesan
All India Institute of Speech and Hearing, India

ABSTRACT

The history of rehabilitation of communication disorder has journeyed from magical-religious conceptualizations through biological-medical approaches to the contemporary rights-based paradigm, wherein the person-in-environment is emphasized. The understanding of its nature and characteristics, classification, etiology, treatment, social perception, and practices, including law-making about the affected persons, have all moved in tandem with the temper of the times. This chapter attempts to outline the salient course of these changes under two sections: (1) changing models and paradigms and (2) impacts on policy programs in areas of health, education, economy, housing, and social security with special reference to the Indian sub-continent. Illustrative domains of social change in areas of education are specifically highlighted with appropriate case vignettes. The endnote raises oncoming challenges, issues, and problems related to communication disorders in the emergent dynamic socio-cultural matrix for generation next parents and children.

INTRODUCTION

The greatest discovery of all times is that people change the world by merely changing their own attitude! – Oprah Winfrey

The concept of normality subsumes adjacent layers of abnormality, sub-normality, and para-normality. People exist in a variety of hues. Differences, disparity, and dissimilarities are the existential reality although similarities, similitude, and sameness are a fostered norm. Social systems are created or carved

DOI: 10.4018/978-1-5225-4955-0.ch015

with the typical in concern. Society thrives on a myth of equality (Stamos, 2013). For example, available footwear, furniture, garments or gadgetry are made on assumed average sizes. Those in outside layers, despite grave personal difficulties, have to perforce take the mainstream or center course (Clarkson and Clarkson, 2016; Ngugi, 1993). To an extent, it is all right to talk of the average, typical and normal for footwear or garments. What about other human attributes and behaviors? The situation can become devastating for the individual. A left-handed in the world of right-handed, dark-skinned among fair complexioned, obese among thin companions, Lilliputian among giants, aggressive among unassertive, introverted among extroverted, a foreigner amidst native speakers, illiterate among literates, the uninitiated among computer savvy are all vivid examples of such a predicament (Koretsky, 2007; Simmons, 2002). Notwithstanding all this, society is made for the supposedly typical. In doing so, all differences are sought to be obliterated.

Stereotyping and Labeling

The easiest way to mask differences is stereotyping. It is an oversimplified, usually pejorative attitude that people hold towards those outside one's own experience of who are different. Persons are often viewed under various stereotypes. There are gender stereotypes, only-child stereotype, or person with disability stereotype. Single children are believed to be bossy, aggressive, selfish and spoiled. They are presumed to have imaginary companions to compensate for their loneliness. Similarly, persons who stutter are viewed as shy, nervous, guarded, self-conscious, anxious, hesitant, introverted and diffident (Crutchfield and Wang, 2016; Klassen, 2001). Persons with disabilities (PWDs) are 'different' from their non-disabled peers, or that they belong to a 'lesser' category, while a successful 'handicapped' person is hailed as 'superhuman'. The burden of disability is viewed as an unending saga of sorrow. Able-bodied persons are considered to be under obligation to help PWDs. Those with intellectual disabilities are considered as 'holy innocents endowed with special grace and are meant to inspire others to value life' (Nario-Redmond, 2010). A stereotype, also erroneous, is the view that disabled is a wheelchair-bound person. This is partly because that is the symbol allotted to them, or also since, many leaders of disabled people's organizations fit into that image (Shakespeare, 2013; 2006).

The problem with stereotypes is that it will implicitly or explicitly influence the self and other perception of the affected as well as people around them. Naming or labeling has the unique power to influence a person. The moment a child is named 'autistic', for example, everyone around will start expecting and viewing every action of that child as an inherent feature of that condition. If the child laughs, then it is viewed as a symptom of autism. If he cries, that is also deemed as characteristic of that condition. Whether he looks the other way or stares at you, clings to his mother, eats or refuses to eat, or play-each and every action are attributed as 'autism' (Green et al. 2005). Many times, implicitly conveyed expectations of others will itself prompt the person to behave in a manner that fulfills their expectations! When a mother keeps telling her child that she is a fussy eater, the child turns out to be one. This phenomenon is called 'self-fulfilling prophecy', 'Pygmalion Effect' or 'Rosenthal Effect'. If a teacher expects enhanced performance from her pupils, then the student's performance will be actually enhanced. The reverse is also true. It is a kind of observer-expectancy effect that works. When people say you are dumb, you feel dumb. This is best exemplified in persons who stutter (Hulit, 2004; p. 198). When a child is repeatedly told that she cannot do it without help or she better not try doing by herself, the child will then never give a try. It cripples her willingness to act. Even as the phone rings, if the stutterer approaches it reluctantly expecting to stutter, he will end up doing exactly the same (Rentschler, 2012; p. 154).

Case Vignette #1

The presenting complaint of a mother in the consulting chamber was that her child is 'autistic', 'hyperactive' and suffering from 'attention deficit disorder'. When confronted as to how she could come to such conclusions even before the consultation had begun, she explained that she had browsed extensively on the net and was convinced about the child's condition. The 5-year old could hardly 'copy-write a paragraph', was 'always overactive and jumpy', 'snatched things from others' and 'never obeyed commands'. It did not matter that the child could sit for hours with gadgets, and never threw any tantrum in front of an intimidating uncle!

Nomenclature

Nomenclature is offering names or terms to denote their existence. It is part of everyday communication. Various semantic categories carry names, such as a table, shirt, rose, dog, nose, etc. The trouble starts when such names gather connotative meanings. For example, being named as 'dwarf', 'idiot', 'imbecile', 'moron', 'retarded', 'drug addict', 'criminal', 'schizophrenic', 'blind', 'deaf', 'mute', or 'crippled' has negative nuances. It upsets self-perception, self-image, and self-esteem. Such terms are best avoided. Names may range from simple descriptions as 'disturbed', 'difficult', 'different', or 'dissimilar' to more serious labels like 'disease', 'disorder', 'illness', 'deviant' or 'delayed'. Of course, each term has a different meaning and context for its use.

Impairment is being propagated as the term to designate any visible structural anatomical loss of physical or sensory organs. Disability refers to the functional inability of an individual to perform any activity in the manner or within the range considered 'normal' for any human being. It is usually a result of impairment. The word 'handicap' is explained as any disadvantage usually resulting or consequence but emanating from the environment of an individual that limits or prevents the fulfillment of a social role that is expected for their age, gender or cultural background (Venkatesan, 2004; Orgogozo, 1994). A person can face handicap without impairment and disability. A girl child made to drop out of school after attaining menarche is an example of this kind. The significance of these terms or their distinctions becomes apparent with these examples. The loss of one's little finger is a visible physical impairment. This may result in a disability which restricts a musician from playing on a stringed instrument, or in typing if one was a typist. However, the same impairment may pose no handicap for an orator or singer. Although the terms: impairment, disability, and handicap have now become old-fashioned, it is continued to be used for its practical utility in uniting various models for explaining the phenomenon (Jones, 2001).

This chapter proceeds to outline the happening course of changes in the field of rehabilitation of persons with communication disorders under two sections: (a) changing models and paradigms; and, (b) impacts on policy programs in areas of health, education, economy, housing and social security with special reference to the Indian sub-continent.

CHANGING MODELS AND PARADIGM SHIFTS

The story of habilitation-rehabilitation of affected individuals can be classified, for ease of explanation, into three models: (a) Magical-Religious Model; (b) Medical Model; and, (c) Rights Based Model. An understanding of these models is actually a history of social attitude change across times. It has ramifications for understanding the whole gamut diagnosis, magnitude, survey, screening, identification, labeling, referral, history taking, causative analysis, diagnosis, counseling, the law as well as handling, treatment, or interventions that go on in the service delivery systems for affected persons with communication disorders.

Magical-Religious Model

Many misconceptions, prejudice, discrimination, stigma, and stereotypes that are customarily attached to PWDs are exemplified by several mythological characters, such as, the 'mean-minded' *Mandira* in Ramayana, who is afflicted by Scoliosis, or the villainy of a paraplegic in *Shakuni* of Mahabharata (Basham, 1924). The role of a helpless gullible blind king is ascribed to Dhritarashtra in the same epic. There are descriptions of involution melancholia experienced by King Dasaratha, father of Lord Rama, following the latter's separation after the abdication of the throne. There is a dramatic illustration of Catatonic Stupor in the petrified Ahalya following the traumatic discovery of an episode of infidelity. There are also positive stereotypes in some characters embodied with the sagacity of the multiply deformed Astavakra, or cerebral palsy in one of Lord Krishna's boyhood buddies (Misra and Paranjpe, 2012; Rao, 2010).

The understanding of causes and treatment of communication disorders can be also drawn from such magical-religious underpinnings in ancient texts. They continue to be staunchly believed by its followers even in contemporary India. A stigma is attached to psychiatry, psychology and mental diseases. While laypersons dread or avoid consulting mental health professionals, it is believed that early rising, fasting, baths, diet, gargling, regulated sleep, body posturing, breathing exercise, observance of rituals, offering prayer, acts of philanthropy, attending spiritual discourse, visiting holy places, and regular performance of some ceremonies can undo the malevolent causative effects of diseases, disorders, disabilities and disturbances in the present birth cycle (Cornelissen, Misra, and Varma, 2014; Manickam, 2010).

A common denominator underlying the Hindu approach to human disabilities is an invocation of the concepts of Karma, Dharma, Moksha, and Reincarnation with a repetitive cycle of births and deaths. This continues till one attains salvation through the performance of good, just, honest, virtuous and selfless deeds. Intended to foster individual discipline and social control, some of its prescriptions recommend rearrangement of home architecture, wearing certain attire or ornaments, fulfillment of marital vows, changing one's name, or adherence to auspicious timings (Veereshwar, 2002; Gupta, 1977; Singh, 1977). If one follows the magical-religious models, it is believed that one's condition is the consequence of a curse or blessings from supernatural forces for the supposedly good or evil deeds committed by the victim in past birth (Bhattacharya, Khanna, and Kohli, 2009). By this view, socio-cultural based causal attributions cover categories like environment, self-blame, super-natural, chance occurrence, or others. It is held, for example, that the oro-facial anomaly characteristic of a person with cleft lip, resembling the mouth of a rabbit or monkey, along with the animal's temperament, is caused by inheritance from the simian clan (Weatherley-White, 2012).

Case Vignette #2

A 9-year old pupil of class four was brought with complaints of frequent episodes of a headache, at times associated with or without vomiting. Consultation with an ophthalmologist ended with a prescription for a pair of spectacles to correct a refractive error of -0.75 diopters. The eye correction was to no avail.

Another round of consultations with physicians and family doctors also proved futile. The family guru recommended the application of certain oils or herbal pastes. With no respite despite all these attempts, someone suggested prayers or making offerings at a religious place. What emerged eventually from a detailed psycho-educational evaluation was that the child with an average level of intellectual functioning had a severe academic lag and his performance was at the level of kindergarten. The daily stress and expectation of academic performance at school and home, repeated class tests, combined with poor grades and frequent teasing by peers, precipitated the headaches. Surprisingly, it escaped everyone's attention that the student's symptoms did not appear during extended vacations.

Interventions for mental ill-health and disability conditions in ancient India are understood as falling under mystical-metaphysical traditions like Buddhism, Yoga, and Bhakti customs as well as medical traditions like Ayurveda, Unani, Siddha, Naturopathy, and Homeopathy (Neki, 1975; Bhugra, 1992). Based on a holistic system of treatment for maintenance Swasthya or good health, the Ayurveda for example prescribe regular use of techniques like wearing precious gems, performing propitiatory rites, early rising, regulated sleep, gargling, fasting, sunbath (Tejopasana) or mud baths (Pruthvipasana), water therapy (Jalopasana), oil massages, or use of herbs, just as Gandharvaveda recommends dance, music, and theatre (Balodhi and Chowdhary, 1986; Dube, 1978; Vahia, 1969; Debsikdar, 1961)

Medical Model

This model insists on biological causes (Miller, Vandome, and McBrewster, 2010). The International Classification of Diseases (ICD-10; WHO, 2008) and Diagnostic and Statistical Model, 5th Revision (DSM-5; APA, 2013) are examples. An extra chromosome is explained as a cause for a type of intellectual disability. A hormone deficiency is clarified as etiology of another type of physical handicap. A neurological insult is assumed to cause a learning disability. Medical models are invoked to explain causes as well as provide limited cures for various disabilities. To put it correctly, disabilities are relatively permanent conditions. Therefore, there can be no 'cure' as there is for diseases, disorders, illness or infections. Although this model succeeded in bringing disabilities to the center stage, it is faulted for the medicalization of disability and reducing the affected person as an unfortunate victim of a disease, deficit or deviant condition. Nowadays, the field of disability-rehabilitation has undergone a sea of change particularly with regard to its perspective on understanding their 'causes' and/or 'management'.

Rights-Based Model

Overriding the above-mentioned models, a contemporary post-millennium rights-based model uses a 'person-in-environment' social perspective (Fougeyrollas and Beauregard, 2001). It argues that human disabilities are not the making or misfortune of an affected gene, faulty chromosome or gestational insults. It is not owing to retaliatory machinations of divine forces for errors committed in one's past life. Rather, it is alleged as the intended or unintended consequence of several barriers imposed by the larger social system on the affected persons. The argument is that society is created and operated in a way that does not take into account the genuine differences among people (Ormerod, 2005; Braddock and Parish, 2001). Going by their tenor, instead of disease based classifications, positivistic health-oriented classifications are invoked, such as, International Classification of Functioning, Disability, and Health: Children and Youth Version (ICF-CY; WHO, 2007).

Impact of the Models

The knowledge, opinions, attitudes, misconceptions, prejudices and/or stereotypes that individuals or societies have about disability-impairment phenomenon depend on which of a model of disability is adopted. One rooted in the magical-religious model would view the disability as a product of one's past misdeeds. He may seek intervention and therapy consultations from astrology, palmistry, nameology, faith healing, etc. Another person moved by the medical model will end up doctor shopping by seeking medicine based cures or laboratory investigations. A comparison and contrast between the three models are exemplified best in the instance of a challenged person with dwarfism. Tradition and popular culture describe them as short, ugly and freakish. In Hindu mythology, *Apasmara* is a dwarf who represented ignorance and epilepsy. He was to be subdued by the mighty Lord Shiva under his feet during a cosmic dance. The dwarf appears as the fifth incarnation of Lord Vishnu as *Vamana,* a short Brahmin with a wooden umbrella, to restore authority over the heavens. Laypersons view them as epitomes of either tragedy or comedy. Going by medical model, dwarfism is caused by growth hormone deficiency. Under the rights-based model, the condition is not a problem with the affected individual. It is a consequence of a society which has not designed itself to accommodate the height needs of such persons. A low height chair or table, switchboard, or door openers would minimize or eliminate the handicap (Adelson, 2005).

A similar predicament is experienced by people with differences in other areas. The left-handed amidst right handed, dark-skinned among fair complexioned, obese in a society which worships being trim and slim, the low scorer of academic grades in a school with premium for high marks, or the slow learner in a neighborhood of multitasking whiz kids-all of them stand the risk of social discrimination, exclusion or even downright rejection. When a common curriculum is prepared for all same-aged students in our schools, it is assumed, albeit erroneously, all pupils in that age group are identical. In reality, no two children are the same. We know that even identical twins are not similar. Ideally, every child requires individualized instruction. This is all the more true for children on the fringe or those at the ends of so-called center (Alur, 2002).

PWDs are frequently victims of denied opportunity rather than inherent inabilities. For centuries, they have been condemned as victims of some supernatural wrath for all the supposedly wrongdoings in a previous birth. They have been segregated from mainstream society, feared, condemned, criticized, laughed, joked, disliked, pitied, sympathized, rejected and relegated to stay indoors. They have been kept away from social contacts fearing their condition could be contagious, or that they are born incapable, or that it was better to leave them to their own fate of things. Thereafter, under medical model, they were continued to be viewed as victims of an unfortunate predicament to known or unknown causes not attributable to past birth. The rights approach argued against these stereotypes. It turned the earlier views upside down. Instead of viewing their predicament as the making or misfortune of the affected individual (Stroman, 2003; Fleischer and Frieda, 2001), it was seen as the intended or unwitting consequences of several barriers imposed by the majority of a larger system on the affected minority (Silvers, 2010). The argument was that society is designed, created or operated in a way without taking into account people who do not meet its perceived norm. Society excludes such persons as disabled, abnormal, subnormal or deviant. To this model, the use of such terms makes no sense. If only barriers in education, employment, urban design, housing, transport, tourism, travel, leisure, and recreation can all be eliminated, then there is no handicap in the real sense of the term (Burnett and Bender-Baker, 2001).

This approach demands a rightful space for one and all. Schools or workspaces are now being mandated to accommodate all types or levels of learners and performers. It is demanded that the differences are not discriminated, branded, nick-named, separated, denied or punished. Rather, accommodations are insisted. Ramps with railings are sought for smooth physical movement and mobility of persons with locomotion difficulties. An easy question paper or an oral test is asked for children with writing disabilities. The provision of extra time is sought for slow learners. A permission to use calculator is claimed for children with arithmetic delays. Above all, the banning of corporal punishment, giving preference for a child over curriculum are some of the positive and proactive measures contemporary governments, and education departments are promoting for optimizing the potentials in these persons with different abilities.

Another impact of rights approach is improving access for these persons. Since handicap is viewed as the making of society, removal of barriers is gathering momentum. Physical barriers are sought to be demolished by the construction of gradient ramps along with stairways, making provision for lifts and elevators, and marking of slippery surfaces. Social attitudinal barriers are being broken. Unfortunately, there are still some who think that a student with cerebral palsy should be made to write by holding a pen in the mouth or that severe physical punishment will make students with learning disabilities correct their spelling mistakes. A few related concepts involving social appraisal termed as 'access audit', 'universal design', 'tourism access' is gaining momentum all over the world including our country (Friedner and Osborne, 2015; 2013; Sharma, Kumar, and Singh, 2013; Kadir and Jamaluddin, 2012; Venkatesan, Jayakaran, Purusotham, and Rafi, 2012). Despite its theoretical strength and attractions associated with egalitarian principles of equality and non-discrimination, there is also a downside of human rights-based approach. It is shown that rights-based discourse having origins in the west will take the time to sink in the east. As pointed, there are challenges of making them operational or transforming them into the real thing (Batliwala, 2007). It is noted that 'rights conflict with one another, rights are vague, rights have exceptions, many situations fall between rights' (Kennedy, 2004).

In recent times, economic models of disability are being floated. They define these conditions in terms of loss of human capital or productivity owing to non-participation in work for the individual, employer, and the nation. This model is used by policymakers to assess opportunity cost and the cost of non-rehabilitation. The presence of one child with permanent disablement in a family will reduce the opportunity for going to work for the mother or leave out of station for the father, and reconcile to home study for a sibling. Application of economic models on disability drastically changes one's perspective of the affected individual as a prospective consumer or customer. For example, when applied to the tourism industry, it necessitates that special packages are made to accommodate such persons.

Integrating Models Approach to Indian Culture

The 3-tier model approach provides a convenient backdrop to sequence and explains the course or development of disability rehabilitation in India. The role of culture in this understanding cannot be ignored. All human beings are part of a culture. Culture refers to the unique ways of life of groups of people. It distinguishes one group from another through its actions. It is the 'sum total of customs, arts, science, political and religious behavior taken as an integrated whole that distinguishes one society from another. Cultural learning is unique to human beings. It is transmitted through certain symbols that do not necessarily or naturally need to have a connection for what they stand. For example, wearing the vermillion on one's forehead or bangles on one's wrist is a symbol of feminine gender in Indian culture. It communicates the marital status of the user. There are several characteristics that are unique to Indian culture. The value attributed to joint over nuclear family, glorification of the mother-child relationship, stress on cooperation, conformity and collectivism than selfishness, competition, conflict, and individualism are unique to our culture. Dependency, especially of women, elderly and children, is considered normal, natural and expected. Overt excessive expression of sexuality is considered taboo (Venkatesan, 2010). Historically, the Indian culture has typically invoked a 'moral model' to define, understand, explain or treat disabilities. Leprosy, one of the visible disabilities in the country since ages, is shown as the making one's evil deeds in past birth. Hence, the victim is rightfully condemned to live in separate colonies. This picture was recast only recently by Christian missionaries who typified such a person as the innocent sinner, a reprobate who had no role in being cast as such. However, unlike in the west, in Indian scenario, there was a plurality of medical contexts with Ayurveda, Siddha, Unani, and other systems of medicine to provide succor to persons with diseases and disabilities (Anand, 2016).

Culture plays a crucial role in naming things, persons, or places. Even today, a dwarf is frequently named as 'Vamana' ('Kulla' or 'Kulli') and the 'hunch-back' is 'Kurmi' resembling the tortoise reminiscent of an avatar of Lord Vishnu in Indian mythology. Similarly, moved by fear, reverence or sentiment, children affected by cleft palate are named as 'Anjaneya' or 'Hanumantha' after the Monkey God with prayers and appeasement by rituals as a cure (Venkatesan, 2015a). It is one thing to be named and called by it, and it is quite another thing to observe how people react to them. In India, people show a surprising disconnect between the two. The author recalls an incident where an intellectually disabled couple was the butt of everyday jokes in a village. However, the same villagers took turns to provide board and lodging to the pair, thereby displaying a rare sense of camaraderie for philanthropic social action. The disjoint between thought, feeling, and action component is an evident feature in the Indian psyche.

Contrast these with typical stereotypes of an 'ideal' western culture that stress on the nuclear family, individualism, competition, and institutionalization of services across age groups. A divorce in India is still viewed as a disgrace and bad name for the family, whereas the typical American would view it as a sign of individual freedom. The father, grandfather or even family guru becomes the point of the first contact for felt individual crises or calamity. A consultation with mental health/rehabilitation professional is deemed unnecessary or stigma that is evaded and avoided or procrastinated. Even if such consultations are sought, discretion demands seeking help in private rather than the public hospital (Venkatesan, 2016b). A delayed speech in children is defended as normal and natural for boys than girls. Chewing or eating Indian gooseberry ever morning for a few months is a recommended cure for stammering. Rubbing a mixture of one tablespoon honey and one teaspoon salt on the tongue is another common cure. Adding cinnamon powder in meals daily is suggested for overcoming bed-wetting. Feeding a spoon of butter thrice a day is considered therapeutic for managing problem behaviors in children-presumably because Lord Krishna loved it as a 'naughty' child! Dispensing culture-bound therapies for communication problems in children come in plenty and for free. Caregivers are bound by social obligation to follow them for fear of a social boycott. Seeking services of professionals is the last resort when matters have worsened beyond limits. Even if it happens, the counselor-counselee dyad is viewed as god-devotee or teacher-pupil (guru-chela) relationship (Manickam, 2010). There are differences even in the counseling expectations, processes, procedures and practices that may be unique to our country. For example, prestige suggestion, often used as adjuvant becomes a rather regular and main course intervention technique in Indian settings. It is common to hear parents seeking to counsel for their wards saying:

He will obey if you tell him to do so!' Some demand secrecy by wanting to consult in the guise of 'friend' or 'uncle' or they just want to 'talk it over'. Many Indian parents proclaim in front of their wards: 'We have tried telling, advising, lecturing, threatening, scolding, bargaining, begging, punishing or even intimidating him to mend his ways…but, to no avail. Hope this counseling would at least put some sense into his head!

Further, it is pointed out that many western models of diagnosis and therapy may not be applicable to an average Indian consumer. Mythology and influence of Hindu epics are deeply and intensely ingrained in the typical Indian psyche. The cultural symbols of Lord Hanuman as bachelor hero, or goddess Lakshmi as the personification of wealth is widespread. Available therapy, if any, which is loaded only on western models, may not succeed in clinical practice. Western psychotherapeutic interventions typically recognize or recommend various depth, duration or degrees of engagement between the clinician and client, such as supportive, re-educative and re-constructive respectively. Given the constraints of time, cost and labor-intensive nature of re-educative and reconstructive therapies combined with the available demand-supply scenario in our country, the most reasonable option left out is to avoid 'deep' therapies. Instead, short-term and supportive individual or group counseling become the wisest option for optimum benefits to clients affected by communication disorders (George and Pothan, 2015). Cultural elements play a significant role at all stages and at every level in the origin, development, pathogenesis, and maintenance of clinical symptoms related to communication disorders. For example, a child with an abrupt psychogenic voice loss is apparently trying to communicate symbolically that s/he has no voice in a given stressful milieu or during an ongoing frustrating experience (Venkatesan, 2016a). Similarly, a teenager with stuttering may require additional training inputs in soft skills and life skills in as much a young woman may need to learn social graces and upper-class cultural etiquettes as a preparation for entry into such a society (Cottrell, 2015). The psychosocial sequel of problems in speech fluency is amply shown as a source of comedy for the public even in movies although its experience is a great personal tragedy. Notwithstanding all this, the person has to bear with regularly given unsolicited advice or suggestions from good intentioned well-wishers pouring out their overflowing sympathies to overcome the stuttering problem.

Case Vignette #3

A 30-year old team head for a software development project consulted for high pitched voice called puberphonia. On phone, he found it embarrassing that listeners addressed him as 'madam' mistaking him for a woman. He suspected that his colleagues could be making fun of him, probably even called him 'queer' or 'weird' owing to feminine voice and mannerisms. At first, he thought that the voice problem could be due to a lump in the throat which needed surgery. When it was not to be so, he grew anxious and worried. He presumed that he was an incomplete man. He doubted if he would be respected by his juniors at the workplace or if ever, he would get married at all. He avoided people, speaking aloud, on phone or on stage. He feared being joked, laughed or ridiculed. He took to bodybuilding and gym assuming it would build his voice as well as body.

IMPACTS ON POLICY AND PROGRAMS

The changing models are also having their impacts on the policy and programs for rehabilitation of persons with communication disorders in the Indian sub-continent. These effects are seen across a wide range of domains including health education, economy, housing and social security to mention only a few.

Changing Laws

Law, jurisprudence, and governance have always evolved in tandem with societal levels or contemporary perspectives on or about disability. The ancient Hindu laws prohibited the blind, deaf, or lame from ascending the throne as king, disallowed them to perform Vedic rites, and excluded them from inheritance (Dutt, 1972; p. 59). Under the magical-religious approach to disability, the then existing 'Lepers Act (1898)' and the now defunct 'Indian Lunacy Act' (1912) used terms like 'asylum', 'lunatic', 'insane', 'unsound mind' or 'idiot' (Dixit, 1998). Moving away from isolation, incarceration, and exclusion, the promulgation of International Year of Disabled Persons (1980) led to movements towards their integration. This was changed into 'Mental Health Act' (1987). More positively flavored terms like 'mentally ill person', 'psychiatric hospital', or 'psychiatric nursing home' were used with an endnote in one of its chapters on the protection of human rights of mentally ill persons. Another related legislation titled 'Persons with Disabilities Equal Opportunities Protection of Rights and Full Participation Act' (1995) followed the medical model to list 'blindness', 'hearing impairment', 'leprosy cured', 'locomotor disability (including 'cerebral palsy'), 'mental retardation' and 'mental illness' as officially recognized disabilities. Autism was still not recognized or included as a separate form of disability in that legislation. It was included later in the National Trust for Autism, Cerebral Palsy, Mental Retardation and Multiple Disabilities' (1999) to ensure that such affected persons receive benefits on their own. An entirely rights-based legislation has now appeared following passage of 'Mental Healthcare Act' (2016) and 'Rights of Persons with Disabilities Act' (2016). The former aims to provide for mental health care and services for persons with mental illness and ensure that they have the right to live with dignity by not being discriminated or harassed. The latter legislation improved on its repealed predecessor by covering 21 categories of disabilities, adding gender specific clauses, the inclusion of private sector, providing all India permit to entitlements, providing the right to free legal aid, etc.

Despite these positive developments, discussions are doing rounds whether these new laws allow PWDs having mental illness to consult in the prevailing scenario of stigma and paucity of mental health services and professionals in the country (Narayan and John, 2017; Ahmed. 2015). Further, given the recognition of disabilities and impairments as a rights-based social problem, there is a growing clamor by rehabilitation professionals to be allowed to independently certify such persons (Goswami, Venkatesan, and Mathew, 2015) over and above or in place of medical practitioners. Attempts are on to move away from official classifications based on medical models like ICD and DSM towards applying rights-based models, such as, ICF-CY for PWDs (de Schipper et al, 2015; Danermark et al. 2010; Jones, Crews, and Danielson, 2010; Battaglia et al. 2004; Simeonsson et al. 2003).

The Impact of Rights-Based Models: An Illustration of Isolation to Inclusion in Educational Settings

An example of the changing scenario of various models vis-à-vis disability habilitation is the isolation to inclusion saga of such affected children in the country. There was a time, not very long ago when these students were isolated or secluded in places usually far away from mainstream society. When an affected child was taken to school, the typical refrain then was: 'Sorry! No admission. You'd better keep him at home'. Then, a scenario of separating or segregation of such children entered when it used to be remarked: 'Sorry! No admission. But, you could probably admit the child to a special school'. Later, there was an era of 'integration', when it was stated: 'Welcome! But you'll have to put extra efforts to adjust or match the child to other kids at school'. The contemporary trend is one of inclusion, wherein, it would probably be said: 'Welcome! We'll adjust ourselves to suit the needs or requirements of your child'.

Contemporary inclusion is not merely a matter of simply providing a seat for the affected children amidst the so-called typical students. Much more than mere physical proximity, it involves even social, attitudinal, instructional and functional inclusion. It is not that the children with different needs have to study the same books or curriculum as the other pupils. It is not to be construed as a running race between equals. Rather, it is to be scheduled as a race that is equitable. As in the long distance racing track, the runners must be stationed such that they are staggered to start at different spots. But they all end up racing the same distance!

Inclusion can and must take place in different hues and at various levels. There can be resource rooms when these students work for few hours according to their talents, interests, and aptitude, trained itinerant teachers visit their homes, shadow teachers follow them during activities requiring high concentration, co-teachers and/or buddies teach by role reversals. Ideally, the teaching is to be individually tailor-made, adjusted to the pace of the student, play-based, functional, child-initiated, developmentally age-appropriate, interactive and activity oriented (Venkatesan, 2015b). Entitlements for benefits and concessions made available through available legislation include exemption from study of additional languages, provision for rest breaks, seating such children in smaller non-distracting rooms, giving extra time, grace marks, oral viva, options for taking alternate subjects, or minimizing portions of study for examinations, issue of question papers with multiple choice, single-word answers, scribe facility, prohibition of holding back, detention, and expulsion from school. Question papers with larger font size are to be given to visually challenged students, There are also rules related to maintaining a zero detention policy, making provision for resource rooms, shadow teachers, partial schooling or use of voice to text conversion software, spell checkers and of not using physical or psychological pressure provoking practices either intended or otherwise.

Source of Solace or Euphemism for Exclusion: The Indian Experience

Even as the country is grappling with the challenge of providing the PWDs their rightful place in society, several vestiges of exclusion, segregation or seclusion of such persons continue even today in contemporary India. Examples like the Dargah of Baba Saeed Ibrahim, a Saudi Arabian King who traveled here 800 years ago, is now a place for the mentally ill to come to pray for sanity is infamous. Other such places include: Mehendipur Balaji Temple in Rajasthan, Hazrat Syed Ali Meera Datar Dargah in Gujarat, Devji Maharaj Mandir, Malajpur, Dattatreya Temple in Gangapur, Nizamuddin Dargah, Delhi, Temple of Muthusamy in Dindigul District, Gunaseelam Vishnu Temple in Trichy, Gora Veerabhadraswamy Temple, Hanumanthapuram, Chennai, Sri Kaleshwar's Ashram, Penukonda, Benny Hinn Ministries of Kolkatta, are all popular places for exorcism of evil spirits or faith healing cures to treat mental illness. While temples, dargahs, and visitations to religious places are deemed as a cure by one class of citizenry, there is another educated elite, who prefer hospital-based western psychiatric treatment. There are, once again, various classes of such treatments available for NRI seeking to dump their chronic mentally ill wards in privileged 5-star level homes on the outskirts of metropolitan cities, as there are also middle to low middle-class government or non-government agencies for the abandonment of such persons. There are also institutions who seek a lifetime non-refundable charge, albeit surreptitiously, to care for the terminally ill.

The movements towards integration in the 1980s led to welcome of the disabled child, for example, into schools, although the onus was still placed on their shoulders to put extra efforts and adjust, achieve or match the other typical kids at school. It continued to be a level playing field. These students would have to sit in the same class, study same subjects, take the same tests or exams, and sit alongside the unaffected students. Such a predicament led to the failure of the special children, which was thrown back at them as due to their disability. In reality, this was not true. Apparently, a hard of hearing or partially sighted student would not be able to perform if seated on the last bench. A child with an intellectual disability would obviously fail to solve arithmetic sums requiring the application of trigonometry, geometry or algebra. Therefore, the argument was brought in that such pupils may be simply relegated to special schools, or within a separate campus in the regular school. The Project on Integrated Education of Disabled, flaunted by National Council of Education Research and Training, New Delhi, in 1980s and 1990s is a testimony to establishing several such now-defunct integrated schools wherein children with disabilities were located within the campus of a regular school although with separate entrance, staff, students, uniform and activities (Azad, 1996).

Inclusion, in the strictest sense of a rights approach, requires not the child but the school, its milieu, curriculum, and teachers to adjust or tune themselves to the requirements of the student with special needs. The changing temper and trend favoring inclusion of PWDs is reflected by recent happenings, such as, promulgation of rights-based laws related to Disabilities (2016) as well as Mental Health Care (2016), announcement on establishing a university for Disability Studies and Rehabilitation Science through an Act of Parliament, enactment of rules for making provisions for benefits and concessions, change of names (Viklangjan to *Divyangjan*) to ensure de-stigmatization, marginalization, and to end discrimination on the grounds of disability. Inclusion is not something that is to be viewed as restricted only to the field of school and education. Its impact is to cut across various life domains including health, work, and vocation, public transport, home, community, parenting, and family. Denial of health facilities or voting is no more allowed as is child marriage as a cure for intellectual disability or mental illness is deemed liable to be punished by current laws. Branding, burying, chaining or administration of electroconvulsive therapy is illegal. Hysterectomy or removal of the uterus without consent was a routine practice on adolescent girls with intellectual disability can result in prosecution. In a landmark decision, the Supreme Court of India recently denied abortion for an unwed intellectually challenged mother who was a victim of sexual abuse. Denial of a job since one is affected by thalassemia is viewed as much as exclusionary practices as disallowing a person with stuttering into the societal club.

While the preceding discourse may give an impression that the changing models and paradigm shifts in the country are having its impact only in the field of education, the ground realities are much more than that. It has influenced other domains of life like housing, economy, health, and social security.

With respect to the housing, contemporary laws, and rules, for example, ensures that extended residential or commercial layouts within the limits of the municipal corporation and/or urban developmental authorities earmark sites meant for community amenities are also distributed for benefit of persons with differential needs. The concept of community access has been adopted in a big way through a national program and 'Accessible India Campaign' (Singh, 2017; p. 56). Built environment access audits to ensure that public buildings and spaces are redesigned or built to render them barrier-free for all persons including those with communication disorders. Railway stations, airports, and bus stands are mandated to make a visual display of departure or arrivals for the benefit of deaf and hard of hearing in as many announcements are insisted for the visually challenged or ramps and railings are required for the locomotion affected. A National Building Code is in place as also Central Public Works Department Guidelines and Space Standards for barrier-free and accessibility are underlined in a recently published document by the Government of India (Ministry of Urban Development, 2016).

In the earlier charity based models, the persons with communication disorders were viewed as a burden and economic liability for the family, community as well as the nation. The changed rights-based perspectives view them as wastage or loss of opportunity and unused human capital including their work hours. Individualized, government supported or consumer self-initiated services and community-based programs are now converted as part of industry initiatives based on corporate social responsibility (Bhattacharya, 2016; p. 50). The rigorous implementation of rules and schemes that guarantee compulsory and minimum employment, the abolition of bonded child and adolescent labor, and vigilance activities against differential payment of wages are some examples of how persons with communication disorders as one of the most vulnerable sections are most liable to be affected. In the area of health, there are enactments that protect these persons from magico-religious treatments like branding, chaining, administration of electric shocks or incarceration, denial of medical treatments, and/or use of practices like hysterectomy. Additionally, there are special courts made available in every district to provide free legal aid, provide guardianship supports, informed self-decision making, guarantee property rights and inheritance, ensure citizenship and voting rights for these persons (Venkatesan, 2015c).

A critical dimension for the Indian sub-continent is the intimate linkage between poverty and disability in the country (Rao, 2009). Disability is explained both as a cause as well as consequence of poverty in the Indian scenario. The intersection of poverty and disability is a two-way process. Poor households without basic food, sanitation, and access to health care add to the burden of disability. The affected persons become viewed as liability thereby resulting in an increase of barriers, reduction of opportunities, exclusion, and marginalization. Their prospects of marriage are reduced and risks of abuse increase. The age-standardized disability prevalence calculated using 2011 census data found higher rates for women, rural dwellers, and members of scheduled castes and tribes (Saika, Bora, Jasilionis, and Shkolnikov, 2016).

Oncoming Trends in Gen-Next Parents and Children

The country is undergoing change following initiation of economic reforms after liberalization, privatization and globalization in a pre-millennium decade (Gupta, 2006). A whole new lot of Generation-Next people born between late 80's and mid 90's have become the youth in this post-millennium era. These young parents of the high tech age are assailed with a changed quality of life, over-optimistic outlooks, have a great many opportunities compared to their previous generation. Their technology has driven lifestyle, working hours and with changed views on finances. Their heroes and role models are different. Their personal concerns, habits, hobbies, tattoos, piercings and appearance, lack of social life, virtual worlds, religious beliefs, and practices are altered even as their views on cohabitation, homosexuality, marriage, divorce, and children are now different. Their outlook on childbirth, adoption, child-rearing and caring, and old age care is varying. In these circumstances, the psycho-social implications of such alterations vis-à-vis communication disorders are also likely to undergo impacts. Given below are few examples.

Affluenza, a term used by critics of consumerism, refer to a metaphorical psychological malaise owing to profoundly dysfunctional parenting supposedly affecting a social class of young wealthy people in a privileged lifestyle showing symptoms which include lack of motivation, feelings of guilt, and sense of isolation (Luthar, 2003). It refers to a new generation which has given them too much and never taught them the consequences of their actions (Oliver, 2007; Graaf, Wann and Naylor, 2005). Such parents offer 'no reasonable boundaries' and convey messages that people beneath them have no intrinsic worth or that money can compensate for everything including for advertently or inadvertently hurting people. The result is greater depression, anxiety, and substance abuse compared to their friends (Luthar and Latendresse, 2005). As applied to infants, toddlers, preschoolers and young children, the result in the pampered child syndrome. More specifically, materialistic conditions made available easily with money spoils the children (Labounty, 2009).

Pampering is the act of indulging or gratifying a desire by going out of the way in an excessive way that it ends up adversely affecting the shaping of the recipient's character, temperament or personality. In the name of 'love', to avoid inconvenience, or seeking to be 'perfect parent', some parents disallow the experience of the slightest struggle in their children. Such children tend to take in everything for granted, lives with loads of money from young age, has always someone paid to do things for him, tend to perceive those without money as inferior, will seek things at any cost without justifying its means, suffer loss of attention or interest in everything beyond a short time, behave stubborn, use expletives and disrespect elders (Bornstein, 2013).

Helicoptering is a form of pathological parenting pattern wherein extremely close attention is paid to their child's experiences and problems. They hover overhead to oversee every detail in their child's life. This distinct form of over-protective, over-bearing and over-controlling parenting seeks to ensure that the child is always on the right path to success on the way paved for them. A contrast is free-range parenting that allows children to function independently with little or no parental supervision.

Other new age terms are the latchkey kid who returns home from school to an empty home because both parents are away at work and the child is often left alone at home without supervision. Concerted cultivation refers to another tendency or style of parenting wherein the kids are perpetually kept engaged in organized activities, such as yoga, child clubs, gardening, pet care, music, soft skill acquisition, dance, drawing, karate, painting, religious practices, and so on. The parent, usually the mother, is full time engaged, busy or ever-burdened transporting the child from one destination to another. The hurried child cannot surely become an achieving child. Growing up fast does not mean going very far in life. The resulting stress may only snap the rubber band stretched beyond limits (Duffy, 2011). Narcissistic parenting involves the practice of some parents who live out their unfulfilled dreams or achievements through their children. They develop vicarious satisfaction with the small achievements of their child. Often, a generation lag in the mother may spur her to overstretch and learn all that is for the child to do so (Clinton and Sibcy, 2006). Parentification is a phenomenon wherein there is role reversal on the part of a child who is obliged to act as a parent to their own parent or their younger siblings. This happens more likely with siblings of children with special needs (Venkatesan and Ravindran, 2011; Chase, 1999; Cicirelli, 1976). Brexting involves the use of gadgets like I-pod, laptops, television, music, speaking on phone, reading or simply staring at a spot on the wall while feeding young children. This practice may be used as means to distract but it is a bad idea since it takes away needed eye contact or face to face conversation with the child. The 'centum' madness refers to the ongoing craze among some schools, teachers, parents, and pupils to score full marks in all subjects of high school and senior secondary examinations. Following the publication of results, every year, several names with their photographs and pass percentages are advertised in newspapers, public hoardings, and handbills across cities in the country. Schools and tutorials vie against one another to take credit for the achievement of the rank holder, while the candidate quietly retreats to boast about own hard work. Official records show high rates of suicide in this age group especially around the time the results are out. The period of preparation for examinations, attending multiple coaching centers for different subjects, taking several surprise class tests, mock exams or practice tutorials online or offline is all undertaken by these youngsters without food, sleep, and socialization. No wonder, students desperately seek ways out of the pressure cooker and dream of escaping into other easy ways through illness presentations including stress-induced communication disorders (Mary, Marslin, Franklin, and Sheeba, 2014; Deb, Chatterjee, and Walsh, 2010; Raakhee and Aparna, 2011).

CONCLUSION

In sum, this chapter sought to outline the history of rehabilitation of PWDs with reference to communication disorders. In doing so it has voyaged through early magical-religious conceptualizations in the Hindu context before explaining the biological-medical approaches doing rounds in a 19th and 20th century. The turn-of-millennium witnessed the contemporary rights-based paradigm wherein the person-in-environment conceptualization is emphasized. It is to be noted that the understanding of nature and characteristics, classification, etiology, treatment, social perception, and practices, including law-making about such affected persons have all along been growing in tandem with the temper of the times. This article has outlined the salient course of these changes with special reference to the Indian sub-continent. Illustrative domains of social change in the area of education are particularly highlighted. The end-note raises oncoming challenges, issues and problems related to communication disorders in the emergent dynamic socio-cultural matrix for generation next parents and children.

REFERENCES

Adelson, B. M. (2005). *Dwarfism: Medical and psychosocial aspects of profound short stature*. Baltimore, MD: The John Hopkins University Press.

Ahmed, R. (2015). *Rights of persons with disability in India*. Chandigarh, India: White Falcon Publishing Solutions.

Alur, M. (2002). 'They did not figure': Policy exclusion of disabled people in India. *International Journal of Inclusive Education*, *6*(2), 101–112. doi:10.1080/13603110110091625

American Psychiatric Association. (2013). *Diagnostic and Statistical Manual of Mental Disorders* (5th ed.). Arlington, VA: Author.

Anand, S. (2016). The models approach to disability scholarship: An assessment of its failings. In N. Ghosh (Ed.), *Interrogating disability in India: Theory and practice* (pp. 23–38). India: Springer. doi:10.1007/978-81-322-3595-8_2

Azad, Y. A. (1996). *Integration of disabled in common schools: A survey-study of IEDC in the country*. New Delhi: National Council of Educational Research and Training.

Balodhi, J. P., & Chowdhary, J. R. (1986). Psychiatric concepts in Atharva Veda: A review. *Indian Journal of Psychiatry*, *28*, 63–68.

Basham, A. L. (1924). *The wonder that was India*. London: Sidgwick and Jackson Press.

Batliwala, S. (2007). When rights go wrong. *Seminar*, *569*, 89–94.

Battaglia, M., Russo, E., Bolla, A., Chiusso, A., Bertelli, S., Pellegri, A., ... Martinuzzi, A. (2004). International Classification of Functioning, Disability, and Health in a cohort of children with cognitive, motor, and complex disabilities. *Developmental Medicine and Child Neurology*, *46*(2), 98–106. doi:10.1111/j.1469-8749.2004.tb00458.x PMID:14974634

Bhattacharya, S., Khanna, V., & Kohli, R. (2009). Cleft lip: The historical perspective. *Indian Journal of Plastic Surgery: Official Publication of the Association of Plastic Surgeons of India*, *42*(3Suppl), S4–S8. doi:10.4103/0970-0358.57180 PMID:19884680

Bhattacharya, T. (2016). Diversity at workplace and education. In N. Ghosh (Ed.), *Interrogating disability in India: Theory and practice* (pp. 39–64). New York: Springer. doi:10.1007/978-81-322-3595-8_3

Bhugra, D. (1992). Psychiatry in ancient Indian texts: A review. *History of Psychiatry*, *3*(10), 167–186. doi:10.1177/0957154X9200301002 PMID:11623029

Bornstein, M. H. (2013). Handbook of parenting (*5th vol.*). Mahwah, NJ: Lawrence Erlbaum Associates, Publishers.

Braddock, D. L., & Parish, S. L. (2001). An institutional history of disability. In Handbook of disability studies (pp. 11-68). Sage Publications. doi:10.4135/9781412976251.n2

Burnett, J. J., & Bender-Baker, H. (2001). Assessing the travel-related barriers of the mobility-disabled consumer. *Journal of Travel Research*, *40*(1), 4–11. doi:10.1177/004728750104000102

Chase, N. D. (Ed.). (1999). *Burdened children: Theory, research, and treatment of Parentification*. New York: Sage Publications.

Cicirelli, V. G. (1976). Siblings teach siblings. In V. L. Allen (Ed.), *Children as teachers: Theory and research in tutoring*. New York: Academic Press. doi:10.1016/B978-0-12-052640-6.50013-3

Clarkson, S., & Clarkson, N. (2016). *Different: The story of an outside the box kid and the mom who loved him*. Tyndale House Publishers.

Clinton, T., & Sibcy, G. (2006). *Loving your child too much: Raise your kids without overindulging, overprotecting or over controlling*. Nashville, TN: Thomas Nelson.

Cornelissen, R. M. M., Misra, G., & Varma, S. (2014). *Foundations and applications of Indian psychology*. Delhi: Pearson.

Cottrell, S. (2015). *Skills for success: Personal development and employability*. New York, NY: Macmillan Education, Palgrave. doi:10.1007/978-1-137-42653-6

Crutchfield, R., & Wang, X. (2016). The perceptions of stereotypes of people who stutter in Hispanic university students. *Clinical Archives of Communication Disorders*, *1*(1), 36–4. doi:10.21849/cacd.2016.00045

Danermark, B., Cieza, A., Gimigliano, F., Granberg, S., Hickson, L., Kramer, S. E., ... Stucki, G. (2010). International classification of functioning, disability, and health core sets for hearing loss: A discussion paper and invitation. *International Journal of Audiology*, *49*(4), 256–262. doi:10.3109/14992020903410110 PMID:20170312

de Schipper, E., Lundequist, A., Coghill, D., de Vries, P. J., Granlund, M., Holtmann, M., ... Singhal, N. (2015). Ability and disability in autism spectrum disorder: A systematic literature review employing the international classification of functioning, disability and health-children and youth version. *Autism Research*, *8*(6), 782–794. doi:10.1002/aur.1485 PMID:25820780

Deb, S., Chatterjee, P., & Walsh, K. (2010). Anxiety among high school students in India: Comparisons across gender, school type, social strata and perceptions of quality time with parents. *Australian Journal of Educational and Developmental Psychology*, *10*, 18–31.

Debsikdar, B. M. (1961). Glimpses of medico-psychological practices in ancient India. *Indian Journal of Psychiatry*, *3*, 250–259.

Dixit, V. (1998). Historical foundations of disability discrimination in classical Hindu Law. *Delhi Law Review*, *12*, 15–16.

Dube, K. C. (1978). Nosology and therapy of mental illness in Ayurveda. *The American Journal of Chinese Medicine: An International Journal of Comparative Medicine East and West*, *6*(3), 209–228. doi:10.1142/S0147291778000289 PMID:383394

Duffy, J. (2011). *The available parent: Expert advice for raising successful, resilient and teens and tweens*. Berkeley, CA: Cleis Press.

Dutt, R. C. (1972). *A history of civilization in ancient India*. New Delhi: Vistar Publishers.

Fleischer, D. Z., & Frieda, Z. (2001). *The disability rights movement: From charity to confrontation*. Philadelphia: Temple University Press.

Fougeyrollas, P., & Beauregard, L. (2001). Disability: An interactive person-environment social creation. In *Handbook of disability studies* (pp. 171-194). Sage Publications.

Friedner, M., & Osborne, J. (2013). Audit bodies: Embodied participation, disability universalism, and accessibility in India. *Antipode*, *45*(1), 43–60. doi:10.1111/j.1467-8330.2012.00990.x

Friedner, M., & Osborne, J. (2015). New disability mobilities and accessibilities in urban India. *City & Society*, *27*(1), 9–29. doi:10.1111/ciso.12054

Goswami, S. P., Venkatesan, S., & Mathew, S. (2015). Disability certification: Issues and concerns. *Journal of All India Institute of Speech and Hearing*, *34*, 1–7.

Graaf, J., Wann, D., & Naylor, T. (2005). *Affluenza: The all-consuming epidemic*. San Francisco: Beret-Koehler Publishers.

Green, S., Davis, C., Karshmer, E., Marsh, P., & Straight, B. (2005). Living stigma: The impact of labeling, stereotyping, separation, status loss, and discrimination in the lives of individuals with disabilities and their families. *Sociological Inquiry*, *75*(2), 197–215. doi:10.1111/j.1475-682X.2005.00119.x

Gupta, K. R. (2006). *Liberalization and globalization of Indian economy* (Vols. 1-2). New Delhi: Atlantic Publishers.

Gupta, S. P. (1977). *Psychotherapy in Indian medicine: With special reference to its philosophical basis*. Bhopal, India: Ajaya Publishers.

Hulit, L. M. (2004). *Straight talk on stuttering: information, encouragement, and counsel for stutterers, caregivers, and speech-language clinicians*. Springfield, IL: Charles C. Thomas Publishers.

Jones, G. C., Crews, J. E., & Danielson, M. L. (2010). Health risk profile for older adults with blindness: An application of the International Classification of Functioning, Disability, and Health framework. *Ophthalmic Epidemiology*, *17*(6), 400–410. doi:10.3109/09286586.2010.528137 PMID:21090913

Jones, R. B. (2001). Impairment, disability, and handicap: Old-fashioned concepts? *Journal of Medical Ethics*, *37*(6), 377–379. doi:10.1136/jme.27.6.377 PMID:11731599

Kadir, S. A., & Jamaluddin, M. (2012). User's satisfaction and perception of the accessibility of public buildings in Putrajaya: Access audit study. *Procedia: Social and Behavioral Sciences*, *50*, 429–441. doi:10.1016/j.sbspro.2012.08.047

Kennedy, D. (2004). *The dark sides of virtue: Reassessing international humanitarianism*. Princeton, NJ: Princeton University Press. doi:10.1515/9781400840731

Klassen, T. R. (2001). Perceptions of people who stutter: Re-assessing the negative stereotype. *Perceptual and Motor Skills*, *92*(2), 551–559. doi:10.2466/pms.2001.92.2.551 PMID:11361320

Koretsky, J. (2007). *The odd one out the Maverick's guide to adult ADD; How to be happy and different*. Plattekill, NY: Vervante.

Labounty, D. (2009). *Affluenza*. Denver, CO: Silver Thought Press.

Luthar, S. S. (2003). The culture of affluence: Psychological costs of material wealth. *Child Development*, *74*(6), 1581–1593. doi:10.1046/j.1467-8624.2003.00625.x PMID:14669883

Luthar, S. S., & Latendresse, S. J. (2005). Children of the Affluent. *Current Directions in Psychological Science*, *14*(1), 49–53. doi:10.1111/j.0963-7214.2005.00333.x PMID:17710193

Manickam, L. S. S. (2010). Psychotherapy in India. *Indian Journal of Psychiatry, 52*(S), S366-S370. doi: 10.4103/0019-5545.69270

Mary, R. A., Marslin, G., Franklin, G., & Sheeba, C. J. (2014). Test anxiety levels of board exam going students in Tamil Nadu. India. *BioMed Research International*, *21*, 1–9. doi:10.1155/2014/578323 PMID:25143938

Miller, F. P., Vandome, A. F., & McBrewster, J. (2010). *The medical model of disability*. VDM Publishing.

Ministry of Urban Development. (2016). *Central public works department guidelines and space standards for barrier-free and accessibility*. New Delhi: Ministry of Urban Development, Government of India.

Misra, G., & Paranjpe, E. A. C. (2012). Psychology in modern India. In *Encyclopedia of the history of psychological theories* (pp. 881–892). New York: Springer.

Narayan, C. L., & John, T. (2017). The Rights of Persons with Disabilities Act, 2016: Does it address the needs of the persons with mental illness and their families. *Indian Journal of Psychiatry*, *59*(1), 17–20. doi:10.4103/psychiatry.IndianJPsychiatry_75_17 PMID:28529356

Nario-Redmond, M. R. (2010). Cultural stereotypes of disabled and non-disabled men and women: Consensus for global category representations and diagnostic domains. *British Journal of Social Psychology*, *49*(3), 471–488. doi:10.1348/014466609X468411 PMID:19793408

Neki, J. S. (1975). Psychotherapy in India: Past, present, and future. *American Journal of Psychotherapy*, *29*(1), 92–100. PMID:1096647

Ngugi, T. O. (1993). *Moving the center: The struggle for cultural freedoms*. Oxford, UK: James Curry Limited.

Oliver, J. (2007). *Affluenza: How to be successful and stay sane*. London: Vermilion, Ebury Publishing.

Orgogozo, J. M. (1994). The concepts of impairment, disability, and handicap. *Cerebrovascular Diseases (Basel, Switzerland)*, *4*(2), 2–6. doi:10.1159/000108531

Ormerod, M. (2005). Understanding access audits and appraisals: An inclusive design approach. *Journal of Building Appraisal*, *1*(2), 140–152. doi:10.1057/palgrave.jba.2940013

Raakhee, A. S., & Aparna, N. (2011). A study on the prevalence of anxiety disorders among higher secondary students. *Education Science and Psychology*, *1*, 33–37.

Rao, A. N. (2009). Poverty and disability in India. *Social Change*, *39*(1), 29–45. doi:10.1177/004908570903900102

Rao, K. (2010). Psychological interventions: From theory to practice. In G. Mishra (Ed.), *Psychology in India: Clinical and Health Psychology* (Vol. 3, pp. 317–360). New Delhi: Indian Council of Social Science Research/Dorling Kindersley.

Rentschler, G. J. (2012). *Here's how to do stuttering therapy*. San Diego, CA: Plural Publishing.

Riva, S., & Antonietti, A. (2010). The application of the ICF-CY model in specific learning difficulties: A case study. *Psychology of Language and Communication*, *14*(2), 37–58. doi:10.2478/v10057-010-0009-2

Saika, N., Bora, J. K., Jasilionis, D., & Shkolnikov, V. M. (2016). Disability divides India: Evidence from the 2011 census. *PLoS One*, *11*(8), E0159809. doi:10.1371/journal.pone.0159809 PMID:27490469

Shakespeare, T. (2006). *Disability rights and wrongs*. London: Routledge.

Shakespeare, T. (2013). *Disability rights and wrongs revisited*. London: Routledge.

Sharma, R., Kumar, M., & Singh, A. (2013). Evaluation of disable friendliness of a railway transport facility in Ludhiana city of Punjab, India. *International Journal on Disability and Human Development: IJDHD*, *12*(3), 333–339. doi:10.1515/ijdhd-2012-0117

Silvers, A. (2010). An essay on modeling: Their social model of disability. In D. C. Ralston & H. O. Justin (Eds.), *Philosophical reflections on disability* (pp. 19–36). London: Springer.

Simeonsson, R. J., Leornardi, M., Lollar, D., Bjorck-Akesson, E., Hollenwerger, J., & Martinuzzi, A. (2003). Applying the International Classification of Functioning, Disability, and Health (ICF) to measure childhood disability. *Disability and Rehabilitation*, *25*(11-12), 602–610. doi:10.1080/0963828031000137117 PMID:12959334

Simmons, R. (2002). *Odd girl out: The hidden culture of aggression in girls*. Boston: Mariner Books Houghton Mifflin Harcourt.

Singh, H. G. (1977). *Psychotherapy in India: From Vedic to modern times*. Agra: National Psychological Corporation.

Singh, S. (2017). Perseverance pays. In S. Halder & L. C. Assaf (Eds.), *Inclusion, disability, and culture: An ethnographic perspective traversing abilities and challenges* (pp. 41–59). New York: Springer International Publishing. doi:10.1007/978-3-319-55224-8_4

Stamos, D. N. (2013). *The myth of universal human rights: Its origin, history, and explanation, along with a more humane way*. New York: Routledge.

Stroman, D. (2003). *The disability rights movement: From deinstitutionalization to self-determination*. University Press of America.

Vahia, N. S. (1969). A therapy based on some concepts prevalent in India. *Indian Journal of Psychiatry*, *11*, 7–14.

Veereshwar, P. (2002). *Indian systems of psychotherapy*. New Delhi: Kalpaz Publications.

Venkatesan, S. (2004). *Children with Developmental Disabilities: A Training Guide for Parents, Teachers and Caregivers*. New Delhi: Sage Publications.

Venkatesan, S. (2010). Cultural factors in clinical assessment: The Indian perspective. *Indian Journal of Clinical Psychology*, *37*(1), 75–85.

Venkatesan, S. (2015a). Socio-Cultural dimensions of cleft lip and palate in India. *Global Journal of Interdisciplinary Social Sciences*, *4*(3), 72–77.

Venkatesan, S. (2015b). Evaluation of teaching objectives earmarked for children with developmental disabilities. *Disabilities and Impairments*, *29*(2), 85–95.

Venkatesan, S. (2015c). Engagement between justice system vis-à-vis persons with intellectual and developmental disabilities. *International Journal of Psychology and Psychiatry*, *3*(1), 30–56. doi:10.5958/2320-6233.2015.00003.6

Venkatesan, S. (2016a). Themes of intrapsychic conflict in communication disorders having a psychogenic origin. *Global Journal of Interdisciplinary Social Sciences*, *5*(2), 20–26.

Venkatesan, S. (2016b). Some cultural aspects of clinical counseling in Indian Context. *Global Journal of Interdisciplinary Social Sciences*, *5*(6), 21–26.

Venkatesan, S., Jayakaran, G. T., Purusotham, P., & Rafi, M. (2012). Disability access audit of public service facilities. *Journal of All India Institute of Speech and Hearing*, *31*, 190–201.

Venkatesan, S., & Ravindran, N. (2011). Attitudes of well siblings of children with developmental disabilities. *Journal of Disability Management and Special Education, 1*(2), 1–23.

Weatherley-White, R. C. A., Eiserman, W., Beddoe, M., & Vanderberg, R. (2005). Perceptions, expectations, and reactions to cleft lip and palate surgeries in native populations: A pilot study in rural India. *The Cleft Palate-Craniofacial Journal, 42*(5), 550–564. doi:10.1597/04-003.1 PMID:16149840

World Health Organization. (2007). *International Classification of Functioning, Disability, and Health: Children and Youth Version*. Geneva: World Health Organization.

World Health Organization. (2008). *The ICD-10 classification of mental and behavioral disorders descriptions and diagnostic guidelines*. Geneva: World Health Organization.

KEY TERMS AND DEFINITIONS

Access: The term refers to the ways in which institutions strive to ensure everyone has equitable opportunities to take full advantage for participation in the society.

Affluenza: A metaphorical psychological malaise owing to profoundly dysfunctional parenting and supposedly affecting a social class of young wealthy people in a privileged lifestyle showing symptoms which include lack of motivation, feelings of guilt, and sense of isolation.

Exclusion: Also called segregation or exclusion, it involves the practice of forcing children with special needs to lead a separate life outside the ambit or purview of regular or mainstream society and settings.

Gen-Next Parents: Demography identifies people by the generation of their birth. Those born in 1910-1920 are designated as born during "the depression era," just as those born during or after the World War II or later. Those born between the 1950s and 1960s belong to the era of baby boomers. The ones from the 1970s are called Generation X. The turn of the century saw the birth of Millennial or Generation Y. The post-millennium births are viewed as Generation Z, who is the gadget-driven youth of the day.

Inclusion: An all-embracing ideology and practice that seeks to provide equal opportunities for full participation of children with different needs by removal of barriers and discrimination.

Integration: The placement of students with special education needs in a regular or mainstream classroom or school settings on the condition that they can fit into the pre-existing structures, attitudes, and an unaltered environment.

Magical-Religious Model: A layperson's viewpoint of disability as the outcome of one's wrong doings in the present or past birth resulting in incurring the wrath of supernatural forces leading to punishments as the currently acquired unfortunate condition.

Medical Model: Arising from the biomedical perception of disability, this model believes in identifying or listing symptoms, categorizing them, making a diagnosis, before seeking to cure them.

Parentification: A phenomenon wherein there is role reversal on the part of a child who is obliged to act as a parent to their own parent or their younger siblings.

Resource Teacher: A specialist who provides instructional planning and support services to students who have different needs within the regular classroom or school settings.

Rights-Based Social Model: Unlike the medical model which views the individual as victim and the core of the problem, the social model views barriers as the source of problems for persons with disabilities.

Chapter 16
Vocational Rehabilitation of Persons With Hearing Impairment:
A Step Towards Inclusive Development

S. Z. H. Zaidi
Amity University – Lucknow, India

Divya Baveja
Amity University – Lucknow, India

ABSTRACT

This chapter focuses on the importance of vocational rehabilitation of persons with hearing impairment to attain the goal of inclusive development and rights of equal opportunities and participation. It deals with the definition of hearing impairment, in terms of ILO and prevailing legislations, the process of vocational rehabilitation, and importance of follow up. The chapter gives special emphasis to different approaches of evaluations of residual capacities, skill training models, and status of employment market along with the scope of entrepreneurial development. It also deals with various issues and challenges in the process of vocational rehabilitation of persons with hearing impairment.

INTRODUCTION

Ears are delicate and have complex mechanisms for many functions and not for just hearing per se. A well-functioning ear can make you hear very soft sounds over a wide range of frequency as well as withstand very loud sounds. It can also discriminate between sounds of varying pitch and intensity and locate the source of a sound. Various reasons of damage to ear like disease process, any physical trauma, exposure to excessive noise, drugs or simply the process of aging, may result in malfunction. This further may result in varying degrees of deafness which is also known as 'Hearing Impairment'.

Hearing impairment may be understood as a partial or complete inability to hear from one or both ears at a desired or even enhanced frequency. It may be congenital or acquired, and temporary or permanent. Hearing impairment is one of the most frequently experienced sensory deficits in the human

DOI: 10.4018/978-1-5225-4955-0.ch016

population, and it affects more than 250 million people worldwide. Its consequences could be reduced capacity to understand speech sounds, communicate, and delay in language development, educational and economic backwardness, social isolation and stigmatization (Singh, 2015). The various types of hearing impairment are described in Table 1(Nagaraja, 2002).

All previous legislation that were enforced to protect the rights of the disabled have included certain disabilities under them. The International Labour Organization defined a disabled person as 'an individual whose prospects of securing, retaining and advancing in suitable employment are substantially reduced as a result of a duly recognized physical, sensory, intellectual or mental impairment' (ILO, 1983).The Persons With Disability (Equal Opportunities, Protection of Rights, and Full Participation) Act, 1995 covered 7 such specific disabilities viz. Blindness, Low Vision, Hearing Impairment, Mental Retardation, Mental Illness, Leprosy-cured and Locomotor disability. Hearing impairment has been defined in the 1995 Acts 'loss of 60dB or more in the better ear for conversational range of frequencies' (The Persons With Disability Equal Opportunities, Protection of Rights, and Full Participations Act, 1995). However, this Act has been revised and replaced by Rights of Persons with Disability Act, 2016. This new Act of 2016 includes 21 conditions under 'Disability' including the 7 conditions that were covered by earlier Persons with Disability Act 1995. Further, the new Act has also expanded the definition of hearing impairment by including both 'deaf' and 'hard of hearing' persons. As such, hearing impairment has been defined as follows:

A - 'Deaf' means persons having 70 dB hearing loss in speech frequencies in both ears, and

B – 'Hard of hearing' means persons having 60 dB to 70 dB hearing loss in speech frequencies. (Rights of Persons with Disabilities Act (2016)

PREVALENCE OF HEARING IMPAIRMENT

Census of India 2011, reported that out of the population of 1,210 million, about 26.8 million persons are 'disabled' which is 2.21% of the total population (Statistical Profile of Disabled Persons in India, 2016). Figure 1 presents the statistics related to the persons with disability. As one can see, hearing impairment accounts for 19% of the disabled population and is the second biggest type of disability.

Table 1. Description of hearing impairment

Degree in *dB	Types of Loss	Onset	Course of Nature
Normal 0-25	Conductive Hearing Loss	Pre-lingual Congenital or before 4-4.5 years	Gradual
Mild 26-40	Mixed Hearing Loss	During development of language	Sudden
Moderate 41-55	Sensorineural Hearing Loss	Post-lingual and after development of language	Fluctuating
Moderately Severe 70-90	Retro Cochlear		Progressive
Severe 71-90	Central deafness	During Adulthood or old age	
Profound 91 +			

*dB-Decibel

Figure 1. Distribution of various disabilities

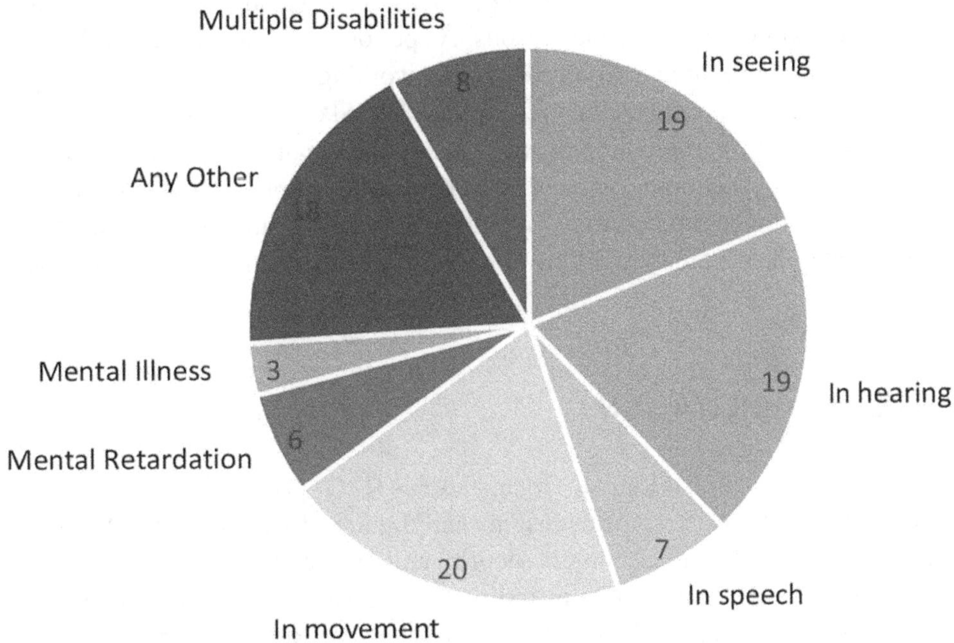

Table 2 presents an overview of the number of persons with disabilities in India, as per the Census 2011 data. Further analysis of the Census Report revealed that though there has been an appreciable improvement in the literacy rate of the general population of India, yet the literacy rate of persons with disability is still considerably low in comparison to the general population which further imposes limitations in their empowerment.

Table 2. Disabled persons in India, census 2011

	Persons	Males	Females
Number (In crores)	2.68	1.5	1.18
Percentage (out of Total Population)	2.21%	1.24%	0.97%

Data from Statistical Profile of Disabled Persons in India, 2016.

Table 3. Literacy status of disabled population in comparison to general population

	Literate		Illiterate		
	General Population	Disabled	General Population	Disabled	
Total Persons	74.04%	55%	25.96%	45%	
Males	Over 80%	62%	Less than 20%	38%	
Females	65.46%	45%	35.54%	55%	

Data from Statistical Profile of Disabled Persons in India, 2016 and Population of India Census 2011

Table 3 presents the data on the literacy status of the disabled population as compared to the general population of India. The poor literacy rate among persons with disabilities is resulting in their limited participation in the workforce as one of the reasons. As per one estimate, about 3 million persons with disabilities belonging to working age are currently not working on regular basis. Analysis of reports available on employment status of persons with disabilities (Statistical Profile of Disabled Persons in India, 2016) revealed that the participation of such group in the main workforce is marginal for various reasons including lack of opportunities, lack of basic education, employable skills and the prejudice attached to their employability and productivity resulting in non-utilization of huge workforce who have full potential to be integrated in main working stream provided suitable training and opportunities are extended.

VOCATIONAL REHABILITATION

Decent work is one of International Labour Organization's (ILO) primary goal for everyone, including Persons with Disabilities. When we promote rights and dignity of Persons with Disability we are empowering individuals, strengthening economic security and in reaching society at large (Shenoy, 2011). Vocational rehabilitation is defined as enabling individuals with either temporary or permanent disability to access, return to, or remain in, employment (British Society of Rehabilitation Medicine, 2000). This definition echoes the one proposed by the ILO which is "Vocational Rehabilitation is a process to enable a disabled person to secure and retain suitable employment" (International Labour Organization, 1998). It is to be understood as a step in the continuous efforts towards the social rehabilitation of any disabled individual, where the aim may be to minimize the functional and psychological, socio-cultural or financial consequences of the disability.

In principle, as explained by ILO (2004), it should cover all services and efforts that contribute in ensuring equality of opportunity in work for people with disabilities and in leading to their integration or reintegration, whichever applicable, to society. It may include vocational guidance, career counselling, vocational training, placement and ergonomic modifications of select jobs to make them disabled-friendly and need-based psychosocial interventions.

The goal of vocational rehabilitation is fostering self-reliance, independence and feelings of self-worth. When given appropriate opportunities, individuals with hearing impairment can become economically productive and contributing citizens of the country. In the time when 'inclusive development' is being emphasized as the right way toward sustainable development, focused efforts for the empowerment of the disabled are essential. The inclusive development consists of ensuring that all marginalized and excluded groups are stakeholders in development processes design, implementation, monitoring and evaluation. It strives to ensure that all sections of the society, including the disabled are valued equally as rights-holding citizens and contribute to the country's developmental issues and strategies. It is based on three principles: accessibility, participation and non-discrimination (International Disability and Development Consortium, 2005).

Economically speaking, nations are battling the global economic crisis, unsteady unemployment trends and inequality. In making efforts for economic growth, it has to be ensured that benefits reach everyone. The inclusive development also focuses on making more comprehensive strategies which will reduce inequality and include diversity.

MODELS FOR REHABILITATION OF INDIVIDUALS WITH HEARING IMPAIRMENT

Disability and Rehabilitation can be explained using various perspectives and models. Few of them are briefly discussed.

Religious-Moral-Spiritual Model/Conventional Model

- It understands disability as a punishment received by an individual or his family by some external force due to any wrong deeds done by the disabled person or someone else in the family in current life or in a previous reincarnation.
- Sometimes it is also attributed to evil spirits for which exorcism or faith healing may be tried, thus putting the disabled in danger and further isolation.
- Rehabilitation efforts are thus done by undoing the so-called sins, pleasing supernatural power, charity in conformity to religious faith or otherwise.

All such efforts have been done to either please supernatural powers or to show sympathy and humility towards persons inflicted with disabilities and not because the disabled is taken as an equal partner of the society. Additionally, the people who help or give charity act as 'pitiful' donors and expect gratitude from the disabled person.

Medical Model

- May also be referred to as the Biological-Inferiority or Functional-Limitation Model.
- Views that disability is a result of the disabled person's physical and/or mental limitations, being largely unrelated to one's social or geographical environment.
- It places the source of the problem within the impaired person and suggests that solutions may be found by treating the physical limitations through medicines, surgical procedures, and fitment of aids and appliances.
- In rehabilitation efforts, the focus is on finding the 'cure' for the disability, and when that inevitably fails, then providing 'care' for the 'incurable' disabled person, consequently, justifying institutionalization and/or segregation.

Psychosocial Model

- It understands disability as a consequence of any environmental, social or attitudinal barriers that may prevent people with impairments from participating maximally in society, therefore removing these is posited to improve the lives of disabled people.
- It seeks solutions outside the disabled person, in his environment.
- Focus on 'equity' rather than on 'equality'.
- It changed the way in which disability was attributed, and has had a huge influence on rehabilitation efforts in terms of anti-discriminatory legislation.

- Rehabilitation efforts are also aimed at changing the psychosocial environment of the disabled person so as to reduce or overcome the barriers in the society. If the problem lies within the environment, then the environment must be changed to cause a solution. For example, if a wheelchair user cannot board a bus limiting his functioning, the bus may be modified to include ramps; or if a hearing impaired cannot hear announcements, the infrastructure may be modified to include important announcements visually on screens.

Economic Model

- It narrows the complex issue of disability to the limitations and restrictions a disabled person can be expected to have, with inferences drawn as to whether and till what extent "flawed" people may be productive.
- Disability is defined by the disabled person's inability to participate in work, with further assessment of the degree to which this impairment may affect an individual's productivity and consequently the economic burden or impact on the individual, his employer and the state. This view may further reinforce the prejudiced beliefs of employers that disabled persons are less productive than their counterparts.
- Policymakers, from this view, assess the distribution of benefits to those who are disabled and hence are unable to participate in work 'fully'.
- Employers may employ less productive disabled persons to enjoy benefits of an image of an organization with community values, for economic reasons and not because of recognition of their rights. Also, they may pay disabled people less.

APPROACH TO VOCATIONAL REHABILITATION WITH PERSONS WITH HEARING IMPAIRMENT

Vocational rehabilitation is based on the multi-disciplinary support consisting of experts from different fields of specialities like neurologists, ENT surgeon, clinical psychologist, speech pathologist, audiologist, special educator, special vocational instructor, communication instructor, placement counsellor, and employment provider. It aims at finding a suitable income generating activity in which person can be suitably inducted and flourish. It is a process involving following steps:

1. Assessment
2. Fitment of assistive devices
3. Communication training
4. Career counseling
5. Skill Training
6. Job placement
7. Follow up

Assessment

Assessment is a process of evaluating the residual capacities of an individual with the objective of unfolding his assets and extent of limitations. It has to be done by an interdisciplinary team mentioned above. A medical specialist evaluates possibilities of organic involvement, the location and extent of the damage, possibilities of correction, and introduction of intervention to arrest any further impairment. He/she may also advise the various work situations which may or may not be convenient and suitable for persons with hearing impairment. The clinical psychologist conducts the detailed assessment to evaluate the mental processes, developmental status, intellectual level, personality correlates, attitude, adaptability etc and prepare a psychological profile. The profile prepared by the clinical psychologist becomes the basic guidelines for providing vocational guidance and counselling in later stages. It also helps in selection of suitable careers and support in enhancing adjustment process in workplace and attitude towards employment, employer, and colleagues etc.

Some popular psychological tests used by Clinical Psychologist are given below:

1. Leiter International Performance Scales or LIPS (Roid & Miller, 1997)
2. Wechsler Intelligence Scales for Children or WISC (Wechsler, 1991)
3. Wechsler Individual Achievement Tests or WIAT (Wechsler, 1992)
4. Universal Nonverbal Intelligence Test or UNIT (Bracken & McCallum, 1998)
5. Vineland Adaptive Behavior Scales (Sparrow, 2011)
6. Carolina Picture Vocabulary Test for Deaf and Hearing Impaired Children (CPVT; Layton & Homes, 1985)
7. Bender Visual Motor Gestalt Test, Second Edition (Bender Gestalt II; Dumond & Willis, 2008)
8. The Halstead-Reitan Battery - performance type tests, (e.g., trails, categories, grip strength) (Reitan & Wolfson, 1985)
9. Draw A Person Test (DAPT; Short, DeOrnellas, & Walrath, 2011)
10. House Tree Person Test (HTP; Buck, 1971)
11. Reynolds Adolescent Adjustment Screening Inventory: RAASI (Reynolds, 2001)
12. Meadow-Kendall Social-Emotional Assessment Inventory for Deaf & Hearing Impaired Students (Meadow, 1980)

In addition to the above, there are many rating scales based on observational techniques for evaluating the mental status, emotional reactions, and adjustment processes. Some of the above-reported tests are having separate norms and specific guidelines for administration on hearing impaired population. Although some of them may not have Indian norms specifically yet they can be used in day to day rehabilitation practice as they are not used to diagnose any specific condition but to assess psychological variables and for profiling their assets, liabilities and residual capacities to arrange their skill training and job placement.

Audiologist assesses the extent of hearing loss and level of Disability. Audiologist's role is also in assisting the ENT Surgeon in exploring the possibilities of the fitment of hearing aids and the possibilities of major surgical intervention. The speech pathologist is a specialist who provides Speech therapy to enhance language development, vocabulary, and verbal expression/communication. Sign language instructor may also be associated here, in planning the speech training with special reference to developing the functional conversational skills required for acquiring a vocational skill and discharging the duties at the workplace.

Assessment to unfold the suitability of the hearing impaired person for induction informal/non-formal education program leading to different certifications is conducted by the special educator. A specific educational need of the individual to facilitate the development of lesson plan, study material, teaching aids, periodical assessment procedure, individualized examination pattern to assure acquiring of functional literacy and preparedness for induction in formal education imparting recognized courses are evaluated.

The special vocational instructor is responsible for evaluating the trainability of the individual for any specific vocation. Special vocational instructor under the guidance of clinical psychologist observes the person with hearing impairment in the real job setting. A series of job samples consisting of operations required in performing a particular job is given to the individual and the performance on these job samples are rated through different rating scales. The vocational instructor also assesses the work traits on the basis of behavior shown by the individual on workstation. Some of the important work traits are endurance, comprehension, safety consciousness, adaptability, fatigue, stress tolerance, resistance, adjustment with colleagues, work environment, regularity, punctuality etc. The profiles prepared by the vocational instructor are used in the selection of a suitable skill set and placement area for the individual.

Fitment of Assistive Devices

Success in vocational rehabilitation requires effective communication skills on the continuous basis. Hearing aids which have been traditionally used since many years have undergone tremendous improvement and upgradation. Based on the recommendation of ENT surgeon and audiologist, the individual being prepared for vocational rehabilitation is provided with suitable hearing aids properly adjusted with frequencies recommended by the experts. They are also trained to adjust with hearing aids and go for periodical maintenance/repair of their device depending upon the financial background and availability of funds. Hearing aids are also provided to individuals under various government schemes either free of cost, or with subsidized rates.

Communication Training

Communication is usually considered to a mean of conveying the message and feelings through words. Words play a very limited role in communicating the message of various types provided the sender is suitably trained and the receiver is suitably sensitized. In the process of communication training, the trainer may use sign language, lips reading or combination of both. However, he would also train his client on job-specific communication skills like sign for tools, sign required for receptionist, signs required for sales and marketing, and for many such job profile/requirements.

Career Guidance and Counselling

Career guidance and counseling is a very important component of vocational rehabilitation where a career counselor tries to match the job profile and profile of the individual and help the client in choosing a career best suited to him. In case of persons with hearing impairment, career guidance and counselling is still more important to prevent the individual from sticking up to the point of no return in the course of his career advancement. In Indian scenario, having limited opportunities the role of career guidance and counselling is not only to provide the information about the jobs available but also to collect the employment market information, explore the future market scenario, conduct job identification studies in the area in which persons with hearing impairment can be trained and placed. Such studies are needed to be based on local employment market from which the persons with hearing impairment belong to and not on the hypothetical basis for the jobs which may not be existing in the area of their normal residency. Beside the career-related information, the career counselor should also be well versed in communication skills to minimize the communication gaps between the client and the information.

Skill Training

Skill training refers to the organized and systematic efforts to train a person suitably so that he may develop ability required for performing a job, operation and earn his livelihood. Skill training also involves the adaptation with different work environments to meet out the vocational challenges. It could be arranged in formal mode by admitting the persons in an institute of different levels depending upon his educational background, the severity of communication problem, aptitude and other psychological parameters, or in non-formal mode, where the training is arranged as per the individual need and his psychosocial profile. All the formal training institutes starting from Industrial training Institute (ITI), Polytechnic to upgraded professional institutes like College of Engineering, Indian Institute of Technology (IIT), National Institute etc. and governed by government have certain seats reserved for persons with hearing impairment provided the applicant is otherwise eligible for admission and has functional conversational ability and could qualify the entrance examination/assessment test. However, in spite of having the reservation of seats and other support systems, the representation of persons with hearing impairment in formal training institutes based on inclusive education and training system has been extremely marginal, mainly because by and large, they do not possess the basic educational qualification required for the higher level of vocational training. Hence, the only alternative left out for the majority of persons with hearing impairment is undergoing non-formal training in places like Vocational Rehabilitation Centres (VRC), other training centres, Vocational Training centres (VTC) run by different Non-Governmental Organizations(NGOs) and apprenticeship training in different workshops. The main principle of arranging such non-formal training is modular-based practical oriented training having minimum involvement of language, and verbal inputs. However, the certificate granted by NGOs and other organizations for non-formal training may endorse the level of skill attained but lack the approval of any regulatory authority.

In order to ease the above limitation, the government of India has launched short-term training programs with the name of Modular Employable Skill Scheme (MES) (Ministry of Labour and Employment, 2008) which has now been transferred to state government. MES is based on short-term operational based training in different vocational skills required in the employment market. The theoretical component of the training is 10% while 90% is practical and workshop training. It is a tri-partite program involving recognized training institutes who would be organizing the day to day training activities, employers who would be appraising the organization with changing employment market and the need for their industry. Employers would also support in skill mapping and in conducting the skill test on completion of training, and regulatory council like National Council of Vocational Training (NCVT)/State Council of Vocational Training (SCVT) will award the certificates to successful candidates. The most popular and employable skill sets for persons with hearing impairment include data entry operator, networking and hardware professionals, fashion technology, fine arts, photography, ceramics related activities, assembly line activities, food craft, printing technology, architectural draftsmanship, horticulture and gardening, interior decoration, and furniture making etc. The above list is only illustrative and not exhaustive. The success of individuals in attaining the skills directly depends upon motivational level, aptitude, family support, and infrastructure facilities (modified workstations and tools) and sensitivity and training of instructional staff. Recently, Planning Commission has identified 20 high growth sectors where the requirement of skilled workforce would be in plenty during years to come and wherein Persons with different physical limitations including hearing impairment can also be trained.

The priority list of 20 high growth sectors is as per following:

1. Automobile and Auto Components
2. Banking/Insurance and Finance services
3. Building and construction industries
4. Chemical and Pharmaceuticals
5. Leather and leather goods
6. Retails
7. Educational and Skill Development Services
8. Electronics and Hardware
9. Food Processing
10. Furniture and Furnishing
11. Gems and Jewellery
12. Healthcare
13. Handloom and Handicraft
14. Business Process Outsourcing
15. Software Service/Hardware Assembly
16. Real Estate
17. Textile/Garments
18. Tourism Hospitality and Travel
19. Transportation and Logistic
20. Packing (Planning Commission of India's report on 12th Five-year plan, 2013)

Job Placement

Placement can be defined as an activity which not only supports the individual in finding an income generating engagement but also sustaining in it and progressing in future. Placement for persons with disabilities has always been a great challenge and a rewarding experience too. Because of change of disability models, the placement scenario has also undergone the drastic change. The concepts like sheltered employment, protected employment or welfare factory etc. have been redefined mainly because of the growing concern about the rights of persons with disabilities, their working abilities, commitment, proven sincerity and of course, expenses required to set up an exclusive workshop or industry for persons with disabilities. Advancement in technology has also brought a revolution in trainability, and employability of persons with disabilities. Persons with hearing impairment in spite of their good physical fitness, motivational level and ability to perform well have not been the first choice for many employers because of their own (employer's) inability to establish effective communications. In order to assure the equal opportunity to persons with disabilities in the employment market, the government of India has identified thousands of jobs available in public and private sectors that can be performed by persons of different types of disabilities. The list of jobs also includes those for the hearing impaired workforce and range from routine jobs to jobs requiring the high level of skills, scientific knowledge, and administrative abilities. All the employers, particularly in government sectors, are governed by different Acts assuring job reservation and placement support. They do not impose any restrictions for employers to recruit persons with hearing impairment even on those jobs which may not be in the list of identified jobs because the identification exercise can never be updated at a pace comparable to the change in employment markets. Beside job reservation and identification of jobs, there are many agencies of the government of India and state government exclusively functioning to promote and arrange placements for them. The organizations like Special Employment Exchange, Vocational Rehabilitation Centres (VRC) for handicapped (now known as National Career Service Centre for Differently Abled), model career centres run by state government and placement divisions working under national institutes for different types of disabilities register the persons with hearing impairment and arrange their placements in different government and private sectors. The preparation for competitive examinations known as Pre Recruitment Tests has also been a point of concern for candidates with hearing impairment. Government agencies like VRC (National Career Service Centre for Differently abled) in collaboration with various banks, staff selection commissions, NGOs have been organizing the pre-recruitment training for briefing them about the knowledge and skills required for qualifying the competitive examinations.

The continuous shrinking and cuts in salaried employment globally have also imposed additional limitations in arranging salaried employment for persons with hearing impairment and with this universal phenomenon, the only alternative left out is to encourage the person with hearing impairment towards self-employment activities. Self-employment as the name suggests means taking up or setting up a program by an entrepreneur individually or in partnership by producing and marketing an item or extending services on fixed or negotiable financial returns in the form of yield or income. Self-employment has not been a preferred mode for many years for various reasons such as lack of awareness of market needs, lack of skills to produce or market a particular item, lack of finance, lack of management skills, lack of marketing skills and salesmanship, and on the top of all, lack of risk taking capacity or entrepreneurship. But now the scenario is changing. There are many government agencies and NGO initiatives focusing on entrepreneurial skill development among person with disabilities which also include hearing impairment at every stage. National Handicap Finance and Development Corporation (NHFDC) set up by the government of India is addressing the issue of financial requirement of self- employment projects of PWD in a big way through its wide net of channelizing agencies functioning in grass root level. NHFDC not only provides the finances in the form of the loan on a highly subsidized rate of interests but also supports pre self-employment vocational skill training to facilitate smooth implementation of project. Central and state government also encourage physically challenged entrepreneurs by procuring their product on the priority basis. There are many persons with hearing impairment who have set up their units of garment making, furniture making workshops, laundry work, automobile service centres and washing plants, gents and ladies' parlors to name a few.

Follow Up

Follow up is the extension of placement activities especially in the sector of placement of PWD. Follow up involves frequent visit of the workplace by the professional member of placement agencies, interaction with employers, supervisors and colleagues and sorting out issues if any. The effective follow up enhances the confidence among employees, employers and co-workers. It also gives a very important feedback to placement agencies as to what extent the persons with hearing impairment has been placed suitably and what changes may be required in future placement efforts. It also gives an insight into the real work challenges and requirements to modify the pre-placement skill training, orientation program and advocacy. In fact, effective placement and follow up open the avenues for future placement and possibilities of success for other candidates. In case of persons with hearing impairment, the follow up is particularly very important in the enhancement of communication between the employee with hearing impairment and his colleagues which ultimately reduces the fear of being isolated of which such persons have been serious victims, which may lead to dropouts, discontinuation and high attrition rate.

Issues and Challenges

Inspite of commitment of government of India, and the United Nation Convention on Rights of Persons with Disability, 2007 Article 27 which recognizes the rights of persons with disability to work on an equal basis with others, this includes the opportunity to gain living by work freely chosen or accepted in the labour market and work environment that is open, intrusive and accessible to persons with disabilities,the representation of persons with disabilities particularly hearing impaired in national workforce is far from satisfactory to the extent that even the quota reserved for this category of candidates could not be filled in many organizations. Private sector companies that are not governed by the reservation policy and are open and flexible in employment recruitment process could also not be assured respectable representation of the persons with hearing impairment in their workforce.

Various studies conducted by different national and international agencies and also individual experiences of employers, recruiting agencies and hearing impaired persons reveal following issues that need to be addressed to assure reasonable sustainable vocational rehabilitation to persons with hearing impairment.

1. The huge gap between the resources, infrastructure and manpower and the number of persons with hearing impairment to be employed in sustainable employment activities.
2. The training and educational requirements of children with pre-lingual deafness and post-lingual deafness are different. Children with pre-lingual deafness are mostly congenital having no understanding of words, meaning and are primarily trained by sign language with visual training aids, whereas children with post-lingual deafness are the victims of acquired deafness. Many of them after the development of their language and having good vocabulary may be communicated with amplified equipment supported with the sign, but there are hardly any vocational training institutes that can bifurcate the training module as per the onset and typology of the hearing loss. This leads to more or less permanent gaps in communication, acquiring of vocational skills and job performance. Employers also may not be equipped enough to appreciate the difference between pre-lingual and post-lingual hearing impaired persons and may undervalue the efficiency of the employees for no fault of both.
3. The area/domain of vocational training is mostly focused on urban-based employment opportunities while the sizable numbers of persons with disabilities are residing in rural or semi-urban areas having very little opportunities of post-training placements resulting in either non-utilization of skill

acquired or underutilization of the trained manpower. For example, desktop publishing and other printing related training can only be utilized in industrial or metropolitan cities and there would hardly be any use of placement in rural areas no matter how well the hearing impaired person has been trained.

4. The workplace, nature of occupation and employer's perception also play an important barrier and causative factor in the feeling of being discriminated resulting in discontinuation of the jobs.
5. No matter what social security schemes any government may frame, accessibility and effectiveness of scheme would directly depend upon the basic education level, awareness, risk-taking attitude, independence and family support in case of persons with hearing impairment. They are trailing behind in almost all the above parameters. Their basic education is still not compatible with the educational level of their counterparts in open employment. They are not aware of various social security schemes, legislation and not easily approachable because of their scattered and remote living vicinity. The skill sets are not being upgraded frequently mainly because of lack of trained instructors required for imparting and upgrading the skills.
6. In spite of the fact that self-employment is perhaps the only long-term solution for the continuous shrinking of salaried pay employment opportunities, yet persons with hearing impairment by and large are not very keen to go for self-employment ventures and there is hardly any facility available exclusively for them for entrepreneurial development. This lack of motivation towards self-employment has many a time proved to be the main cause of failures of many governments sponsored schemes promoting self-employment.
7. The assistive devices are either beyond the easy approach of common hearing impaired persons due to its scarcity/short of supply or beyond financial reach. The devices provided by different agencies either free of cost or in subsidized rates have not been very long lasting and require continuous maintenance and repair which may not be available or accessible easily.

SOLUTIONS AND RECOMMENDATIONS

1. There cannot be a second opinion that no one would disagree or show any resistance to the efforts of assuring full participation and integration of persons with hearing impairment with mainstream workforce but some deep-seated biases and stereotypes about their efficacy, productivity and employability are still persisting which require intensive desensitization and advocacy by showcasing their employability through various media.
2. Intensive training of school teachers of so-called normal schools and vocational instructors in communication skills for both pre-lingual deaf students and post-lingual deaf students would ease the problem of attaining basic education required for acquiring marketable vocational skills.
3. Area-based employment market and job surveys would help in providing vocational guidance and career counselling with special reference to the locality and usual residency.
4. Accessibility to the social security schemes and awareness about rights of the person with hearing impairment may elevate the motivational levels and drives toward vocational independence.
5. Effective implementation of different legislations and accountability of its implementing agencies would also be helpful in the integration of persons with hearing impairment with the workforce.

CONCLUSION

Vocational rehabilitation of persons with hearing impairment is not only an important step in the entire management of persons with hearing impairment but the ultimate outcome of entire rehabilitation exercise. In a country like India, where more than 26 million persons are inflicted with hearing impairment, they cannot be left unattended particularly when they possess all the qualities, abilities, personality traits and potential to become a productive member of workforce par excellence to their fellow citizens, provided suitable education and training is inculcated, positive attitude and accommodative environment is created and advancement in technology in skill development and training and job-related assistive devices are made available.

REFERENCES

Bracken, B. A., & McCallum, R. S. (1998). *Universal nonverbal intelligence test.* Riverside Publishing Company.

Buck, J. N. (1971). The house-tree-person (HTP) manual supplement: Administration and interpretation of the HTP test. *Western Psychological Services.*

Disabled Persons in India. (2016). *A statistical profile.* Social Statistics Division, Ministry of Statistics and Program Implementation, Government of India.

Dumond, R., & Willis, J. O. (2008). Bender Visual-Motor Gestalt Test (2nd ed.). Encyclopedia of Special Education.

International Disability and Development Consortium. (2005). *Inclusive Development and the Comprehensive and Integral International Convention on the Protection and Promotion of the Rights and Dignity of Persons with Disabilities.* Author.

International Labour Organization. (1998). Vocational rehabilitation and employment of disabled persons. In *International Labour Conference, 86th Session.* ILO.

Layton, T. L., & Holmes, D. W. (1985). *Carolina picture vocabulary test for dead and hearing impaired children (CPVT).* PRO-ED Inc.

Meadow, K. P. (1980). *Meadow/Kendall Social-Emotional Assessment Inventory for Deaf Students: Manual.* Academic Press.

Nagaraja, M. N. (2002). Challenges in Vocational & Technical Education of PWHI. In *Proceeding of Challenges in Vocational & Technical Education to persons with disabilities.* Mumbai: Seminar at Ali Yavar Jung National Institute of Hearing Handicapped.

Planning Commission of India. (2013). *Report on 12th Five year Plan.* New Delhi: Government of India.

Reitan, R. M., & Wolfson, D. (1985). *The Halstead-Reitan neuropsychological test battery: Theory and clinical interpretation* (Vol. 4). Reitan Neuropsychology.

Reynolds, W. M. (2001). *Reynolds adolescent adjustment screening inventory: RAASI: Professional manual*. Psychological Assessment Resources.

Rights of Persons With Disabilities Act. (2016). Ministry of Law and Justice, Government of India.

Roid, G. H., & Miller, L. J. (1997). *Leiter international performance scale-revised: Examiners manual*. Wood Dale, IL: Stoelting.

Shenoy, M. (2011). *Persons with disability and the India labour market: Challenges and Opportunities Geneva*. International Labour Organization.

Short, C., DeOrnellas, K., & Walrath, R. (2011). Draw-A-Person Test. In S. Goldstein & J. A. Naglieri (Eds.), *Encyclopedia of Child Behavior and Development* (pp. 523–524). New York: Springer.

Singh, V. (2015). Hearing in India: All aspects. *Online Journal of Otolaryngology*, *5*(1), 39–70.

Skill Development Initiative. (2008). *Modular Employable Skills Scheme*. Ministry of Labour and Employment, Government of India.

Sparrow, S. S. (2011). Vineland adaptive behavior scales. In *Encyclopedia of clinical neuropsychology* (pp. 2618–2621). New York: Springer. doi:10.1007/978-0-387-79948-3_1602

The Persons with Disability (Equal Opportunities, Protection of Rights, and Full Participations) Act. (1995). Ministry of Law, Justice and Company Affairs, Government of India.

Vocational Rehabilitation and Employment (Disabled Persons) Convention. (1983). (*No. 159*). International Labour Organization.

Vocational Rehabilitation - the way forward: Report of a working party. (2000). London: British Society of Rehabilitation Medicine.

Wechsler, D. (1991). *Wechsler Intelligence Scale for Children* (3rd ed.). San Antonio, TX: Psychological Corp.

Wechsler, D. (1992). *Wechsler Individual Achievement Tests*. San Antonio, TX: Psychological Corp.

Wood, N., & Dockrell, J. (2010). Psychological assessment procedures for assessing deaf or hard-of-hearing children. *Educational and Child Psychology*, *27*(2), 11.

KEY TERMS AND DEFINITIONS

Acquired Disability: Getting some disability after birth.

Advocacy: The act of speaking up for others.

Anxiety: Fear reactions for unknown reasons.

Assistive Listening Device: Equipment like hearing aids that help in listening by amplifying the pitch/tone.

Audiogram: A graphic status obtained from electronic equipment depicting hearing thresholds.

Audiometer: Electronic equipment measuring the threshold of hearing.

Barrier-Free Environment: A physical environment where any person with any physical limitations such as those of locomotion, vision, or hearing can live and function independently.

Communication: The process of conveying one's thoughts and feelings through gestures or words.

Communication Disorders: A condition that is characterized by the inability to use a communication medium to successfully convey to others, one's thoughts, feelings, beliefs, etc.

Counselling: It is a professional technique to help an individual in understanding and solving his problems of different natures.

Disability: A status caused by physical or mental impairment and resultant functional limitations.

Evaluation: A process of assessing assets and liabilities of an individual objectively to the extent possible.

Hearing Impaired: A person who cannot hear the sound even those with amplified pitch/tone, and whose hearing threshold is higher than the normal hearing threshold.

On-the-Job Training: Arranging skill training in real shop floor or actual working conditions.

Open Employment: Placement of an individual in salaried employment without any special consideration, relaxation, and by open competitions.

Self-Advocacy: Speaking up for oneself.

Sign Language: A method of communication by using different symbolic signs by using fingers and facial expressions in place of words.

Social Exclusion: Excluding persons due to a range of reasons determined and influenced by culture, communities, attitudes, etc.

Social Inclusion: Including all persons regardless of any dividing factors to the social fabric of life. There are various types of inclusion; full, partial and mainstreaming. It is a process that requires deliberate actions.

Social Model of Disability: First introduced in 1976, the model seeks to place responsibility on society to enable inclusion and to actively engage in eradicating barriers that subscribe to exclusion of people with disabilities.

Special Vocational Instructor: A vocational instructor who is trained for imparting vocational training and transferring the skills to persons with disabilities.

Vocational Evaluation: Assessment of an individual to evaluate his physical and mental potentials/abilities to acquire specific skills related to different vocations.

Work Study: A method of analyzing different operations involved in performing a specific work sample.

Chapter 17
Speech Therapy for Children Who Stutter:
A Systematic Review

Divya Seth
All India Institute of Speech and Hearing, India

Santosh Maruthy
All India Institute of Speech and Hearing, India

ABSTRACT

This chapter aims to investigate and evaluate the evidence available for stuttering treatment research in children who stutter (CWS) and provide a qualitative review of the same. Studies were considered for review if (1) they were behavioral intervention of stuttering for children, (2) participants were in the age range of 2-18 years, and (3) the outcomes reported assessed stuttering. Twenty-seven studies were obtained through an electronic search of databases covering two approaches and 10 techniques. The analysis of these studies revealed that direct approaches have a stronger evidence base in comparison to the indirect approaches. The most popular approach with maximum studies is the early intervention Lidcombe program. The commonly used outcome measures included the percentage of syllables stuttered, syllables per minute, and severity rating scales. The conclusion drawn from the review suggest that evidence base to support behavioral intervention of CWS exists for a limited number of intervention techniques and among them very few exploring the long-term effects of the intervention.

INTRODUCTION

Stuttering is defined as the disturbance or interruption in the effortless flow of speech. The core features of stuttering as described by Van Riper (1971, 1982) include: (a) sound or syllable repetitions, (b) sound prolongations, and (c) blocks. These core behaviours seem to be involuntary for a person, unlike secondary behaviours that are learned or acquired, often an individual's response or reaction to his or her stuttering. Secondary behaviours can further be classified as either escape or avoidance behaviours. Escape behaviours are said to occur when a person tries to terminate the stutter. These include eye blinks,

DOI: 10.4018/978-1-5225-4955-0.ch017

head nods and interjections like "uh". Avoidance behaviours are a result of anticipating the stutter and recalling associated negative experiences. To avoid the stutter the person may resort to behaviours which he or she used earlier as escape mechanism (Guitar, 2014).

As suggested in the literature, stuttering is considered to be a highly prevalent disorder both in children and adults. Yairi and Ambrose (2013) in their review reported significantly higher prevalence of stuttering in preschool children (3.46%) when compared to school-age and high-school children (0.84%). It is also observed that in majority of the individuals, the onset of stuttering is during the preschool period i.e., between 2 to 5 years of age (Andrews and Harris, 1964; Bernstein-Ratner and Silverman, 2000; Geetha, Mahesh, and Swathy, 2015; Guitar, 2014; Johnson and Associates, 1959; Yairi and Ambrose, 1992a, 2005) and the risk of developing stuttering reduces with increase in age (Craig, Hancock, Tran, Craig, and Peters, 2002). This decline in prevalence rate with advancing age is attributed to two factors: first, the low incidence rate after the age of 4 years and second, spontaneous recovery in a significant group of children (Yairi and Seery, 2015). The natural, spontaneous, or recovery without any treatment in young children is considered to be one of the remarkable aspects of stuttering (Yairi and Seery, 2015). A wide range of recovery rates from 30 to 89% have been reported in the literature (Bryngelson, 1938; Craig et al., 2002; Johnson and Associates, 1959; Wingate, 1976; Yairi and Ambrose, 1992b).

Though a large group of these children recover on their own, there still remains a significant number who continue to stutter and these children are at an increased risk of psycho-social problems. Children who stutter (CWS) are reported to be more sensitive, anxious, fearful, introverted and withdrawn (Embrechts, Ebben, Franke, and van de Poel, 2000; Fowlie and Cooper, 1978; Oyler, 1996). They are also known to have more negative quality of mood (Howell et al., 2004; Johnson, Walden, Conture, and Karrass, 2010) and a negative attitude towards communication (Guttormsen, Kefalianos, and Næss, 2015; Kawai, Healey, Nagasawa, and Vanryckeghem, 2012; Vanryckeghem, Hylebos, Brutten, and Peleman, 2001). Moreover, this negative attitude is noticed as early as the preschool age (Clark, Conture, Frankel, and Walden, 2012; Vanryckeghem and Brutten, 2007; Vanryckeghem, Vanrobayes, and De Niels, 2015). The negative attitude towards communication is said to diminish with age in children who do not stutter (CWNS) (Clark et al., 2012; Vanryckeghem and Brutten, 1996) unlike CWS where this relation is strengthened with increase in age (Clark et al., 2012; Kawai et al., 2012; Vanryckeghem et al., 2001). In addition, a direct relation is reported between the severity of stuttering and negative communication attitude (Kawai et al., 2012; Vanryckeghem et al., 2001; Vanryckeghem and Brutten, 1996). Clark et al. (2012) proposed that the early onset of such negative attitude towards communication negatively influences the child's "ability to establish normally fluent speech-language planning and production".

Along with the CWS, the peers and parents are also reported to have negative attitude towards speech of CWS (Langevin and Hagler, 2004; Langevin, Packman, and Onslow, 2009, 2010; Onslow, Attanasio, and Harrison, 2003; Vanryckeghem, 1995; Yairi, 1983). It is also suggested that the vulnerable temperament of CWS makes them more susceptible to stuttering and diminishes their chances of recovery (Conture, 1991, 2001; Guitar, 1998; Zebrowski and Conture, 1998). Some of the other effects of stuttering on CWS include teasing and bullying by peers (Blood and Blood, 2004, 2007; Davis, Howell, and Cooke, 2002; Hugh-Jones and Smith, 1999; Onslow et al., 2003; Packman, Onslow, and Attanasio, 2003), reduced social acceptance (Davis et al., 2002), difficulty "fitting-in" at school (Evans, Healey, Kawai, and Rowland, 2008) and making friends (Hartford and Leahy, 2007). These further reinforce the feeling of shame and embarrassment (Iverach and Rapee, 2014), loss of self-confidence, depression and low self-esteem in CWS (Hawker and Bolton, 2000; Hugh-Jones and Smith, 1999; Mooney and Smith, 1995). CWS are also reported to have behavioural, emotional and social difficulties to a greater extent than CWNS and these can occur as early as 3 years of age (McAllister, 2016). These findings necessitate the assessment of speech associated attitude even in preschool and kindergarten CWS and target these during intervention (Conture, 2001; Zebrowski and Kelly, 2002). Further, early intervention not only prevents or reduces the impact of these psycho-social challenges; it also ensures a better and faster recovery with increased chance of maintenance of fluency skills.

Though early intervention has been indicated in the literature, treatment techniques for CWS were relatively late to appear when compared to AWS. This was mainly because of the belief that children would recover naturally. The last three decades have witnessed a significant shift in trend and a substantial increase in clinical and theoretical research in CWS. The present study aims to investigate and evaluate the stuttering treatment research in CWS till date. The present study is a qualitative review. It provides a brief introduction to the popular intervention programs and summarizes the evidence base for the same.

METHOD

- **Inclusion Criteria:** The studies included in this review were selected through a systematic search of the literature in PubMed, Google Scholar, and core journals in the field of speech and hearing. Some amount of gray literature is also included. The search was restricted to original papers written in English and those published in peer-reviewed journals. All the studies included were pertaining to stuttering intervention in CWS. Intervention here refers to the behavioural management of stuttering in children which includes manipulation of the environmental factors or the speech production characteristics of CWS or both. The study designs included were: case reports, longitudinal and cross-sectional designs. All the studies had CWS as participants in the age range of 2;4 to 18 years. Studies published up to April 2017 were considered.
- **Study Retrieval:** The search was conducted using the following keywords- stuttering intervention in CWS, stuttering, stammering, dysfluency, therapy, intervention, behavioural management, children who stutter, preschoolers, school-age, efficacy, and effectiveness.
- **Study Selection:** Initially the studies were screened based on the title and the abstract. These studies were further screened for the relevance of their contents with regard to the present review. Finally, a total of 27 studies were shortlisted and are included in the present review.
- **Data Extraction:** Each of the studies was further analyzed in terms of following characteristics (a) research design; (b) participant; (c) intervention; and (d) outcome.

RESULTS

Therapeutic interventions for early childhood stuttering is believed to stem from two different philosophies of direct and indirect intervention. The indirect approaches are the ones which target the child's environment and behaviour of people present in the environment. On the other hand, direct intervention approaches involve direct contact between the child and the clinician, where the CWS are directly subjected to treatment. This kind of an approach focuses on modifying the speech production characteristics of CWS. Further, many clinicians have used a combined or mixed approach wherein they include principles from both direct and indirect methods. As mentioned earlier a substantial amount of research is done exploring the potential of direct and indirect approach which will be discussed in the later sections of this chapter. However, there is no evidence base available for the combined or mixed approach. Table 1 lists the various treatment programs under each of the approaches.

There are several other techniques like EVMS Fluency Shaping Program, Hollin's Precision Fluency Shaping, Computer Aided Fluency Establishment Training, the Van Riper Program, biofeedback techniques, cognitive-behaviour therapy, self-help therapy programs and many online and offline software tools which are more popular in intervention for AWS. To our knowledge there is no evidence base for these techniques with respect to intervention of CWS. Therefore, these have not been included further in the chapter.

Both direct and indirect approaches dominated at different points of time. Indirect approach preceded the direct approach of treatment as per the literature. This was due to the emergence of Diagnosogenic theory and the demands and capacity model (DCM) which believed that stuttering was caused by the external environmental factors. Later, theories focusing on laryngeal dynamics and speech motor control system of individuals who stutter, suggested a deficit in the speech system of an individual which became an internal factor. This led to the advent of direct treatment approach. The present study attempts to put forth a brief description of the major techniques under the two approaches and a collective view of the evidence base available for the same.

Indirect Approaches

The indirect approach is believed to have emerged in late 1930s as a combined influence of Diagnosogenic theory (Johnson, 1942) and some aspects of psychogenic theories of stuttering (Bloodstein, 1975, 1981). Indirect approach focuses on parents and the environment, and is often referred to as "hands off

Table 1. Techniques for Intervention in CWS

Indirect Approaches	Direct Approaches	Mixed Approaches
Group play therapy (Wakaba, 1983)	Regulated breathing (Azrin and Nunn, 1974)	Preschool fluency development program (Culp, 1984)
Teaching and facilitating mother-child interaction therapy (Wyatt, 1969)	The Monterey Fluency Program (Ryan and Ryan, 1983, 1995)	The intensive stuttering therapy program (Hasbrouck et al., 1987)
Parent-focused treatment (Yaruss, Coleman, and Hammer, 2006)	Rhythmic speech timing (Coppola and Yairi, 1982)	Fluency facilitation (Jones-Prus, 1980)
The Demands and Capacities Model (Franken, Kielstra- Van der Schalk, -and Boelens, 2005) – RESTART	Speech Restructuring (Shine, 1984)	
Parent-child interaction therapy (Rustin, Botterill, and Kelman, 1996)	The comprehensive stuttering program (Kully and Boberg, 1991)	
	The Fluency rules program (Runyan and Runyan, 1986)	
	The Stuttering Intervention Program (Pindzola, 1987)	
	Speech Motor Training (Riley and Riley, 1984)	
	The Lidcombe program (Jones et al., 2005)	
	Westmead program (Trajkowski et al., 2009)	

the child" philosophy (Yairi and Seery, 2015). The primary recipients of the treatment in this approach include people who closely interact with CWS (e.g., parents, other family members, and teachers). It is presumed that working to improve the emotional well being, attitudes and behaviour of these significant people will positively influence the child's speech. In addition it is also believed that environmental conditions influence speech related behaviours of an individual.

In the initial phases of indirect approach, researchers proposed psychotherapy for parents with neurotic personalities (Glasner, 1949; Glauber, 1958). They attributed pathological mother-child relationship to the emotional conflict in children, later exhibited as stuttering. However, psychotherapy for parents did not gain much popularity and soon faded as a treatment option. Parent counselling then emerged as a popular approach which assumed the Diagnosogenic theory as the probable cause for developmental stuttering. Johnson (1948) strongly believed in the Diagnosogenic theory and promoted parent counselling as treatment which aimed at reducing parents' negative responses/reactions to a child's stutter. Schuell (1949) and Brown (1949) further supported parent counselling and proposed similar counselling approaches. However, evidence base for this approach is limited. In this review, 5 studies providing evidence base for three of the techniques under the indirect approach are reported. Table 2 summarizes the details about these studies and the following section discusses the findings of the same.

- **Wakaba's Group Play Therapy:** A single study was published by Wakaba back in 1983. This group play therapy method included one hour of group play therapy and aimed to reduce stuttering and improve social adaptation in CWS. All CWS attended twenty-one sessions of group play therapy. It also included counselling sessions for mothers of CWS wherein they were instructed to work on improving family environment and mother-child relationship. A follow-up evaluation was also conducted at 6 months and 5 years duration. Post-therapy and on follow-up sessions improvement was observed in both fluency skills and social adaptation of CWS.
- **Demands-Capacity Model (DCM) Treatment or RESTART Approach (Franken Et Al., 2005):** DCM treatment or RESTART approach is based on a theoretical model which considers

Figure 1. Figure depicting Indirect approach or "hands off the child philosophy" where environmental factors are manipulated. The recipients of the treatment include parents (in most cases) along with caregivers and teachers.

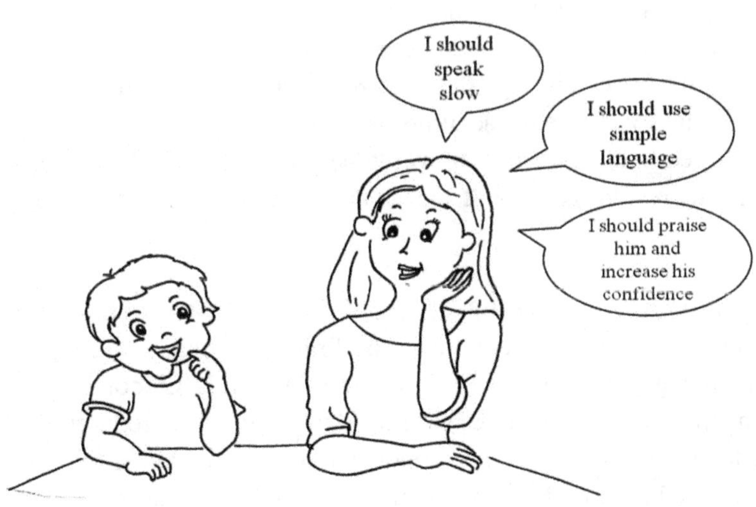
I should speak slow
I should use simple language
I should praise him and increase his confidence

Table 2. Details of design, participant, treatment and outcome measures of studies included under the indirect approach

Author(s)/ Year	Country of Origin	Study Design	Technique/ Program Used	N	Age Range (Years; Months)	Duration of Tx	Outcome Measures	Follow-Up	Results
Wakaba (1983)	Japan	QED	Group play therapy	3	4;6 – 5;3	5 months	• Stuttering frequency • Social maturity age (SMA)	6 months and 5 years	<1% stuttering in all 3 CWS Significant improvement in SMA
Franken et al. (2005)	Netherlands	RCT	DCM LP	23	< 6;0	12 weeks	• % SS • SR • Parent perception and acceptance	-	%SS reduced as follows: LP- 7.2% to 3.7%. DCM- 7.9% to 3.1%
de Sonneville-Koedoot et al. (2015)	Netherlands	RCT	DCM LP	177	3;0 – 6;3	NS	• % SS • SR • HRQoL • Emotional and Behavioural problems • Speech attitude	18 months	%SS reduced in both groups similarly Parent rating of severity- greater decline in LP group
Millard, Nicholas, and Cook. (2008)	England	QED	PCIT	6	3;3 – 4;10	12 weeks	% Stuttering (cusum analysis) SR	12 months	4/6 CWS improved significantly (SR of 0 or 1) and discharged 2/6 CWS- direct therapy
Millard, Edwards, and Cook (2009)	England	QED	PCIT	10	3;7 – 4;11	24 weeks	% Stuttering (cusum analysis)	6 months	
Sawyer et al. (2017)	United States of America	QED	Parent focused slow relaxed speech	17	2;7 – 5;6	3 weeks	%SS Articulation Rate Response time latency	-	

Note: Tx = Treatment; N = sample size; RCT = Randomized Controlled Trial; QED = Quasi Experimental Design; DCM = Demands and Capacity model; LP = Lidcombe program; PCIT = Parent Child Interaction Therapy; %SS = Percentage of syllables stuttered; SR = Severity Rating; HRQoL = Health Related Quality of Life; NS = Not specified.

stuttering as a multifactorial disorder (Gregory, Campbell, Gregory, and Hill, 2003; Smith and Kelly, 1997; Starkweather, 1997). It is based on the Demands and Capacity theory which believes that when the demands on a child exceed his/her capacity, they lead to a breakdown resulting in stuttering. The demands here refer to the physical, linguistic, psychological, and/or environmental factors. Thus, the treatment aims to manipulate factors related to the child and the environment which are believed to be influencing the speech fluency. The rationale behind this approach is to reduce the demands set by the environment (e.g., instructing parents to reduce their rate of speech) and by the child him- or herself (e.g., desensitize the child for dysfluency), and increase the child's capacities for fluent speech (e.g., accurate and effortless age-appropriate speech motor movements). It is believed that these, in turn, would help establish a balance between the demands and capacities gradually resulting in fluent speech (Sonnekville-Koedoot, Adams, Stolk, and Franken, 2015).

Two recent investigations compared the efficacy of RESTART program with direct treatment approaches. The first one is a pilot study conducted by Franken, Schalk, and Boelens (2005) comparing outcomes of two treatment programs – RESTART treatment and Lidcombe program. Their findings revealed that both the treatments were effective and led to a significant reduction in the dysfluencies and the severity. A satisfaction measure was also conducted for parents in the two treatment groups and no differences were observed in terms of treatment outcome satisfaction i.e., in both the groups parents were equally satisfied with the outcomes. In another investigation by de Sonneville-Koedoot et al. (2015) direct treatment i.e. Lidcombe program was found to have caused a relatively rapid reduction in dysfluencies during the initial three months of the treatment when compared to the RESTART approach. In addition, they found that the group who underwent Lidcombe program treatment had better outcome than those who were subjected to RESTART approach. However, on follow-up after 18 months both the groups had similar performance with no significant between group differences. A focused group discussion was conducted with 13 speech-language pathologists working throughout Netherlands. All the professionals agreed to the effectiveness of RESTART approach and suggested that it is unique and effective in terms of reducing the tempo of speech and communication, facilitating turn taking, and in training parents to modify their communication style (de Sonneville-Koedoot, Adams, Stolk, and Franken, 2015).

- **Parent-Child Interaction Therapy (PCIT) Approach (Rustin, Botterill, and Kelman, 1996):** This program was developed at Michael Palin Centre for Stammering Children in London. This program entrusts the multifactorial model of stuttering. To reiterate, this model believes that stuttering is triggered and sustained by various motor, physiological, linguistic and developmental child variables and how these interact with their environment. The program includes a detailed pre-treatment assessment followed by a 6 once-a-week clinic sessions and later a 6-week period of home consolidation. The program encourages discussion and acknowledgment of stuttering by the parents. It further guides them to manage the child's stuttering behaviour and improve their own skills. In contrast to other structured intervention programs this one is a relatively flexible approach and has undergone several modifications based on clinical experience, parent feedback and research evidence (Kelman and Nicholas, 2008). A recent modification was proposed by Millard, Nicholas, and Cook (2008) which includes both management and interaction strategies. Management strategies involve breaking down the target into smaller achievable steps, explicitly explaining these to the child and reinforcing and rewarding target behaviours. It empowers parents to be the decision maker; they are the ones who decide upon the targets and the strategies.

Two research investigations provide some account on the effectiveness of PCIT. Millard et al. (2008) conducted a longitudinal multiple single-subject study and reported that 4 out of 6 children had significant reduction in their stuttering with both parents. One of the other two children reduced his stuttering with the father but not with the mother and the other child didn't show any significant reduction of stuttering with either of the parents. Both these children were recommended for direct therapy 6 weeks post PCIT and follow-up assessments revealed improvement highlighting the combination of direct and indirect treatments. Another successive investigation by Millard, Edwards, and Cook (2009) revealed significant reduction in stuttering in all the children who received therapy. 4 out of 6 children showed significant reduction in stuttering by the end of therapy phase attributing the reduction to the therapy. However, two of the children reached a significant level of reduction in stuttering by the end of the follow-up phase and not the therapy phase, thus indicating possible extraneous factors for improvement.

Another recent investigation reported reduction in stuttering of CWS when their parents were asked to use a slow relaxed speech (Sawyer, Matteson, Ou, and Nagase, 2017). In this study the parents were trained to use a slow relaxed speech i.e., reduce their rate of speech while interacting with the child. The study was conducted in three 1-hour sessions spread over three weeks. Parents were instructed to use similar speech as a part of home-training as well. Post intervention assessment revealed that parents were able to follow a slow rate of speech and there was a significant reduction in the dysfluencies for 70% of the participants. Three of the children had dysfluencies like CWNS.

Direct Approaches

Direct approaches are considered to be more popular in terms of clinical practice especially in Europe and America. Late 19th century and early decades of 20th century witnessed a plethora of programs advocating direct approach for stuttering intervention. These programs focused on fluency enhancement instead of stuttering modification. Techniques which became popular in Europe included speech breathing and easy phonation (Emil-Behnke, 1947), music and singing, coordinating speech with body movements in a rhythmic pattern (Pichon and Borel-Maisonny, 1937), talking in unison (Kingdon-Ward, 1941) and shadowing (Marland, 1957). Motorically oriented approaches were dominant in contrast to the linguistic approaches. On the other side, majority of the practitioners in the United States believed stuttering to be a result of neurological dysfunction and preferred a non-speech approach. They focused on manipulating neurological and muscular functions. Based on the rationale behind the cerebral dominance theory (Travis, 1931), Johnson (1934) proposed retraining handedness as a cure to stuttering. Few significant others suggested to strengthen oral structures and movements and conducted drills for specific speech movements in CWS (Young and Hawk, 1955). Thus, with the evolution in attitudes and beliefs, some of these techniques became more popular while others dissolved with time and new techniques emerged every decade. Table 3 provides details of 21 studies available as evidence base for direct treatment approach.

It can be observed from Table 3 that in contrast to the indirect approach, direct approach has more evidence base. However, there are few techniques which have much higher evidence while there are others which haven't received the same amount of scrutiny. Hereunder is a brief explanation of the techniques listed in Table 3 and the existing evidence for the same.

- **Programmed Traditional Approach:** This approach consists of eight steps which include identification, cancellation, pull-out, prolongation and fluent speech step. In Ryan and Ryan (1983) study, this approach was found to be effective, however internal characteristics of the approach increased the operation time of the technique. In specific the participants faced great difficulty in identifying the stutters and when identified it became a challenge to modify it.
- **Delayed Auditory Feedback (DAF):** In this approach the individual who stutters receives his or her own speech with an initial delay of 250 ms. This delay is gradually decreased to zero in 50 ms steps. The rationale is that the delayed feedback would result in slow prolonged speech which in turn would reduce stuttering. Ryan and Ryan (1983) reported significant reduction in stuttering with the use of DAF and it was found that DAF needed least number of therapy hours when compared to other methods used in the study.
- **Pause:** It is a time-out program which included a range of pause time or time-outs than a single pause time. In Ryan and Ryan (1983) study the pause times used were: 10s, 7s, 3s, 1s, no pause, and fluent speech. The treatment was carried out at three levels- reading, monologue, and conversation. A total of 21 steps were involved. They suggested that this technique was very effective to eliminate stuttering in those with severe stuttering. The limitation of this technique was that it highly depended on client's ability to learn to speak fluently without any guidance.
- **Gradual Increase in Linguistic Complexity of Utterance (GILCU):** It is a structured program for fluency shaping based on the principles of operant conditioning. The program begins with establishing fluency at word level and gradually moves to connected speech. In Ryan and Ryan (1983) study, GILCU was reported to have yielded the best results compared to the other three approaches (Programmed Traditional, DAF, and Pause).

Table 3. Details of design, participant, treatment and outcome measures of studies included under the direct approach

Author(s)/ Year	Country of Origin	Study Design	Technique/ Program Used	N	Age Range (Years; Months)	Duration of Tx	Outcome Measures	Follow-Up	Results	Limitations
Ryan and Ryan (1983)	USA	QED	• Programmed traditional • DAF • Pause • GILCU	16	7;0 – 18;0	NS	• SW/M • WS/M • Total sessions/hours • % Talk time • Total no. of days	9 months	Skills could be transferred in all 4 conditions. DAF- least therapy hours GILCU- best overall results On follow-up SW/M rate reduced from 8.1 to 0.8	
Ryan and Ryan (1995)	USA	RCT	• DAF • GILCU	20	7;0 – 17;0	NS	• SW/M • WS/M • %SS	14 months	23/24 CWS improved Initially better generalization with GILCU On follow-up similar performance of 2 groups. Reduction from 7.9 SW/M to 0.8 SW/M	Small sample size considering the wide age range
Onslow et al. (1994)	Australia	RCT	• Parent-administered RCS operant program	23 (18-EG; 5 – RG)	2;4 – 4;10	NS	• %SS • SPM • Parent surveys	-	12/18 CWS – median %SS < 1 on 12 month follow-up	
Lincoln et al. (1996)	Australia	RCT	• Parent administered RCS operant program	11	6;10 – 12;4	NS	• % SS • SPM • Parent surveys	12 months	Around 1% SS post treatment On follow-up 1%SS maintained	
Riley and Ingham (2000)	USA	RCT	• SMT • ELU • RG	21	3;8 – 8;4	NS	%SS	-	%SS (pre- to post-therapy) SMT: 7.8 to 4.61 ELU: 4.25 to 1.89	
Trajkovski et al. (2009)	Australia	Case study	STS	3	3;5 – 3;11	35 weeks	%SS	-	Stuttering reduced for all three children below the baseline level	
Trajkovski et al. (2011)	Australia	QED	STS	17	3;0 – 3;9	NS	• %SS • Tx time • Speech quality • Parent SR	12 months	Reduction of %SS from 6% pre-therapy to 1.3% post therapy On follow-up it reduced to 0.2%SS	
Andrews et al. (2016)	Australia	QED	STS	22	6;0 -6;11	NS	• %SS • SR • Situation avoidance • Participant satisfaction • Impact of stuttering • Speech rhythmicity	12 months	Dysfluencies reduced from 8.4% SS to 2.5% SS At both 6 and 12 months 1.9% SS was maintained	
Harris et al. (2002)	Australia	RCT	LP	23	2;0 – 4;11	12 weeks	%SS	-	Stuttering reduced twice in treatment group than the control group	
Wilson et al. (2004)	Australia	Case study	LP – Telehealth	5	3;5 – 5;7	CB	• %SS • SPM • Efficacy measures	12 months	4/5 CWS had <2%SS and maintained it on follow-up 1/5 CWS – relapsed Overall telehealth delivery – more no. of sessions than std. LP	
Jones et al. (2008)	Australia	RCT	LP	20	3;5 – 7;0	Follow-up investigation	• %SS • Parent questionnaire	-	Zero or near zero %SS in all but one child	
Lattermann et al. (2008)	Germany	RCT	LP	45	3;0 – 5;11	CB	• %SS • SR	-	%SS (pre to post-therapy) At home: 6.9% to 1.6% At clinic: 6.8% to 3.6%	
Lewis et al. (2008)	Australia	RCT	LP – Telehealth	22	3;0 – 6;0	CB	• %SS • Tx time • Parent satisfaction	-	%SS (pre- to post therapy) EG: 6.7% to 1.1% RG: 4.5% to 1.9%	
Koushik et al. (2009)	Canada	RCT	LP	11	6;8 – 10;8	CB	• %SS • SPM	9 – 187 weeks	Pre treatment: 9.2% SS Follow-up: 1.9% SS	

continued on following page

Table 3. Continued

Author(s)/ Year	Country of Origin	Study Design	Technique/ Program Used	N	Age Range (Years; Months)	Duration of Tx	Outcome Measures	Follow-Up	Results	Limitations
Miller and Guitar (2009)	USA	RCT	LP	15	2;5 – 5;9	CB	• %SS • SSI-3 scores	12 months	No. of sessions to clear Stage 1 ranged between 6 -44 sessions Pretreatment % SS = 12.6 SSI 3 Score = 24.9 Follow up % SS = 0.5 SSI 3 Score = 3.5	
Bakhtiar and Packman (2009)	Iran	Case study	LP	1	8;11	CB	• %SS • Parent SR	-	Stage 1 completed – 13 weeks %SS < 1 and SR = 1 (within and beyond clinic)	
O'Brian et al. (2013)	Australia	RCT	LP	57	2;7 – 6;4	CB	• %SS • Parent SR • Tx time	-	1.7% SS post 9 months of treatment	
Arnott et al. (2014)	Australia	RCT	LP	54	3;5 – 11;0	CB	• SLP hrs / child • Tx time • %SS • Parent SR • Exit Questionnaire	18 months	SLP hours to reach stage 2 Group: 9.2 hours Individual: 14.3 hr No difference in fluency scores between the two groups on follow-up	
Guitar et al. (2015)	USA	RCT	LP	14	3;4 -6;2	CB	• %SS • SSI-3 scores	24 months	An avg of 16.8 sessions to complete Stage 1 (almost stutter free speech) Pretreatment % SS = 9.61 Follow up %SS = 0.48	
Vong, Wilson, and Lincoln (2016)	Malaysia	Case study	LP	4	3;3 -4;9	CB	• %SS • SPM • Parent SR	-	2/4 CWS near zero level of stuttering post 12 months treatment 1/4 CWS – withdrew from Tx 1/4 CWS – Completed Stage 1; Relapsed in Stage 2	Due to convenience based sampling, more females were there than males in contrast to the prevalence rate as per literature
Bridgman et al. (2016)	Australia	RCT	LP	49	3;5 – 11;0	CB	• %SS • Parent SR • Tx time • Parent perception	18 months	Pre randomization % SS RG= 4.0 EG = 3.8 9 months post randomization % SS RG = 1.0 EG = 1.7 On follow-up %SS RG = 0.7 EG = 0.8	

Note: Tx = Treatment; N = sample size; QED = Quasi-Experimental Design; RCT = Randomized Controlled Trial; DAF = Delayed Auditory Feedback; GILCU = Gradual Increase in Length and Complexity of Utterance; NS = Not specified; SW/M = Stuttered words per minute; WS/M = Words spoken per minute; %SS = Percentage of syllables stuttered; RCS = Response Contingent Stimulation; SPM = Syllables per minute; SMT = Speech Motor Training; ELU = Extended Length of Utterance; RG = Reference group; STS = Syllable timed speech; SR = Severity Rating; LP = Lidcombe program; CB = Criterion based; SSI-3 = Stuttering Severity Instrument -3.

- **Speech Motor Training (SMT):** As the name suggests, this approach involves motor coordination, formulation of sentences, and auditory processing. Initially, the participant is trained to produce nonsense syllables with increasing complexity and gradually he/she moves to connected speech controlling the number of syllables and speech rate.
- **Extended Length of Utterance (ELU):** This approach focuses on gradually increasing the length of verbal output. This is combined with the principles of Operant conditioning. Treatment begins

with establishment of fluency at sound level and then proceeding to mono- and multisyllabic words followed by phrases, monologue and finally conversation.

The literature search unravelled a single study by Ryan and Ingham (2000) which compared the effectiveness of SMT and ELU. They found that both SMT and ELU showed a significant reduction in stuttering. On comparing the two approaches, it was found that ELU had a greater effect and showed greater reduction in stuttering when compared to SMT.

- **Syllable-Timed Speech or Westmead Program (Trajkowski, 2009):** This approach demands one to speak with equal stress across syllables. It follows a rhythmic pattern wherein each syllable is said to a rhythmic beat. This approach is based on the assumption that reducing the linguistic stress in turn reduces the load on one's speech motor control system. This is particularly helpful in CWS whose system otherwise is prone to get perturbed as the linguistic stress demands increase. Literature reports this technique to be effective for children as young as 3-5 years of age (Trajkovski et al., 2009, 2011). In their study, they reported that the post treatment CWS achieved <2% dysfluencies which reduced to 0.2% SS on a follow-up evaluation after 12 months. In another recent investigation by Andrew and colleagues (2016) in school age CWS, it was found that the dysfluencies reduced significantly to 2.5% SS from a pre-treatment percentage of 8.4. They also conducted two follow-up evaluations at 6 months and 12 months respectively where they found that a constant of 1.9% SS was maintained.
- **Lidcombe Program (Jones et al., 2005):** It is a parent delivered early intervention program based on the principles of operant conditioning. It uses verbal contingencies for both stutter and stutter-free responses. It has two phases. Phase I is the establishment phase where parents visit clinic on a weekly basis and carry out the therapy session. Clinician acts like a passive observer and provides feedback and suggestions at the end of each session. The second phase is the maintenance phase where the frequency of clinic visits is reduced. The outcome measures included in this program are %SS, severity ratings by parents and clinicians, and stutters per minute of speaking time (SMST).

Lidcombe program is one of the most popular early intervention programs in the present era which has a strong evidence base documented in three phases. Phase I was preliminary investigation evaluating the efficacy of a new treatment approach. Phase II took a leap and included larger sample size and investigated the likelihood and relative size of a treatment effect. Phase III included the randomized controlled trials. The program is designed specifically for preschool children and is found to be effective in reducing stuttering in them (Harris et al., 2002; Jones et al., 2008; Latterman et al., 2008; Miller and Guitar, 2009; O'Brian et al., 2013; Guitar et al., 2015, and Bridgman et al., 2016).

In most of these studies, improvement seen was found to be maintained even on follow-up after 12 months. Another study included school age children and found a significant reduction in dysfluencies from 9.2% SS during pre-treatment assessment to 1.9% SS on follow-up assessment (Koushik et al., 2009). Further, overcoming the challenge of speech therapy services limited to few geographical locations, tele-health delivery of treatment has been introduced. Two studies in this regard have shown significant evidence with respect to effectiveness of program through distant mode (Wilson et al., 2004; Lewis et al., 2008). The program is also found to be effective even when delivered as group therapy (Arnott et al., 2014). They reported that children in the group therapy session needed only 9.2 hours

Figure 2. Illustration of Direct treatment – Lidcombe program. Figure (a) Mother-child interaction in clinic session with clinician as passive observer; (b) Mother-child in a structured conversation at home; and (c) Mother-child in an unstructured conversation at home.

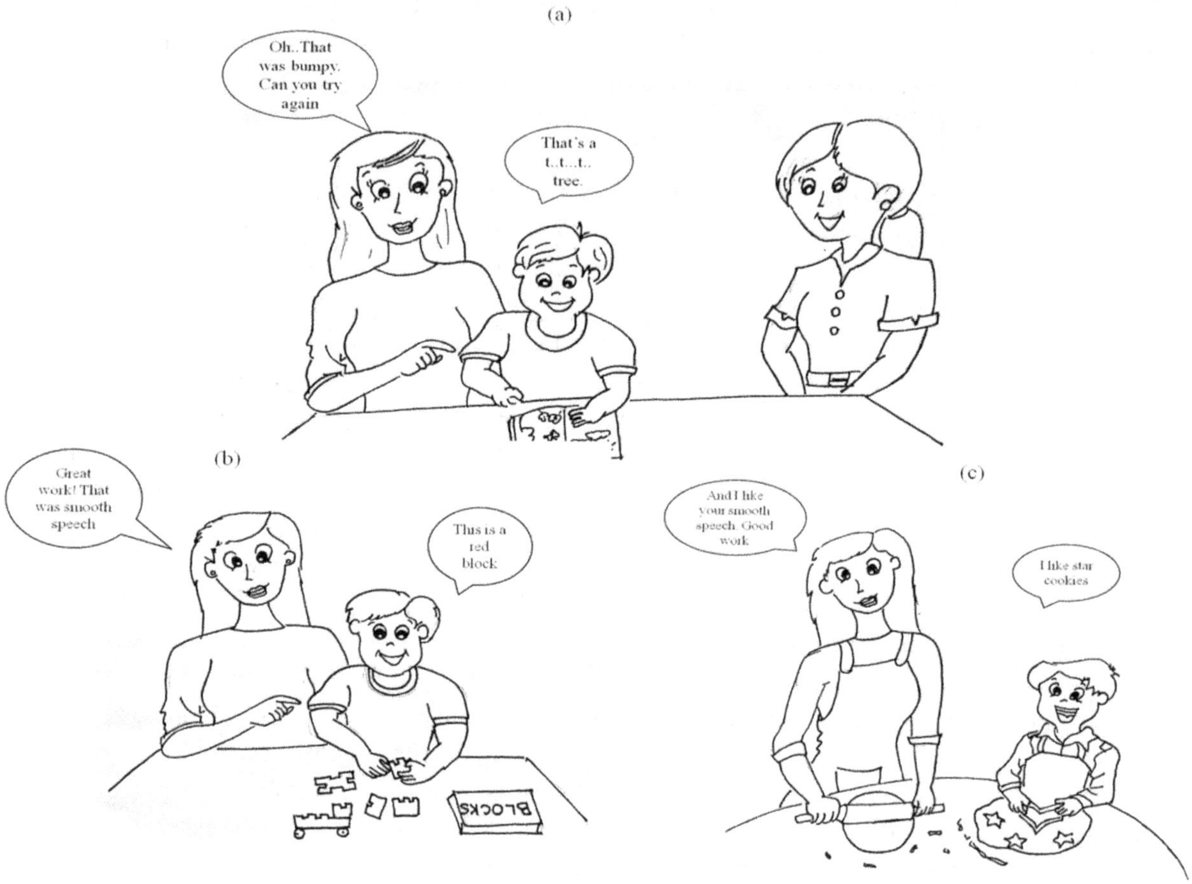
(a)
Oh..That was bumpy. Can you try again
That's a t..t..t.. tree.
(b)
Great work! That was smooth speech
This is a red block
(c)
And I like your smooth speech. Good work
I like star cookies

to enter the maintenance phase when compared to children receiving individual session who took 14.3 hours to achieve the same. The two groups were equivocal in terms of their fluency scores on a 9-month follow up. Apart from group design, single subject case studies are also reported in literature and the findings are in consensus with other studies (Wilson et al., 2008; Bakhtiar and Packman, 2009; Vong, Wilson, and Lincoln, 2016). In a recent meta-analysis of randomized controlled evidence for the treatment (Onslow, Jones, Menzies, O'Brian, and Packman, 2012) it was found that, those who received the Lidcombe Program treatment had 7.5 times the odds of recovering from stuttering at 9 months compared with those who received no treatment.

DISCUSSION

A total of twenty seven studies were identified and included in the present review. It is observed that the last few decades provide substantial evidence supporting early intervention of CWS. Further, early intervention has brought significant reduction in the stuttering of CWS with changes being maintained even on long-term follow ups. It is also observed that the associated psycho-social problems also tend to reduce and have a relatively lesser impact on quality of life in case of early intervention. Thus, this review reiterates and strongly recommends early intervention for better outcomes.

It is also noted that direct approach has significantly stronger literature support and evidence base in contrast to the indirect approach (Refer to Figure 1). Considering the strong support for direct approaches one might assume that direct approach is more effective than the indirect approach. One should do a critical analysis of the available evidence before making any concrete assumptions. It is true that only a handful of studies have explored the potential of indirect treatment approach, but this small constellation of research investigations has shown promising outcomes (Franken et al., 2005; de Sonneville-Koedoot et al., 2015; Millard et al., 2008, 2009). It is understood that indirect approaches are more flexible and less structured in comparison to the direct approach. This flexibility allows the parents and/or caregivers and the children themselves to be at ease, and helps reduce the linguistic and cognitive load on the child. Among the indirect approaches PCI and DCM were found to be the popular intervention programs. Both these programs are similar in several aspects. PCI focuses on promoting and modifying the aspects of interaction between the parent and the child while in DCM parent-child interaction is only a component. Both the programs are reported to be helpful in facilitating fluency in CWS, but due to the involvement of multiple components, what exactly leads to reduction of stuttering remains unclear (Sawyer et al., 2017).

In contrast to the indirect approaches, growing body of literature is observed for direct treatment approach. But even among the direct approaches, it was seen that few intervention programs have significant number of research studies to support their validity (for example Lidcombe program), while few others have received very less attention. Not all treatment programs have received the same amount of scrutiny, however this does not warrant the efficiency of these approaches. Some of the approaches haven't been successful to draw the attention of speech scientists but are highly recommended in textbooks and clinical anecdotes. One such approach is Response Cost treatment based on the principles of operant conditioning which is highly recommended and practiced by clinicians all over the world. If these approaches need to be promoted on a larger scale and recommended under the banner of evidence based practice, future research needs to certify the effectiveness of these. Only a few studies have followed up CWS for greater than 12 months duration. Even though a vast body of literature exists on treatment based investigations in persons who stutter (PWS), there is limited evidence on the efficacy and long-term outcomes of these intervention approaches, especially in CWS. Moreover, RCT will provide a clear insight into the effectiveness of these approaches. Thus, there is a need for future investigations with stronger research designs and long-term follow-ups to increase the credibility of the intervention.

Though the need for an early and intensive intervention program is realized, few challenges are still faced. In developing countries like India, still the number of children who need intervention is much higher than the number of clinicians. Further, speech-language therapy services are concentrated in few major cities/towns. There is still a major group of children who are not able to avail these services, especially for a longer duration. In such cases, the indirect approaches offer brighter avenues wherein parents can be trained to monitor and practice techniques at home with weekly or monthly clinic visits. As mentioned earlier, some of the researchers have investigated the efficacy of telehealth delivery of Lidcombe program and found it to be equally effective. The telehealth delivery of intervention not only overcomes the barriers of geographically restricted services but also is cost-effective. With the continual advancement in the networking technology and the widespread use of smartphones and laptops, this

Figure 3. Proportion of direct and indirect treatment approaches among the 27 studies reported in the present review

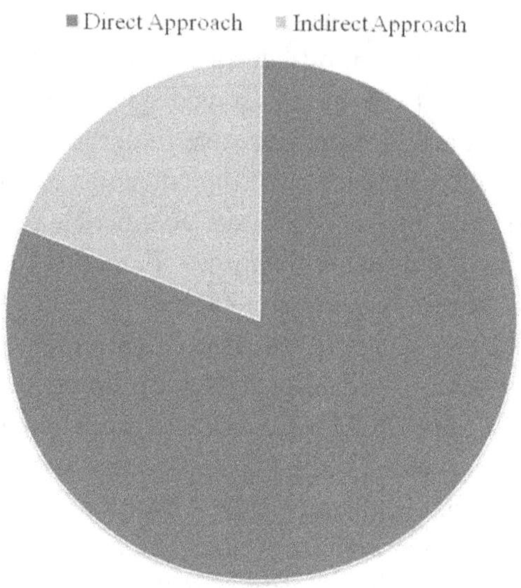

mode of intervention is believed to have a strong potential. Thus, future research investigating efficacy of other approaches or interventions delivered through this mode would unravel their effectiveness.

Another important observation made was that significant amount of attention is given to few specific outcome variables, whereas few others are often not incorporated. The most commonly used outcome measures in the studies included in the present review include %SS and SPM. Though these are the essential measures, these aren't the sole ways to assess a child's speech. Some of the intervention programs like Lidcombe use daily severity rating by both parents and clinicians which has proved to be an efficient measure and it help improve parents' understanding of their child's speech and instil confidence in them to manage their child's stuttering better. In addition few others have included measures like parent satisfaction, impact of stuttering and attitude of CWS and others. To reiterate from the literature, stuttering is said to lead to several psycho-social problems for CWS as early as preschool age. Still limited evidence base exists for any pre- and post-treatment changes in these factors. Thus, it is recommended to include %SS, SR, SPM, and naturalness rating as core outcome measures. In addition to these, inclusion of some social parameters like quality of life (QoL), self and perception/attitude of others towards the speech of CWS, personality characteristics of CWS, and the impact of stuttering on the CWS and their family, as outcome measures would strengthen the evidence base. These would also help combat psycho-social challenges and improve quality of life both for CWS and their families.

Accessibility of evidence base to all practicing clinicians is another issue of concern. If clinicians are to employ principles of evidence base practice to select appropriate intervention approach for CWS, it is essential for them to have access to empirical data of clinical outcomes. More efforts are needed to improve the accessibility of such data.

Further it is observed that there are only a handful of studies investigating the effect of bi-/multilingualism on stuttering, with most of them considering AWS as subjects. However, the estimated population of bilinguals in the world is approximately 50% (Grosjean, 2010) and it is found that approximately 1%

of the world's population has stuttering (Bloodstein and Ratner, 2008). Considering the changing trend of developmental milestones, neuroplasticity and the ability of young children to acquire new languages rapidly and with greater proficiency when compared to adults, it will be interesting to study multilingual issues in these young individuals. Investigating the effect of treatment in different languages and comparison across languages will be essential in decision making and selecting the target language(s) for intervention in case of bi-/multilingual CWS. Research investigations on these lines especially in CWS are suggested to enhance our understanding of this multi-faceted disorder.

SUMMARY AND CONCLUSION

The review of literature has proven early intervention as a boon for CWS. Both direct and indirect treatment approaches have proven their potential. However, not all techniques have received same amount of attention. On one hand techniques like Lidcombe program, Syllable timed speech and PCIT have been repeatedly subjected to scrutiny while on the other, techniques like Response Cost, Fluency Rules Program and many others are yet to be explored for their credibility. A lack of longitudinal studies, randomised controlled trials and long-term follow ups is also observed. It is believed that RCT with long-term follow-ups and greater sample size would provide a better insight into the nature and recovery pattern of the disorder. In addition, practicing clinicians need to be encouraged to have more systematic documentation and these clinical reports can be a major source of "practice-based evidence".

Though there is a consensus about early intervention for stuttering, there are several barriers preventing this. These include lack of services in all cities/towns, lesser clinicians in proportion to the children in the need of therapy/intervention and working parents unable to attend regular therapy sessions. It is suggested that in this era of advanced science and technology, telehealth delivery of intervention services would prove to be a boon to overcome these barriers. However, evidence base for the effectiveness of these services is limited and hence is recommended as future goals.

Another major issue has been the accountability of the intervention. Selection of adequate and appropriate outcome variables is essential to determine the efficacy of any treatment program/technique. Inclusion of %SS, SPM, SR and naturalness rating as core behaviours and other social parameters like QoL, attitude and impact of stuttering on CWS and their families as secondary outcomes will provide a holistic view. Further it will be interesting to explore the stuttering characteristics, response to intervention and prognosis in monolingual versus bi-/multilingual children. It is also suggested that cultural adaptations of the techniques and intervention programs should be implemented and investigated for any differences in the outcome measures in comparison to the standard form.

In the light of several issues and factors associated with intervention one should remember that any one specific approach or technique can never include or manage all aspects of treatment. Moreover, even a technique with a strong evidence base might not be able to cater to the needs of all CWS. A clinician needs to understand the evidence base practice and consider it to be a starting point that would help them to shape their own approach and practice.

REFERENCES

Andrews, C., O'Brian, S., Onslow, M., Packman, A., Menzies, R., & Lowe, R. (2016). Phase II trial of a syllable-timed speech treatment for school-age children who stutter. *Journal of Fluency Disorders*, *48*, 44–55. doi:10.1016/j.jfludis.2016.06.001 PMID:27498894

Andrews, G., & Harris, M. (1964). *The syndrome of stuttering: Clinics in developmental medicine*. London: Spastics Society Medical Education and Information Unit in association with Heinemann Medical Books.

Arnott, S., Onslow, M., O'Brian, S., Packman, A., Jones, M., & Block, S. (2014). Group Lidcombe program treatment for early stuttering: A randomized controlled trial. *Journal of Speech, Language, and Hearing Research: JSLHR*, *57*(5), 1606–1618. doi:10.1044/2014_JSLHR-S-13-0090 PMID:24824991

Azrin, N. H., & Nunn, R. G. (1974). A rapid method of eliminating stuttering by a regulated breathing approach. *Behaviour Research and Therapy*, *12*(4), 279–286. doi:10.1016/0005-7967(74)90002-3 PMID:4447567

Bakhtiar, M., & Packman, A. (2009). Intervention with the Lidcombe Program for a bilingual school-age child who stutters in Iran. *Folia Phoniatrica et Logopaedica*, *61*(5), 300–304. doi:10.1159/000241880 PMID:19786790

Bernstein-Ratner, N., & Silverman, S. (2000). Parental perceptions of children's communicative development at stuttering onset. *Journal of Speech, Language, and Hearing Research: JSLHR*, *43*(5), 1252–1263. doi:10.1044/jslhr.4305.1252 PMID:11063245

Blood, G. W., & Blood, I. M. (2004). Bullying in adolescents who stutter: Communicative competence and self-esteem. *Contemporary Issues in Communication Science and Disorders*, *31*, 69–79.

Blood, G. W., & Blood, I. M. (2007). Preliminary study of self-reported experience of physical aggression and bullying of boys who stutter: Relation to increased anxiety. *Perceptual and Motor Skills*, *104*(3suppl), 1060–1066. doi:10.2466/PMS.104.3.1060-1066 PMID:17879638

Bloodstein, O. (1975). Stuttering as tension and fragmentation. In J. Eisenson (Ed.), *Stuttering: A second symposium* (pp. 1-96). New York: Harper and Row.

Bloodstein, O. (1981). *A Handbook on Stuttering*. Chicago: The National Easter Seal Society.

Bloodstein, O., & Ratner, N. B. (2008). *A Handbook on Stuttering*. Clifton Park, NY: Delmar Cengage Learning.

Bridgman, K., Onslow, M., O'Brian, S., Jones, M., & Block, S. (2016). Lidcombe program webcam treatment for early stuttering: A randomized controlled trial. *Journal of Speech, Language, and Hearing Research: JSLHR*, *59*(5), 932–939. doi:10.1044/2016_JSLHR-S-15-0011 PMID:27617680

Brown, S. (1949). Advising parents of early stutterers. *Pediatrics*, *4*(2), 170–175. PMID:18137839

Bryngelson, B. (1938). Prognosis of stuttering. *The Journal of Speech Disorders*, *3*(2), 121–123. doi:10.1044/jshd.0302.121

Clark, C. E., Conture, E. G., Frankel, C. B., & Walden, T. A. (2012). Communicative and psychological dimensions of the KiddyCAT. *Journal of Communication Disorders*, *45*(3), 223–234. doi:10.1016/j.jcomdis.2012.01.002 PMID:22333753

Conture, E. G. (1991). Young stutterers' speech production: A critical review. In H. F. M. Peters, W. Hulstijn, & C. W. Starkweather (Eds.), *Speech motor control and stuttering* (pp. 365–384). Amsterdam: Elsevier/Excerpta Medica.

Conture, E. G. (2001). *Stuttering: Its nature, diagnosis, and treatment.* Boston, MA: Allyn and Bacon.

Coppola, V. A., & Yairi, E. (1982). Rhythmic speech training with preschool stuttering children: An experimental study. *Journal of Fluency Disorders*, *7*(4), 447–457. doi:10.1016/0094-730X(82)90020-1

Craig, A., Hancock, K., Tran, Y., Craig, M., & Peters, K. (2002). Epidemiology of stuttering in the community across the entire life span. *Journal of Speech, Language, and Hearing Research: JSLHR*, *45*(6), 1097–1206. doi:10.1044/1092-4388(2002/088) PMID:12546480

Culp, D. M. (1984). The preschool fluency development program: Assessment and treatment. In M. Peins (Ed.), *Contemporary approaches in stuttering therapy* (pp. 39–72). Boston: Little, Brown.

Davis, S., Howell, P., & Cooke, F. (2002). Sociodynamic relationships between children who stutter and their non-stuttering classmates. *Journal of Child Psychology and Psychiatry, and Allied Disciplines*, *43*(7), 939–947. doi:10.1111/1469-7610.00093 PMID:12405481

de Sonneville-Koedoot, C., Adams, S. A., Stolk, E. A., & Franken, M. C. (2015). Perspectives of clinicians involved in the RESTART-Study: Outcomes of a focus group. *American Journal of Speech-Language Pathology*, *24*(4), 708–716. doi:10.1044/2015_AJSLP-14-0215 PMID:26363127

de Sonneville-Koedoot, C., Stolk, E., Rietveld, T., & Franken, M. C. (2015). Direct versus indirect treatment for preschool children who stutter: The RESTART randomized trial. *PLoS One*, *10*(7), e0133758. doi:10.1371/journal.pone.0133758 PMID:26218228

Embrechts, M., Ebben, H., Franke, P., & van de Poel, C. (2000). Temperament: A comparison between children who stutter and children who do not stutter. In H. G. Bosshardt, J. S. Yaruss, & H. F. M. Peters (Eds.), *Proceedings of the 3rd World congress on fluency disorders, in Nyborg, Denmark* (pp. 557–562). Nijmegen, The Netherlands: Nijmegen University Press.

Emil-Behnke, K. (1947). *Stammering: Its nature, causes, and treatment.* London: Williams and Norgate.

Evans, D., Healey, E. C., Kawai, N., & Rowland, S. (2008). Middle school students' perceptions of a peer who stutters. *Journal of Fluency Disorders*, *33*(3), 203–219. doi:10.1016/j.jfludis.2008.06.002 PMID:18762062

Fowlie, G. M., & Cooper, E. B. (1978). Traits attributed to stuttering and non-stuttering children by their mothers. *Journal of Fluency Disorders*, *3*(4), 233–246. doi:10.1016/0094-730X(78)90023-2

Franken, M. C., Kielstra-Van der Schalk, C. J., & Boelens, H. (2005). Experimental treatment of early stuttering: A preliminary study. *Journal of Fluency Disorders*, *30*(3), 189–199. doi:10.1016/j.jfludis.2005.05.002 PMID:16023710

Geetha, Y. V., Mahesh, S., & Swathy, A. (2015). AIISH Survey of Fluency Disorders. Unpublished Project funded by AIISH Research Fund, Mysuru.

Glasner, P. (1949). Personality characteristics and emotional problems in stutterers under the age of five. *The Journal of Speech and Hearing Disorders*, *14*(2), 135–138. doi:10.1044/jshd.1402.135 PMID:18144389

Glauber, P. (1958). Stuttering and personality dynamics. In J. Eisenson (Ed.), *Stuttering: A symposium* (pp. 71–120). New York, NY: Harper and Row.

Gregory, H. H., Campbell, J. H., Gregory, C. B., & Hill, D. G. (2003). *Stuttering therapy: Rationale and procedures*. Boston, MA: Allyn and Bacon.

Grosjean, H. (2010). *Bilingual: Life and reality*. Cambridge, MA: Harvard University Press. doi:10.4159/9780674056459

Guitar, B. (1998). *Stuttering: An integrated approach to its nature and treatment*. Baltimore, MD: Williams and Wilkins.

Guitar, B. (2014). *Stuttering- An integrated approach to its nature and treatment* (4th ed.). Baltimore, MD: Lippincott Williams and Wilkins.

Guitar, B., Kazenski, D., Howard, A., Cousins, S. F., Fader, E., & Haskell, P. (2015). Predicting treatment time and long-term outcome of the Lidcombe program: A replication and reanalysis. *American Journal of Speech-Language Pathology, 24*(3), 533–544. doi:10.1044/2015_AJSLP-13-0156 PMID:26125134

Guttormsen, L. S., Kefalianos, E., & Naess, K. B. (2015). Communication attitudes in children who stutter: A meta-analytic review. *Journal of Fluency Disorders, 46*, 1–14. doi:10.1016/j.jfludis.2015.08.001 PMID:26365773

Harris, V., Onslow, M., Packman, A., Harrison, E., & Menzies, R. (2002). An experimental investigation of the impact of the Lidcombe program on early stuttering. *Journal of Fluency Disorders, 27*(3), 203–214. doi:10.1016/S0094-730X(02)00127-4 PMID:12371348

Hartford, E., & Leahy, M. M. (2007). The perceptions of primary school children of a person who stutters. In J. Au-Yeung, & M. M. Leahy (Eds.), *Proceedings of the 5th world congress on fluency disorders* (pp. 223–229). Dublin, Ireland: The International Fluency Association.

Hasbrouck, J. M., Doherty, J., Mehlman, M. A., Nelson, R., Randle, B., & Whitaker, R. (1987). Intensive stuttering therapy in a public school setting. *Language, Speech, and Hearing Services in Schools, 18*(4), 330–343. doi:10.1044/0161-1461.1804.330

Hawker, D. S., & Bolton, M. J. (2000). Twenty years' research on peer victimization and psychosocial maladjustment: A meta-analytic review of cross-sectional studies. *Journal of Child Psychology and Psychiatry, and Allied Disciplines, 41*(4), 441–455. doi:10.1111/1469-7610.00629 PMID:10836674

Howell, P., Davis, S., Patel, H., Cuniffe, P., Downing-Wilson, D., Au-Yeung, J., . . . Peters, H. F. M. (2004). Fluency development and temperament in fluent children and children who stutter. In A. Packman, A. Meltzer, and H. F. Peters (Eds.), *Theory, research and therapy in fluency disorders. Proceedings of the 4th world congress on fluency disorders* (pp. 250–256). Montreal, Canada: Nijmegen University Press.

Hugh-Jones, S., & Smith, P. K. (1999). Self-reports of short- and long-term effects of bullying on children who stammer. *The British Journal of Educational Psychology, 69*(2), 141–158. doi:10.1348/000709999157626 PMID:10405616

Iverach, L., & Rapee, R. (2014). Social anxiety disorder and stuttering: Current status and future directions. *Journal of Fluency Disorders, 40*, 69–82. doi:10.1016/j.jfludis.2013.08.003 PMID:24929468

Johnson, K., Walden, T., Conture, E., & Karrass, J. (2010). Spontaneous regulation of emotions in preschool-age children who stutter: Preliminary findings. *Journal of Speech, Language, and Hearing Research: JSLHR*, *53*(6), 1478–1495. doi:10.1044/1092-4388(2010/08-0150) PMID:20643793

Johnson, W. (1934). *Stuttering in the preschool child (Child Welfare Pamphlets No. 37)*. Iowa City, IA: University of Iowa.

Johnson, W. (1942). A study of onset and development of stuttering. *The Journal of Speech Disorders*, *7*(3), 251–257. doi:10.1044/jshd.0703.251

Johnson, W. (1948). Stuttering. In W. Johnson, S. Brown, J. Curtis, C. Edney, & J. Keaster (Eds.), *Speech handicapped school children*. New York, NY: Harper and Row.

Johnson, W., & ... (1959). *The onset of stuttering: Research findings and implications*. Minneapolis, MN: University of Minnesota.

Jones, M., Onslow, M., Packman, A., O'Brian, S., Hearne, A., Williams, S., ... Schwarz, I. (2008). Extended follow up of a randomized controlled trial of the Licombe program of early stuttering intervention. *International Journal of Language & Communication Disorders*, *43*(6), 649–661. doi:10.1080/13682820801895599 PMID:18608610

Jones, M., Onslow, M., Packman, A., Williams, S., Ormond, T., Schwarz, I., & Gebski, V. (2005). Randomised controlled trial of the Lidcombe Programme of Early Stuttering Intervention. *British Medical Journal*, *331*(7518), 659–661. doi:10.1136/bmj.38520.451840.E0 PMID:16096286

Jones-Prus, D. (1980). Training fluency as a motor skill in the treatment of dysfluent children. *Human Communication*, *5*, 75–86.

Kawai, N., Healey, E. C., Nagasawa, T., & Vanryckeghem, M. (2012). Communication attitudes of Japanese school-age children who stutter. *Journal of Communication Disorders*, *45*(5), 348–354. doi:10.1016/j.jcomdis.2012.05.004 PMID:22796115

Kelman, E., & Nicholas, A. (2008). *Practical intervention for early childhood stammering: Palin PCI Approach*. Milton Keynes, UK: Speechmark Publishing.

Kingdon-Ward, W. (1941). Stammering. London: Hamilton.

Koushik, S., Shenker, R., & Onslow, M. (2009). Follow-up of 6-10 year old stuttering children after Lidcombe Program treatment: A Phase I trial. *Journal of Fluency Disorders*, *34*(4), 279–290. doi:10.1016/j.jfludis.2009.11.001 PMID:20113771

Kully, D., & Boberg, E. (1991). Therapy for school-age children. *Seminars in Speech and Language*, *12*(4), 291–300. doi:10.1055-2008-1064230

Langevin, M., & Hagler, P. (2004). Development of a scale to measure peer attitudes toward children who stutter. In A. K. Bothe (Ed.), *Evidence-based treatment of stuttering: Empirical bases and clinical applications* (pp. 139–170). Mahwah, NJ: Erlbaum.

Langevin, M., Packman, A., & Onslow, M. (2009). Peer responses to stuttering in the preschool setting. *American Journal of Speech-Language Pathology*, *18*(3), 264–276. doi:10.1044/1058-0360(2009/07-0087) PMID:19332523

Langevin, M., Packman, A., & Onslow, M. (2010). Parent perceptions of the impact of stuttering on their preschoolers and themselves. *Journal of Communication Disorders*, *43*(5), 407–423. doi:10.1016/j.jcomdis.2010.05.003 PMID:20599207

Latterman, C., Euler, H. A., & Neumann, K. (2008). A randomized control trial to investigate the impact of the Lidcombe program on early stuttering in German-speaking preschoolers. *Journal of Fluency Disorders*, *33*(1), 52–65. doi:10.1016/j.jfludis.2007.12.002 PMID:18280869

Lewis, C., Packman, A., Onslow, M., Simpson, J. A., & Jones, M. (2008). A Phase II trial of telehealth delivery of the Lidcombe Program of Early Stuttering Intervention. *American Journal of Speech-Language Pathology*, *17*(2), 139–149. doi:10.1044/1058-0360(2008/014) PMID:18448601

Lincoln, M., Onslow, M., Lewis, C., & Wilson, L. (1996). A clinical trial of an operant treatment for school-age children who stutter. *American Journal of Speech-Language Pathology*, *5*(2), 73–85. doi:10.1044/1058-0360.0502.73

Marland, P. (1957). Shadowing: A contribution to the treatment of stuttering. *Folia Phoniatrica*, *9*(4), 242–245. doi:10.1159/000262784 PMID:13480408

McAllister, J. (2016). Behavioural, emotional and social development of children who stutter. *Journal of Fluency Disorders*, *50*, 23–32. doi:10.1016/j.jfludis.2016.09.003 PMID:27865227

Millard, S. K., Edwards, S., & Cook, F. M. (2009). Parent-child interaction therapy: Adding to the evidence. *International Journal of Speech-Language Pathology*, *11*(1), 61–76. doi:10.1080/17549500802603895

Millard, S. K., Nicholas, A., & Cook, F. M. (2008). Is parent-child interaction therapy effective in reducing stuttering? *Journal of Speech, Language, and Hearing Research: JSLHR*, *51*(3), 636–650. doi:10.1044/1092-4388(2008/046) PMID:18506041

Miller, B., & Guitar, B. (2009). Long-term outcome of the Lidcombe program for early stuttering intervention. *American Journal of Speech-Language Pathology*, *18*(1), 42–49. doi:10.1044/1058-0360(2008/06-0069) PMID:18845699

Mooney, S., & Smith, P. K. (1995). Bullying and the child who stammers. *British Journal of Special Education*, *22*(1), 24–27. doi:10.1111/j.1467-8578.1995.tb00907.x

O'Brian, S., Iverach, L., Jones, M., Onslow, M., Packman, A., & Menzies, R. (2013). Effectiveness of the Lidcombe program for early stuttering in Australian communities clinics. *International Journal of Speech-Language Pathology*, *15*(6), 593–603. doi:10.3109/17549507.2013.783112 PMID:23691980

Onslow, M., Andrews, C., & Lincoln, M. (1994). A control/experimental trial of an operant treatment for early stuttering. *Journal of Speech, Language, and Hearing Research: JSLHR*, *37*(6), 1244–1259. doi:10.1044/jshr.3706.1244 PMID:7877284

Onslow, M., Attanasio, J., & Harrison, E. (2003). Parents talk about the Lidcombe Program. In M. Onslow, A. Packman, & E. Harrison (Eds.), *The Lidcombe Program of early stuttering intervention: A clinician's guide* (pp. 193–206). Austin, TX: Pro-Ed.

Onslow, M., Jones, M., Menzies, R., O'Brian, S., & Packman, A. (2012). Stuttering. In P. Sturmey & M. Hersen (Eds.), Handbook of evidence-based practice in clinical psychology (pp. 185 – 207). Hoboken, NJ: Wiley.

Oyler, M. E. (1996). Vulnerability in stuttering children. *Dissertation Abstracts International*, *56*, 3374.

Packman, A., Onslow, M., & Attanasio, J. (2003). The timing of early intervention with the Lidcombe Program. In M. Onslow, A. Packman, & E. Harrison (Eds.), *The Lidcombe Program of early stuttering intervention: A clinician's guide* (pp. 41–55). Austin, TX: Pro-Ed.

Pichon, E., & Borel-Maisonny, S. (1937). *Stuttering, its nature and treatment*. Paris, France: Masson.

Pindzola, R. (1987). *Stuttering intervention program: Age 3 to grade 3*. Austin, TX: Pro-Ed.

Pindzola, R. (1999). *The stuttering intervention program. In The handbook of early stuttering intervention* (pp. 119–138). London: Singular Publishing Inc.

Riley, G. D., & Ingham, J. C. (2000). Acoustic duration changes associated with two types of treatment for children who stutter. *Journal of Speech, Language, and Hearing Research: JSLHR*, *43*(4), 965–978. doi:10.1044/jslhr.4304.965 PMID:11386482

Riley, G. D., & Riley, J. (1984). A component model for treating stuttering in children. In M. Peins (Ed.), *Contemporary approaches in stuttering therapy* (pp. 123–172). Boston: Little, Brown.

Runyan, C. M., & Runyan, S. E. (1986). A fluency rules therapy program for young children in the public schools. *Language, Speech, and Hearing Services in Schools*, *17*(4), 276–284. doi:10.1044/0161-1461.1704.276

Rustin, L., Botterill, W., & Kelman, E. (1996). *Assessment and therapy for young dysfluent children: Family interaction*. London: Whurr.

Ryan, B. P., & Ryan, B. V. K. (1983). Programmed stuttering therapy for children: Comparison of four establishment programs. *Journal of Fluency Disorders*, *8*(4), 291–321. doi:10.1016/0094-730X(83)90011-6

Ryan, B. P., & Ryan, B. V. K. (1995). Programmed stuttering treatment for children: Comparison of two establishment programs through transfer, maintenance, and follow-up. *Journal of Speech and Hearing Research*, *38*(1), 61–75. doi:10.1044/jshr.3801.61 PMID:7731220

Sawyer, J., Matteson, C., Ou, H., & Nagase, T. (2017). The effects of parent-focused slow relaxed speech intervention on articulation rate, response time latency, and fluency in preschool children who stutter. *Journal of Speech, Language, and Hearing Research: JSLHR*, *60*(4), 794–809. doi:10.1044/2016_JSLHR-S-16-0002 PMID:28289751

Schuell, H. (1949). Working with parents of stuttering children. *The Journal of Speech and Hearing Disorders*, *14*(3), 251–254. doi:10.1044/jshd.1403.251 PMID:18137760

Shine, R. E. (1984). Assessment and fluency training and the young stutterer. In M. Peins (Ed.), *Contemporary approaches in stuttering therapy* (pp. 173–216). Boston: Little, Brown.

Smith, A., & Kelly, E. (1997). Stuttering: A dynamic, multifactorial model. In R. F. Curlee & G. M. Siegel (Eds.), *Nature and treatment of stuttering: New directions* (pp. 97–127). Boston, MA: Allyn and Bacon.

Starkweather, C. (1997). Therapy for younger children. In R. F. Curlee & G. M. Siegel (Eds.), *Nature and treatment of stuttering: New directions* (pp. 257–292). Boston, MA: Allyn and Bacon.

Trajkovski, N., Andrews, C., Onslow, M., Packman, A., O'Brian, S., & Menzies, R. (2009). Using syllable-timed speech to treat preschool children who stutter: A multiple baseline experiment. *Journal of Fluency Disorders*, *34*(1), 1–10. doi:10.1016/j.jfludis.2009.01.001 PMID:19500711

Trajkovski, N., Andrews, C., Onslow, M., Packman, A., O'Brian, S., & Menzies, R. (2011). A phase II trial of the Westmead Program: Syllable-timed speech treatment for pre-school children who stutter. *International Journal of Speech-Language Pathology*, *13*(6), 500–509. doi:10.3109/17549507.2011.578660 PMID:22070727

Travis, L. E. (1931). *Speech Pathology*. New York: Appleton-Century.

Van Riper, C. (1971). *The nature of stuttering*. Englewood Cliffs, NJ: Prentice-Hall.

Van Riper, C. (1982). *The nature of stuttering* (2nd ed.). Englewood Cliffs, NJ: Prentice-Hall.

Vanryckeghem, M. (1995). The Communication Attitude Test: A concordancy investigation of stuttering and non-stuttering children and their parents. *Journal of Fluency Disorders*, *26*(2), 191–203. doi:10.1016/0094-730X(94)00021-K

Vanryckeghem, M., & Brutten, G. J. (1996). The relationship between communication attitude and fluency failure of stuttering and non-stuttering children. *Journal of Fluency Disorders*, *21*(2), 109–118. doi:10.1016/0094-730X(96)00015-0

Vanryckeghem, M., & Brutten, G. J. (2007). *Communication attitude test for preschool and kindergarten children who stutter*. San Diego, CA: Plural Publishing.

Vanryckeghem, M., Hylebos, C., Brutten, G. J., & Peleman, M. (2001). The relationship between communication attitude and emotion of children who stutter. *Journal of Fluency Disorders*, *26*(1), 1–15. doi:10.1016/S0094-730X(00)00090-5

Vanryckeghem, M., Vanrobayes, S., & De Niels, T. (2015). The KiddyCAT: A test-retest reliability investigation. *Cross-Cultural Communication*, *11*(4), 10–16.

Vong, E., Wilson, L., & Lincoln, M. (2016). The Lidcombe program of early stuttering intervention for Malaysian families: Four case studies. *Journal of Fluency Disorders*, *49*, 29–39. doi:10.1016/j.jfludis.2016.07.003 PMID:27638190

Wakaba, Y. Y. (1983). Group play therapy for Japanese children who stutter. *Journal of Fluency Disorders*, *8*(2), 93–118. doi:10.1016/0094-730X(83)90023-2

Wilson, L., Onslow, M., & Lincoln, M. (2004). Telehealth adaptation of the Lidcombe program of early stuttering intervention: Five case studies. *American Journal of Speech-Language Pathology*, *13*(1), 81–93. doi:10.1044/1058-0360(2004/009) PMID:15101816

Wingate, M. (1976). *Stuttering: Theory and treatment*. New York, NY: Wiley.

Wyatt, G. L. (1969). *Language learning and communication disorders in children*. New York: Free Press.

Yairi, E. (1983). The onset of stuttering in two- and three-year-old children: A preliminary report. *The Journal of Speech and Hearing Disorders*, *48*(2), 171–177. doi:10.1044/jshd.4802.171 PMID:6621009

Yairi, E., & Ambrose, N. (1992a). Onset of stuttering in preschool children: Selected factors. *Journal of Speech and Hearing Research*, *35*(4), 782–788. doi:10.1044/jshr.3504.782 PMID:1405533

Yairi, E., & Ambrose, N. (1992b). A longitudinal study of stuttering in children: A preliminary report. *Journal of Speech and Hearing Research*, *35*(4), 755–760. doi:10.1044/jshr.3504.755 PMID:1405530

Yairi, E., & Ambrose, N. (2005). *Early childhood suttering*. Austin, TX: Pro-Ed.

Yairi, E., & Ambrose, N. (2013). Epidemiology of stuttering: 21st century advancements. *Journal of Fluency Disorders*, *38*(2), 66–87. doi:10.1016/j.jfludis.2012.11.002 PMID:23773662

Yairi, E., & Seery, C. H. (2015). *Stuttering: Foundations and Clinical Applications* (2nd ed.). Upper Saddle River, NJ: Pearson Education, Inc.

Yaruss, J. S., Coleman, C., & Hammer, D. (2006). Treating preschool children who stutter: Description and preliminary evaluation of a family-focused treatment approach. *Language, Speech, and Hearing Services in Schools*, *37*(2), 118–136. doi:10.1044/0161-1461(2006/014) PMID:16646215

Young, E., & Hawk, S. (1955). *Moto-kinesthetic speech training*. Standford, CA: Stanford University.

Zebrowski, P., & Conture, E. G. (1998). Influence of nontreatment variables on treatment effectiveness for school age children who stutter. In A. Cordes & R. Ingham (Eds.), *Treatment efficacy for stuttering: A search for empirical bases* (pp. 293–310). San Diego, CA: Singular.

Zebrowski, P., & Kelly, E. (2002). Manual of stuttering intervention. Singular Publishing Group, Thomson Learning.

KEY TERMS AND DEFINITIONS

Blocks: A type of dysfluency where the production of a sound/syllable/word is completely seized and the articulators are fixed in a specific articulatory position.

Dysfluency: A disruption in the smooth flow/production of speech. These are of two types: stuttering like dysfluencies (SLDs), which include repetitions, prolongation, and blocks; and other dysfluencies (ODs), which include pauses, interjections, and revisions.

Efficacy: The extent to which a specific intervention, procedure, regimen, or service produces a beneficial result under ideally controlled conditions when administered or monitored by experts.

Gray Literature: Materials and research produced by organizations outside of the traditional commercial or academic publishing and distribution channels. These include reports (annual, research, technical, project, etc.), working papers, and government documents.

Intervention: It refers to the actions performed to modify behavior, emotional state, or feelings of an individual.

Outcome Measures: Variables which measure the effect of a something. In case of intervention using a specific therapy technique, it is the effect of that particular technique on an individual's behavior.

Prolongation: A type of dysfluency in which an individual prolongs/elongates/drags a specific phoneme/syllable.

Repetitions: A type of dysfluency in which an individual repeats a syllable/partial word/complete word/phrase several times disrupting the flow of speech.

Stuttering: A speech disorder characterized by disruption in smooth flow of speech.

APPENDIX: ABBREVIATIONS

AWS: Adults who stutter
CB: Criterion Based
CWNS: Children who do not stutter
CWS: Children who stutter
DAF: Delayed Auditory Feedback
DCM: Demands and Capacity Model
ELU: Extended Length of Utterance
GILCU: Gradual Increase in Length and Complexity of Utterance
HRQoL: Health-Related Quality of Life
LP: Lidcombe Program
PCIT: Parent-Child Interaction Therapy
PWS: Persons who stutter
QED: Quasi-Experimental Design
RCS: Response Contingent Stimuli
RCT: Randomised Controlled Trial
SMST: Stutters per minute of speaking time
SMT: Speech Motor Training
SPM: Syllables per minute
SR: Severity Rating
SSI-3: Stuttering Severity Instrument -3
STS: Syllable Timed Speech

Chapter 18
Manual for Adult Aphasia Therapy

S. P. Goswami
All India Institute of Speech and Hearing, India

Rachel V.
All India Institute of Speech and Hearing, India

ABSTRACT

This chapter is a treatment manual developed to aid professionals working in the field of rehabilitation of persons with aphasia in India. It is clinically field tested and has proved to be effective in the treatment of persons with fluent and non-fluent aphasia. This chapter provides a brief and comprehensive overview of the manual, information on its contents, and an outline about its use in clinical settings. The reader can also develop an understanding of how to assess baseline, document progress, and systematically record the outcomes of therapy. This chapter is a clinically invaluable therapy material for speech-language pathologists working in the country.

INTRODUCTION

Aphasia is a language disorder acquired by damage to the linguistic areas of the brain, which leads to deficits of varying degree in comprehension, expression, repetition, naming, reading and writing. It is a multimodal language disorder resulting from traumatic brain injury, brain tumour, infection, and surgical removal of brain tissue or more commonly stroke (Hallowell and Chapey, 2008). According to WHO (2012), around one-sixth of the entire population suffer stroke during their lifetime, out of which 30% have a residual language impairment (aphasia). Though aphasia is majorly a language disorder, persons with aphasia (PWA) can have associated problems in aspects of cognition, physical, emotional/ psychological, social and swallowing. Speech-Language Pathologists (SLP's) are key member in the communication rehabilitation of PWA. Aphasiologists have described number of therapy techniques and approaches towards rehabilitation of persons with aphasia, based on their views of the underlying impairment. Controlled research and treatment efficacy studies in the recent years have provided evidence towards the efficacy of the aphasia treatment techniques mentioned in the literature. Though researchers have been successful in systematically documenting the positive outcomes of the treatment efficacy studies, the variability in these research have been the stimuli used.

DOI: 10.4018/978-1-5225-4955-0.ch018

Stimuli used for language therapy of PWA form an essential material in rehabilitation. Despite the importance on understanding how stimulus used affect outcome of intervention programs, there are few relevant studies. The therapy resources available for an SLP providing rehabilitative services for PWA in India are limited if not any. Majority of them refer to studies and manuals prepared for western population. To mention a few in western context, Manual for the Aphasic Patient by Longerich (1968), An Auditory and Verbal Task Hierarchy by Ross and Spencer (1980); and Manual of Aphasia and Aphasia Therapy (third edition) by Helm-Estabrooks and Albert (2004). The dearth of resources available in the country led to the development of MAAT.

The *Manual for Adult Aphasia Therapy* (MAAT) was developed for use with Kannada speaking individuals with Aphasia, ages 18 to 89. It is a therapy manual for Speech Language Pathologists working with Persons with Aphasia (PWA), to systematically train and track the progress from baseline assessment. The manual consists of stimuli under five domains of language: Functional Communication, Comprehension and Expression, Repetition, Naming and Reading and Writing. MAAT-K is a compilation of therapy manuals: *Manual for Adult Non-Fluent Aphasia Therapy in Kannada* (MANAT-K) (Venugopal and Goswami, 2008) and *Manual for Adult Fluent Aphasia Therapy in Kannada* (MAFAT-K) (Chaitra and Goswami, 2009). These manuals focused mainly on providing materials for therapy purposes. Later, MANAT-K and MAFAT-K were modified and field tested on persons with non-fluent and fluent aphasia by Goswami, Shanbal, Navitha and Samasthitha, (2010) and Goswami, Shanbal, Chaitra and Ranjini (2011) respectively. To improve the ease towards management of people with aphasia and for commercialization, MANAT-K and MAFAT-K were combined and developed as the *Manual for Adult Aphasia Therapy in Kannada* (MAAT-K). This manual was computerized to improve ease of documentation as *Computerized Version of Manual for Adult Aphasia Therapy in Kannada (CV-MAAT K)* (Goswami, Renuka, and Kruthi 2013). This software has five major domains namely functional communication, repetition, comprehension and expression, naming and reading and writing. Each of these domains consists of graded sub-sections. They have computerized culturally relevant pictures. The scoring patterns of the manuals have been retained and are semi-automatic. This software enables the clinician mediated aphasia therapy to be carried out.

The five major domains of the MAAT-K contains sub-sections and cover a series of activities which can be carried out by the clinicians to fortify a wide range of responses from the Person with Aphasia (PWA). MAAT-K has proved to be clinically invaluable as it provides structured guidelines and materials to provide evidence-based therapy for persons with aphasia.

To improve the scope and utility of the MAAT-K, the manual is also developed in six other languages as MAAT-6 (Tamil, Telugu, Malayalam, Marathi, Hindi and English) (Goswami, Thomas, and Rachel, 2015) as a project under Department of Science and Technology at All India Institute of Speech and Hearing, Mysore. According to 2011 census report on languages in India, Hindi is considered the official language of the country, with English being the provisional official language and used widely across the country. And, along with Hindi; Tamil, Telugu, Marathi and Malayalam are among the 22 Eighth scheduled languages in the country. These languages also cover most of the regions and population across India. Therefore, therapy manuals were developed in these languages to enhance uniformity in aphasia therapy and documentation. SLP/clinicians across the country are encouraged to develop and adapt the manual in their native language to suit the needs of persons with aphasia in the region.

The clinical utility of MAAT has been established by field testing each of these individual manuals. Field testing is the process of manually administering the developed manual/ software/ protocol to check for its validity/outcome measure. In the field of communication rehabilitation, where there are number of techniques and approaches developed, and also where the characteristics of each patient with communication impairment is unique, field testing is of utmost importance as it helps to assess, if the developed material works equally well across the range of severities and domains. The outcome of field testing also helps to make necessary changes to the manuals developed, if any. A key step in the process of field testing the manual is for correct outcome prior release to its end users. MAAT has been field tested on fluent and non-fluent persons with aphasia and it is proven to be useful and effective. MAAT can be used with any standard therapy techniques available for PWA. It provides guidance for SLP's to progress through the course of rehabilitation. The use of MAAT reduces the time required for an SLP in creating a stimulus material individually for each PWA. With these field-tested manuals, SLP's can provide better and effective rehabilitation for persons with aphasia.

PURPOSE

The purpose of the *Manual for Adult Aphasia Therapy* is to provide a treatment guide for speech-language pathologists/ student clinicians working with PWA. MAAT provides a set of stimuli under five linguistic domains (Functional Communication, Comprehension and Expression, Repetition, Naming and Reading and Writing) that are affected in PWA. It enables speech-language pathologists to easily establish a baseline status of the five linguistic domains and provide therapy for the affected domain. It can be used with any severity of aphasia. The manual provides stimuli ranging in complexity and has provision to present the stimuli through different modes of communication namely, visual, auditory and orthographic modes, based on the need of PWA and severity of aphasia. The baseline assessment yields information on domain specific-strengths and weakness and provides a clear direction for the SLP to initiate therapy. The main domains of the manual are based on research and clinical evidence of linguistic impairments in PWA in these five areas of language which also differentiates the different types of aphasia. Hence, this manual covers stimuli under these language domains. The manual provides simple scoring system, which makes it easy to score responses under each category, the simplicity in scoring system allows for easy comparison and documentation across sessions. Therefore, allowing for systematic recording of progress through therapy.

RATIONALE

The manual for adult aphasia therapy is developed based on the principles of Life Participation Approach to Aphasia (LPAA; Chapey et al., 2000). This is a psychosocial and functional approach towards intervention of communication impairments in persons with aphasia. The focus of this approach is to improve functional communication for activities of daily living and to improve independent and functional living within the means and ability of an individual. The advocates of this approach encourage researchers and clinicians to focus on immediate and long-term real-life goals of PWA and their life partners/ people surrounding them and also to assist PWA to achieve active social participation. Therefore, treatment based on LPAA has to facilitate the achievement of life goals. The treatment does not view communication impairment as a barrier instead focuses on any modality through which PWA can communicate. The activities based on the approach need not be communication oriented, rather any activity that will enhance PWA participate in his/her environment.

Based on the principles of LPAA, the manual consists of ecologically valid stimuli and activities. The stimuli proposed are those that are from the functional environment of the PWA. These are words and pictures that frequently appear in daily life. As the explicit goal of this approach is to enhance the life participation, the stimuli chosen and the hierarchy in which it is arranged is in the order that it enhances the participation of the PWA in the real-life situations, irrespective of their severity. The activities in the manual are graded in difficulty level (Level I, Level II, and Level III); this allows the participation of PWA irrespective of his/her communication impairment. As mentioned in this approach, the stimuli in the manual also target the personal and the environmental factors of an individual. The first section in the manual is "functional communication". The goal of this domain is to get PWA started with some form of communication. It does not focus solely on verbal communication rather on any mode where PWA is able to communicate his/her needs. The subsections of this domain consist of activities of daily living (brushing, eating, dressing etc) and activities of independent living (bank transaction, post office, bus-stand/ railway station). Initially, clinician-assisted activities are carried out until PWA are able to execute the task independently. Once, the individual is able to perform the task successfully, the task is introduced to tasks with increasing level of difficulty. Finally, the core aim of this approach is to make the individual fully functional in the society. This is facilitated by MAAT as the domains in the manual focus on the overall areas that could be affected in PWA, including reading, writing and functional arithmetic skills.

With the overwhelming literature available on different approaches for the treatment of PWA the concern remains on the stimuli that can be used with such approaches and techniques. For research purposes, SLP's generally adopt stimuli from standard assessment tests or customize a stimulus list based on stimulus familiarity and semanticity ratings. MAAT was not developed as, nor is it recommended as, an exhaustive manual of stimulus for use with adult aphasia therapy. The treatment material can be easily customized to suit the individual needs of PWA. The therapy with MAAT should assist in the adult aphasia therapy following standard assessment procedures. As the PWA progress with therapy with the manual; SLP can modify and accommodate stimuli that are functional in the PWA's environment. The stimuli in each of the MAAT are based on the rating on 20 parameters consisting of 5 point rating scale (adapted from Field testing of MANAT-K, Goswami, et al., 2010) by 10 SLP's who are also native speakers of the language. The stimuli in MAAT are clear and culturally appropriate colour pictures painted by a professional artist. This enhances the ecological validity of the stimulus manual. The word stimuli are in the form of black and white cards.

MAAT is appropriate for Kannada, English, Hindi, Malayalam, Marathi, Tamil or Telugu speaking adults with aphasia as a result of stroke, traumatic brain injury or dementia in the age range of 18-89 years. The complete kit consists of

- **The Therapy Manual:** The manual provides directions for administering and presenting stimuli, scoring and evaluation percentage of improvement. It provides progression criteria for introducing each language domain in order to obtain optimum results.
- **5 Booklets:** Three booklets with pictures and two booklets with letters/ words (Booklets 1, 2, 3, 4, 5). Booklets 1, 2 and 3 contain picture stimuli related to Functional Communication, Comprehension and Expression and Naming domains; Booklets 4 and 5 are word booklets for Repetition and Reading and Writing domain.
- Treatment recording sheets.
- Overall communication Profile analysis form.

LINGUISTIC DOMAINS OF MAAT

Aphasia can be severe to an extent that a PWA finds it difficult to communicate their basic needs or it might be mild. It can cause difficulties in comprehension of language, affect expressive speech, lead to impairment of word retrieval in speech, in some it might compromise the ability to read or write. However, in most cases, aphasia affects more than one aspect of communication, while less severely affected channel is accessible for limited communication exchange. It is in the hands of a speech-language pathologist to assess the functional residue in each domain and undermine the communication impairments in PWA. The goal of intervention is to help PWA maximize the quality of life through the compensatory use of communication strength in one domain to de-block impairment in other channels of communication. Below is a brief description of the domains and sub-sections of MAAT.

1. Functional communication (FC)
2. Repetition (R)
3. Comprehension and expression(C and E)
4. Naming (N)
5. Reading and writing (RandW)

Each of these domains is further sub-divided into several sub-sections. As these five linguistic domains form the core areas affected in persons with aphasia, the stimuli in MAAT are sectioned in these domains.

Functional Communication

Functional communication is the ability to successfully communicate a message via spoken, written or through non-verbal modality. It helps to communicate basic needs. The initial goal in the rehabilitation of PWA is to achieve functional communication. Difficulties in communication can impinge on a person's participation in the society and lead to social isolation, mental and emotional changes, problems in adjustments of interpersonal relations, lack of independence and return to their workplace (Cruice, Worrall, Murison, and Hickson, 2003). Activities of daily living and activities of independence form an essential part of functional communication in PWA as it prepares him/her to face real-life situations with minimal assistance. Treatment of PWA should focus on bridging the language skills and adaptations into the real-life needs (La Pointe, 2005).

From a socio-linguistic perspective, functional communication is an important aspect of communication. Functional communication is one of the initial goals of language intervention in PWA. After baseline assessment, it is imperative to work on functional communication skills, unless the level of functional communication is sufficiently good to carry out communication and function independently. In this domain, aspects related to daily living such as nouns, common verbs which are basic and applicable in day-to-day life are included. The eight aspects covered under functional skills are:

1. Responding to own name
2. Recognition of family members
3. Recognition of familiar objects
4. Comprehension of simple verbal commands
5. Comprehension of action verbs

6. Functional verbal language
7. Activities of Daily Living (ADL)
8. Activities of independent living (AOI)

The stimuli are presented via combination of auditory and gestural mode or through auditory mode alone, based on the condition of the PWA. Even a head nod, eye blink or gestures are acceptable responses as the goal is to get the person with aphasia to communicate. Therefore, this domain uses total communication strategies where every accessible means of communication by PWA are used to convey the message. This increases the communicative competence and confidence of PWA. As the PWA starts to show progress in communicating, the goal of intervention is increased in difficulty level in order to achieve verbal responses if it is within the purview of the individual's ability.

The stimuli in this domain can be used with any aphasia intervention technique that focuses on improving functional communication. For example: Promoting Aphasic's Communicative Effectiveness (PACE) by Davis and Wilcox (1991) where the main focus is on the mode through which the information is conveyed and not on the accuracy of information content. The clinician and the PWA equally participate as senders and receivers of new information.

Repetition

Repetition refers to the ability to reproduce elements of speech sounds after an auditory presentation. It is the most elementary mechanism at the core of spoken language. Goodglass and Kaplan (1983) reported that repetition in PWA could be affected at any of the three points in the process: at the level of recognition, may fail to grasp sounds as words; at the level of articulation in spite of demonstrating that the person knows the meaning of the word; failure due to selective dissociation between auditory input and speech output. Therefore, some aspect of repetition is usually affected in all aphasic groups. While it is preserved in persons with anomic aphasia, it is affected in persons with Broca's aphasia, Wernicke's Aphasia, Global Aphasia. Difficulty in repetition is the most striking characteristic feature of persons with conduction aphasia, while their comprehension and expression is preserved when compared to other types of aphasia. Whereas, persons with trans-cortical sensory and trans-cortical motor aphasia have parrot-like repetition skills where, though repetition is preserved, comprehension of repeated word/phrase is impaired. Therefore, repetition of language is one skill which needs to be worked on in most PWA.

The manual provides stimuli to work on production of a range of repetition tasks. This domain aims at improving the repetition abilities of PWA at word and sentence level. The subsections of this domain are:

1. Equivocal response
2. Automatic speech
3. Egocentric stimuli
4. Environmental stimuli
5. Phrases

The hierarchical arrangement of stimuli in this domain assists in a stepwise improvement of repetition skills in PWA. Starting with equivocal response where, the clinician and the PWA articulate the word together and gradually the clinician fades off. Automatic speech is the production of word sequences which are produced with least cognitive stress. It is the simplest form of repetition of over-learnt sequences (days of the week, months of year, alphabets etc); it is usually preserved in most PWA, if it is not; it is easier for the PWA to repeat such sequence. This in-turn motivates PWA and provides a positive outlook towards prognosis of his/her communication skills. The sub-sections of egocentric stimuli, environmental stimuli and repetition of phrases consists of stimuli that are most frequently produced in everyday communication, it also consists of sentences with increasing mean length of utterance. This enables the clinicians/ SLPs to systematically work on improving repetition skills in PWA.

Initially, the stimuli are presented through combination of auditory and graphic modality. As the person improves through this mode, the graphic stimuli are removed and the PWA is expected to carry out repetition tasks with auditory presentation of stimuli. The stimuli in this domain can be used with aphasia therapy techniques that utilize repetition as their core component, example: Melodic Intonation Therapy (Albert, Sparks, and Helm, 1973), Response Elaboration Task (Kearns, 1985) etc.

Comprehension and Expression

Almost every person with aphasia exhibits some impairment in understanding a speaker's message (Pierce and Patterson, 1996). Varying level of deficits in comprehension and expression can be found in PWA. The nature of comprehension and expression deficit in an individual also helps in differentiating different types of aphasia. It is observed that auditory comprehension is better preserved in persons with non-fluent aphasia than fluent type. The speech of persons with non-fluent aphasia is characterised by loss of syntax and often appears telegraphic due to the omission of functional grammatical markers, but the semanticity of speech is maintained to an extent. In persons with fluent aphasia, verbal expression is semantically inappropriate and paraphasic, agrammatism/ paragrammatism can also be accompanied. In MAAT, stimuli for comprehension and expression are combined as a single domain. However, the SLP has to work on comprehension first and move on to expression, or work on both simultaneously as need may be.

The focus of this section is to improve comprehension and expression abilities at various linguistic levels; to improve communication of PWA through verbal/ non-verbal mode, by reducing apraxic errors, perseveration, jargon utterance and paraphasias. In case of persons with non-fluent aphasia, along with working on enhancing the comprehension skills, additional emphasis should be given on their verbal expression. In persons with fluent aphasia, receptive language skills are more affected than expressive skills. The main sub-sections in this domain with stimuli and tasks for its sub components (e.g. semantic level: vocabulary, antonyms, synonyms, semantic contiguity etc) are mentioned below.

1. Semantic level
2. Syntax level
3. Discourse level
4. Advanced Discourse level

As the areas of comprehension and expression encompass a larger part of language each of these sub-sections are further divided into sub-categories in order to cover major components of language. At the semantic level, the sub-categories include comprehension and expression at gross phoneme level, fine phonemic level and at word level. At word level comprehension and expression are worked on vocabulary of various lexical categories, antonyms, synonyms, syntagmatic and paradigmatic relations, semantic similarity, semantic contiguity and semantic anomaly. The tasks for comprehension requires PWA to point at the correct picture and the tasks for expression requires PWA to name the picture that is pointed by the clinician and gradually produce an automatic response.

Similar to the previous domains, the stimuli are placed with increasing difficulty level. For example, the category of finer phonemic level consists of Level I and Level II; the task in Level I is to identify finer phonemic difference in bisyllabic words and Level II is finer phonemic difference in trisyllabic/ polysyllabic words. Similarly, the other categories of semantic level have stimuli arranged under level I and level II.

Sub-section of syntax consists of seven sub-categories: PNG (Person, Number, and Gender) markers, tenses, answering polar questions, following body part commands, following commands with visual stimuli (one, two and multiple step commands), identification of objects described by function and sentence types(six types of sentence types). Once PWA progresses on the various sub-categories of syntax, more advanced level of language is introduced, that is, comprehension and expression of discourse and advanced discourse level. The categories at this level include picture description, narration and spontaneous speech. During discourse level tasks, PWA is expected to listen intently to the passage read by the clinician. Once passage is read, clinician re-reads the passage with missing components and PWA is expected to fill in the missing parts of the passage/ story. In another task, the passage is read and PWA is expected to listen intently and answer the questions based on the passage. The stimuli for this task are presented at three levels of increasing semantic and syntactic complexity. However, the clinician/SLP is free to select any other passage as stimulus depending on the literacy level of person with aphasia.

The main aim of this domain is to induce use of complete sentences, accurate grammar, cohesive discourse, appropriate topic initiation and maintenance. Thus, the tasks and sub-sections in this domain cover every aspect of verbal communication. In achieving these skills, the expression domain also aids in reducing linguistic errors that are usually present in aphasic speech (Paraphasias, neologisms, circumlocution and jargon utterances). The scoring of these linguistic errors during discourse tasks follows a five-point rating scale (0 = no error and 4 = very frequently occurring).

The stimuli in this domain is presented via combination of auditory, visual and graphic modality and as PWA progresses, it is presented through auditory and visual mode and finally through auditory mode alone. Similarly, for tasks of comprehension, pointing is accepted as a response, gradually as expression is worked upon, pointing is combined with verbal responses and finally PWA is expected to respond verbally. Progression at each level depends on the ability of PWA.

The stimuli in this domain of MAAT can be used with any language therapy technique for persons with aphasia, as the core principle of each technique is to improve comprehension and expression of language.

Naming

Naming difficulties/Anomia forms the core symptom of all persons with aphasia. Even after substantial recovery, PWA tends to have some form of word retrieval difficulty. This is usually observed during discourse where PWA struggles to retrieve words or might exhibit circumlocution to compensate for word retrieval difficulty. Anomia might be found in different classes of words or lexical category or in responsive speech. Therefore, it is of utmost importance to identify at what level the impairment lies and to work on it. The bulk of studies published in aphasiology consist of treatment studies to improve word retrieval or naming [to name a few (Chapey, 2008; Kiran and Basetto, 2008; Basso, Marangolo,

Piras, and Galluzzi, 2001)]. Therefore, to have a manual as MAAT helps bring uniformity in the treatment outcome studies.

This domain targets the core symptom of all persons with aphasia, especially the anomic aphasia. It is sub-divided into three sub-sections as listed below:

1. Confrontation naming (objects and picture naming)
2. Lexical generative naming (Phoneme fluency, word fluency, category specific, semantic mapping)
3. Responsive naming

During confrontation naming task, the clinician presents a picture or an object to PWA and ask "what is this?" or "can you name this?" and PWA is expected to answer. The clinician can initially provide as many cues as possible and gradually fade the cues as PWA improves. Lexical generative naming sub-section contains various tasks that require PWA to generate naming against competing neighbour words. For example, during phoneme fluency task of letter /b/, PWA is supposed to name items that start with the phoneme /b/ alone and exclude words that do not start with /b/ but compete with target word. The task increases the cognitive load, in turn improving word retrieval in PWA with intensive therapy. Responsive naming task is carried out by asking PWA to respond to the question asked by the clinician. It is also identification of objects described by function. This sub-section helps improve word retrieval in discourse (e.g. if the target word is "Pen". Clinician questions- What do you write with?)

The stimuli in this domain is presented with a cueing hierarchy i.e., named without any cues = 5, named with rhyming cues = 4, named with orthographic cues = 3, named with semantic cue = 2, named with phonemic cues =1 and no response with all the cues = 0.

Example: During a confrontation naming task, if the target response is "Pen", the cues could include the following:

Show the picture of the target stimulus and ask "what is this?"

"It sounds like 'Hen' (Rhyming cue- score 4)

Show the written form of the target stimulus (orthographic cue- score 3)

"What do you do with it?" / "Show me what you do with it?" / "You write with it. It is ..." (Semantic cue- score 2)

"It is /p/..." (Phonemic cue- score 1)

"It is pen"

The stimuli in the naming domain of MAAT cover a range of lexical categories and words that are frequently encountered in daily conversation or are essential in daily life. The stimuli in this domain are vital in improving the subtle impairments that are present in the speech of PWA. The stimuli in this domain can be used with any treatment technique that targets treating word retrieval in PWA.

Reading and Writing

As the main emphasis in aphasia rehabilitation is to improve the overall quality of communication, it is essential to work on reading and writing skills, especially on functional reading and writing skills in cases of persons with severe aphasia. Persons who have auditory comprehension deficit (e.g., Wernicke's aphasia) have comparable deficits in reading comprehension (Porrazzo, 1975). Thus, treatment programs targeting auditory processing skills invariably aid in improved performance across the entire language continuum including reading. Whithworth, Webster, and Howard (2005) stated that PWA finds written words easier to understand than spoken words.

Writing can pose a problem for PWA, following stroke affecting the dominant limb. Therefore, as a result of hemiplegia, they may have to shift to writing with non-dominant hand, due to which they may be unwilling to use writing as a facilitator or alternate mode of communication. They may also present with alexia/agraphia depending on the site of lesion. Hence, persons with aphasia present a wide range of reading and writing difficulties.

This domain aims at providing stimuli to improve reading and writing abilities in PWA at functional as well as advanced level. A sub-section on arithmetic skills is also included in order to train functional usage of money and other mathematical concepts. This domain is sub-divided into four sub-sections as listed below:

1. Functional reading and writing
2. Advanced reading
3. Advanced writing
4. Arithmetic skills

Functional reading and writing sub-section aims at helping PWA recognize one's own name, reading time, reading signboards and reading newspaper headlines. Writing also progresses in a hierarchy; starting from copy writing to writing on dictation to spontaneous writing. Advanced reading and writing sub-sections provide stimuli for literate PWA, wherein the goals of language therapy focus on the vocational training/ placement. In this subsection, the task is to achieve recognition of all the alphabets and reading bi-tri and polysyllabic words and non-words and finally reading at phrases and sentence level. The sub-section of arithmetic skills aims at improving basic mathematical skills required for independent living of PWA. In this level, clinician works on basic addition, subtraction, multiplication and other concepts necessary for banking, money concept, counting and functional mathematics used in everyday life. The stimuli for each task are systematically presented in the manual. The stimuli in each sub-section of this domain are presented in three levels of increasing difficulty (Level I, Level II and Level III).

Scoring

The scoring of responses throughout all the activities of the five domains follows a simple three-point scoring system as listed:

- 0= No response/ incorrect response/ unintelligible.
- ½= partially correct and intelligible response.
- 1= fully correct and intelligible response.

In addition to this, details of scoring are provided specifically under each sub-section. The naming domain provides a cueing hierarchy with specific scoring as mentioned under the naming domain. The discourse sub-section of comprehension and expression domain also has a scoring system to calculate other linguistic errors.

Once the raw score is obtained for each section, it can be converted into percentage by adding the raw scores and dividing it by the total number of stimuli presented (averaging) and multiplying it by 100.

$$Percentage\ score\ of\ each\ subsection = \frac{PWA's\ raw\ score}{Total\ score\ of\ the\ section} \times 100$$

USE OF MAAT IN CLINICAL SETTING

The first step in using this manual for aphasia therapy following detailed clinical assessment is to conduct a baseline assessment with this manual. The baseline assessment is carried out by administering all the domains of this manual on PWA. Start with assessment on functional communication domain by presenting the stimuli and tasks under each subsection of this domain till the level where PWA is able to respond based on his/her severity and type of aphasia. Similarly, carry out baseline assessment for each domain up to the level at which PWA is able to respond accurately. Once this initial assessment is carried out, the clinician/ the SLP has baseline level and scores of their patient with aphasia. Clinicians may take up to two sessions to conduct baseline assessment based on the ability of PWA. After the baseline assessment clinicians can follow the progression criteria mentioned in the Manual for Adult Aphasia Therapy in order to achieve considerable improvement in overall communication with this manual. The progression criteria provided also assist in choosing goals for therapy after baseline assessment. The details of progression criteria are adapted from Manual for Adult Fluent Aphasia Therapy in Kannada, MAFAT-K (Chaitra and Goswami, 2009) and are as follows.

- Begin with functional communication and comprehension domains simultaneously. When the total score in each of these domains reaches 50%, move to the next level.
- The activities of the repetition and activities of functional reading and writing domain should be introduced now. When a score of 25% in repetition, functional reading and writing is achieved and 75% in functional communication and comprehension, each, proceed to the next level.
- When the person with aphasia scores 100% on both functional communication, comprehension and 50% on repetition, functional reading and writing move to the next level.
- The activities in expression should be introduced now. When 25% score in the expression domain, 75% in repetition and 100% on functional reading and writing is reached move to the next level.
- The activities in expression should be continued till a score of 75% is achieved. Naming should be introduced and worked on till 75% score is achieved. Move to the next level.
- The advanced reading, writing and arithmetic skills should be introduced now and worked upon till 75% of the score is achieved.
- At the end of the manual, it is expected that in each domain, the performance of person with aphasia is 75% or above and in overall 90% and above.
- **Note**: To generalize the learnt skills, it is advised that in every session clinician takes up activities from each domain even though he/she would have achieved a score of 75% or more in that particular domain.

The progression criteria is organised in order to achieve simultaneous improvement across all domains of language. It is also based on the evidence of prognosis exhibited by PWA. In this order, PWA establishes functional communication skills from the beginning of language intervention and gradually improves his/her overall communication skills. An exemplar of scoring and documenting the responses of PWA using this manual is depicted in *Appendix 1*.

At every level of therapy with MAAT, the clinician is expected to provide appropriate repair strategies to assist PWA respond. There are a set of repair strategies that as presented in MAAT that can be used by the clinician to improve the overall communication skills. The repair strategies range from repetition, self-correction, and cueing to rephrasing and use of alternative communication strategy.

- **Stimulus Presentation Hierarchy:** The stimulus presentation under each domain follows a stimulus presentation hierarchy, which are individually mentioned at every level. It is presented in order to assist PWA respond favourably. Following the stimulus hierarchy also depends on the ability of each PWA; it is expected that stimulus be presented through the modality that is likely to elicit a response from PWA.
    - Combination of auditory, visual/orthographic and gesture (A+V/O+G)
    - Combination of auditory and gesture (A+G)
    - Auditory (A)
- **Expected Response:** Initially any meaningful response communicated by the person with aphasia is acceptable and not restricted. But, as PWA gradually progresses through the therapy, the response mode is expected to be stringent and he/she is expected to produce a verbal response if it is achievable by PWA. Acceptable mode of response is as follows:
    - Eye blinking (EB)
    - Head nod (HN)
    - Hand movement (HM)
    - Verbal utterances: partial or complete meaningful (VU)
- **Documentation with MAAT:** Responses of PWA are recorded on a treatment recording sheet. The MAAT provides a systematic treatment recording sheet (A template is provided in *Appendix 2*) which eases the process of documenting the responses and comparing the progress across sessions. This recording sheet is comprehensive in nature and provides detailed information on the therapy technique used, the repair strategies applied, nature of stimulus presentation and mode of response by PWA. It also provides information on the number of trials taken to produce the target and raw and/or percentage scores.

MAAT also consists of a profile analysis form (an exemplar is provided in *Appendix 3*). This form provides a visual depiction of PWA's performance. The clinician is required to shade the columns based on responses in terms of percentage across each domain. More the shaded area, the better is the performance. With this form, the performance of PWA can be recorded at specified intervals which allows for visual comparison of improvement across intervals.

CONCLUSION

Manual for Adult Aphasia Therapy (MAAT) is a therapy manual for use with persons with aphasia. It is a valuable therapy tool in Indian context for professionals working in the field of rehabilitation of persons with aphasia. It was initially field tested and developed in Kannada. It is available in six other Indian languages and has been field tested in each of these language and has proved to be clinically effective in treating PWA. The manuals provide easy guide for speech-language pathologists and student clinicians to initiate and progress through language therapy for persons with aphasia. Caregivers of PWA can also be trained to improve the communication abilities using the manual. MAAT covers stimuli under the five linguistic domains (Functional Communication, Comprehension and Expression, Repetition, Naming and Reading and Writing) which are affected in persons with aphasia to varying degrees.

The uniqueness of MAAT is its flexibility for use with any therapy technique or approach and the ease with which PWA can be accommodated into therapy irrespective of the aphasia type, severity and the individual's functional abilities. The manual is very comprehensive and guides the clinicians with ease to employ the manual on PWAs. The progression criteria mentioned in the manual is based on the clinical and empirical evidence and hence, directs the clinicians on a systematic timeline to introduce appropriate language domain at proper intervals of the therapy, based on the progress shown by each PWA. Clinicians across the country can also customise the stimuli according to individual needs of PWA, which in turns increases the ecological validity of the manual. The repair strategies provided in the manual assists the clinicians and the caregivers to use apt communication strategies to obtain maximum output from PWA. Further, the use of this manual will lead to a systematic and uniform approach of clinicians towards PWA across the country. It will assist a standardized documentation of outcome of evidence-based clinical data/research. Hence, Manual for Adult Aphasia Therapy is a clinically invaluable therapy material for speech-language pathologists working in the country.

ACKNOWLEDGMENT

Authors acknowledge the financial aid and support provided by All India Institute of Speech and Hearing Research Fund for the projects titled "Manual for Adult Non-fluent Aphasia therapy in Kannada (MANAT-K)" and "Field Testing Manual for Adult Fluent Aphasia Therapy in Kannada (MAFAT-K)" [sanction No: SH/CDN/ARF/3.69/2010-11]; the outcome of which was "Manual for Adult Aphasia Therapy in Kannada (MAAT-K)". Authors also acknowledge Department of Science and Technology Government of India for financial support vide reference No. SR/CSI/75/2011 (c) Dated: 22/02/2012 under cognitive science research initiative (CSRI) to carry out the project titled "Development of Manual for Adult Fluent and Non-Fluent aphasia Therapy in Hindi, English, Tamil, Telugu, Malayalam and Marathi (MAAT-6)".

REFERENCES

Albert, M. L., Sparks, R. W., & Helm, N. A. (1973). Melodic intonation therapy for aphasia. *Archives of Neurology*, *29*(2), 130–131. doi:10.1001/archneur.1973.00490260074018 PMID:4717723

Basso, A., Marangolo, P., Piras, F., & Galluzzi, C. (2001). Acquisition of new words in normal subjects. A suggestion for treatment of anomia. *Brain and Language*, *77*(1), 45–49. doi:10.1006/brln.2000.2422 PMID:11247655

Chaitra, S., & Goswami, S. P. (2009). *Manual for Adult Fluent Aphasia Therapy in Kannada (MAFAT-K). Articles based on Dissertation done at AIISH.* All India Institute of Speech and Hearing, Mysore, India.

Chapey, R. (2008). Language intervention strategies in aphasia and related neurogenic communication disorders. Philadelphia, PA: Lippincott Williams and Wilkins.

Chapey, R., Duchan, J. F., Elman, R. J., Garcia, L. J., Kagan, A., Lyon, J. G., & Simmons-Mackie, N. (2000). Life participation approach to aphasia: A statement of values for the future. *ASHA Leader*, *5*(3), 4–6. doi:10.1044/leader.FTR.05032000.4

Cruice, M., Worrall, L., Murison, R., & Hickson, L. (2003). Finding a focus for quality of aphasia: Social and emotional health, and psychological well-being. *Aphasiology*, *17*(4), 333–353. doi:10.1080/02687030244000707

Davis, G. A., & Wilcox, M. J. (1991). Incorporating parameters of natural conversation in aphasia treatment. In R. Chapey (Ed.), *Language intervention strategies in adult aphasia*. Baltimore, MD: Williams and Wilkins.

Goodglass, H., & Kaplan, E. (1983). *The Assessment of Aphasia and Related Disorder* (2nd ed.). Philadelphia: Lea and Febiger.

Goswami, S. P. R., & Kruthi, G. (2013). Computerized Version of Manual for Adult Aphasia Therapy in Kannada. Mysore: All India Institute of Speech and Hearing.

Goswami, S. P., Jayashree, C. S., Samasthitha S., Navitha U., Chaitra, S., & Ranjini, M. (2011). Manual for Adult Aphasia Therapy in Kannada (MAAT-K). Mysore: All India Institute of Speech and Hearing.

Goswami, S. P., Shanbal, J. C., Navitha, U., & Samasthitha, S. (2010). Field testing of Manual for Adult Non Fluent Aphasia Therapy. All India Institute of Speech and Hearing, Mysore, India. Unpublished AIISH Research Fund project.

Goswami, S. P., Thomas, P., & Rachel, V. (2015). Development of manual for Adult Fluent and Non Fluent Aphasia therapy in Hindi, English, Tamil, Telugu, Malayalam and Marathi. Unpublished Project funded by the Department of Science and Technology, New Delhi.

Government of India, Ministry of Home Affairs. (n.d.). *List of languages in the Eighth Schedule*. Retrieved from http://mha.nic.in/hindi/sites/upload_files/mhahindi/files/pdf/Eighth_Schedule.pdf

Hallowell, B., & Chapey, R. (2008). Introduction to language intervention strategies in adult aphasia. In R. Chapey (Ed.), *Language intervention strategies in aphasia and related neurogenic communication disorders* (5th ed.; pp. 3–19). Philadelphia: Lippincott Williams and Wilkins.

Helms-Estabrooks, N., & Albert, M. L. (2014). *Manual of Aphasia and Aphasia Therapy* (3rd ed.). Austin, TX: PRO-ED.

Kearns, K. P. (1985). Response elaboration training of patient initiated utterances. In R. H. Brookshire (Ed.), *Clinical Aphasiology* (p. 15). Minneapolis, MN: BRK Publishers.

Kiran, S., & Bassetto, G. (2008). Evaluating the effectiveness of semantic based treatment for naming disorders in aphasia: What works? *Seminars in Speech and Language*, *29*(1), 71–82. doi:10.1055-2008-1061626 PMID:18348093

La Pointe, L. L. (2005). Foundations: Adaptation, Accomodation, Aristos. In L. L. La Pointe (Ed.), *Aphasia and related neurogenic language disorders* (pp. 1–18). New York: Thieme Medical.

Language in India. (2014). *Census of India 2011 towards a bright future.* Retrieved from http://www.languageinindia.com/feb2014/censusofindia2011data.pdf

Longerich, M. C. (1968). *Manual for the Aphasia Patient*. New York: Macmillan Company.

Pierce, S. R., & Patterson, P. J. (1996). Treatment of auditory comprehension impairment. In G. L. Wallace (Ed.), *Adult Aphasia Rehabilitation*. Butterworth-Heinemann.

Porrazzo, A. S. (1975). *Evaluation and treatment of reading deficits in aphasic patients*. Paper presentation at the fifth conference on clinical aphasiology, Santa Fe, NM.

Ross, D., & Spencer, S. (1980). *Aphasia Rehabilitation-An Auditory and Verbal Task Hierarchy*. Charles C. Thomas.

Venugopal, M. B., & Goswami, S. P. (2008). *Manual for Adult Non-fluent Aphasia Therapy-in Kannada. In Student Research* (Vol. 3, pp. 181–189). Mysore: All India Institute of Speech and Hearing.

Whithworth, A., Webster, J., & Howard, D. (2005). *A cognitive neuropsychological approach to assessment and treatment of aphasia. A clinicians guide*. East Sussex, UK: Psychology Press.

World Health Organization. (2012). *World Stroke Day*. Retrieved from http://www.who.int/cardiovascular_diseases/media/events/stroke_day/en/

KEY TERMS AND DEFINITIONS

Agrammatism: Speech characterized by lack of functional words and contains only content words. It is commonly present in persons with non-fluent aphasia.

Ecological Validity: Ecological validity of the stimulus refers to the similarity of stimulus and material to real life things and situations.

Equivocal Response: In the context of the manual it refers to the simultaneous verbal production of the response by the clinician and the person with aphasia.

Paradigmatic Relations: These are relations that linguistic units share because they may be substituted by another (e.g., dog: animal; crow: bird).

Paragrammatism: Speech characterized by grammatically incorrect sentences. It is present in persons with fluent aphasia.

Psycho-Social Approach: It is directed towards looking at how aphasia affects persons with aphasia psychologically and the influence it has on their social participation and how it is related to the mental and physical ability.

Syntagmatic Relations: These are words that come in a sequence or parallel with each other to create meaning (e.g., milk, white, hair, and black).

APPENDIX 1

Name of the person with aphasia: XX
Case No.: XX
Age/gender: 60yrs/M
Date: DD/MM/YYYY
Provisional Diagnosis: Transcortical motor aphasia
Session No.: 1
Clinician: XX

APPENDIX 2

Table 1. An exemplar depicting the use of treatment recording sheet with cueing hierarchy

Activity	Stimulus Number	Stimulus Mode	Response Mode	Target Response	No. of Trials										% Correct Responses	Final Percentage
					1	2	3	4	5	6	7	8	9	10		
	1.	A+V	Verbal	Chair	1 (5)										100%	
	2.	A+V	Verbal	Door	0 (2)	0 (2)	½ (3)	½ (1)	1 (1)	1 (5)	1				57.14%	
Functional Communication-Recognition of familiar objects-Level 1	3.	A+V	Verbal	Window	½ (2)	½ (2)	1 (1)	1 (5)	1						80%	79.92%
	4.	A+V	Verbal	Table	½ (2)	1 (1)	1 (5)	1							87.5%	
	5.	A+V	Verbal	Fan	0 (1)	1 (5)	1 (5)	1							75%	
	1.	A+V	Verbal	Red	0 (1)	1									50%	
	2.	A+V	Verbal	Green	1/2	1/2	1								66.66%	
Naming-Confrontation naming-Picture naming-Level 9	3	A+V	Verbal	Yellow	0 (3)	0 (2)	½ (2)	½ (1)	½ (5)	½					33.33%	59.99%
	4.	A+V	Verbal	Blue	1 (5)										100%	
	5.	A+V	Verbal	Orange	0 (1)	1									50%	

Note: A= Auditory mode V = Visual G= Graphic
Scoring=Total score/No. of trials used x 100
Score sheet applicable for all sections except advanced discourse level under the domain Comprehension and Expression
If cueing hierarchy is not used mention the technique used separately.

Name of the Person With Aphasia:
Case No.:
Age/Gender:
Date:
Provisional Diagnosis:
Session No.:
Clinician:

APPENDIX 3

Name of the Person With Aphasia: XX
Case No.: XX
Age/Gender: 60yrs/M
Date: DD/MM/YYYY
Provisional Diagnosis: Transcortical motor aphasia
Clinician: XX
Number of Sessions Attended.: 15

Table 2. Treatment recording sheet template

Activity	Stimulus Number	Stimulus Mode	Response Mode	Target Response	No. of Trials										% Correct Responses
					1	2	3	4	5	6	7	8	9	10	

Table 3. An exemplar depicting the use of profile analysis form of the overall communication skills for persons with aphasia

Improvement in Terms of Percentage	Functional Communication Domain								Repetition Domain					Comprehension and Expression Domain								Naming Domain			Reading and Writing Domain			
75% and above																												
51-75%																												
26-50%																												
0-25%																												
Activities	1	2	3	4	5	6	7	8	1	2	3	4	5	1	2	3	4	**1**	2	3	4	1	2	**3**	1	2	3	4

Note: The clinician shades the columns for the responses in terms of percentage across each domain. This signifies that more the shaded area the better is the performance.

Chapter 19
Selective Mutism:
Understanding and Management

Charu Kriti
National University of Study and Research in Law, India

ABSTRACT

Selective mutism is a disorder that is characterized by a failure to speak in certain social settings, like the school, while speaking normally in other settings, like home. The settings in which the failure to speak occur are those where speech is expected from the individual. It is a disorder that onsets in childhood, and if left untreated, may go well into adolescence. For a very long time, this disorder has been overlooked and understudied. Though rare, the disorder may pose a potential threat to the social and academic development of a child suffering from it. The DSM-5 has classified selective mutism as an anxiety disorder. The present chapter intends to cover the psychosocial approach to the disorder, the diagnostic criteria, the etiology, the treatment of the disorder, and the management by respective caregivers. An analysis of case studies has also been given in the chapter.

INTRODUCTION

Burson (2006) stated, "At home, Grace was outgoing, funny and bossy to her little sisters. It was just the opposite at school: She was withdrawn, her face a blank stare. She didn't utter a single word to anyone."

Colborn (2017) reported, "At home, Nola is a talkative, high energy child, even as a toddler she would always be making noises. Lately, she would become quiet in public situations and her parents think she is just being shy."

There have been many more stories like these. Parents have reported that their usually talkative children have suddenly shown signs of absolute mutism in certain situations. The entire demeanor of the child changes and she or he shows a drastically different set of behavior patterns in such situations. Quoting a

DOI: 10.4018/978-1-5225-4955-0.ch019

parent, "she went to school that day and came back a different kid" (Burson, 2006). These are instances of what has been called Selective Mutism by the DSM-5 (APA/American Psychiatric Association, 2013).

Selective Mutism is a psychological disorder which has gone unnoticed, misdiagnosed and overlooked for a long time. It is only in the last decade that this particular condition has been talked of at length. It is strange that though the initial reference of selective mutism goes back to over 125 years ago, it is as late as 2006, after the publication of an article called "Behind the wall of silence" by Newsday, that streamlined discussions started (Burson, 2006).

DEFINING AND UNDERSTANDING SELECTIVE MUTISM

History of Selective Mutism

It was back in 1877 that a German physician called Adolph Kussmaul used the term '*aphasia voluntaria*' to describe children who 'refused' to speak though they could speak normally. Kussmaul used the term after he reported three clinical cases with similar symptoms (Jainer, Quasim, & Davis, 2001). In 1934, a child psychologist from Switzerland called Mortis Tramer used the term 'elective mutism' for the first time to describe "a fascinating group of children, whose talking is confined to familiar situations" (Kolvin, Trowell, Le Couteur, Baharaki, & Morgan, 1997). Going by both the terms, it can be seen that the understanding was of a voluntary act of refusing to speak, which would mean it was an oppositional behavior (Noelle, 2017).

The same understanding is reflected in the diagnostic criteria given by the earlier versions of the Diagnostic and Statistical Manual (DSM). The third editions of the Diagnostic and Statistical Manual (DSM-III and DSM-III-R) explained elective mutism in terms of "refusal to speak". This was changed in the fourth edition of DSM, where it was recognized as an *inability to speak* (Noelle, 2107). The diagnostic criteria given in DSM-III (APA, 1980) talks of "continuous *refusal* to speak in almost all social settings", while the diagnostic criteria given in DSM-III-R (APA, 1987) updated it to "*persistent refusal* to speak in one or more social settings". In contrast, after the publication of DSM-IV in 1994, the diagnostic criterion read "*failure* to speak in specific social situations".

There are other differences between the elective mutism as described in the third editions (DSM-III and DSM-III-R) of the Diagnostic and Statistical Manuals (APA, 1980, 1987) and the selective mutism as described in the subsequent editions, i.e., DSM-IV (APA, 1994), DSM-IV-TR (APA, 2000) and DSM 5 (APA, 2013). Some instances would be the predisposing factors and differential diagnosis.

According to both the third editions of the DSM (APA, 1980; 1987), maternal overprotection, speech disorders, mental retardation and trauma were possible predisposing factors for the onset of selective mutism. These factors were, however, removed in the subsequent editions of the DSM (DSM-IV, DSM-IV-TR & DSM-5). Similarly, the third editions stated that the 'refusal' to speak could be differentially diagnosed as developmental disorders, while the later editions (DSM-IV & DSM-IV-TR) list speech abnormalities and social anxiety disorder as differential diagnosis for selective mutism. DSM-5 (APA, 2013) lists a differential diagnosis of communication disorders, social anxiety and psychotic disorders like schizophrenia and autism spectrum disorders.

Symptoms of Selective Mutism

The common symptoms that have been observed in individuals with selective mutism are:

- Inability to speak in social situations
- Normal speech in a comfortable or well-known environment, like home.
- Withdrawal from people around them.
- Anxiety, nervousness, shyness, awkwardness in the presence of people.
- Changed physical conditions like stiffening of body, rigidity or blankness of expressions, tightening of muscles, clenching of fists, avoiding eye contact when in the company of others.
- None of these behaviors is shown when in the company of parents, siblings or immediate family.

Prevalence of Selective Mutism

Like any other psychological disorder, selective mutism works differently for different people. The level and intensity of mutism differ. According to Oerbeck, Manassis, Overgaard, and Kristensen (2016), "Different individuals may increase or lessen symptoms considerably within the same situation." Amir (2005) stated, "The social skills among children affected by selective mutism vary greatly." Some children speak in the presence of peers in school, but not in the presence of any adult (teachers, caregivers, nurse). Some speak only to particular peers they identify as friends, but not to others. It has also been noted that [s]ome will occasionally be able to whisper to a best friend at school" (Oerbeck et al., 2016).

There is a difference in the level of interaction with peers as well. Some children communicate easily with peers; others interact but not necessarily communicate, while a third type is entirely withdrawn in any kind of social settings (Amir, 2005). Oerbeck et al. (2016) further stated, "while some use nonverbal communication effectively, others are non-communicative and might not even laugh or cough in front of others. The latter are often unable to express their needs (going to the toilet, hunger, thirst, or pain), highlighting the potential seriousness of this condition."

DSM-5 explains that the ambit of selective mutism also extends to social behavior, where children may feel too anxious and not indulge in any kind of social interaction which requires a reciprocal exchange with other children, thereby causing impairment in social interaction. Over time, this may also lead to social isolation of the children with selective mutism. These children also hesitate in speaking in front of or to the teacher. They often abstain from communicating at all, so the teacher is usually unaware of their personal or academic needs. This, in turn, may also impair the academic development of the children suffering from selective mutism (APA, 2013).

Despite many reports to the contrary, there is no difference in the prevalence of the disorder on the basis of either ethnicity (race) or gender (APA, 2013). The International Classification of Diseases -10 (ICD-10) also states that the frequency of occurrence of the disorder is relatively same in both the sexes (WHO/World Health Organization, 1992). The ICD-10 further states that the manifestation of the disorder usually occurs in early childhood (WHO, 1992).

Based on the criteria given by the text revision of the Diagnostic and Statistical Manual's fourth edition (DSM-IV-TR), certain epidemiologic studies were conducted. The results of the same gave substantive data on the extent and prevalence of selective mutism. One study reported 0.6% prevalence in preschoolers, while another reported 0.69% in children between 4 to 5 years of age (Sadock & Sadock, 2007).

In an advice sheet for parents on selective mutism, the Sussex Community NHS Trust reported that one in every 150 students suffers from selective mutism. However, the prevalence of selective mutism is less than 1% in mental health (Elizur & Perednik, 2003). Yet, it is possible that selective mutism in schools may be higher, since it is in the classroom where impairment in verbal conversation is most likely to be observed (Bergman, Piacentini, & McKracken, 2002; Kumpulainen, Rasanen, Raaska, & Somppi, 1998).

Diagnostic Criteria of Selective Mutism

The ICD-10 classification of mental and behavioral disorders still calls it elective mutism (F94.0) and it falls under F94-Disorders of social functioning with onset specific to childhood and adolescence (WHO, 1992). However, in the beta draft of ICD-11, which is yet to be published, the name is changed to selective mutism (6B36) and it is included under anxiety and fear-related disorders. The ICD also specifically marks down the characteristics of the disorder as "emotionally determined selectivity in speaking" (WHO, 1992).

Selective Mutism was called Elective Mutism till the revision version of the third edition of the diagnostic and statistical manual (DSM-III-R) (APA, 1987). In 1994, when the fourth edition (DSM-IV) came out, the name was changed to selective mutism. In the ongoing fifth edition (DSM-5), it has been defined as *"consistent failure to speak in specific social situations in which there is an expectation to speak (e.g., at school) despite speaking in other situations"* (APA, 2013).

It must be noted that emphasis has been placed on those 'social situations' in which it is expected of the child to speak and on the fact that children suffering from selective mutism show speaking behavior in other situations. As reported in the case studies at the beginning of the chapter, children suffering from selective mutism speak like any other child in the comfortable environment of their homes. But when put in a new situation, the same children fail to interact with people around them.

It is a childhood disorder, the symptoms of which are first seen when the child leaves the protected environment of his or her home, and has the first interaction with the society as he or she joins school. The DSM-5 clearly states that a diagnosis of selective mutism cannot be made in case of failure to speak in the first month of joining school, as the reason could simply be the child's difficulty in adjustment to a new environment. It is important that in situations where there is a necessity to speak, like academic

Table 1. The diagnostic criteria and the comorbid disorders of selective mutism as per DSM-5 (APA, 2013)

Diagnostic Criteria 312.23 (F94.0)
• Consistent failure to speak in specific social situations in which there is an expectation for speaking (e.g., at school) despite speaking in other situations. • The disturbance interferes with educational or occupational achievement or with social communication. • The duration of the disturbance is at least 1 month (not limited to the first month of school). • The failure to speak is not attributable to a lack of knowledge of, or comfort with, the spoken language required in the social situation. • The disturbance is not better explained by a communication disorder (e.g., childhood-onset fluency disorder) and does not occur exclusively during the course of autism spectrum disorder, schizophrenia, or another psychotic disorder.
Comorbid Disorders
• Social anxiety disorder, followed by separation anxiety disorder and specific phobia • Oppositional behaviors • Speech and language deficiencies • Subtle learning disabilities or difficulty processing information

and social settings, there must be a significant impairment in speaking. Children are more likely to be affected by the disorder as compared to adults (APA, 2013).

Misdiagnosis

The epidemiological studies show that selective mutism is one of the less prevalent disorders occurring in childhood. The awareness for the same is, for much of the same reason, not as it ought to be. Thus, many a times, the diagnosis is either delayed, for lack of recognition or an incorrect diagnosis is made. Probably the most common form of misdiagnosis in the case of selective mutism is the child being shy. According to reports, not only parents but doctors and psychologists also at times have concluded that it's just a bout of shyness on being put in a new situation, which the child would eventually grow out of.

The example given at the beginning of the chapter of the 4-year-old girl called Nola states that though in her case there was a very sudden onset of the disorder, for a very long time her parents thought it to be mere shyness. Her mother stated that she had always been talkative. In fact, even as a toddler, she would be making different kind of sounds. Thus, when she entered school and she stopped talking all of a sudden, the parents did not immediately jump to the conclusion of the possibility of some kind of disorder.

Based on evidences of different case studies, this has been seen that the more sudden the onset and more drastic the change in the speaking behavior (where the child goes from being talkative to absolutely silent in social settings), more readily do the parents take the change to be mere shyness. Because of this, many times a late diagnosis of selective mutism is made. But it has to be remembered that different children differ in their intensity of mutism, their choice of people that they wish to communicate verbally to and their symptoms of the disorder.

However, misconstrued shyness is by far not the only cause for misdiagnosis of selective mutism. There are several disorders of which a differential diagnosis can be made in the place of selective mutism. It can be speculated whether these disorders could be one of the reasons why selective mutism is usually misdiagnosed. According to the DSM-5 (APA, 2013), the differential diagnosis of selective mutism could be anything among communication disorders, neurodevelopmental disorders, social anxiety disorders or psychotic disorders like schizophrenia.

For instance, selective mutism needs to be distinguished from language disorder, childhood onset fluency disorder, social communication disorder or speech sound disorder (APA, 2013). Yet, in some rare cases, children with selective mutism have had a history of delay in achieving speech related developmental milestones. Since the symptoms for some of the abovementioned communication disorders might overlap with speech delays, leading to misconstruing the symptoms, and misdiagnosis.

However, there is clear demarcation of what can and should be diagnosed as selective mutism in both DSM-5 and ICD-10. The diagnostic criteria in DSM 5 clearly states that the disorder must not be explained as a symptom for psychotic disorders or communication disorders. For example, children with autism may have problems is communicating in social situations. Such children will not be able to speak appropriately in any social condition. This must not be confused as selective mutism, because in the latter, the inability to speak is only in certain social situations (APA, 2013).

Similarly, sometimes the comorbid disorders overshadow the symptoms of selective mutism. The most common comorbid disorders are social anxiety disorder, specific phobia or separation anxiety disorder. Anxiety in social situations and social withdrawal are symptoms common to both social anxiety disorder as well as selective mutism. Hence, in cases where these symptoms exist, along with the symptoms specific to selective mutism, it is advised that a diagnosis of both social anxiety and selective mutism is made (APA, 2013).

Apart from this, it is also important for a correct diagnosis of selective mutism that the failure of speaking should only be attributed to discomfort and anxiety in social situations. If the person does not speak a particular language or does not feel comfortable in speaking the said language, it cannot be termed as selective mutism (APA, 2013). Children who move to a new location, (town, state or country) where a different language is spoken or a varied dialect of the native language is used, cannot be diagnosed to be selectively mute if the cause is not knowing or lacking fluency in the language. However, if there is adequate understanding of the new language but there still persists a failure or refusal to speak, the child can be diagnosed with selective mutism (APA, 2013).

An explanation on this point can be made by the case study that Leben (n.d.) talked about in the paper on the case study of a 10-year-old Korean boy. The boy in question was a first born. His family had moved to California when he was three years of age. Once he joined school he showed signs of some behavioral problems which were diagnosed and re-diagnosed. The first diagnosis was autism. This was later changed to pervasive developmental disorder. Finally, when he was nine years of age, he was diagnosed with Selective Mutism and Emotional Disturbance.

Hence, it can be safely said that cultural differences play an important role in the onset of selective mutism. Children of immigrant parents usually find themselves in situation where the lack of knowledge of the native language poses a big problem. However, mere lack of knowledge does not amount to selective mutism. Even in the case mentioned above, the Korean boy would speak to his parents in both Korean as well as English. So his failure to speak in social situations was not because he did not understand the language or lacked knowledge of the language spoken in the place he had migrated to. And in such a situation, a diagnosis of selective mutism is in order.

Etiology of Selective Mutism

Till date, no consensus has been reached over the topic of etiology for selective mutism (Camposano, 2011). There are different approaches taken by different schools of psychology, which assign the cause to this ailment of varied factors. On one hand is the view of the psychoanalysts who state that selective mutism is a result of unresolved internal conflicts (Cohen, Chavira, & Stein, 2006), while on the other are behavioral therapists who believe that varied environmental events, both antecedent and consequent produce mute behavior (Kratchowill, 1981).

Family system theorists hold the view that a family with faulty relations may also lead to children developing selective mutism (Anstendig, 1998). Early theorists, on the contrary, were of the opinion that childhood trauma or major life events (abuse or death of loved ones) may act as a prominent factor in triggering selective mutism (Dow, Sonies, Schieb, Moss, & Leonard, 1995). However, this point has been countered in recent studies that state that the association of childhood trauma with the development of the disorder is rare (Gray, Jordan, Ziegler, & Livingstone, 2002; Steinhausen & Juzi, 1996; Dummit et al., 1997).

Modern research suggests that selective mutism is an anxiety related disorder, or at least there is often a co-occurrence with anxiety (Black & Uhde, 1995; Vecchio & Kearney, 2007). Cunningham, McHolm, and Boyle (2006) specified social phobia as the anxiety disorder to which selective mutism could be linked. The DSM-5 (APA, 2013) also enumerates the most common comorbid conditions to be other anxiety disorders. The most common of these is social anxiety disorder, closely followed by separation anxiety disorder and finally, specific phobia.

Also, children with selective mutism have shown signs of oppositional behaviors, although oppositional behavior may only be seen in those social situations where speech is expected or required. In some children with selective mutism, a delay in achieving the communication milestone or any type of communication disorder has also been reported. There is also some support for the idea that children with the disorder are more socially anxious than children without it (Wicks-Nelson & Israel, 2013). However, the relationship between selective mutism and social anxiety remains unclear (Viana, Biedel, & Rabian, 2009; Yeganeh, Biedel, Turner, Pina, & Silverman, 2003).

Other causes of selective mutism include a combination of environmental factors and genetics in the development of the disorder (Sulkowski, Pence, Carlson, & Storch, 2014). Maladaptive family environment, a family history of adjustment problems, dysfunctional patterns of reinforcement or distress due to cultural or linguistic acculturation are some forms of environmental factors that play a role in the onset of the disorder (Viana et al, 2009).

The Psychosocial Aspect of Selective Mutism

Children with selective mutism have different behavioral reactions. However, there is a range of emotional and behavioral problems that can be generalized as the reaction of children with selective mutism. This has been discussed by Burson (2006) in the article "Behind the wall of silence". He stated, "Children who have selective mutism, have the ability to speak and communicate at home and in other situations where they feel safe and comfortable. Their anxiety kicks in most often at school and in other places where they feel they are expected to talk and interact with others. Some freeze up, their bodies stiffen, their faces go blank, and they avoid eye contact. While the cause is unclear, experts say that there might be a genetic predisposition to develop selective mutism in many children and teens. Some children may also have other underlying problems, such as speech and language deficiencies, subtle learning disabilities or difficulty in processing information."

In addition to this, as stated earlier, broken families have also been taken to be a cause for the onset of selective mutism. When the psychosocial causes for mutism or any anxiety related disorder are explored, it is found that family, being the primary agency of socialization, plays a key role. Children with selective mutism appear to be uncomfortable, uneasy, nervous, socially awkward, clingy, withdrawn and sometimes even aggressive.

It would appear that if a child's home and family were disrupted by some major crises, his personal social adjustment would be apt to be adversely affected (Koch, 1961). A study showed that preschool children from broken homes show more anxiety. Between 1932 and 1952, the percentage of under 18 years old individuals who were affected by divorce increased from 41% to 60% (Burchinal, 1964).

Furthermore, anxiety is also said to be inheritable. There is research based evidence in favor of anxiety disorders running in the family (Camposano, 2011). The parents whose children suffer from selective mutism may themselves suffer from moderate to severe anxiety (Kristersen & Torgersen, 2001). In a survey, it was found that in almost 33% of the cases there was at least one family member suffering from social anxiety disorder and in 12% of the cases, family members suffered from selective mutism itself (Schwartz, Freedy, & Sheridan, 2006). In addition, any history of shyness, social isolation, and social anxiety in either of the parents may play a role in the onset of selective mutism (APA, 2013). Sadock and Sadock (2007) were of the view that like any anxiety disorder, the genetic contribution in the onset of the disorder is quite prominent.

The genetic aspect, to an extent, invites the application of the *diathesis-stress model* of psychopathology (Weiner, 1977). Baron (2015) sates, "Mental disorders result from the joint effect of two influences: a predisposition for a given disorder (diathesis) and stressors in the individual's environment that tend to activate or stimulate the predisposition or vulnerability." In the case of selective mutism, the inheritability works as the diathesis, where the child has a genetic predisposition to develop mutism.

The starting of school works as the stressor, where taken away from the comfortable surroundings of his or her home, the child finds himself or herself in a new, awkward and sometimes, even traumatic situations.There is also a sudden increase in the amount of social interaction. At the same time, performance tasks, such as reading aloud is also assigned to them which adds to the stress (APA, 2013). Experts say that while the cause for selective mutism is unclear, many children and teens with the disorder have a genetic predisposition to it (Burson, 2006). Kimble (1990) stated, "the greater an individual's vulnerability, the lesser the stress required to induce a pathological reaction."

Assessment of Selective Mutism

Once the child enters a continuous social life away from home, and social interaction starts, the symptoms of selective mutism become clear in those children who have a predisposition to the same. Hence, one of the most prominent prerequisites for managing this disorder is an early diagnosis. Since the behavior shown by children is not what is expected, it is better to have a correct diagnosis made at the earliest (Schwartz et al., 2006).

The assessment of selective mutism might include a speech-language assessment of the child. Since the child himself or herself is incapable of speaking, reports are collected from the parents and the teachers of the child suffering from selective mutism. The Selective Mutism Questionnaire (SMQ) developed by Bergman, Keller, Wood, Piacentini, and McCraken (2001) is one such questionnaire that asks the parents to rate the child on the frequency of communication at home and in public settings and the teacher's report on communication in school (Shipon-Blum, 2009).

Other ways of speech- language assessment is record reviews and structured interviews (Vecchio & Kearney, 2007), functional assessment (Shipon-Blum, 2009) in which people who know the child well are interviewed and the frequency of communication is recorded and non-standardized testing like videotaping the child at home so that an analysis of the language sample of the child could be done (Shipon-Blum, 2009). Another such non-standardized testing procedure is the Strong narrative analysis procedure (SNAP) developed by Strong, Mayer, and Mayer (1998). Based on the assessment, the treatment can be scheduled as soon as the diagnosis is done.

Treatment Approaches for Selective Mutism

It has been found that the sooner the diagnosis is made, more effective is the prognosis. If left unattended, it would lead to the child developing non-verbal conditioned responses, becoming a habit, with little or no chances to break. Since the etiology is so diverse and varied, the treatment for selective mutism also requires similar variety and different approaches. Similar to the etiology, the treatment, too, is different for different schools of psychology.

However, a positive psychology based basic framework of goals can be prepared for different kind of treatment programs. The first and foremost goal should be to lessen the anxiety associated with selective mutism, along with teaching coping mechanisms to handle the anxiety (Shipon-Blum, 2007). The mechanisms used for the same would be those involved in *subjective well-being* which would include systematic breathing techniques, teaching relaxation skills and practicing meditation. Another goal would be inducing self-esteem and boosting confidence of the child in social situations. The ultimate goal would be a psychosocial one, where an increase in verbal communication in the previously anxiety-arousing situation would be sought.

Psychodynamic Approach

Cline and Baldwin (1994) described mutism as a defense mechanism used by the child, where the child prefers mutism over expressing the true feelings towards the parents directly. This approach also holds the view that the cause of mutism lies in the internal unresolved conflict of the child (Kratochowill, 1981). Thus, the initial attempt at treatment derives from the psychodynamic approach, which focuses more on the origin than the disorder (Cohen et al., 2006).

An attempt was made to study the child's psychosexual development (Cline & Baldwin, 1994). The effectiveness of this approach was questioned in the same. The major concern raised was that since the disorder has been linked to anxiety, the techniques used by the psychodynamic approach wherein the child would be pressurized to speak about his or her thoughts and emotions will overwhelm the him or her instead of reducing the anxiety (Camposano, 2011). Moreover, this approach is not even cost-effective.

Behavioral Approach

This school of thought recognizes selective mutism as a coping mechanism due to anxiety and aims at treating it by reducing anxiety and increasing verbal communication (Camposano, 2011). Different mechanisms and techniques are employed for achieving the desired results. Shaping, self-modeling, stimulus generalization, escape and avoidance procedure, contingency management, and systematic desensitization are some of these techniques.

- *Shaping*, or ritual sound approach as it is also known, is the most commonly used approach. It uses gradually changing the quality of the response given by the child (Richburg & Cobia, 1994). Successive approximation to a behavior is reinforced as the response gets closer to the target behavioral goal. Richburg and Cobia (1994) explained the steps of shaping and stated, "the child is first reinforced for making nonverbal responses, then for making certain sounds, and finally for speaking at least one word.
- *Self-modeling* is a two-part process. The first part involves using a recorder, either audio or video, in which the child answering questions in a comfortable environment is recorded. As the second step, the tape is edited, to make it appear as if the child is speaking in other social situations, usually in the anxiety causing situations, like school. The child listens to or views the tape repeatedly. This process is also repeated in the presence of others (family members or peers). The purpose is to make the child comfortable about hearing his or her own voice in the presence of company. This is followed by the child answering questions orally, initially alone and then in the presence of other people.

- *Stimulus generalization* derives the reinforcing answers from the shaping technique, with the difference that the reinforcement is given for verbal responses given in the presence of different stimuli like new peers, adults or new situations (Shriver, Segool, & Gortmaker, 2011). The target goal here is based on the stimulus fading procedure, which focuses on where, when and with whom is the child communicating.
- *Escape-avoidance procedure* requires the child to utter at least one word before leaving that particular setting. This is then combined with positive reinforcements. Once speech has been initiated, the stimulus fading technique is employed, combined with positive reinforcements, to produce generalized speech in the anxiety causing environments (Kratchowill, 1981).
- *Contingency management* talks of the technique where the child is encouraged to practice and engage in verbalization instead of using non-verbal gestures for communication, and each attempt at verbalization by the child is positively reinforced (Camposano, 2011). Based on Skinner's theory of learning, it can be understood that behavior can be learned if the behavior is immediately followed by positive reinforcement (Morgan, King, Weisz, & Schopler, 1993). This technique is usually coupled with systematic desensitization, which shall be dealt with in the next portion.
- *Systematic desensitization*, the basic idea underlying this technique was that a fear or anxiety-inducing situation, when presented to an individual, with relaxation combined with that situation, results in lessening the anxiety or fear. Benson (1968) reported on the process of systematic desensitization "by repeating feared situations during an antagonistic state of relaxation, the degree of anxiety can be reduced until the fear-arousing stimulus loses its former intensity. In essence, the technique represents the substitution of the relaxation response for a maladaptive neurotic habit."

Cognitive Behavioral Approach

Though behavioral techniques used to treat selective mutism have yielded effective results, it does contain certain flaws. One of the most prominent of such flaws that has been pointed out in subsequent research is that it does not pay any attention to the anxiety-inducing and the anxiety causing thoughts of the individual suffering from the disorder. In response to this criticism, CBT or the cognitive-behavioral approach has been offered as a substitute (Camposano, 2011).

CBT fulfills the requirement of targeting anxious thoughts, and restructuring them, thereby lessening the mutism causing anxiety. CBT is a practical and action-based form of treatment that includes and uses many other techniques like systematic desensitization and stimulus fading (Camposano, 2011). In addition to these techniques, the CBT incorporates anxiety management education. Camposano (2011) elucidated that, "for the purpose of the therapy, both children and their parents develop a specific set of skills to address the thoughts, physiological responses, and behavior associated with anxiety."

The primary step involved in CBT is assessment. Before an intervention can be planned, it is necessary that certain basic information is collected and some factors are identified. A basic framework, like what kind of verbal behavior is to be shaped, what aids would be used, what stimuli need to be introduced and how stimuli will be introduced (Shriver et al., 2011) and the likes must be ascertained. The first step has to be to *assess* the level of anxiety and the factors that are responsible for it.

In 2009, Shipon-Blum developed a continuum in which absolute non-communication was put at one end and initiating verbal communication lay at the other end. In between were different levels of nonverbal and verbal communication. Once the assessment is done, the next step of intervention is usually training the children in relaxation techniques like breathing or muscle relaxation. Then this technique is coupled with the anxiety causing situations, which would be elevated every time the intervention would start.

The steps of behavioral approach and CBT are similar in these initial steps. However, once the behavior aspect has been assessed and addressed, the restructuring of the anxiety causing thoughts becomes the next step. A common technique used here is *cognitive restructuring* which works at minimizing the negative automatic thoughts that lead to mutism. Drawing a distinction from the psychodynamic approach of addressing the origin and not the mutism, CBT aims to alter the underlying thought process and root out mutism from the anxiety that causes it. However, it poses a similar drawback to that of psychodynamic approach.

This approach, too, requires the client to express the feelings of anxiety unambiguously. However, in case of selective mutism, the child is at a loss of verbalizing his or her emotions, thereby defeating the conventional functioning of CBT. In addition, a counselor's office falls under the criterion of new and uncomfortable situation or setting, thus adding to the problem. However, in cases where nonverbal methods of communication can be used to substitute verbal methods, the process of cognitive restructuring works well towards the development of a pragmatic thinking process in the child.

The level to which cognitive behavioral therapy is effective can be seen by the following example of an eight-year-old boy who was taken for treatment when his mother noticed that throughout his school life so far, he had only uttered one complete phrase, that too, in a bout of sheer frustration. He was put on medication by his psychiatrist. But the medication alone was not very effective.

Eventually he was referred to therapy. A 21-session cognitive behavioral treatment program was provided for the boy himself as well as his family members. By the end of the treatment, his symptoms were almost gone and he could no longer be diagnosed with selective mutism. Treatment gains were maintained at a 6-month follow-up (Wicks-Nelson & Israel, 2013). Cognitive- behavioral therapy has been said to be the best possible treatment plan for selective mutism. Coupled with pharmacological treatment it yields effective results.

Exposure Therapy

Neither behavioral approach nor cognitive-behavioral approach can be used to an optimum level without the assistance and aid of exposure-based therapy. In 2014, Sulkowski et al. presented a case study on "Treatment of selective mutism with exposure therapy". Special emphasis was paid to increasing parental involvement, where the parents and caregivers were given psychoeducation in the beginning. This was followed by graded exposure therapy.

Similar to the techniques used in the former two approaches, exposure therapy involves first, confronting an anxiety- provoking stimulus. This is followed by experiencing the ensuing anxiety or stress by the subject.Finally, the subject is prevented from engaging anxiety reductive rituals like reassurance seeking, avoidance, etc. to lessen the anxiety (Sulkowski et al., 2014). The procedure that was used included development of an exposure therapy hierarchy, similar to that of systematic desensitization, in which each of the stressors was ranked on the basis of level of distress it caused. The therapy began with mild to moderate level of stressors, moving out to the high level of stressors. The study highlighted the importance of evaluating the efficacy of exposure therapy as a technique to treat selective mutism.

A case study reported by Sulkowski et al. (2014) shows the extent of effectiveness of exposure therapy in treating selective mutism. The case was one of the common ones in children suffering from selective mutism. The child in question showed absolutely no signs of speaking in front of people who were not his immediate family. There were no developmental delays otherwise. During assessment done on the child which was done only after he consented to it, it was found that anxiety disorders ran in his family. During his treatment he was prescribed certain dosage of drugs. However, once exposure therapy was included he showed signs of improvement.

This case could be used to elicit two conclusions. One, family history of anxiety also plays a role in the onset of selective mutism. It works as a genetic predisposition for the development of the disorder. This has been explained as the diathesis-stress model. And two, the efficacy of exposure theory as an intervention program has been reported to be good. A combination of this kind of therapy along with medication yields successful results.

Family Therapy

As explained in the psychosocial aspect of selective mutism, dysfunction within the families usually lies at the base of development of mutism in the children. Studies have been conducted which have reported children with selective mutism coming from divorced and broken families (Viana et al., 2009). It is, therefore, necessary that along with the individual treatment of the child with selective mutism, there is family counseling or therapy combined, for optimum results. The most important function that a family therapy would serve in such cases is that cooperation of the parents and involvement in therapy sessions will make the child comfortable, confident and more willing to engage in therapy.

In addition, this technique helps in making the parents aware of the situation. Because selective mutism is usually misconstrued as shyness on the child's part, parents are quite unaware of the symptoms of the disorder. Parent involvement is a key ingredient in the treatment success (Sharkey & McNicholas, 2008). For an effective treatment, it is necessary that there is an understanding and acceptance from the parents and other members of the family who are included in therapy.

Pharmacological Approach

It is not often that the researcher would resort to pharmacological techniques. The effectiveness of pharmacological treatment in the case of selective mutism is still highly debatable. Yet, there are times when the anxiety levels of the child are so high that some pharmacological aid is needed to lessen the anxiety levels so that other therapeutic techniques yield effective results. Schneier (2003) said, "The best-established treatments of social anxiety are cognitive behavioral therapy and serotonin reuptake inhibitors."

Selective serotonin reuptake inhibitors or SSRIs are considered to be best-established drugs for treating social anxiety disorder. Controlled trials of SSRI administration has shown efficacy for paroxetine, sertraline, and fluvoxamine. Apart from SSRIs, monoamine oxidase inhibitors or MAOs may also be prescribed. It is to be remembered that pharmacological treatment is not the primary mode of treatment. Instead, this method is used to facilitate cognitive behavioral therapy or any other intervention (Kumpulainen et al., 1998).

Multimodal Approach

It can be said that the complexity of the disorder makes it difficult to pinpoint one approach of treatment and name it as the most effective treatment pattern to manage selective mutism. The data available for successful treatment of selective mutism is scarce (Sadock & Sadock, 2007). Despite this, evidence from different case studies show that in some cases pharmacological treatment involving prescription of SSRIs has yielded positive results (Oerbeck et al., 2016). Cognitive behavior therapies combined with pharmacological treatment has also been an effective treatment schedule in some cases (Wicks-Nelson & Israel, 2013). However, these are individual references and the evidence to all of this is limited. Thus, the best treatment option can be 'eclectic approach' which would combine all the above-mentioned different approaches and tailor-made special treatment schedule according to each individual (Camposano, 2011).

Sadock and Sadock (2007) also assert that a multimodal approach is the best direction to follow. They state that a treatment program should be framed in such a manner that includes therapy, preferably cognitive behavioral therapy, and prescription of SSRIs along with psychoeducation for the family. As the first-line treatment, cognitive behavioral therapy serves the purpose. The family therapy can assist in effective treatment. And though SSRIs were medication for social anxiety and phobia, they are accepted when psychosocial interventions alone do not prove to be sufficient to manage selective mutism (Sadock & Sadock, 2007).

Role of School Personnel and Educators

Though parents and immediate family have an important responsibility to understand and seek treatment for a child with selective mutism, an equal responsibility falls on the child's teachers. Since the onset of the disorder has been stated to be once the child enters school, it falls to the teachers to recognize the symptoms and make the necessary intimations and references. Also, an understanding of the level of anxiety of the child is required from the teacher. It is not necessary that the teacher, per se, has an expertise in child psychology or psychopathology. However, it is important that the child is referred to the school psychologist timely.

In addition to this, a proper treatment program would include the parents, school psychologist, and the teachers to be a part of the treatment schedule. Even when the program has been planned, it falls on the teacher to execute it at certain levels, like assisting in reinforcing verbal behaviors in classrooms or participating in a video recording of the child (Camposano, 2011).

Usually, the counselor or therapist creates a stepwise strategy for teachers to deal with the children with this disorder. The first direction given to the teacher is to remove the pressure from the child to necessarily speak. If the child is forced to speak in the uncomfortable situation, he or she might develop a hostile attitude towards the teacher. It is important that the child should feel comfortable in the company of the teacher. The teacher must try and break the anxious barrier of the child gently.

Once the child develops a comfort zone in the teacher's presence, the latter should proceed and ask forced choice questions or open-ended questions. Any question with a yes/no response must be avoided as it gives the child an opportunity to resort to nonverbal communication like nodding or shaking of head. The teacher should be patient with the child. The child must not be hurried to answer or made conscious. He or she should be given time to respond according to his or her convenience. If the child is taking too long to respond, the question must be repeated in a gentle manner.

Once the child responds, his or her answer should be repeated so that he or she gets comfortable with listening of the response too. This reinforces the verbal response, thereby strengthening the speaking behavior. Each response must be followed by praise or encouragement on the teacher's part. The teacher has to continuously boost the morale of the child to continue speaking.

Apart from these steps, the teacher must also make sure that the child does not face any kind of humiliation or mockery at the hand of the peers, as it may lead to relapse of the condition. Shipon-Blum (2009) stated, "A nurturing, comforting classroom environment and flexibility within the classroom schedule and setting are important factors which affect the efficacy of any treatment for selective mutism."

CONCLUSION

There is ample evidence to support that selective mutism has gone unnoticed, unrecognized, and misdiagnosed for a long time. However, the present state of research has brought focus to this issue and a lot of initiative has been made in the field. The purpose of all these research is to find the best possible treatment for selective mutism. The disorder is treatable and the prognosis offered is very effective if there is an early diagnosis. There are other factors that play a role in the onset and development of the disorder, like individual differences, which would directly affect the efficacy of any intervention. Thus, the need for awareness in parents, teachers, educators, caregivers, and close family is a prerequisite. Along with proper treatment, a nurturing and comfortable environment at home, in school and other social settings is also needed. For optimum results, a multifaceted approach that includes different kinds of settings, with a combined usage of the different therapeutic techniques (including pharmacology), along with involvement of parents, family members, teachers, peers and caregivers, all put together seems to be the best shot at approaching the treatment for selective mutism.

REFERENCES

American Psychiatric Association. (1980). *Diagnostic and Statistical Manual of Mental Disorder* (3rd ed.). Washington, DC: Author.

American Psychiatric Association. (1987). *Diagnostic and Statistical Manual of Mental Disorder* (3rd Ed., Revised). Washington, DC: Author.

American Psychiatric Association. (1994). *Diagnostic and Statistical Manual of Mental Disorder* (4th ed.). Washington, DC: Author.

American Psychiatric Association. (2000). *Diagnostic and Statistical Manual of Mental Disorder* (4th Ed., Text Revision). Washington, DC: Author.

American Psychiatric Association. (2013). *Diagnostic and Statistical Manual of Mental Disorder* (5th ed.). Washington, DC: Author.

Amir, D. (2005). Re-finding the voice: Music therapy with a girl who has selective mutism. *Nordic Journal of Music Therapy*, *14*(1), 67–77. doi:10.1080/08098130509478127

Anstendig, K. (1998). Selective Mutism: A review of treatment literature by modality from 1908-1996. *Psychotherapy (Chicago, Ill.)*, *35*(3), 381–390. doi:10.1037/h0087851

Baron, R. A. (2015). Mental Disorders: Their Nature and Causes. In Psychology (5th ed.). Delhi: Dorling Kindersley (India) Pvt. Ltd.

Benson, S. L. (1968). Systematic desensitization in the treatment of phobic reactions. *The Journal of General Education*, *20*(2), 119–130.

Bergman, R. L., Keller, M., Wood, J., Piacentini, J., & McCracken, J. (2001). *Selective Mutism Questionnaire (SMQ): Development and findings.* Poster session presented at the American Academy of Child and Adolescent Psychiatry, Honolulu, HI.

Bergman, R. L., Piacentini, J., & McKracken, J. T. (2002). Prevalence and description of selective mutism in a school based sample. *Journal of the American Academy of Child and Adolescent Psychiatry*, *41*(8), 938–946. doi:10.1097/00004583-200208000-00012

Black, B., & Uhde, T. (1995). Psychiatric characteristics of children with selective mutism: A pilot study. *Journal of the American Academy of Child and Adolescent Psychiatry*, *34*(7), 847–856. doi:10.1097/00004583-199507000-00007

Burchinal, L. G. (1964). Characteristics of adolescents from unbroken, broken and reconstituted families. *Journal of Marriage and the Family*, *26*(1), 44–51. doi:10.2307/349375

Burson, P. (2006). Behind the wall of silence. *Newsday.* Retrieved from http://www.newsday.com/lifestyle/advice/behindawallofsilence-1.590417

Camposano, L. (2011). Silent Suffering: Children with Selective Mutism. *The Professional Counselor*, *1*(1), 46–56. doi:10.15241/lc.1.1.46

Cline, T., & Baldwin, S. (1994). *Selective mutism in children*. San Diego, CA: Singular.

Cohen, S. L., Chavira, D. A., & Stein, M. B. (2006). Practical Review: Psychosocial interventions for children with selective mutism: A critical evaluation of the literature from 1990- 2005. *Journal of Child Psychology and Psychiatry, and Allied Disciplines*, *47*(11), 1085–1097. doi:10.1111/j.1469-7610.2006.01662.x

Colborn, S. (2017). *Selective mutism handout*. Retrieved from http://www.sbbh.pitt.edu/files/pdf/Selective%20Mutism%20Handout.pdf

Cunningham, C. E., McHolm, A. E., & Boyle, M. H. (2006). Social phobia, anxiety, oppositional behavior, social skills and self-concept in children with specific selective mutism, generalized mutism and community controls. *European Child & Adolescent Psychiatry*, *15*(5), 245–255. doi:10.100700787-006-0529-4

Dow, S. P., Sonies, B. C., Schieb, D., Moss, S. E., & Leonard, H. L. (1995). Practical guidelines for the treatment and assessment of selective mutism. *Journal of the American Academy of Child and Adolescent Psychiatry*, *34*(7), 836–846. doi:10.1097/00004583-199507000-00006

Dummit, E. S. III, Klein, R. G., Tancer, N. K., Asche, B., Martin, J., & Fairbanks, J. A. (1997). Systematic assessment of 50 children with selective mutism. *Journal of the American Academy of Child and Adolescent Psychiatry, 36*(5), 653–660. doi:10.1097/00004583-199705000-00016

Elizur, Y., & Perdnik, R. (2003). Prevalence and description of selective mutism in immigrant and native families: A controlled study. *Journal of the American Academy of Child and Adolescent Psychiatry, 42*(12), 1451–1459. doi:10.1097/00004583-200312000-00012

Gray, R. M., Jordan, C. M., Ziegler, R. S., & Livingstone, R. B. (2002). Two sets of twins with selective mutism: Neuropsychological findings. *Child Neuropsychology, 8*(1), 41–51. doi:10.1076/chin.8.1.41.8717

Jainer, A. K., Quasim, M., & Davis, M. (2001). *Elective mutism: A case study*. Retrieved September from http://www.aimuse.it/wp/wp-content/uploads/2015/11/Jainer-Quasim-Davis-Elective-Mutism-Case-Study-UK-2002.pdf

Kimble, G. A. (1990). Mother Nature's Bag of tricks is small. *Psychological Science, 1*(1), 36–41. doi:10.1111/j.1467-9280.1990.tb00062.x

Koch, M. B. (1961). Anxiety in preschool children from Broken Homes. *Merrill-Palmer Quarterly of Behavior and Development, 7*(4), 225–231.

Kolvin, I., Trowell, J., Le Couteur, A., Baharaki, S., & Morgan, J. (1997). The origin of selective mutism: Some strategies in attachment and bonding research. *Occasional Papers-Association of Child Psychology and Psychiatry, 14,* 17-26.

Kratchowill, T. (1981). *Selective Mutism: Implications of Research and Treatment*. Hillsdale, NJ: Lawrence Erlbaum.

Kristersen, H., & Torgersen, S. (2001). MCMI-II personality traits and symptoms traits in parents of children with selective mutism: A case control study. *Journal of Abnormal Psychology, 110*(4), 648–652. doi:10.1037/0021-843X.110.4.648

Kumpulainen, K., Rasanen, E., Raaska, H., & Somppi, V. (1998). Selective mutism among second graders in elementary school. *European Child & Adolescent Psychiatry, 7*(1), 24–29. doi:10.1007007870050041

Leben, N. (n.d.). *Selective Mutism: A Case Study of a 10 Year Old Korean Boy and Applicable Play Therapy Techniques*. Retrieved from http://www.playtherapygames.com/HTML/SelectiveMutism_NormaLeben.pdf

Morgan, C. T., King, R. A., Weisz, J. R., & Schopler, J. (1993). Principles of learning. In Introduction to Psychology (7th ed.). New Delhi: Tata McGraw-Hill Publishing Company Limited.

Noelle, T. (2017). *Selective Mutism: Frozen in Silence*. Retrieved from https://www.nami.org/Blogs/NAMI-Blog/January-2017/Selective-Mutism-Frozen-in-Silence

Oerbeck, B., Manassis, K., Overgaard, K. R., & Kristensen, H. (2016). Selective Mutism. In IACAPAP e-Textbook of Child and Adolescent Mental Health (pp. 1-23). Geneva: International Association for Child and Adolescent Psychiatry and Allied Professions.

Richburg, M. L., & Cobia, D. C. (1994). Using behavioral techniques to treat elective mutism: A case study. *Elementary School Guidance & Counselling*, *28*(3), 214–220.

Sadock, B. J., Kaplan, H. I., & Sadock, V. A. (2007). Selective Mutism. *Annals of Clinical Psychiatry*, *10*, 4475–4483.

Schneier, F. R. (2003). Social anxiety disorder is common, underdiagnosed, impairing and treatable. *British Medical Journal*, *327*(7414), 515–516. doi:10.1136/bmj.327.7414.515

Schwartz, R. H., Freedy, A. S., & Sheridan, M. J. (2006). Selective mutism: Are primary care physicians missing the silence? *Clinical Pediatrics*, *45*(1), 43–48. doi:10.1177/000992280604500107

Sharkey, L., & McNicholas, F. (2008). 'More than a 100 years of silence', elective mutism: A review of the literature. *European Child & Adolescent Psychiatry*, *17*(5), 255–263. doi:10.100700787-007-0658-4

Shipon-Blum, E. (2007). *When the words just won't come out: Understanding selective mutism*. Jenkintown, PA: Selective Mutism Group-Childhood Anxiety Network.

Shipon-Blum, E. (2009). *What can we do to assess and treat selective mutism*. Retrieved from www.asha.org/Events/convention/handouts/2009/2296_Shipon-Blum_Elisa/

Shriver, M. D., Segool, N., & Gortmaker, V. (2011). Behavior Observation for linking assessment to treatment for selective mutism. *Education & Treatment of Children*, *34*(3), 389–411. doi:10.1353/etc.2011.0023

Steinhausen, H., & Juzi, C. (1996). Elective Mutism: An analysis of 100 cases. *Journal of the American Academy of Child and Adolescent Psychiatry*, *35*(5), 606–614. doi:10.1097/00004583-199605000-00015

Strong, C. J., Mayer, M., & Mayer, M. (1998). *The strong narrative assessment procedure (SNAP)*. Thinking Publications.

Sulkowski, M. L., Pence, S. L., Carlson, J. S., & Storch, E. A. (2014). Treating Selective mutism with exposure therapy: A Case Study. *Annals of Psychotherapy*.

Vecchio, J., & Kearney, C. A. (2007). Assessment and treatment of a Hispanic youth with Selective Mutism. *Clinical Case Studies*, *6*(1), 34–43. doi:10.1177/1534650106290393

Viana, G. A., Biedel, D. C., & Rabian, B. (2009). Selective Mutism: A review and integration of the last 15 years. *Clinical Psychology Review*, *29*(1), 57–67. doi:10.1016/j.cpr.2008.09.009

Weiner, H. (1977). *Psychobiology and Human diseases*. New York: Elsevier.

Wicks-Nelson, R., & Israel, A. C. (2013). Anxiety and related disorders. In Abnormal Child and Adolescent Psychology with DSM-V Updates (8th ed.; pp. 114-117). Pearson Education Inc.

World Health Organization. (1992). *The ICD-10 classification of mental and behavioural disorders: Clinical descriptions and diagnostic guidelines*. Geneva, UK: World Health Organization.

Yeganeh, R., Biedel, D. C., Turner, S. M., Pina, A. A., & Silverman, W. K. (2003). Clinical distinctions between selective mutism and social phobia: An investigation of childhood psychopathology. *Journal of Adolescent and Child Psychiatry*, *43*, 605–612.

KEY TERMS AND DEFINITIONS

Contingency Management: A technique where the individual is positively reinforced for indulging in the desired behavior instead of the behavior substitute that the individual has created for himself or herself.

Escape-Avoidance Procedure: A technique where, when the individual is not willing to go through the modification process in its entirety, he or she is allowed to leave only after making at least one display of the desired behavior.

Selective Mutism: A form of communication disorder where the individual fails to speak in a social setting, where speech is expected. The individual is capable of speech and speaks normally in the presence of close family members.

Self-Modeling: Another behavior modification technique where the individual model his or her own behavior.

Shaping: A technique used in behavior therapy. Here the individual is made to make several attempts to master the desired behavior. The behavior is strengthened by reinforcements, as it gets closer to perfection.

Stimulus Generalization: The desired behavior is reinforced in the presence of different stimuli and different situations.

Systematic Desensitization: This technique is used in behavior modification. The individual is presented with anxiety-inducing stimuli and the presentation is combined with relaxation, thereby leading to a pairing of relaxation and the anxiety-arousing stimuli.

Compilation of References

Abbeduto, L., Seltzer, M. M., Shattuck, P., Krauss, M. W., Orsmond, G., & Murphy, M. M. (2004). Psychological well-being and coping in mothers of youths with autism, Down syndrome, or fragile X syndrome. *American Journal of Mental Retardation*, *109*(3), 237–254. doi: PMID:15072518

Abd-Elfattah, H. M., Abdelazeim, F. H., & Elshennawy, S. (2015). Physical and cognitive consequences of fatigue: A review. *Journal of Advanced Research*, *6*(3), 351–358. doi:10.1016/j.jare.2015.01.011 PMID:26257932

Abraham, A. (1990). Behavior modification in institutionalized mentally retarded children: Case reports. *Journal of Personality and Clinical Studies*, *6*(1), 124–126.

Abraham, A., Mishra, H., & Kumaraiah, V. (1989). The effectiveness of behavior modification in institution-based mentally retarded children. *Journal of Personality and Clinical Studies*, *5*(3), 153–160.

Adelson, B. M. (2005). *Dwarfism: Medical and psychosocial aspects of profound short stature*. Baltimore, MD: The John Hopkins University Press.

Affoo, R. H., Foley, N., Rosenbek, J., Shoemaker, K. J., & Martin, R. E. (2013). Swallowing dysfunction and autonomic nervous system dysfunction in Alzheimer's disease: A scoping review of the evidence. *Journal of the American Geriatrics Society*, *61*(12), 2203–2213. doi:10.1111/jgs.12553 PMID:24329892

Afshan, Y. (2009, February 26). Fresh concessions for dyslexic students. *The Hindu*. Retrieved from http://www.hindu.com/2009/02/26/stories/2009022659340400.htm

Ahearn, W. H., Castine, T., Nault, K., & Green, G. (2001). An assessment of food acceptance in children with autism or pervasive developmental disorder-not otherwise specified. *Journal of Autism and Developmental Disorders*, *31*(5), 505–511. doi:10.1023/A:1012221026124 PMID:11794415

Ahmed, R. (2015). *Rights of persons with disability in India*. Chandigarh, India: White Falcon Publishing Solutions.

Alagiakrishnan, K., Bhanji, R. A., & Kurian, M. (2013). Evaluation and management of oropharyngeal dysphagia in different types of dementia: A systematic review. *Archives of Gerontology and Geriatrics*, *56*(1), 1–9. doi:10.1016/j.archger.2012.04.011 PMID:22608838

Albert, M. L., Sparks, R. W., & Helm, N. A. (1973). Melodic intonation therapy for aphasia. *Archives of Neurology*, *29*(2), 130–131. doi:10.1001/archneur.1973.00490260074018 PMID:4717723

Allport, G. W. (1937). *Personality: A psychological interpretation*. Oxford, UK: Holt.

Alur, M. (2002). 'They did not figure': Policy exclusion of disabled people in India. *International Journal of Inclusive Education*, *6*(2), 101–112. doi:10.1080/13603110110091625

Ambert, A. (1992). *The effect of children on parents*. New York: Haworth Press.

American Psychiatric Association (APA) (Ed.). (2000). Diagnostic and statistical manual of mental disorders, fourth edition, text revision (DSM-IV-TR).Washington, DC: American Psychiatric Association.

American Psychiatric Association. (1980). *Diagnostic and Statistical Manual of Mental Disorder* (3rd ed.). Washington, DC: Author.

American Psychiatric Association. (1994). *Diagnostic and statistical manual of mental disorders (DSM-IV)*. Washington, DC: American Psychiatric Association.

American Psychiatric Association. (2013). *Diagnostic and statistical manual of mental disorders* (5th ed.). Arlington, VA: American Psychiatric Publishing.

American Psychiatric Association. (2013). *Diagnostic and Statistical Manual of Mental Disorders* (5th ed.). Washington, DC: Author.

American Speech Hearing Association. (2008). *Communication facts*. Rockville, MD: ASHA, Science and Research Department.

American Speech-Language-Hearing Association (ASHA). (1993). Definitions of communication disorders and variations. *ASHA. Supplement*, *35*(c10), 40–41. PMID:8097650

Amir, D. (2005). Re-finding the voice: Music therapy with a girl who has selective mutism. *Nordic Journal of Music Therapy*, *14*(1), 67–77. doi:10.1080/08098130509478127

Anand, S. (2016). The models approach to disability scholarship: An assessment of its failings. In N. Ghosh (Ed.), *Interrogating disability in India: Theory and practice* (pp. 23–38). India: Springer. doi:10.1007/978-81-322-3595-8_2

Andra, M. L., & Thomas, A. M. (1998). The influence of parenting stress and socioeconomic disadvantage on therapy attendance among parents and their behaviour disordered preschool children. *Education & Treatment of Children*, *27*, 195–208.

Andreasen, A., Stenager, E., & Dalgas, U. (2011). The effect of exercise therapy on fatigue in multiple sclerosis. *Multiple Sclerosis Journal*, *17*(9), 1041–1054. doi:10.1177/1352458511401120 PMID:21467189

Andrews, G., & Harris, M. (1964). *The syndrome of stuttering: Clinics in developmental medicine*. London: Spastics Society Medical Education and Information Unit in association with Heinemann Medical Books.

Andrews, C., O'Brian, S., Onslow, M., Packman, A., Menzies, R., & Lowe, R. (2016). Phase II trial of a syllable-timed speech treatment for school-age children who stutter. *Journal of Fluency Disorders*, *48*, 44–55. doi:10.1016/j.jfludis.2016.06.001 PMID:27498894

Aniah, U., Kumaraiah, V., & Mishra, H. (1991). Behavior modification in self-help skills of mentally retarded children. *Journal of Personality and Clinical Studies*, *7*(1), 15–19.

Anjana, A. V., & Shanbal, J. (2010). Cognitive communication assessment protocol for persons with dementia-Malayalam (Part B, VIII, pp. 12-28). Mysore: Students Research at All India Institute of Speech and Hearing.

Ansari, P., Gorji, Y., & Shafie, B. (2013). An empirical study on the effect of speech therapy with cognitive behavior therapy on reducing the severity of stuttering and anxiety. *Management Science Letters*, *3*(12), 2957–2962. doi:10.5267/j.msl.2013.11.001

Anstendig, K. (1998). Selective Mutism: A review of treatment literature by modality from 1908-1996. *Psychotherapy (Chicago, Ill.)*, *35*(3), 381–390. doi:10.1037/h0087851

Antia, S. D., Jones, P., Luckner, J., Kreimeyer, K. H., & Reed, S. (2011). Social outcomes of students who are deaf and hard of hearing in general education classrooms. *Exceptional Children*, *77*(4), 489–504. doi:10.1177/001440291107700407

Antony, F., Venkatesan, S., Jayarama, G., & Gupta, S. K. (2013). Impact of an educational program about learning disability on primary school teachers. *Periyar University Journal of Psychology*, *1*(1), 83–87.

Appell, J., Kertesz, A., & Fisman, M. (1982). A study of language functioning in Alzheimer patients. *Brain and Language*, *17*(1), 73–91. doi:10.1016/0093-934X(82)90006-2 PMID:7139272

Armstrong, T. S., & Gilbert, M. R. (2012). Practical strategies for management of fatigue and sleep disorders in people with brain tumors. *Neuro-Oncology*, *14*(suppl 4), 65–72. doi:10.1093/neuonc/nos210 PMID:23095832

Arnott, S., Onslow, M., O'Brian, S., Packman, A., Jones, M., & Block, S. (2014). Group Lidcombe program treatment for early stuttering: A randomized controlled trial. *Journal of Speech, Language, and Hearing Research: JSLHR*, *57*(5), 1606–1618. doi:10.1044/2014_JSLHR-S-13-0090 PMID:24824991

Aronson, A. E. (1990). *Clinical voice disorders-An interdisciplinary approach*. New York: University of Cambridge.

Aronson, A. E., & Bless, D. M. (2009). *Voice Disorders of Structural Origin. In Clinical Voice Disorders* (4th ed.; pp. 24–38). New York: Thieme Med Pub.

Arvedson, J., & Brodsky, L. (2002). *Pediatric Swallowing and Feeding*. New York, NY: Singular.

Ash, S., Moore, P., Antani, S., McCawley, G., Work, M., & Grossman, M. (2006). Trying to tell a tale discourse impairments in progressive aphasia and frontotemporal dementia. *Neurology*, *66*(9), 1405–1413. doi:10.1212/01.wnl.0000210435.72614.38 PMID:16682675

Assal, F., & Cummings, J. L. (2003). Cortical and frontosubcortical dementias. *Dementia: Presentations, Differential Diagnosis, and Nosology*, 3-30.

Au, R., Albert, M. L., & Obler, L. K. (1988). The relation of aphasia to dementia. *Aphasiology*, *2*(2), 161–173. doi:10.1080/02687038808248901

Ayuse, T., Ishitobi, S., Yoshida, H., Nogami, T., Kurata, S., Hoshino, Y., & Oi, K. (2010). The mandible advancement may alter the coordination between breathing and the non-nutritive swallowing reflex. *Journal of Oral Rehabilitation*, *37*(5), 336–345. doi:10.1111/j.1365-2842.2010.02067.x PMID:20337868

Azad, Y. A. (1996). *Integration of disabled in common schools: A survey-study of IEDC in the country*. New Delhi: National Council of Educational Research and Training.

Azrin, N. H., & Nunn, R. G. (1974). A rapid method of eliminating stuttering by a regulated breathing approach. *Behaviour Research and Therapy*, *12*(4), 279–286. doi:10.1016/0005-7967(74)90002-3 PMID:4447567

Bachman, L. F. (1990). *Fundamental consideration in language testing*. Oxford, UK: Oxford University Press.

Bader, C. A., & Niemann, G. (2010). Dysphagia in children with cerebral palsy-fiber optic-endoscopic findings. *Laryngo-Rhino- Otologie*, *89*(2), 90–94. doi:10.1055-0029-1237348 PMID:19728257

Baerentsen, K. B., Stødkilde-Jørgensen, H., Sommerlund, B., Hartmann, T., Damsgaard-Madsen, J., Fosnaes, M., & Green, A. C. (2010). An investigation of brain processes supporting meditation. *Cognitive Processing*, *11*(1), 57–84. doi:10.100710339-009-0342-3 PMID:19876663

Bahia, M. M., & Chun, R. Y. S. (2014). Quality of life in aphasia: Differences between fluent and non-fluent aphasic augmentative and alternative communication users. *Audiology - Communication Research*, *19*(4), 352–359. doi:10.1590/S2317-64312014000300001353

Bailey, D. B., Hebbeler, K., Spiker, D., Scarborough, A., Mallik, S., & Nelson, L. (2005). Thirty-six- month outcomes for families of children who have disabilities and participated in early intervention. *Pediatrics*, *116*(6), 1346–1352. doi:10.1542/peds.2004-1239 PMID:16322157

Bailey, D. B., & Simeonsson, R. J. (1988). *Family assessment in early intervention.* Merrill Publishing Company.

Bajpai, N. (2011). *Business research methods.* New Delhi, India: Pearson Education.

Baker-Ericzén, M. J., Brookman-Frazee, L., & Stahmer, A. (2005). Stress levels and adaptability in parents of toddlers with and without autism spectrum disorders. *Research and Practice for Persons with Severe Disabilities*, *30*(4), 194–204. doi:10.2511/rpsd.30.4.194

Baker, J. (2003). Psychogenic voice disorders and traumatic stress experience: A discussion paper with two case reports. *Journal of Voice*, *17*(3), 308–318. doi:10.1067/S0892-1997(03)00015-8 PMID:14513954

Baker, J., Ben-Tovim, D., Butcher, A., Esterman, A., & McLaughlin, K. (2013). Psychosocial risk factors which may differentiate between women with FVD, Organic Voice Disorder and a Control group. *International Journal of Speech-Language Pathology*, *15*(6), 547–563. doi:10.3109/17549507.2012.721397 PMID:23075157

Bakhtiar, M., & Packman, A. (2009). Intervention with the Lidcombe Program for a bilingual school-age child who stutters in Iran. *Folia Phoniatrica et Logopaedica*, *61*(5), 300–304. doi:10.1159/000241880 PMID:19786790

Ball, M. J. (2005). *Clinical Sociolinguistics*. Oxford, UK: Blackwell Publishing. doi:10.1002/9780470754856

Balodhi, J. P., & Chowdhary, J. R. (1986). Psychiatric concepts in Atharva Veda: A review. *Indian Journal of Psychiatry*, *28*, 63–68.

Bamford, O., Taciak, V., & Gewolb, I. H. (1992). The relationship between rhythmic swallowing and breathing during suckle feeding in term neonates. *Pediatric Research*, *31*(6), 619–624. doi:10.1203/00006450-199206000-00016 PMID:1635825

Barac, R., & Bialystok, E. (2011). Cognitive development of bilingual children. *Language Teaching*, *44*(01), 36–54. doi:10.1017/S0261444810000339

Barlow, J. H., Cullen-Powell, L. A., & Cheshire, A. (2006). Psychological well-being among mothers of children with cerebral palsy. *Early Child Development and Care*, *176*(3-4), 421–428. doi:10.1080/0300443042000313403

Baron, R. A. (2015). Mental Disorders: Their Nature and Causes. In Psychology (5th ed.). Delhi: Dorling Kindersley (India) Pvt. Ltd.

Barrett, K. C., Ashley, R., Strait, D. L., & Kraus, N. (2013). Art and science: How musical training shapes the brain. *Frontiers in Psychology*, *4*. doi:10.3389/fpsyg.2013.00713 PMID:24137142

Basham, A. L. (1924). *The wonder that was India.* London: Sidgwick and Jackson Press.

Bashir, A. S., Wiig, E. H., & Abrams, J. C. (1987). Language disorders in childhood and adolescence: Implications for learning and socialization. *Pediatric Annals*, *16*(2), 145–156. doi:10.3928/0090-4481-19870201-08 PMID:3562098

Basso, A., Marangolo, P., Piras, F., & Galluzzi, C. (2001). Acquisition of new words in normal subjects. A suggestion for treatment of anomia. *Brain and Language*, *77*(1), 45–49. doi:10.1006/brln.2000.2422 PMID:11247655

Batliwala, S. (2007). When rights go wrong. *Seminar*, *569*, 89–94.

Battaglia, M., Russo, E., Bolla, A., Chiusso, A., Bertelli, S., Pellegri, A., ... Martinuzzi, A. (2004). International Classification of Functioning, Disability, and Health in a cohort of children with cognitive, motor, and complex disabilities. *Developmental Medicine and Child Neurology*, *46*(2), 98–106. doi:10.1111/j.1469-8749.2004.tb00458.x PMID:14974634

Bauer, A., & Kulke, F. (2004). Language Exercises for dinner: Aspects of aphasia management in family settings. *Aphasiology*, *18*(12), 1135–1160. doi:10.1080/02687030444000570

Bayles, K. A., & Tomoeda, C. K. (1993). *Arizona battery for communication disorders of dementia*. Tucson, AZ: Canyonlands Publishing.

Bayles, K. A., & Tomoeda, C. K. (1994). *FLCI: Functional Linguistic Communication Inventory*. Canyonlands Publishing, Incorporated.

Bayles, K. A., Tomoeda, C. K., Montgomery, E. B., Cruz, R. F., & Azuma, T. (2000). The relation of mental status to performance on lexical-semantic tasks in Parkinson's disease. *Advances in Speech Language Pathology*, *2*(2), 67–75. doi:10.3109/14417040008996792

Bećirević, M., & Dowling, M. (2010). *Inclusion or illusions? Policies and practices for children with disabilities and their families in Bosnia and Herzegovina and Bulgaria* (Unpublished doctoral dissertation). The Open University, London, UK.

Beck, A., Virudhagirinathan, B. S., Santosham, S., & Begum, F. J. (2014). Developing cognitive behavior therapy training in India: Using the Kolb learning cycle to address challenges in applying trans-cultural models of mental health and mental health training. *International Review of Psychiatry (Abingdon, England)*, *26*(5), 572–578. doi:10.3109/09540261.2014.918024 PMID:25343633

Beckman, P. A. (1983). Influence of selected child characteristics on stress in families of handicapped infants. *American Journal of Mental Deficiency*, *88*(2), 150–156. PMID:6227240

Beebe, D. W. (2011). Cognitive, behavioral, and functional consequences of inadequate sleep in children and adolescents. *Pediatric Clinics of North America*, *58*(3), 649–665. doi:10.1016/j.pcl.2011.03.002 PMID:21600347

Beilby, J. M., Byrnes, M. L., & Young, K. N. (2012). The experiences of living with a sibling who stutters: A preliminary study. *Journal of Fluency Disorders*, *37*(2), 135–148. doi:10.1016/j.jfludis.2012.02.002 PMID:22531288

Beitchman, J., & Brownlie, E. (2010). Language development and its impact on children's psychosocial and emotional development. In Encyclopedia of language and literacy development (rev. ed.; pp. 1-8). Montreal, Quebec: Centre of Excellence for Early Childhood Development and Strategic Knowledge Cluster on Early Child Development.

Bella, G. P., Garcia, M. C., & Spadari-Bratfisch, R. C. (2011). Salivary cortisol, stress, and health in primary caregivers (mothers) of children with cerebral palsy. *Psychoneuroendocrinology*, *36*(6), 834–842. doi:10.1016/j.psyneuen.2010.11.005 PMID:21146316

Belleville, S., Peretz, I., & Malenfant, D. (1996). Examination of the working memory components in normal aging and in dementia of the Alzheimer type. *Neuropsychologia*, *34*(3), 195–207. doi:10.1016/0028-3932(95)00097-6 PMID:8868277

Benfer, K. A., Weir, K. A., & Boyd, R. N. (2012). Clinimetrics of measures of oropharyngeal dysphagia for preschool children with cerebral palsy and neurodevelopmental disabilities: A systematic review. *Developmental Medicine and Child Neurology*, *54*(9), 784–795. doi:10.1111/j.1469-8749.2012.04302.x PMID:22582745

Benson, D. F. (1979). *Aphasia, alexia, and agraphia* (Vol. 1). Churchill Livingstone.

Benson, S. L. (1968). Systematic desensitization in the treatment of phobic reactions. *The Journal of General Education*, *20*(2), 119–130.

Bentley, K. J. (1987). Major legal and ethical issues in behavioral treatment: Focus on institutionalized mental patients. *Behavioral Sciences & the Law*, *5*(3), 359–372. doi:10.1002/bsl.2370050309

Ben-Zeev, S. (1977). The influence of bilingualism on cognitive strategy and cognitive development. *Child Development*, *48*(3), 1009–1018. doi:10.2307/1128353

Bercow, J. (2008). The Bercow report: A review of services for children and young people (0-19) with speech, language and communication needs. Nottingham, UK: DCSF Publications.

Bergman, R. L., Keller, M., Wood, J., Piacentini, J., & McCracken, J. (2001). *Selective Mutism Questionnaire (SMQ): Development and findings.* Poster session presented at the American Academy of Child and Adolescent Psychiatry, Honolulu, HI.

Bergman, R. L., Piacentini, J., & McKracken, J. T. (2002). Prevalence and description of selective mutism in a school based sample. *Journal of the American Academy of Child and Adolescent Psychiatry*, *41*(8), 938–946. doi:10.1097/00004583-200208000-00012

Berkman, N. D., Wallace, I., Watson, L., Coyne-Beasley, T., Cullen, K., Wood, C., & Lohr, K. N. (2015). *Screening for speech and language delays and disorders in children age 5 years or younger: A systematic review*. Rockville, MD: Agency for Healthcare Research and Quality.

Berlin, C. I., Hood, L. J., Morlet, T., Rose, K., & Brashears, S. (2003). Auditory Neuropathy/Dys-Synchrony: Diagnosis and Management. *Developmental Disabilities Research Reviews*, *9*(4), 225–231. doi:10.1002/mrdd.10084 PMID:14648814

Berlin, C. I., Hood, L. J., Morlet, T., Wilensky, D., Li, L., Mattingly, K. R., ... Frisch, S. A. (2010). Multi-site diagnosis and management of 260 patients with auditory neuropathy/dys-synchrony (auditory neuropathy spectrum disorder). *International Journal of Audiology*, *49*(1), 30–43. doi:10.3109/14992020903160892 PMID:20053155

Berlin, C. I., Hood, L., Morlet, T., Den, Z., Goforth, L., Tedesco, S., ... Keats, B. (2000). The search for auditory neuropathy patients and connexin 26 patients in schools for the deaf. *ARO Abstracts*, *23*, 23–24.

Berlin, C. I., Hood, L., & Rose, K. (2001). On renaming auditory neuropathy as auditory dys-synchrony. *Audiology Today*, *13*, 15–17.

Berlin, C. I., Jeanfreau, J., Hood, L., Morlet, T., & Keats, B. (2001). Managing and renaming auditory neuropathy as part of a continuum of auditory dys-synchrony. *ARO Abstracts*, *24*, 137.

Berninger, V. W., & Abbott, R. D. (1994). Redefining learning disabilities: Moving beyond aptitude–achievement discrepancies to failure to respond to validated treatment protocols. In G. R. Lyon (Ed.), *Frames of reference for the assessment of learning disabilities: New views on measurement issues* (pp. 163–184). Baltimore, MD: P.H. Brookes.

Bernstein-Ratner, N., & Silverman, S. (2000). Parental perceptions of children's communicative development at stuttering onset. *Journal of Speech, Language, and Hearing Research: JSLHR*, *43*(5), 1252–1263. doi:10.1044/jslhr.4305.1252 PMID:11063245

Bess, F. H., Dodd-Murphy, J., & Parker, R. A. (1998). Children with minimal sensorineural hearing loss: Prevalence, educational performance, and functional status. *Ear and Hearing*, *19*(5), 339–354. doi:10.1097/00003446-199810000-00001 PMID:9796643

Bess, F. H., & Hornsby, B. W. Y. (2014). The complexities of fatigue in children with hearing loss. *Perspectives on Hearing and Hearing Disorders in Childhood*, *24*(2), 25. doi:10.1044/hhdc24.2.25

Betts, J., Mckay, J., Maruff, P., & Anderson, V. (2006). The development of sustained attention in children: The effect of age and task load. *Child Neuropsychology*, *12*(3), 205–221. doi:10.1080/09297040500488522 PMID:16837396

Bhasi, S. (2003*). Remediation for arithmetic disorders-A neuropsychological perspective* (Unpublished doctoral dissertation). Department of Clinical Psychology, NIMHANS, Bangalore.

Bhat, J. S., Kumar, K., & Sinha, S. K. (2007). Auditory Neuropathy/Dys-synchrony In School-aged Hearing-impaired Children: A South Indian Perspective. *Asia Pacific Journal of Speech, Language and Hearing*, *10*(3), 157–164. doi:10.1179/136132807805297512

Bhattacharya, L., Chaudari, B., Saldanha, D., & Menon, P. (2013). Cognitive behavior therapy. *Medical Journal of DY Patil University*, *6*(2), 132–138. doi:10.4103/0975-2870.110294

Bhattacharya, S., Khanna, V., & Kohli, R. (2009). Cleft lip: The historical perspective. *Indian Journal of Plastic Surgery: Official Publication of the Association of Plastic Surgeons of India*, *42*(3Suppl), S4–S8. doi:10.4103/0970-0358.57180 PMID:19884680

Bhattacharya, T. (2016). Diversity at workplace and education. In N. Ghosh (Ed.), *Interrogating disability in India: Theory and practice* (pp. 39–64). New York: Springer. doi:10.1007/978-81-322-3595-8_3

Bhola, P., Hirisave, U., & Kapur, M. (1997). Self perception and learning environment in children with scholastic skill disorder. In R. Hegde, S. Malhotra & L. P. Shah (Eds.), Research endevours in child and adoloscent psychiatry in India. Goa: Indian Association for child and Adolescent Mental Health.

Bhugra, D. (1992). Psychiatry in ancient Indian texts: A review. *History of Psychiatry*, *3*(10), 167–186. doi:10.1177/0957154X9200301002 PMID:11623029

Bialystok, E. (1999). Cognitive complexity and attentional control in the bilingual mind. *Child Development*, *70*(3), 636–644. doi:10.1111/1467-8624.00046

Bialystok, E. (2001). *Bilingualism in development: Language, literacy, and cognition*. Cambridge, UK: Cambridge University Press. doi:10.1017/CBO9780511605963

Bialystok, E. (2009). Claiming evidence from non-evidence: A reply to Morton and Harper. *Developmental Science*, *12*(4), 499–501. doi:10.1111/j.1467-7687.2009.00868.x PMID:19635076

Bialystok, E., Craik, F., & Luk, G. (2008). Cognitive control and lexical access in younger and older bilinguals. *Journal of Experimental Psychology. Learning, Memory, and Cognition*, *34*(4), 859–873. doi:10.1037/0278-7393.34.4.859 PMID:18605874

Bialystok, E., & Viswanathan, M. (2009). Components of executive control with advantages for bilingual children in two cultures. *Cognition*, *112*(3), 494–500. doi:10.1016/j.cognition.2009.06.014 PMID:19615674

Bickel, C., Pantel, J., Eysenbach, K., & Schröder, J. (2000). Syntactic comprehension deficits in Alzheimer's disease. *Brain and Language*, *71*(3), 432–448. doi:10.1006/brln.1999.2277 PMID:10716871

Billings, A. G., & Moos, R. H. (1982). Stressful life event and symptoms: A longitudinal model. *Health Psychology*, *1*(2), 99–117. doi:10.1037/0278-6133.1.2.99

Bishop, S. L., Richler, J., Cain, A. C., & Lord, C. (2007). Predictors of perceived negative impact in mothers of children with autism spectrum disorder. *American Journal of Mental Retardation*, *112*(6), 450–461. doi:10.1352/0895-8017(2007)112[450:POPNII]2.0.CO;2 PMID:17963436

Black, L. I., Vahratian, A., & Hoffman, H. J. (2015). Communication disorders and use of intervention services among children aged 3–17 years: United States (DHHS Publication No. 2015–1209). Washington, DC: U.S. Government Printing Office.

Black, L. I., Vahratian, A., & Hoffman, H. J. (2015). Communication disorders and use of intervention services among children aged 3-17 years: United States, 2012. NCHS data brief, no 205. Hyattsville, MD: National Center for Health Statistics.

Black, A. P., & Baker, M. (2011). The impact of parent advocacy groups, the Internet, and social networking on rare diseases: The IDEA League and the IDEA League United Kingdom example. *Epilepsia*, *52*(2), 102–104. doi:10.1111/j.1528-1167.2011.03013.x PMID:21463291

Black, B., & Uhde, T. (1995). Psychiatric characteristics of children with selective mutism: A pilot study. *Journal of the American Academy of Child and Adolescent Psychiatry*, *34*(7), 847–856. doi:10.1097/00004583-199507000-00007

Blessing, M. (n.d.). *Meaning of family*. Retrieved from http://family.lovetoknow.com/about-family-values/meaning-family

Blom Johansson, M. (2012). *Aphasia and Communication in Everyday Life: Experience of persons with aphasia, significant others, and speech-language pathologists* (Doctoral Thesis). Uppsala: Acta Universitatis Uppsaliensis.

Blood, G. W., & Blood, I. M. (2004). Bullying in adolescents who stutter: Communicative competence and self-esteem. *Contemporary Issues in Communication Science and Disorders*, *31*, 69–79.

Blood, G. W., & Blood, I. M. (2007). Preliminary study of self-reported experience of physical aggression and bullying of boys who stutter: Relation to increased anxiety. *Perceptual and Motor Skills*, *104*(3suppl), 1060–1066. doi:10.2466/PMS.104.3.1060-1066 PMID:17879638

Bloodstein, O. (1975). Stuttering as tension and fragmentation. In J. Eisenson (Ed.), *Stuttering: A second symposium* (pp. 1-96). New York: Harper and Row.

Bloodstein, O. (1981). *A Handbook on Stuttering*. Chicago: The National Easter Seal Society.

Blumenfeld, H. K., & Marian, V. (2007). Constraints on parallel activation in bilingual spoken language processing: Examining proficiency and lexical status using eye-tracking. *Language and Cognitive Processes*, *22*(5), 633–660. doi:10.1080/01690960601000746

Boksem, M. A. S., Meijman, T. F., & Lorist, M. M. (2005). Effects of mental fatigue on attention: An ERP study. *Brain Research. Cognitive Brain Research*, *25*(1), 107–116. doi:10.1016/j.cogbrainres.2005.04.011 PMID:15913965

Bolarinwa, O. A. (2015). Principles and methods of validity and reliability testing of questionnaire used in social and health science researches. *The Nigerian Postgraduate Medical Journal*, *22*(4), 195–201. doi:10.4103/1117-1936.173959 PMID:26776330

Bornstein, M. H. (2013). Handbook of parenting (*5th vol.*). Mahwah, NJ: Lawrence Erlbaum Associates, Publishers.

Borson, S., Scanlan, J., Brush, M., Vitaliano, P., & Dokmak, A. (2000). The Mini-Cog: A cognitive 'vital signs' measure for dementia screening in multi-lingual elderly. *International Journal of Geriatric Psychiatry*, *15*(11), 1021–1027. doi: PMID:11113982

Bor, W., Sanders, M. R., & Markie-Dadds, C. (2002). The effects of Triple P-Positive Parenting Program on preschool children with co-occurring disruptive behaviour and attentional/hyperactive difficulties. *Journal of Abnormal Child Psychology*, *30*(6), 571–587. doi:10.1023/A:1020807613155 PMID:12481972

Bos-Clark, M., & Carding, P. (2011). Effectiveness of voice therapy in functional dysphonia: Where are we now? *Current Opinion in Otolaryngology & Head & Neck Surgery*, *19*(3), 160–164. doi:10.1097/MOO.0b013e3283448f85 PMID:21330925

Bose, A., McHugh, T., Schollenberger, H., & Buchanan, L. (2009). Measuring quality of life in aphasia: Results from two scales. *Aphasiology*, *23*(7–8), 797–808. doi:10.1080/02687030802593189

Bowers, L. (2002). An audit of referrals of children with autistic spectrum disorder to the dietetic service. *Journal of Human Nutrition and Dietetics*, *15*(2), 141–144. doi:10.1046/j.1365-277X.2002.00345.x PMID:11972743

Boyse, K. (2009). Siblings with Siblings with Special Needs. *Your Child Development & Behavior Resources*. Retrieved September 14, 2017, from http://www.med.umich,edu/yourchild/topics/specneed.htm

Bozoki, A., Giordani, B., Heidebrink, J. L., Berent, S., & Foster, N. L. (2001). Mild cognitive impairments predict dementia in nondemented elderly patients with memory loss. *Archives of Neurology*, *58*(3), 411–416. doi:10.1001/archneur.58.3.411 PMID:11255444

Bracken, B. A., & McCallum, R. S. (1998). *Universal nonverbal intelligence test*. Riverside Publishing Company.

Braddock, D. L., & Parish, S. L. (2001). An institutional history of disability. In Handbook of disability studies (pp. 11-68). Sage Publications. doi:10.4135/9781412976251.n2

Brandt, H. E., Deliens, L., Steen, J. T. V. D., Ooms, M. E., Ribbe, M. W., & Wal, G. V. (2005). The last days of life of nursing home patients with and without dementia assessed with the palliative care outcome scale. *Palliative Medicine*, *19*(4), 334–342. doi:10.1191/0269216305pm1018oa PMID:15984506

Bray, M. (2006). Language and communication in young people with learning difficulties. In J. Clegg & J. Ginsborg (Eds.), *Language and social disadvantage: Theory into practice* (pp. 106–121). London, UK: John Wiley and Sons Ltd.

Breslau, N., Staruch, K. S., & Mortimer, E. A. (1982). Psychological distress in mothers of disabled children. *American Journal of Diseases of Children*, *136*, 682–686. PMID:6213143

Bridgman, K., Onslow, M., O'Brian, S., Jones, M., & Block, S. (2016). Lidcombe program webcam treatment for early stuttering: A randomized controlled trial. *Journal of Speech, Language, and Hearing Research: JSLHR*, *59*(5), 932–939. doi:10.1044/2016_JSLHR-S-15-0011 PMID:27617680

Brinton, B., & Fugiki, M. (2006). Social intervention for children with language impairment: Factors affecting efficacy. *Communication Disorders Quarterly*, *28*(1), 39–41. doi:10.1177/15257401060280010501

Broadbent, D. E. (1969). *Perception and communication*. Oxford, UK: Pergamon Press.

Bromley, J., Hare, D. J., Davison, K., & Emerson, E. (2004). Mothers supporting children with autistic spectrum disorders: Social support, mental health status and satisfaction with services. *Autism*, *8*(4), 409–423. doi:10.1177/1362361304047224 PMID:15556959

Brown, S. (1949). Advising parents of early stutterers. *Pediatrics*, *4*(2), 170–175. PMID:18137839

Bruck, M. (1986). Social and emotional adjustments of learning disabled children: A review of the issues. In S. J. Ceci (Ed.), *Handbook of cognitive, social, and neuropsychological aspects of learning disabilities* (pp. 361–380). Hillsdale, NJ: Erlbaum.

Brust, J. C., Shafer, S. Q., Richter, R. W., & Bruun, B. (1976). Aphasia in acute stroke. *Stroke*, *7*(2), 167–174. doi:10.1161/01.STR.7.2.167 PMID:1265809

Bryngelson, B. (1938). Prognosis of stuttering. *The Journal of Speech Disorders*, *3*(2), 121–123. doi:10.1044/jshd.0302.121

Bschor, T., Kühl, K. P., & Reischies, F. M. (2001). Spontaneous speech of patients with dementia of the Alzheimer type and mild cognitive impairment. *International Psychogeriatrics*, *13*(3), 289–298. doi:10.1017/S1041610201007682 PMID:11768376

Bu'Lock, F., Woolridge, M. W., & Baum, J. D. (1990). Development of co-ordination of sucking, swallowing and breathing: Ultrasound study of term and preterm infants. *Developmental Medicine and Child Neurology*, *32*(8), 669–678. doi:10.1111/j.1469-8749.1990.tb08427.x PMID:2210082

Buckingham, J., Wheldall, K., & Wheldall, R. B. (2013). Why poor children are more likely to become poor readers: The school years. *Australian Journal of Education*, *57*(3), 190–213. doi:10.1177/0004944113495500

Buck, J. N. (1971). The house-tree-person (HTP) manual supplement: Administration and interpretation of the HTP test. *Western Psychological Services.*

Burchinal, L. G. (1964). Characteristics of adolescents from unbroken, broken and reconstituted families. *Journal of Marriage and the Family*, *26*(1), 44–51. doi:10.2307/349375

Burke, M. M., & Hodapp, R. M. (2016). The Nature, Correlates, and Conditions of Parental Advocacy in Special Education. *Exceptionality*, *24*(3), 137–150. doi:10.1080/09362835.2015.1064412

Burklow, K. A., Phelps, A. N., Schultz, J. R., McConnell, K., & Rudolph, C. (1998). Classifying complex pediatric feeding disorders. *Journal of Pediatric Gastroenterology and Nutrition*, *27*(2), 143–147. doi:10.1097/00005176-199808000-00003 PMID:9702643

Burnett, J. J., & Bender-Baker, H. (2001). Assessing the travel-related barriers of the mobility-disabled consumer. *Journal of Travel Research*, *40*(1), 4–11. doi:10.1177/004728750104000102

Burns, N., & Grove, S. K. (2009). *The Practice of Nursing Research: Appraisal, Synthesis, and Generation of Evidence.* St Louis, MO: Saunders Elsevier.

Burns, R. C., & Kaufman, S. H. (1972). *Actions, Styles, and Symbols in Kinetic Family Drawings (KFD): An Interpretive Manual.* New York: Brunner/Mazel.

Burson, P. (2006). Behind the wall of silence. *Newsday.* Retrieved from http://www.newsday.com/lifestyle/advice/behindawallofsilence-1.590417

Busatto, C. (2007). *Solidary governance for creating inclusive societies.* Paper presented at the Expert Group Meeting on Creating Inclusive Society: Practical Strategies to Promote Social Integration, Paris, France.

Buschke, H., Kuslansky, G., Katz, M., Stewart, W. F., Sliwinski, M. J., Eckholdt, H. M., & Lipton, R. B. (1999). Screening for dementia with the memory impairment screen. *Neurology*, *52*(2), 231–231. doi:10.1212/WNL.52.2.231 PMID:9932936

Butterworth, B. (2005). The development of arithmetical abilities. *Journal of Child Psychology and Psychiatry, and Allied Disciplines*, *46*(1), 3–18. doi:10.1111/j.1469-7610.2004.00374.x PMID:15660640

Callanan, C. R. (1990). *Since owen.* Baltimore, MD: Johns Hopkins University Press.

Campbell, F. K. (2009). *Contours of ableism: The production of disability and abledness.* London, New York: Palgrave Macmillan. doi:10.1057/9780230245181

Camposano, L. (2011). Silent Suffering: Children with Selective Mutism. *The Professional Counselor*, *1*(1), 46–56. doi:10.15241/lc.1.1.46

Caraballo, R. H., Cejas, N., Chamorro, N., Kaltenmeier, M. C., Fortini, S., & Soprano, A. M. (2014). Landau–Kleffner syndrome: A study of 29 patients. *Seizure*, *23*(2), 98–104. doi:10.1016/j.seizure.2013.09.016 PMID:24315829

Cardon, L. R., Smith, S. D., Fulker, D. W., Kimberling, W. J., Pennington, B. F., & DeFries, J. C. (1994). Quantitative trait locus for reading disability on chromosome 6. *Science*, *266*(5183), 276–279. doi:10.1126cience.7939663 PMID:7939663

Caron, C. J. J. M., Pluijmers, B. I., Joosten, K. F. M., Mathijssen, I. M. J., Van Der Schroeff, M. P., Dunaway, D. J., ... Koudstaal, M. J. (2015). Feeding difficulties in craniofacial microsomia: A systematic review. *International Journal of Oral and Maxillofacial Surgery*, *44*(6), 732–737. doi:10.1016/j.ijom.2015.02.014 PMID:25771070

Carter, I. (2013). Advocacy for children with disabilities: Issues and strategies. In *Special needs parenting: Working together for success, monograph II*. Retrieved March 13, 2017, from http://www.adoption.ca/uploads/Image/Monograph2-Irene-FINAL.pdf

Casas, M. J., Kenny, D. J., & McPherson, K. A. (1994). Swallowing/ventilation interactions during oral swallow in normal children and children with cerebral palsy. *Dysphagia*, *9*(1), 40–46. doi:10.1007/BF00262758 PMID:8131424

Catsambis, S., & Beveridge, A. (2001). *Neighborhood and school influences on the family life and mathematics performance of eighth-grade students*. Retrieved from http://www.csos.jhu.edu/ crespar/techReports/Report54.pdf

Cazden, C. B. (1974). Play and metalinguistic awareness: One dimension of language experience. *The Urban Review*, *7*(1), 28–39. doi:10.1007/BF02223202

CDC - Diagnosis - Chronic Fatigue Syndrome (CFS). (n.d.). Retrieved September 15, 2016, from http://www.cdc.gov/cfs/diagnosis/index.html

Census of India. (2011). *Measurement of Disability through census, National Experiences*. Office of the Registrar general and Census Commissioner, New Delhi, India. Retrieved October 27th, 2017, from https://unstats.un.org/unsd/demographic-social/meetings/2016/bangkok--disability-measurement-and-statistics/Session-6/India.pdf

Census of India. (2013). *Disabled population by type of Disability, age, and sex*. Office of the Registrar General and Census Commissioner.

Center for Educational Research and Innovation (CERI) (Ed.). (2004). *Equity in education: Students with disabilities, learning difficulties and disadvantages*. Paris: OECD Publication Service.

Chaitra, S., & Goswami, S. P. (2009). *Manual for Adult Fluent Aphasia Therapy in Kannada (MAFAT-K). Articles based on Dissertation done at AIISH*. All India Institute of Speech and Hearing, Mysore, India.

Chandan, H. S., Prabhu, P., & Deepthi, M. (2013). Prevalence and characteristics of tinnitus in individuals with auditory neuropathy spectrum disorder. *Hearing, Balance and Communication*, *11*(4), 214–217. doi:10.3109/21695717.2013.821755

Chapey, R. (2008). Language intervention strategies in aphasia and related neurogenic communication disorders. Philadelphia, PA: Lippincott Williams and Wilkins.

Chapey, R., Duchan, J. F., Elman, R. J., Garcia, L. J., Kagan, A., Lyon, J. G., & Simmons-Mackie, N. (2000). Life participation approach to aphasia: A statement of values for the future. *ASHA Leader*, *5*(3), 4–6. doi:10.1044/leader.FTR.05032000.4

Chapey, R., Duchan, J. F., Elman, R. J., Garcia, L. J., Kagan, A., Lyon, J. G., & Simmons-Mackie, N. (2001). Life participation approach to aphasia: A statement of values for the future. In R. Chapey (Ed.), *Language intervention strategies in aphasia and related neurogenic communication disorders* (pp. 235–245). Baltimore, MD: Lippincott, Williams and Wilkins.

Chase, N. D. (Ed.). (1999). *Burdened children: Theory, research, and treatment of Parentification*. New York: Sage Publications.

Chatoor, I. (2009). Sensory food aversions in infant and toddlers. *Journal of Zero to Three*, *29*(3), 43–49.

Chatterjee, M. (2009). *Indian teachers still not trained to tackle dyslexia*. Retrieved from http://www.daijiworld.com/news/news_disp.asp?n_id=65148

Chee, M. W. L. (2006). Dissociating language and word meaning in the bilingual brain. *Trends in Cognitive Sciences*, *10*(12), 527–529. doi:10.1016/j.tics.2006.09.009 PMID:17049907

Cheong, J. L., Doyle, L. W., Burnett, A. C., Lee, K. J., Walsh, J. M., Potter, C. R., ... Spittle, A. J. (2017). Association between moderate and late preterm birth and neurodevelopment and social-emotional development at age 2 years. *JAMA Pediatrics*, *171*(4), e164805–e164805. doi:10.1001/jamapediatrics.2016.4805 PMID:28152144

Cherney, L. R., Shadden, B. B., & Coelho, C. A. (1998). *Analyzing discourse in communicatively impaired adults*. Gaithersburg, MD: Aspen Publishers, Inc.

Chorney, D. B., Detweiler, M. F., Morris, T. L., & Kuhn, B. R. (2008). The interplay of sleep disturbance, anxiety, and depression in children. *Journal of Pediatric Psychology*, *33*(4), 339–348. doi:10.1093/jpepsy/jsm105 PMID:17991689

Christian, L. M., & Dillman, D. A. (2004). The influence of graphical and symbolic language manipulations on responses to self-administered questions. *Public Opinion Quarterly*, *68*(1), 58–81. doi:10.1093/poq/nfh004

Chunco, R. (2011). The effects of massage on pain, stiffness, and fatigue levels associated with ankylosing spondylitis: A case study. *International Journal of Therapeutic Massage & Bodywork*, *4*, 12–17. PMID:21589691

Cian, C., Barraud, P. A., Melin, B., & Raphel, C. (2001). Effects of fluid ingestion on cognitive function after heat stress or exercise-induced dehydration. *International Journal of Psychophysiology*, *42*(3), 243–251. doi:10.1016/S0167-8760(01)00142-8 PMID:11812391

Cian, C., Koulmann, N. A. P., Raphel, C., Jimenez, C., & Melin, B. (2000). Influences of variations in body hydration on cognitive function: Effect of hyperhydration, heat stress, and exercise-induced dehydration. *Journal of Psychophysiology*, *14*, 29–36. doi:10.1027//0269-8803.14.1.29

Cicirelli, V. G. (1976). Siblings teach siblings. In V. L. Allen (Ed.), *Children as teachers: Theory and research in tutoring*. New York: Academic Press. doi:10.1016/B978-0-12-052640-6.50013-3

Clancy, K. J., & Hustad, K. C. (2011). Longitudinal changes in feeding among children with cerebral palsy between the ages of 4 and 7 years. *Developmental Neurorehabilitation*, *14*(4), 191–198. doi:10.3109/17518423.2011.568467 PMID:21732803

Clark, C. E., Conture, E. G., Frankel, C. B., & Walden, T. A. (2012). Communicative and psychological dimensions of the KiddyCAT. *Journal of Communication Disorders*, *45*(3), 223–234. doi:10.1016/j.jcomdis.2012.01.002 PMID:22333753

Clark, M., Isaacks-Downton, G., Wells, N., Redlin-Frazier, S., Eck, C., Hepworth, J. T., & Chakravarthy, B. (2006). Use of preferred music to reduce emotional distress and symptom activity during radiation therapy. *Journal of Music Therapy*, *43*(3), 247–265. doi:10.1093/jmt/43.3.247 PMID:17037953

Clarkson, S., & Clarkson, N. (2016). *Different: The story of an outside the box kid and the mom who loved him*. Tyndale House Publishers.

Cline, T., & Baldwin, S. (1994). *Selective mutism in children*. San Diego, CA: Singular.

Clinton, T., & Sibcy, G. (2006). *Loving your child too much: Raise your kids without overindulging, overprotecting or over controlling*. Nashville, TN: Thomas Nelson.

Cogher, L., Savage, E., & Smith, M. F. (1992). *Cerebral palsy. The child and young person*. London: Chapman & Hall Medical.

Cohen, L., Manion, L., & Morrison, K. (2000). *Research methods in education*. London, UK: Routledge. doi:10.4324/9780203224342

Cohen, S. L., Chavira, D. A., & Stein, M. B. (2006). Practical Review: Psychosocial interventions for children with selective mutism: A critical evaluation of the literature from 1990- 2005. *Journal of Child Psychology and Psychiatry, and Allied Disciplines*, *47*(11), 1085–1097. doi:10.1111/j.1469-7610.2006.01662.x

Cohen, S. M., Kim, J., Roy, N., Asche, C., & Courey, M. (2012). Prevalence and causes of dysphonia in a large treatment-seeking population. *The Laryngoscope*, *122*(2), 343–348. doi:10.1002/lary.22426 PMID:22271658

Colborn, S. (2017). *Selective mutism handout.* Retrieved from http://www.sbbh.pitt.edu/files/pdf/Selective%20Mutism%20Handout.pdf

Cole, B. A. (2004). *Mother–Teachers: Insights into Inclusion.* London: David Fulton.

Collie, A., Maruff, P., & Currie, J. (2002). Behavioral characterization of mild cognitive impairment. *Journal of Clinical and Experimental Neuropsychology*, *24*(6), 720–733. doi:10.1076/jcen.24.6.720.8397 PMID:12424647

Collins, M. S., Kyle, R., Smith, S., Laverty, A., & Roberts, S., and Eaton- Evans, J. (. (2003). Coping with the unusual family diet: Eating behavior and food choices of children with Down's syndrome, autistic spectrum disorders or cri du chat syndrome and comparison groups of siblings. *Journal of Learning Disabilities*, *7*, 137–155. doi:10.1177/1469004703007002004

Comeau, L., Cormier, P., Grandmaison, E., & Lacroix, D. (1999). A longitudinal study of phonological processing skills in children learning to read in a second language. *Journal of Educational Psychology*, *91*(1), 29–43. doi:10.1037/0022-0663.91.1.29

Cone-Wesson, B., & Rance, G. (2000). *Auditory neuropathy: A brief review*. Retrieved August 6, 2014, from http://journals.lww.com/co-otolaryngology/Abstract/2000/10000/Auditory_neuropathy__a_brief_review.12.aspx

Conti-Ramsden, G., Botting, N., Simkin, Z., & Knox, E. (2001). Follow-up of children attending infant language units: Outcomes at 11 years of age. *International Journal of Language & Communication Disorders*, *36*(2), 207–219. doi:10.1080/13682820010019883 PMID:11344595

Conture, E. G. (1991). Young stutterers' speech production: A critical review. In H. F. M. Peters, W. Hulstijn, & C. W. Starkweather (Eds.), *Speech motor control and stuttering* (pp. 365–384). Amsterdam: Elsevier/Excerpta Medica.

Conture, E. G. (2001). *Stuttering: Its nature, diagnosis, and treatment*. Boston, MA: Allyn and Bacon.

Cook, B. G., Tankersley, M., Cook, L., & Landrum, T. J. (2000). Teachers' attitudes toward their included students with disabilities. *Exceptional Children*, *67*(1), 115–135. doi:10.1177/001440290006700108

Cooke, R. J., Ford, A., Werkman, S., Conner, C., & Watson, D. (1993). Postnatal growth in infants born between 700 and 1,500g. *Journal of Pediatric Gastroenterology and Nutrition*, *16*(2), 130–135. doi:10.1097/00005176-199302000-00006 PMID:8450378

Coppola, V. A., & Yairi, E. (1982). Rhythmic speech training with preschool stuttering children: An experimental study. *Journal of Fluency Disorders*, *7*(4), 447–457. doi:10.1016/0094-730X(82)90020-1

Cordini, K. L., Oda, E. Y., & Furlanetto, L. M. (2005). Qualidade de vida de pacientes com história prévia de AVE: Observação de casos. *Arquivos de Neuro-Psiquiatria*, *54*(4).

Cornelissen, R. M. M., Misra, G., & Varma, S. (2014). *Foundations and applications of Indian psychology*. Delhi: Pearson.

Cornish, E. (1998). A balanced approach towards healthy eating in autism. *Journal of Human Nutrition and Dietetics*, *11*(6), 501–509. doi:10.1046/j.1365-277X.1998.00132.x

Cornish, E. (2002). Gluten and casein free diets in autism: A study of the effects on food choice and nutrition. *Journal of Human Nutrition and Dietetics*, *15*(4), 261–269. doi:10.1046/j.1365-277X.2002.00372.x PMID:12153499

Cosco, N., Moore, R., & Islam, M. (2010). Behaviour mapping: A method for linking preschool physical activity and outdoor design. *Medicine and Science in Sports and Exercise*, *42*(3), 513–519. doi:10.1249/MSS.0b013e3181cea27a PMID:20068497

Costa, A., Hernández, M., & Sebastián-Gallés, N. (2008). Bilingualism aids conflict resolution: Evidence from the ANT task. *Cognition*, *106*(1), 59–86. doi:10.1016/j.cognition.2006.12.013 PMID:17275801

Cottrell, S. (2015). *Skills for success: Personal development and employability*. New York, NY: Macmillan Education, Palgrave. doi:10.1007/978-1-137-42653-6

Couper, M. P. (2000). Web-based surveys: A Review of Issues and Approaches. *Public Opinion Quarterly*, *64*, 464–494. doi:10.1086/318641 PMID:11171027

Couriel, J. M., Bisset, R., Miller, R., Thomas, A., & Clarke, M. (1993). Assessment of feeding problems in neurodevelopmental handicap: A team approach. *Archives of Disease in Childhood*, *69*(5), 609–613. doi:10.1136/adc.69.5.609 PMID:7504911

Crabtree, S. A. (2007). Maternal perceptions of care-giving of children with developmental disabilities in the United Arab Emirates. *Journal of Applied Research in Intellectual Disabilities*, *20*(3), 247–255. doi:10.1111/j.1468-3148.2006.00327.x

Craig, A., Hancock, K., Tran, Y., Craig, M., & Peters, K. (2002). Epidemiology of stuttering in the community across the entire life span. *Journal of Speech, Language, and Hearing Research: JSLHR*, *45*(6), 1097–1206. doi:10.1044/1092-4388(2002/088) PMID:12546480

Crawford, S. D., Couper, M. P., & Lamias, M. J. (2001). Web surveys: Perception of burden. *Social Science Computer Review*, *19*(2), 146–162. doi:10.1177/089443930101900202

Creswell, J. W. (2005). *Educational research: Planning, conducting, and evaluating quantitative and qualitative research* (2nd ed.). Upper Saddle River, NJ: Pearson Education.

Crinion, J., Turner, R., Grogan, A., Hanakawa, T., Noppeney, U., Devlin, J. T., ... Price, C. J. (2006). Language Control in the Bilingual Brain. *Science*, *312*(5779), 1537–1540. doi:10.1126cience.1127761 PMID:16763154

Cruce, M., Hill, R., Worrall, L., & Hickson, L. (2010). Conceptualising quality of life for older people with aphasia. *Aphasiology*, *24*(3), 327–347. doi:10.1080/02687030802565849

Cruice, M., Worrall, L., & Hickson, L. (2006). Quantifying aphasic people's social lives in the context of their non-aphasic peers. *Aphasiology*, *20*(12), 1210–1225. doi:10.1080/02687030600790136

Cruice, M., Worrall, L., Murison, R., & Hickson, L. (2003). Finding a focus for quality of aphasia: Social and emotional health, and psychological well-being. *Aphasiology*, *17*(4), 333–353. doi:10.1080/02687030244000707

Crutchfield, R., & Wang, X. (2016). The perceptions of stereotypes of people who stutter in Hispanic university students. *Clinical Archives of Communication Disorders*, *1*(1), 36–4. doi:10.21849/cacd.2016.00045

Culley, W. J., & Middleton, T. O. (1969). Caloric requirements of mentally retarded children with and without motor dysfunction. *The Journal of Pediatrics*, *75*(3), 380–384. doi:10.1016/S0022-3476(69)80262-3 PMID:5804183

Culp, D. M. (1984). The preschool fluency development program: Assessment and treatment. In M. Peins (Ed.), *Contemporary approaches in stuttering therapy* (pp. 39–72). Boston: Little, Brown.

Cummings, J. L., & Benson, D. F. (1992). *Dementia: A clinical approach*. Butterworth-Heinemann Medical.

Cummings, L. (2014). *The Communication Disorders Workbook*. Cambridge, UK: Cambridge University Press. doi:10.1017/CBO9781107295117

Cummins, J. (1978). Bilingualism and the development of metalinguistic awareness. *Journal of Cross-Cultural Psychology, 9*(2), 131–149. doi:10.1177/002202217892001

Cunningham, C. E., McHolm, A. E., & Boyle, M. H. (2006). Social phobia, anxiety, oppositional behavior, social skills and self-concept in children with specific selective mutism, generalized mutism and community controls. *European Child & Adolescent Psychiatry, 15*(5), 245–255. doi:10.100700787-006-0529-4

Cunningham, R., & Ward, C. D. (2003). Evaluation of training programme to facilitate conversation between people with aphasia and their partners. *Aphasiology, 17*(8), 687–707. doi:10.1080/02687030344000184

Cuskelly, M., & Gunn, P. (2006). Adjustment of Children who have a sibling with Down syndrome: Perspectives of Mothers, Fathers and Children. *Journal of Intellectual Disability Research, 50*(12), 912–925. doi:10.1111/j.1365-2788.2006.00922.x PMID:17100952

Dahaene, S., & Cohen, L. (2011). The unique role of the visual word form area in reading. *Trends in Cognitive Sciences, 15*(6), 254–262. doi:10.1016/j.tics.2011.04.003 PMID:21592844

Dalal, A. K., & Pandey, N. (1999). Cultural Beliefs and Family Care of the Children with Disability. *Psychology and Developing Societies, 11*(1), 55–75. doi:10.1177/097133369901100103

Dallas, E., Stevenson, J., & McGurk, H. (1993). Cerebral-palsied children's interactions with siblings-I. Influence of severity of disability, age and birth order. *Journal of Child Psychology and Psychiatry, and Allied Disciplines, 34*(5), 621–647. doi:10.1111/j.1469-7610.1993.tb01062.x PMID:8340436

Dalrymple, J. (2005). Constructions of child and youth advocacy: Emerging issues in advocacy practice. *Children & Society, 19*(1), 3–15. doi:10.1002/chi.828

Danermark, B., Cieza, A., Gimigliano, F., Granberg, S., Hickson, L., Kramer, S. E., ... Stucki, G. (2010). International classification of functioning, disability, and health core sets for hearing loss: A discussion paper and invitation. *International Journal of Audiology, 49*(4), 256–262. doi:10.3109/14992020903410110 PMID:20170312

Danforth, S. (2008). John Dewey's contributions to an educational philosophy of intellectual disability. *Educational Theory, 58*(1), 45–62. doi:10.1111/j.1741-5446.2007.00275.x

Daniel, L. T., Gupta, S., & Sagar, R. (2013). Effect of educational module on knowledge of primary school teachers regarding early symptoms of childhood psychiatric disorders. *Indian Journal of Psychological Medicine, 35*(4), 368. doi:10.4103/0253-7176.122228 PMID:24379497

Daniels, S. K. (2000). Swallowing apraxia: A disorder of the Praxis system? *Dysphagia, 15*(3), 159–166. doi:10.1007004550010019 PMID:10839830

Daniels, S. K., Brailey, K., Priestly, D. H., Herrington, L. R., Weisberg, L. A., & Foundas, A. L. (1998). Aspiration in patients with acute stroke. *Archives of Physical Medicine and Rehabilitation, 79*(1), 14–19. doi:10.1016/S0003-9993(98)90200-3 PMID:9440410

Darley, F. L. (1982). *Aphasia*. WB Saunders Company.

Das, J. P. (1973). How to teach retardates to control their behavior. *Indian Journal of Mental Retardation, 6*(1), 5–20.

Davidoff, B. E. (2017). AAC with energy-earlier. *ASHA Leader, 22*(1), 48–53. doi:10.1044/leader.FTR2.22012017.48

Davidoff, L. (2006). The sibling relationship and sibling incest in historical context. In P. Coles (Ed.), *Sibling relationships* (pp. 17–48). London: Karnac Books, Ltd.

Davis, G. A. (1986). Pragmatics and treatment. In R. Chapey (Ed.), *Language intervention strategies in adult aphasia* (pp. 251–265). Baltimore, MD: Williams and Wilkins.

Davis, G. A., & Wilcox, M. J. (1991). Incorporating parameters of natural conversation in aphasia treatment. In R. Chapey (Ed.), *Language intervention strategies in adult aphasia*. Baltimore, MD: Williams and Wilkins.

Davis, S., Howell, P., & Cooke, F. (2002). Sociodynamic relationships between children who stutter and their non-stuttering classmates. *Journal of Child Psychology and Psychiatry, and Allied Disciplines*, *43*(7), 939–947. doi:10.1111/1469-7610.00093 PMID:12405481

Dawes, P., Emsley, R., Cruickshanks, K. J., Moore, D. R., Fortnum, H., Edmondson-Jones, M., ... Munro, K. J. (2015). Hearing loss and cognition: The role of hearing AIDS, social isolation and depression. *PLoS One*, *10*(3), e0119616. doi:10.1371/journal.pone.0119616 PMID:25760329

De Caroli, M. E., & Sagone, E. (2013). Siblings and disability: A study on social attitudes toward disabled brothers and sisters. *Procedia: Social and Behavioral Sciences*, *93*, 1217–1223. doi:10.1016/j.sbspro.2013.10.018

de Kieviet, J. F., Piek, J. P., Aarnoudse-Moens, C. S., & Oosterlaan, J. (2009). Motor development in very preterm and very low-birth-weight children from birth to adolescence: A meta-analysis. *Journal of the American Medical Association*, *302*(20), 2235–2242. doi:10.1001/jama.2009.1708 PMID:19934425

de Schipper, E., Lundequist, A., Coghill, D., de Vries, P. J., Granlund, M., Holtmann, M., ... Singhal, N. (2015). Ability and disability in autism spectrum disorder: A systematic literature review employing the international classification of functioning, disability and health-children and youth version. *Autism Research*, *8*(6), 782–794. doi:10.1002/aur.1485 PMID:25820780

De Silva, P. (1984). Buddhism and behavior modification. *Behaviour Research and Therapy*, *22*(5), 661–678. doi:10.1016/0005-7967(84)90129-3 PMID:6517830

de Sonneville-Koedoot, C., Adams, S. A., Stolk, E. A., & Franken, M. C. (2015). Perspectives of clinicians involved in the RESTART-Study: Outcomes of a focus group. *American Journal of Speech-Language Pathology*, *24*(4), 708–716. doi:10.1044/2015_AJSLP-14-0215 PMID:26363127

de Sonneville-Koedoot, C., Stolk, E., Rietveld, T., & Franken, M. C. (2015). Direct versus indirect treatment for preschool children who stutter: The RESTART randomized trial. *PLoS One*, *10*(7), e0133758. doi:10.1371/journal.pone.0133758 PMID:26218228

Deater-Deckard, K., Pinkerton, R., & Scarr, S. (1996). Child care quality and children's behavioral adjustment: A four-year longitudinal study. *Journal of Child Psychology and Psychiatry, and Allied Disciplines*, *37*(8), 937–948. doi:10.1111/j.1469-7610.1996.tb01491.x PMID:9119941

Deb, S., Chatterjee, P., & Walsh, K. (2010). Anxiety among high school students in India: Comparisons across gender, school type, social strata and perceptions of quality time with parents. *Australian Journal of Educational and Developmental Psychology*, *10*, 18–31.

Debsikdar, B. M. (1961). Glimpses of medico-psychological practices in ancient India. *Indian Journal of Psychiatry*, *3*, 250–259.

Deepthi, G., Padmavathi, N., Philip, R. R., & Kavitha, R. R. (2015). Effect of structured teaching program on knowledge regarding specific learning disabilities among primary school teachers. *International Journal of Psychiatric Nursing*, *1*(1), 69–72. doi:10.5958/2395-180X.2015.00017.1

Dehaene, S., Piazza, M., Pinel, P., & Cohen, L. (2003). Three parietal circuits for number processing. *Cognitive Neuropsychology*, *20*(3-6), 487–506. doi:10.1080/02643290244000239 PMID:20957581

Del Giudice, E., Staiano, A., Capano, G., Romano, A., Florimonte, L., Miele, E., ... Crisanti, A. F. (1999). Gastrointestinal manifestations in children with cerebral palsy. *Brain & Development*, *21*(5), 307–311. doi:10.1016/S0387-7604(99)00025-X PMID:10413017

Deltenre, P., Mansbach, A., Bozet, C., Christiaens, F., Barthelemy, P., Paulissen, D., & Renglet, T. (1999). Auditory neuropathy with preserved cochlear microphonics and secondary loss of otoacoustic emissions. *Audiology*, *38*(4), 187–195. doi:10.3109/00206099909073022 PMID:10431904

DeLuca, J., Johnson, S. K., Ellis, S. P., & Natelson, B. H. (1997). Cognitive functioning is impaired in patients with chronic fatigue syndrome devoid of psychiatric disease. *Journal of Neurology, Neurosurgery, and Psychiatry*, *62*(2), 151–155. doi:10.1136/jnnp.62.2.151 PMID:9048715

Démonet, J. F., Taylor, M. J., & Chaix, Y. (2004). Developmental dyslexia. *Lancet*, *363*(9419), 1451–1460. doi:10.1016/S0140-6736(04)16106-0 PMID:15121410

Dervishaliaj, E., & Murati, E. (2014). Families of children with developmental disabilities: Perceptions and experiences of adolescent siblings of children with developmental disabilities. *European Scientific Journal*, *10*(2), 129–142.

Desa, U. (2015). World population prospects: The 2015 revision, key findings and advance tables. New York: United Nations.

Desmond, D. W., Moroney, J. T., Sano, M., & Stern, Y. (2002). Mortality in patients with dementia after ischemic stroke. *Neurology*, *59*(4), 537–543. doi:10.1212/WNL.59.4.537 PMID:12196645

Dew, A., Baladin, S., & Llewellyn, G. (2008). The psychosocial impact in siblings of people with lifelong physical disability: A review of the literature. *Journal of Developmental and Physical Disabilities*, *20*(5), 485–507. doi:10.100710882-008-9109-5

Diamond, K. E., & Hong, S. Y. (2010). Young children's decisions to include peers with physical disabilities in play. *Journal of Early Intervention*, *32*(3), 163–177. doi:10.1177/1053815110371332

Dietrich, M., Abbott, K. V., Gartner-Schmidt, J., & Rosen, C. A. (2008). The frequency of perceived stress, anxiety, and depression in patients with common pathologies affecting voice. *Journal of Voice*, *22*(4), 472–488. doi:10.1016/j.jvoice.2006.08.007 PMID:18395419

Dijkstra, T., Grainger, J., & van Heuven, W. J. B. (1999). Recognition of cognates and interlingual homographs: The neglected role of phonology. *Journal of Memory and Language*, *41*(4), 496–518. doi:10.1006/jmla.1999.2654

Dillman, D. A., Smyth, J. D., & Christian, L. M. (2009). *Internet, mail and mixed-mode surveys: The tailored design method*. Hoboken, NJ: Wiley.

Disabled Persons in India. (2016). *A statistical profile*. Social Statistics Division, Ministry of Statistics and Program Implementation, Government of India.

Divyashree, M. S., Divyashree, G., Sudha, P. N., & Jain, S. (2014). Categorical perception in musicians and non musicians. *Proceedings of International Symposium on Frontiers of Research on Speech and Music*.

Dixit, V. (1998). Historical foundations of disability discrimination in classical Hindu Law. *Delhi Law Review*, *12*, 15–16.

Dobbelsteyn, C., Peacocke, S. D., Blake, K., Crist, W., & Rashid, M. (2008). Feeding difficulties in children with CHARGE syndrome: Prevalence, risk factors, and prognosis. *Dysphagia*, *23*(2), 127–135. doi:10.100700455-007-9111-6 PMID:18027028

Dobbs, B. M., Dobbs, A. R., & Kiss, I. (2001). Working memory deficits associated with chronic fatigue syndrome. *Journal of the International Neuropsychological Society*, *7*(3), 285–293. doi:10.1017/S1355617701733024 PMID:11311029

Donovan, W. L., Leavitt, L. A., & Walsh, R. O. (1990). Maternal self-efficacy: Illusory control and its effect on susceptibility to learned helplessness. *Child Development*, *61*(5), 1638–1647. doi:10.2307/1130771 PMID:2245753

Dormans, J. P., & Pelligrino, L. (Eds.). (1998). *Caring for children with cerebral palsy: A team approach*. Baltimore, MD: Paul H. Brookes Publishing Co.

Dorrian, J., Roach, G. D., Fletcher, A., & Dawson, D. (2007). Simulated train driving: Fatigue, self-awareness and cognitive disengagement. *Applied Ergonomics*, *38*(2), 155–166. doi:10.1016/j.apergo.2006.03.006 PMID:16854365

Dow, S. P., Sonies, B. C., Schieb, D., Moss, S. E., & Leonard, H. L. (1995). Practical guidelines for the treatment and assessment of selective mutism. *Journal of the American Academy of Child and Adolescent Psychiatry*, *34*(7), 836–846. doi:10.1097/00004583-199507000-00006

DSE. (1994). *Functional Assessment Checklist for Programming. Secunderabad.* Department of Special Education, National Institute for the Mentally Handicapped.

Dube, K. C. (1978). Nosology and therapy of mental illness in Ayurveda. *The American Journal of Chinese Medicine: An International Journal of Comparative Medicine East and West*, *6*(3), 209–228. doi:10.1142/S0147291778000289 PMID:383394

Duffy, J. (2011). *The available parent: Expert advice for raising successful, resilient and teens and tweens*. Berkeley, CA: Cleis Press.

Dummit, E. S. III, Klein, R. G., Tancer, N. K., Asche, B., Martin, J., & Fairbanks, J. A. (1997). Systematic assessment of 50 children with selective mutism. *Journal of the American Academy of Child and Adolescent Psychiatry*, *36*(5), 653–660. doi:10.1097/00004583-199705000-00016

Dumond, R., & Willis, J. O. (2008). Bender Visual-Motor Gestalt Test (2nd ed.). Encyclopedia of Special Education.

Dutt, R. C. (1972). *A history of civilization in ancient India*. New Delhi: Vistar Publishers.

Dwolatzky, T., Whitehead, V., Doniger, G. M., Simon, E. S., Schweiger, A., Jaffe, D., & Chertkow, H. (2003). Validity of a novel computerized cognitive battery for mild cognitive impairment. *BMC Geriatrics*, *3*(1), 4. doi:10.1186/1471-2318-3-4 PMID:14594456

Dyson, L. L. (1997). Fathers and mothers of school-age children with developmental disabilities: Parental stress, family functioning, and social support. *American Journal of Mental Retardation*, *102*(3), 267–279. doi: PMID:9394135

Easterling, C. S., & Robbins, E. (2008). Dementia and dysphagia. *Geriatric Nursing*, *29*(4), 275–285. doi:10.1016/j.gerinurse.2007.10.015 PMID:18694703

Eddy, L., & Cruz, M. (2007). The relationship between fatigue and quality of life in children with chronic health problems: A systematic review. *Journal for Specialists in Pediatric Nursing*, *12*(2), 105–114. doi:10.1111/j.1744-6155.2007.00099.x PMID:17371554

Edwards, D., Hahn, M., Baum, C., & Dromerick, A. (2006). The impact of mild stroke on meaningful activity and life satisfaction. *Journal of Stroke and Cerebrovascular Diseases, 15*(4), 151–157. doi:10.1016/j.jstrokecerebrovasdis.2006.04.001 PMID:17904068

Ehrenkranz, R. A., Younes, N., Lemons, J. A., Fanaroff, A. A., Donovan, E. F., Wright, L. L., ... Papile, L.-A. (1999). Longitudinal growth of hospitalized very low birth weight infants. *Pediatrics, 104*(2), 280–289. doi:10.1542/peds.104.2.280 PMID:10429008

Eisenhower, A. S., Baker, B. L., & Blacher, J. (2005). Preschool children with intellectual disability: Syndrome specificity, behaviour problems, and maternal well-being. *Journal of Intellectual Disability Research, 49*(9), 657–671. doi:10.1111/j.1365-2788.2005.00699.x PMID:16108983

Ekberg, O., Hamdy, S., Woisard, V., Wuttge–Hannig, A., & Ortega, P. (2002). Social and psychological burden of dysphagia: Its impact on diagnosis and treatment. *Dysphagia, 17*(2), 139–146. doi:10.100700455-001-0113-5 PMID:11956839

Elias, R. (2014). *Dyslexic Learners: An Investigation into the Attitudes and Knowledge of Secondary School Teachers in New Zealand* (Unpublished dissertation). University of Auckland, New Zealand.

Elizur, Y., & Perdnik, R. (2003). Prevalence and description of selective mutism in immigrant and native families: A controlled study. *Journal of the American Academy of Child and Adolescent Psychiatry, 42*(12), 1451–1459. doi:10.1097/00004583-200312000-00012

Embrechts, M., Ebben, H., Franke, P., & van de Poel, C. (2000). Temperament: A comparison between children who stutter and children who do not stutter. In H. G. Bosshardt, J. S. Yaruss, & H. F. M. Peters (Eds.), *Proceedings of the 3rd World congress on fluency disorders, in Nyborg, Denmark* (pp. 557–562). Nijmegen, The Netherlands: Nijmegen University Press.

Emerson, E., & Hatton, C. (2007). *The Mental Health of Children & Adolescents with Learning Disabilities in Britain.* Retrieved on May 5, 2017, from http://www.lancaster.ac.uk/staff/emersone/FASSWeb/Emerson_07_FPLD_MentalHealth.pdf

Emerson, L., Fear, J., Fox, S., & Sanders, E. (2012). Parental engagement in learning and schooling: Lessons from research. A report by the Australian Research Alliance for Children and Youth (ARACY) for the Family-School and Community Partnerships Bureau, Canberra.

Emil-Behnke, K. (1947). *Stammering: Its nature, causes, and treatment.* London: Williams and Norgate.

Engell, B., Hütter, B. O., Willmes, K., & Huber, W. (2003). Quality of life in aphasia: Validation of a pictorial self-rating procedure. *Aphasiology, 17*(4), 383–396. doi:10.1080/02687030244000734

Eriksson, K., Hartelius, L., & Saldert, C. (2016). On the diverse outcome of communication partner training of significant others of people with aphasia: An experimental study of six cases. *International Journal of Language & Communication Disorders, 51*(4), 402–414. doi:10.1111/1460-6984.12216 PMID:26947265

Erkin, G., Culha, C., Ozel, S., & Kirbiyik, E. G. (2010). Feeding and gastrointestinal problems in children with cerebral palsy. *International Journal of Rehabilitation Research. Internationale Zeitschrift fur Rehabilitationsforschung. Revue Internationale de Recherches de Readaptation, 33*(3), 218–224. doi:10.1097/MRR.0b013e3283375e10 PMID:20216224

Estes, A., Munson, J., Dawson, G., Koehler, E., Zhou, X.-H., & Abbott, R. (2009). Parenting stress and psychological functioning among mothers of preschool children with autism and developmental delay. *Autism, 13*(4), 375–387. doi:10.1177/1362361309105658 PMID:19535467

Evans, D., Healey, E. C., Kawai, N., & Rowland, S. (2008). Middle school students' perceptions of a peer who stutters. *Journal of Fluency Disorders, 33*(3), 203–219. doi:10.1016/j.jfludis.2008.06.002 PMID:18762062

Ewles, G., Clifford, T., & Minnes, P. (2014). Predictors of advocacy in parents of children with autism spectrum disorders. *Journal on Developmental Disabilities*, *20*(1), 73–82.

Eyberg, S. M., Nelson, M. M., & Boggs, S. R. (2008). Evidence-based psychosocial treatments for children and adolescents with disruptive behavior. *Journal of Child Clinical and Adolescent Psychology*, *37*(1), 215–257. doi:10.1080/15374410701820117 PMID:18444059

Fabian, E. S. (2007). Counselor advocacy for access: Addressing the challenges of disability. In C. C. Lee (Ed.), *Counseling for social justice* (pp. 75–94). Alexandria, VA: APA.

Fallone, G., Acebo, C., Arnedt, J. T., Seifer, R., & Carskadon, M. A. (2001). Effects of acute sleep restriction on behavior, sustained attention, and response inhibition in children. *Perceptual and Motor Skills*, *93*(1), 213–229. doi:10.2466/pms.2001.93.1.213 PMID:11693688

Fan, X., & Chen, M. (1999). Parental involvement and students' academic achievement: A meta-analysis. Arlington, VA: National Science Foundation, National Center for Education Statistics. ED430048.

Fan, X., Zhou, Q., Liu, Z., & Xie, F. (2015). Electroencephalogram assessment of mental fatigue in visual search. *Bio-Medical Materials and Engineering*, *26*(s1), S1455–S1463. doi:10.3233/BME-151444 PMID:26405908

Farri, A., Accornero, A., & Burdese, C. (2007). The social importance of Dysphagia: Its impact on diagnosis and therapy. *Acta Otorhinolaryngologica Italica*, *27*(2), 83–86. PMID:17608136

Farrugia, D. (2009). Exploring stigma: Medical knowledge and the stigmatisation of parents of children diagnosed with autism spectrum disorder. *Sociology of Health & Illness*, *31*(7), 1011–1027. doi:10.1111/j.1467-9566.2009.01174.x PMID:19659737

Featherstone, H. (1980). *A difference in the family: Living with a disabled child.* New York, NY: Penguin Books.

Feng, X., Diamond, A., & Bialystok, E. (2007). Manipulating information in working memory: An advantage for bilinguals. *Proceedings of Biennial meeting of the Society for Research in Child Development.*

Ferguson, A., & Armstrong, E. (2009). *Researching communication disorders*. New York, NY: Palgrave Macmillan. doi:10.1057/9780230594340

Ferrans, C. E., & Powers, M. J. (1985). Quality of life index: Development and psychometric properties. *Advances in Nursing Science*, *8*(1), 15–24. doi:10.1097/00012272-198510000-00005 PMID:3933411

Fiedler, R., Simpson, L., & Clark, M. (2005). *Parents and families of children with disabilities*. Englewood Cliffs, NJ: Pearson Prentice Hall.

Field, D., Garland, M., & Williams, K. (2003). Correlates of specific childhood feeding problems. *Journal of Paediatrics and Child Health*, *39*(4), 299–304. doi:10.1046/j.1440-1754.2003.00151.x PMID:12755939

Fiez, J. A., & Petersen, S. E. (1998). Neuroimaging studies of word reading. *Proceedings of the National Academy of Sciences of the United States of America*, *95*(3), 914–921. doi:10.1073/pnas.95.3.914 PMID:9448259

Fiez, J. A., Raichle, M. E., Miezin, F. M., Petersen, S. E., Tallal, P., & Katz, W. F. (1995). PET studies of auditory and phonological processing: Effects of stimulus characteristics and task demands. *Journal of Cognitive Neuroscience*, *7*(3), 357–375. doi:10.1162/jocn.1995.7.3.357 PMID:23961866

Findlay, S. M. (2008). The tired teen: A review of the assessment and management of the adolescent with sleepiness and fatigue. *Paediatrics & Child Health*, *13*(1), 37–42. doi:10.1093/pch/13.1.37 PMID:19119351

Finke, E. H., McNaughton, D. B., & Drager, K. D. (2009). All children can and should have the opportunity to learn: General education teachers' perspectives on including children with autism spectrum disorder who require AAC. *Augmentative and Alternative Communication*, *25*(2), 110–122. doi:10.1080/07434610902886206 PMID:19444682

Finnie, N. R. (1997). *Handling the young cerebral palsied child at home* (3rd ed.). London: Butterworth-Heinemann.

Fjorback, L. O. (2012). Mindfulness and bodily distress. *Danish Medical Journal*, *59*, B4547. PMID:23171754

Flanagan, J. C. (1978). A research approach to improving our quality of life. *The American Psychologist*, *33*(2), 138–147. doi:10.1037/0003-066X.33.2.138

Fleischer, D. Z., & Frieda, Z. (2001). *The disability rights movement: From charity to confrontation*. Philadelphia: Temple University Press.

Florian, V., & Findler, L. (2001). Mental health and marital adaptation among mothers of children with cerebral palsy. *The American Journal of Orthopsychiatry*, *71*(3), 358–367. doi:10.1037/0002-9432.71.3.358 PMID:11495338

Fogle, P. T. (2017). *Essentials of communication sciences and disorders*. Burlington, MA: Jones and Bartlett Learning.

Folstein, M. F., Folstein, S. E., & McHugh, P. R. (1975). "Mini-mental state": A practical method for grading the cognitive state of patients for the clinician. *Journal of Psychiatric Research*, *12*(3), 189–198. doi:10.1016/0022-3956(75)90026-6 PMID:1202204

Forrester-Jones, R., Carpenter, J., Coolen-Schrijner, P., Cambridge, P., Tate, A., Beecham, J., ... Wooff, D. (2006). The social networks of people with intellectual disability living in the community 12 years after resettlement from long-stay hospitals. *Journal of Applied Research in Intellectual Disabilities*, *19*(4), 285–295. doi:10.1111/j.1468-3148.2006.00263.x

Fougeyrollas, P., & Beauregard, L. (2001). Disability: An interactive person-environment social creation, Chapter 6 under part 1: The shaping of disability studies as a field. In G. L. Albrecht, K. D. Seelman, & M. Bury (Eds.), *Handbook of disability studies* (pp. 171-194). Sage Publications.

Fougeyrollas, P., & Beauregard, L. (2001). Disability: An interactive person-environment social creation. In *Handbook of disability studies* (pp. 171-194). Sage Publications.

Fowlie, G. M., & Cooper, E. B. (1978). Traits attributed to stuttering and non-stuttering children by their mothers. *Journal of Fluency Disorders*, *3*(4), 233–246. doi:10.1016/0094-730X(78)90023-2

Francis, D. J., Shaywitz, S. E., & Steubing, K. K. (1994). Measurement of change: Assessing behavior over time and within a developmental context. In G. R. Lyon (Ed.), *Frames of reference for the assessment of learning disabilities: New views on measurement issues* (pp. 29–58). Baltimore, MD: Paul H. Brookes.

Francis, W. S. (1999). Analogical transfer of problem solutions within and between languages in Spanish–English bilinguals. *Journal of Memory and Language*, *40*(3), 301–329. doi:10.1006/jmla.1998.2610

Frankel, E. B., Gold, S., & Ajodhia, A. (2010). International preschool inclusion: Bridging the gap between vision and practices. *Young Exceptional Children*, *13*(5), 2–16. doi:10.1177/1096250610379983

Franken, M. C., Kielstra-Van der Schalk, C. J., & Boelens, H. (2005). Experimental treatment of early stuttering: A preliminary study. *Journal of Fluency Disorders*, *30*(3), 189–199. doi:10.1016/j.jfludis.2005.05.002 PMID:16023710

Frazee, C. (2002). *Thumbs up! Inclusion, rights and equality as experienced by youth with disabilities* (Working paper). Toronto, Canada: Laidlaw Foundation.

Fredenburg, H. A., & Silverman, M. J. (2014). Effects of cognitive-behavioral music therapy on fatigue in patients in a blood and marrow transplantation unit: A mixed-method pilot study. *The Arts in Psychotherapy*, *41*(5), 433–444. doi:10.1016/j.aip.2014.09.002

Fredericks, D. W., Carr, J. E., & Williams, W. L. (1998). Overview of the treatment of rumination disorder for adults in a residential setting. *Journal of Behavior Therapy and Experimental Psychiatry*, *29*(1), 31–40. doi:10.1016/S0005-7916(98)00002-0 PMID:9627823

Freedman, M., & Oscar-Berman, M. (1986). Comparative neuropsychology of cortical and subcortical dementia. *The Canadian Journal of Neurological Sciences*, *13*(S4), 410–414. doi:10.1017/S0317167100037008 PMID:3791055

Friedner, M., & Osborne, J. (2013). Audit bodies: Embodied participation, disability universalism, and accessibility in India. *Antipode*, *45*(1), 43–60. doi:10.1111/j.1467-8330.2012.00990.x

Friedner, M., & Osborne, J. (2015). New disability mobilities and accessibilities in urban India. *City & Society*, *27*(1), 9–29. doi:10.1111/ciso.12054

Friehe, M. J., Bloedow, A., & Hesse, S. (2003). Counseling families of children with communication disorders. *Communication Disorders Quarterly*, *24*(4), 211–220. doi:10.1177/15257401030240040701

Fuchs, L. S., & Fuchs, D. (1998). Treatment validity: A unifying concept for reconceptualizing the identification of learning disabilities. *Learning Disabilities Research & Practice*, *13*, 204–219.

Fuchs, S. L., Fuchs, D., Compton, L. D., Powell, R. S., Seethaler, P. M., Capizzi, A. M., ... Fletcher, J. M. (2006). The cognitive correlates of third – grade skill in arithmetic, algorithmic computation and arithmetic word problems. *Journal of Educational Psychology*, *98*(1), 29–43. doi:10.1037/0022-0663.98.1.29

Gallagher, J. J., Beckman, P., & Cross, A. H. (1983). Families of handicapped children: Sources of stress and its amelioration. *Exceptional Children*, *50*(1), 10–19. doi:10.1177/001440298305000102 PMID:6226529

Gallagher, P. A., & Powell, T. H. (1989). *Topics in early childhood special education: Families in special education.* PRO-ED, Inc.

Ganale, S. A. (2014). A study on association among sleep pattern, sleep disturbance and problem behavior in persons with developmental disabilities. *International Journal of Behavioral Research and Psychology*, *2*(2), 18–26. doi:10.19070/2332-3000-140005

Gandevia, S. C. (2001). Spinal and supraspinal factors in human muscle fatigue. *Physiological Reviews*, *81*(4), 1725–1789. doi:10.1152/physrev.2001.81.4.1725 PMID:11581501

Gandevia, S. C. (2012). Some central and peripheral factors affecting human motoneuronal output in neuromuscular fatigue. *Sports Medicine (Auckland, N.Z.)*, *13*(2), 93–98. doi:10.2165/00007256-199213020-00004 PMID:1561512

Garcia, L. J., & Joanette, Y. (1997). Analysis of conversational topic shifts: A multiple case study. *Brain and Language*, *58*(1), 92–114. doi:10.1006/brln.1997.1871 PMID:9184097

Garralda, M. E., & Rangel, L. (2002). Annotation: Chronic Fatigue Syndrome in children and adolescents. *Journal of Child Psychology and Psychiatry, and Allied Disciplines*, *43*(2), 169–176. doi:10.1111/1469-7610.00010 PMID:11902596

Geary, D. C. (2004). Mathematics and learning disabilities. *Journal of Learning Disabilities*, *37*(1), 4–15. doi:10.1177/00222194040370010201 PMID:15493463

Gedo, J. E. (1988). Disorders of communication: Language, affects, and vegetative signs. In *The mind in disorder: Psychoanalytic models of pathology* (pp. 177–186). Lawrence Erlbaum Associates.

Gee, J. P. (1999). *An introduction to discourse analysis: Theory and practice*. London: Routledge.

Geetha, Y. V., Mahesh, S., & Swathy, A. (2015). AIISH Survey of Fluency Disorders. Unpublished Project funded by AIISH Research Fund, Mysuru.

Gerber, P. J. (2001). Learning disabilities: A life-span approach. In D. P. Hallahan & B. K. Keogh (Eds.), *Research and global perspectives in learning disabilities* (pp. 167–180). Mahwah, NJ: Erlbaum.

Germer, C. K., Siegel, R. D., & Fulton, P. R. (Eds.). (2005). *Mindfulness and psychotherapy*. New York: Guilford Press.

Gersten, R., Chard, D. J., Jayanthi, M., Baker, S. K., Morphy, P., & Flojo, J. (2009). Mathematics instruction for students with learning disabilities: A meta-analysis of instructional components. *Review of Educational Research, 79*(3), 1202–1242. doi:10.3102/0034654309334431

Geschwind, N. (1965). Disconnexion syndromes in animals and man. *Brain, 88*(3), 585–585. doi:10.1093/brain/88.3.585 PMID:5318824

Geschwind, N. (1975). The apraxias: Neural mechanisms of disorders of learned movement: The anatomical organization of the language areas and motor systems of the human brain clarifies apraxic disorders and throws new light on cerebral dominance. *American Scientist, 63*(2), 188–195. PMID:1115438

Gewolb, I. H., Vice, F. L., Schweitzer-Kenney, E. L., Taciak, V. L., & Bosma, J. F. (2001). Developmental patterns of rhythmic suck and swallow in preterm infants. *Developmental Medicine and Child Neurology, 43*(1), 22–27. doi:10.1017/S0012162201000044 PMID:11201418

Ghosh, M., Shah, A. H., Dhir, K., & Merchant, K. F. (2008). Behavior in children with Down syndrome. *Indian Journal of Pediatrics, 75*(7), 685–689. doi:10.100712098-008-0129-z PMID:18716736

Gillam, R. B., Marquardt, T. P., & Martin, F. N. (2011). *Communication sciences and disorders: From science to clinical practice* (2nd ed.). Sudbury, MA: Jones and Bartlett Publishers.

Gisel, E. G., & Patrick, J. (1988). Identification of children with cerebral palsy unable to maintain a normal nutritional state. *Lancet, 1*(8580), 283–286. doi:10.1016/S0140 6736(88)90360-1 PMID:2893092

Glasner, P. (1949). Personality characteristics and emotional problems in stutterers under the age of five. *The Journal of Speech and Hearing Disorders, 14*(2), 135–138. doi:10.1044/jshd.1402.135 PMID:18144389

Glass, A. T., & Maddox, G. L. (1992). The quality and quantity of social support: Stroke recovery as a psycho-social transition. *Social Science & Medicine, 34*(11), 1249–1261. doi:10.1016/0277-9536(92)90317-J PMID:1641684

Glauber, I. P. (1982). *Stuttering: A psychoanalytic understanding*. New York: Human Sciences Press.

Glauber, P. (1958). Stuttering and personality dynamics. In J. Eisenson (Ed.), *Stuttering: A symposium* (pp. 71–120). New York, NY: Harper and Row.

Goldfarb, R. (2006). Operant conditioning and programmed instruction in aphasia rehabilitation. *The Journal of Speech and Language Pathology, Applied Behavior Analysis, 1*(1), 56–65. doi:10.1037/h0100186

Goldfried, M. R., & Cstonguay, L. G. (1993). Behaviour therapy: Redefining strengths and limitations. *Behavior Therapy, 24*(4), 505–526. doi:10.1016/S0005-7894(05)80315-6

Goodglass, H., & Kaplan, E. (1972). *Boston Diagnostic Aphasia Examination*. Philadelphia: Lea and Febiger.

Goodglass, H., & Kaplan, E. (1983). *The Assessment of Aphasia and Related Disorder* (2nd ed.). Philadelphia: Lea and Febiger.

Goodglass, H., & Kaplan, E. (1983). *The Assessment of Aphasia and Related Disorders* (2nd ed.). Philadelphia: Lea and Febiger.

Goodley, D. (2005). Empowerment, self-advocacy, and resilience. *Journal of Intellectual Disabilities*, *9*(4), 333–343. doi:10.1177/1744629505059267 PMID:16330487

Goodley, D. (2016). *Disability Studies. An Interdisciplinary Introduction (2nd ed.).* London: SAGE Publications Ltd.

Gosselin, P. A., & Gagné, J. P. (2010). Use of dual-task paradigm to measure listening effort. *Canadian Journal of Speech-Language Pathology and Audiology*, *34*, 43–51.

Goswami, S. P. R., & Kruthi, G. (2013). Computerized Version of Manual for Adult Aphasia Therapy in Kannada. Mysore: All India Institute of Speech and Hearing.

Goswami, S. P., Jayashree, C. S., Samasthitha S., Navitha U., Chaitra, S., & Ranjini, M. (2011). Manual for Adult Aphasia Therapy in Kannada (MAAT-K). Mysore: All India Institute of Speech and Hearing.

Goswami, S. P., Shanbal, J. C., Navitha, U., & Samasthitha, S. (2010). Field testing of Manual for Adult Non Fluent Aphasia Therapy. All India Institute of Speech and Hearing, Mysore, India. Unpublished AIISH Research Fund project.

Goswami, S. P., Thomas, P., & Rachel, V. (2015). Development of manual for Adult Fluent and Non Fluent Aphasia therapy in Hindi, English, Tamil, Telugu, Malayalam and Marathi. Unpublished Project funded by the Department of Science and Technology, New Delhi.

Goswami, S. P., Venkatesan, S., & Mathew, S. (2015). Disability certification: Issues and concerns. *Journal of All India Institute of Speech and Hearing*, *34*, 1–7.

Goswami, U. (1999). The Relationship between Phonological Awareness and Orthographic Representation in Different Orthographies. In M. Harris & G. Hatano (Eds.), *Learning to Read and Write: A Cross-Linguistic Perspective*. New York: Cambridge University Press.

Government of India, Ministry of Home Affairs. (n.d.). *List of languages in the Eighth Schedule*. Retrieved from http://mha.nic.in/hindi/sites/upload_files/mhahindi/files/pdf/Eighth_Schedule.pdf

Graaf, J., Wann, D., & Naylor, T. (2005). *Affluenza: The all-consuming epidemic*. San Francisco: Beret-Koehler Publishers.

Gray, D. E. (2002). Everybody just freezes. Everybody is just embarrassed: Felt and enacted stigma among parents of children with high functioning autism. *Sociology of Health & Illness*, *24*(6), 734–749. doi:10.1111/1467-9566.00316

Gray, R. M., Jordan, C. M., Ziegler, R. S., & Livingstone, R. B. (2002). Two sets of twins with selective mutism: Neuropsychological findings. *Child Neuropsychology*, *8*(1), 41–51. doi:10.1076/chin.8.1.41.8717

Green, J., & Thorogood, N. (2004). *Qualitative Methods for Health Research*. London: Sage.

Green, S., Davis, C., Karshmer, E., Marsh, P., & Straight, B. (2005). Living stigma: The impact of labeling, stereotyping, separation, status loss, and discrimination in the lives of individuals with disabilities and their families. *Sociological Inquiry*, *75*(2), 197–215. doi:10.1111/j.1475-682X.2005.00119.x

Gregory, H. H., Campbell, J. H., Gregory, C. B., & Hill, D. G. (2003). *Stuttering therapy: Rationale and procedures*. Boston, MA: Allyn and Bacon.

Gresham, F. M. (2002). Responsiveness to intervention: An alternative approach to the identification of learning disabilities. In R. Bradley, L. Danielson, & D. Hallahan (Eds.), *Identification of learning disabilities: Research to practice* (pp. 467–519). Mahwah, NJ: Erlbaum.

Gresham, F. M., & Reschly, D. J. (1986). Social skill deficits and low peer acceptance of mainstreamed learning disabled children. *Learning Disability Quarterly*, *9*(1), 23–32. doi:10.2307/1510398

Griffith, J. P., & Zarrouf, F. A. (2008). A systematic review of chronic fatigue syndrome: Don't assume it's depression. *Primary Care Companion to the Journal of Clinical Psychiatry*, *10*(02), 120–128. doi:10.4088/PCC.v10n0206 PMID:18458765

Grosjean, H. (2010). *Bilingual: Life and reality*. Cambridge, MA: Harvard University Press. doi:10.4159/9780674056459

Groves, R. M., Fowler, F. J., Couper, M. P., Lepkowski, J. M., Singer, E., & Tourangeau, R. (2011). *Survey methodology* (2nd ed.). Toronto, Canada: John Wiley and Sons Inc.

Grunau, R. E., Whitfield, M. F., Petrie-Thomas, J., Synnes, A. R., Cepeda, I. L., Keidar, A., ... Johannesen, D. (2009). Neonatal pain, parenting stress and interaction, in relation to cognitive and motor development at 8 and 18 months in preterm infants. *Pain*, *143*(1), 138–146. doi:10.1016/j.pain.2009.02.014 PMID:19307058

Guillette, E. A. (1998). An anthropological evaluation of preschool children exposed to the toxic effects of pesticides in Mexico. *Environmental Health Perspectives*, *106*(6), 347–353. doi:10.1289/ehp.98106347 PMID:9618351

Guitar, B. (1998). *Stuttering: An integrated approach to its nature and treatment*. Baltimore, MD: Williams and Wilkins.

Guitar, B. (2014). *Stuttering- An integrated approach to its nature and treatment* (4th ed.). Baltimore, MD: Lippincott Williams and Wilkins.

Guitar, B., Kazenski, D., Howard, A., Cousins, S. F., Fader, E., & Haskell, P. (2015). Predicting treatment time and long-term outcome of the Lidcombe program: A replication and reanalysis. *American Journal of Speech-Language Pathology*, *24*(3), 533–544. doi:10.1044/2015_AJSLP-13-0156 PMID:26125134

Gunter, C. D., & Koenig, M. A. (2011). Communication development and disorders for partners in service. Oxfordshire, UK: Plural Publishing.

Guo, W., Ren, J., Wang, B., & Zhu, Q. (2015). Effects of relaxing music on mental fatigue induced by a continuous performance task: Behavioral and ERPs evidence. *PLoS One*, *10*(8), e0136446. doi:10.1371/journal.pone.0136446 PMID:26305353

Gupta, K. R. (2006). *Liberalization and globalization of Indian economy* (Vols. 1-2). New Delhi: Atlantic Publishers.

Gupta, S. K. (2015). Management of communication disorders: A clinical perspective. *International Journal of Psychology and Psychiatry*, *3*(1), 80–93. doi:10.5958/2320-6233.2015.00006.1

Gupta, S. K. (2016). The efficacy of cognitive behavior therapy in an adult who stutters. *Indian Journal of Psychiatry*, *58*(4), 477–778. doi:10.4103/0019-5545.196726 PMID:28197011

Gupta, S. P. (1977). *Psychotherapy in Indian medicine: With special reference to its philosophical basis*. Bhopal, India: Ajaya Publishers.

Gupta, V. B. (2007). Comparison of parenting stress in different developmental disabilities. *Journal of Developmental and Physical Disabilities*, *19*(4), 417–425. doi:10.100710882-007-9060-x

Guttormsen, L. S., Kefalianos, E., & Naess, K. B. (2015). Communication attitudes in children who stutter: A meta-analytic review. *Journal of Fluency Disorders*, *46*, 1–14. doi:10.1016/j.jfludis.2015.08.001 PMID:26365773

Hackworth, R. S. (2007). The effect of vocal hygiene and behavior modification instruction on the self-reported vocal health habits of public school music teachers. *International Journal of Music Education*, *25*(1), 20–28. doi:10.1177/0255761407074889

Haddow, J. E., Palomiki, G. E., Allan, W. C., Williams, J. R., Knight, G. J., Gagnon, J., & Klein, R. Z. (1999). Maternal thyroid deficiency during pregnancy and subsequent development of the child. *The New England Journal of Medicine, 341*(8), 549–555. doi:10.1056/NEJM199908193410801 PMID:10451459

Haig-Ferguson, A., Tucker, P., Eaton, N., Hunt, L., & Crawley, E. (2009). Memory and attention problems in children with chronic fatigue syndrome or myalgic encephalopathy. *Archives of Disease in Childhood, 94*(10), 757–762. doi:10.1136/adc.2008.143032 PMID:19001478

Hallowell, B. (2017). The WHO ICF and its relevance to acquired neurogenic communication disorders. In *Aphasia and other acquired neurogenic language disorders: A guide for clinical excellence* (pp. 69–65). San Diego, CA: Plural Publishing.

Hallowell, B., & Chapey, R. (2008). Introduction to language intervention strategies in adult aphasia. In R. Chapey (Ed.), *Language intervention strategies in aphasia and related neurogenic communication disorders* (5th ed.; pp. 3–19). Philadelphia: Lippincott Williams and Wilkins.

Hamzat, T. K., & Mordi, E. L. (2007). Impact of caring for children with cerebral palsy on the general health of their caregivers in an African community. *International Journal of Rehabilitation Research. Internationale Zeitschrift fur Rehabilitationsforschung. Revue Internationale de Recherches de Readaptation, 30*(3), 191–194. doi:10.1097/MRR.0b013e3281e5af46 PMID:17762763

Hanasoge, S., Ahmed, A., & Jain, S. (2017). Effect of subjective fatigue on the academic performance of children and its relation with working memory. *Proceedings of Indian Speech and Hearing Association Conference.*

Hancock, S., & McNaughton, L. (1986). Effects of fatigue on ability to process visual information by experienced orienteers. *Perceptual and Motor Skills, 62*(2), 491–498. doi:10.2466/pms.1986.62.2.491 PMID:3503256

Harris, V., Onslow, M., Packman, A., Harrison, E., & Menzies, R. (2002). An experimental investigation of the impact of the Lidcombe program on early stuttering. *Journal of Fluency Disorders, 27*(3), 203–214. doi:10.1016/S0094-730X(02)00127-4 PMID:12371348

Hartford, E., & Leahy, M. M. (2007). The perceptions of primary school children of a person who stutters. In J. Au-Yeung, & M. M. Leahy (Eds.), *Proceedings of the 5th world congress on fluency disorders* (pp. 223–229). Dublin, Ireland: The International Fluency Association.

Hartley, L. L. (1995). *Cognitive-communicative abilities following brain injury: A functional approach.* San Diego, CA: Singular Publishing Group.

Hasbrouck, J. M., Doherty, J., Mehlman, M. A., Nelson, R., Randle, B., & Whitaker, R. (1987). Intensive stuttering therapy in a public school setting. *Language, Speech, and Hearing Services in Schools, 18*(4), 330–343. doi:10.1044/0161-1461.1804.330

Hastings, R. P. (2005). Child behaviour problems and partner mental health as correlates of stress in mothers and fathers of children with autism. *Journal of Intellectual Disability Research, 47*(4-5), 231–237. doi:10.1046/j.1365-2788.2003.00485.x PMID:12787155

Hastings, R. P., & Brown, T. (2002). Behavior problems of children with autism, parental self-efficacy, and mental health. *American Journal of Mental Retardation, 107*(3), 222–232. doi: PMID:11966335

Hastings, R. P., & Johnson, E. (2001). Stress in UK families conducting intensive home-based behavioral intervention for their young child with autism. *Journal of Autism and Developmental Disorders, 31*(3), 327–336. doi:10.1023/A:1010799320795 PMID:11518485

Hawker, D. S., & Bolton, M. J. (2000). Twenty years' research on peer victimization and psychosocial maladjustment: A meta-analytic review of cross-sectional studies. *Journal of Child Psychology and Psychiatry, and Allied Disciplines, 41*(4), 441–455. doi:10.1111/1469-7610.00629 PMID:10836674

Hawley, J. A., & Reilly, T. (1997). Fatigue revisited. *Journal of Sports Sciences, 15*, 245–246. PMID:9232549

Hawley, K. M., & Welsz, J. R. (2003). Child, parent, and therapist (dis) agreement on target problems in outpatient therapy: The therapist's dilemma and its implications. *Journal of Consulting and Clinical Psychology, 71*(1), 62–70. doi:10.1037/0022-006X.71.1.62 PMID:12602426

Haynes, S. C., Masuda, A., Bissett, R., Lucoma, J., & Guerrero, L. F. (2004). DBT, FAP, and ACT: How empirically oriented are the new behavior therapy technologies? *Behavior Therapy, 35*(1), 35–54. doi:10.1016/S0005-7894(04)80003-0

Haynes, S. N., O'Brien, W. H., & Kaholokula, J. K. (2011). *Behavioral assessment and case formulation.* John Wiley and Sons.

Haynes, W. O., Moran, M. J., & Pindzola, R. H. (2006). *Communication disorders in the classroom: An introduction for professionals in school settings.* London, UK: Jones and Bartlett Publishers International.

He, A., & Young, R. (1998). Language proficiency interviews: A discourse approach. In R. Young & W. He (Eds.), *Talking and Testing: Discourse approaches to the assessment of oral proficiency* (pp. 1–24). Philadelphia: John Benjamins. doi:10.1075ibil.14.02he

Hegde, M. N., & Freed, D. (2011). Assessment of communication disorders in adults. Oxfordshire, UK: Plural Publishing.

Hegde, M. N. (2007). *Hegde's pocket guide to communication disorders.* Boston, MA: Thomson Delmar Learning.

Hegde, M. N., & Gierut, J. (1979). The operant training and generalization of pronouns and a verb form in a language delayed. *Journal of Communication Disorders, 12*(1), 23–34. doi:10.1016/0021-9924(79)90018-2 PMID:422745

Heins, M. J., Knoop, H., Burk, W. J., & Bleijenberg, G. (2013). The process of cognitive behaviour therapy for chronic fatigue syndrome: Which changes in perpetuating cognitions and behaviour are related to a reduction in fatigue? *Journal of Psychosomatic Research, 75*(3), 235–241. doi:10.1016/j.jpsychores.2013.06.034 PMID:23972412

Helms-Estabrooks, N., & Albert, M. L. (2014). *Manual of Aphasia and Aphasia Therapy* (3rd ed.). Austin, TX: PRO-ED.

Henderson, A. T., & Mapp, K. L. (2002). *The impact of school, family and community connections on student achievement.* Annual Synthesis 2002, Southwest Educational Development Laboratory. Retrieved from https://www.sedl.org/connections/resources/evidence.pdf

Hensch, T. K. (2004). Critical period regulation. *Annual Review of Neuroscience, 27*(1), 549–579. doi:10.1146/annurev.neuro.27.070203.144327 PMID:15217343

Herholz, S. C., & Zatorre, R. J. (2012). Musical training as a framework for brain plasticity: Behavior, function, and structure. *Neuron, 76*(3), 486–502. doi:10.1016/j.neuron.2012.10.011 PMID:23141061

Herring, S., Gray, K., Taffe, J., Tonge, B., Seeney, D., & Einfeld, S. (2006). Behaviour and emotional problems in toddlers with pervasive developmental disorders and developmental delay: Associations with parental mental health and family functioning. *Journal of Intellectual Disability Research, 50*(12), 874–882. doi:10.1111/j.1365-2788.2006.00904.x PMID:17100948

Hersen, M. (2006). *Handbook of behavioral assessment.* Boston: Academic Press.

Hess, R., Molina, A., & Kozleski, E. B. (2006). Until somebody hears me: Parental voice and advocacy in special education decision-making. *British Journal of Special Education, 33*(3), 148–157. doi:10.1111/j.1467-8578.2006.00430.x

Hetu, R., Riverin, L., Lalande, N., Getty, L., & St-Cyr, C. (1988). Qualitative analysis of the handicap associated with occupational hearing loss. *British Journal of Audiology*, *22*(4), 251–264. doi:10.3109/03005368809076462 PMID:3242715

Hevezi, J. A. (2016). Evaluation of a meditation intervention to reduce the effects of stressors associated with compassion fatigue among nurses. *Journal of Holistic Nursing*, *34*(4), 343–350. doi:10.1177/0898010115615981 PMID:26598000

Hewitt, L. (2014). Social anxiety and pragmatics in autism spectrum disorders: Cognitive behavioral therapy and its relation to speech-language pathology. *Perspectives on Language Learning and Education*, *21*(1), 5–12. doi:10.1044/lle21.1.5

Hick, C. B., & Tharpe, A. M. (2002). Listening effort and fatigue in school-age children with and without hearing loss. *Journal of Speech, Language, and Hearing Research: JSLHR*, *45*(3), 573–584. doi:10.1044/1092-4388(2002/046) PMID:12069009

Hilari, K., Byng, S., Lamping, D. L., & Smith, S. C. (2003). Stroke and aphasia quality of life scale-39 (SAQOL-39). *Stroke*, *34*(8), 1944–1950. doi:10.1161/01.STR.0000081987.46660.ED PMID:12855827

Hirst, M. (1985). Young adults with disabilities: Health, employment and financial costs for family carers. *Child: Care, Health and Development*, *11*(5), 291–307. doi:10.1111/j.1365-2214.1985.tb00471.x PMID:2934179

Hitch, G. J., & McAuley, E. (1991). Working memory in children with specific arithmetical learning difficulties. *British Journal of Psychology*, *82*(3), 375–386. doi:10.1111/j.2044-8295.1991.tb02406.x PMID:1954527

Hobart, J. C., Williams, S. L., Moran, K., & Thompson, A. J. (2016). Quality of life measurement after stroke: Uses and abuses of the SF-36. *Stroke*, *33*(5), 1348–1356. doi:10.1161/01.STR.0000015030.59594.B3 PMID:11988614

Hockey, R. (2013). *The psychology of fatigue: Work, effort and control*. Cambridge, UK: Cambridge University Press. doi:10.1017/CBO9781139015394

Hodapp, R. M., Ricci, L. A., Ly, T. M., & Fidler, D. J. (2003). The effects of the child with Down syndrome on maternal stress. *British Journal of Developmental Psychology*, *21*(1), 137–151. doi:10.1348/026151003321164672

Hodges, J. R., Erzinçlioğlu, S., & Patterson, K. (2006). Evolution of cognitive deficits and conversion to dementia in patients with mild cognitive impairment: A very-long-term follow-up study. *Dementia and Geriatric Cognitive Disorders*, *21*(5-6), 380–391. doi:10.1159/000092534 PMID:16601329

Hoffman, Ch. D., Sweeney, D. P., Lopez-Wagner, M. C., Hodge, D., Nam, C. Y., & Botts, B. H. (2008). Children with autism: Sleep problems and mothers' stress. *Focus on Autism and Other Developmental Disabilities*, *23*(3), 155–165. doi:10.1177/1088357608316271

Holmes, T. H., & Rahe, R. H. (1967). The social readjustment rating scale. *Journal of Psychosomatic Research*, *11*(2), 213–218. doi:10.1016/0022-3999(67)90010-4 PMID:6059863

Holroyd, J. (1974). The questionnaire on resources and stress: An instrument to measure family response to a handicapped family member. *Journal of Community Psychology*, *2*(1), 92–94. doi:

Holtzer, R., Shuman, M., Mahoney, J. R., Lipton, R., & Verghese, J. (2010). Cognitive fatigue defined in the context of attention networks. *Neuropsychology, Development, and Cognition. Section B, Aging, Neuropsychology and Cognition*, *18*(1), 108–128. doi:10.1080/13825585.2010.517826 PMID:21128132

Horner, J., Alberts, M. J., Dawson, D. V., & Cook, G. M. (1993). Swallowing in Alzheimer's disease. *Alzheimer Disease and Associated Disorders*, *8*(3), 177–189. PMID:7986487

Horner, J., & Massey, E. W. (1988). Silent aspiration following stroke. *Neurology*, *38*(2), 317–319. doi:10.1212/WNL.38.2.317 PMID:3340301

Horner, J., Massey, E. W., Riski, J. E., Lathrop, D. L., & Chase, K. N. (1988). Aspiration following stroke: Clinical correlates and outcome. *Neurology*, *38*(9), 1359–1362. doi:10.1212/WNL.38.9.1359 PMID:3412582

Hornman, J., de Winter, A. F., Kerstjens, J. M., Bos, A. F., & Reijneveld, S. A. (2016). Emotional and behavioral problems of preterm and full-term children at school entry. *Pediatrics*, *137*(5), e20152255. doi:10.1542/peds.2015-2255 PMID:27244786

Hornsby, B. W. Y., & Kipp, A. M. (2016). Subjective ratings of fatigue and vigor in adults with hearing loss are driven by perceived hearing difficulties not degree of hearing loss. *Ear and Hearing*, *37*(1), e1–e10. doi:10.1097/AUD.0000000000000203 PMID:26295606

Hothschild, A. (1979). Emotion work, feeling rules and social structure. *American Journal of Sociology*, *85*(3), 551–575. doi:10.1086/227049

Howell, P., Davis, S., Patel, H., Cuniffe, P., Downing-Wilson, D., Au-Yeung, J., . . . Peters, H. F. M. (2004). Fluency development and temperament in fluent children and children who stutter. In A. Packman, A. Meltzer, and H. F. Peters (Eds.), *Theory, research and therapy in fluency disorders. Proceedings of the 4th world congress on fluency disorders* (pp. 250–256). Montreal, Canada: Nijmegen University Press.

Huang, H. S., & Hanley, J. R. (1994). Phonological awareness and visual skills in learning to read Chinese and English. *Cognition*, *54*(1), 73–98. doi:10.1016/0010-0277(94)00641-W PMID:7851080

Hudson, H. M., Daubert, C. R., & Mills, R. H. (2000). The interdependency of protein-energy malnutrition, aging and dysphagia. *Dysphagia*, *15*(1), 31–38. doi:10.1007004559910007 PMID:10594256

Hugh-Jones, S., & Smith, P. K. (1999). Self-reports of short- and long-term effects of bullying on children who stammer. *The British Journal of Educational Psychology*, *69*(2), 141–158. doi:10.1348/000709999157626 PMID:10405616

Hulit, L. M. (2004). *Straight talk on stuttering: information, encouragement, and counsel for stutterers, caregivers, and speech-language clinicians*. Springfield, IL: Charles C. Thomas Publishers.

Hutton, J. L., Pharoah, P. O., Cooke, R. W., & Stevenson, R. C. (1997). Differential effects of preterm birth and small gestational age on cognitive and motor development. *Archives of Disease in Childhood. Fetal and Neonatal Edition*, *76*(2), F75–F81. doi:10.1136/fn.76.2.F75 PMID:9135284

Indla, R., Indla, V., & Singh, T. (2008). Impact of disability of mentally retarded persons on their parents. *Indian Journal of Psychological Medicine*, *30*(2), 98–104. doi:10.4103/0253-7176.48482

International Disability and Development Consortium. (2005). *Inclusive Development and the Comprehensive and Integral International Convention on the Protection and Promotion of the Rights and Dignity of Persons with Disabilities*. Author.

International Labour Organization. (1998). Vocational rehabilitation and employment of disabled persons. In *International Labour Conference, 86th Session*. ILO.

Irish Association of Speech and Language Therapists (IASLT). (2007). *Specific speech and language impairment in children: Definition, service provision and recommendations for change*. Dublin, Ireland: Author.

Ishii, A., Tanaka, M., & Watanabe, Y. (2014). Neural mechanisms of mental fatigue. *Reviews in the Neurosciences*, *25*, 469–479. PMID:24926625

Iverach, L., & Rapee, R. (2014). Social anxiety disorder and stuttering: Current status and future directions. *Journal of Fluency Disorders*, *40*, 69–82. doi:10.1016/j.jfludis.2013.08.003 PMID:24929468

Izzo, C. V., Weissberg, R. P., Kasprow, W. J., & Fendrich, M. (1999). A longitudinal assessment of teacher perceptions of parent involvement in children's education and school performance. *American Journal of Community Psychology*, *27*(6), 817–839. doi:10.1023/A:1022262625984 PMID:10723536

Jain, H., Usha, M. N., & Jain, S. (2017). Effect of physical and mental fatigue on working memory skills and speech perception in noise. Proceedings of Indian Speech and Hearing Association, 2017.

Jainer, A. K., Quasim, M., & Davis, M. (2001). *Elective mutism: A case study*. Retrieved September from http://www.aimuse.it/wp/wp-content/uploads/2015/11/Jainer-Quasim-Davis-Elective-Mutism-Case-Study-UK-2002.pdf

Jain, M., & Passi, G. R. (2005). Assessment of a modified mini-mental scale for cognitive functions in children. *Indian Pediatrics*, *42*, 907–991. PMID:16208050

Jain, S., Kashyap, S., & Vinutha, M. M. (2016). Effect of musical training on perception of temporal fine structure cues in children. *Proceedings of International Symposium on Frontiers of Research on Speech and Music.*

Jaradat, N. A. (n.d.). *Attitudes of intellectual disability children's siblings toward intellectual disability*. Retrieved from http://www.zu.edu.jo/MainFile/Profile_Dr_UploadFile/Researcher/Files/ResearchFile_4051_7_50.pdf

Jason, L. A., Boulton, A., Porter, N. S., Jessen, T., Njoku, M. G., & Friedberg, F. (2010). Classification of myalgic encephalomyelitis/chronic fatigue syndrome by types of fatigue. *Behavioral Medicine (Washington, D.C.)*, *36*(1), 24–31. doi:10.1080/08964280903521370 PMID:20185398

Jena, S. P. K. (2008). *Behavior therapy: Techniques, research, and applications*. New Delhi: Sage Publications.

Jeyachandran, P., Vimala, K., & Kumar, S. (1992). *Madras Developmental Programming System* (5th ed.). Madras: Vijay Human Services.

Jijo, P. M., & Yathiraj, A. (2012). Audiological Characteristics and Duration of the Disorder in Individuals with Auditory Neuropathy Spectrum Disorder (ANSD) - A Retrospective Study. *Journal of Indian Speech and Hearing Association*, *26*(1), 17–26.

Jijo, P. M., & Yathiraj, A. (2013). Audiological findings and aided performance in individuals with auditory neuropathy spectrum disorder (ANSD)-A retrospective study. *Journal of Hearing Science*, *3*(1), 18–26.

Joanette, Y., & Brownell, H. H. (Eds.). (1993). *Narrative discourse in neurologically impaired and normal aging adults*. San Diego, CA: Singular Publishing Group.

Johansson, B., Bjuhr, H., & Rönnbäck, L. (2012). Mindfulness-based stress reduction (MBSR) improves long-term mental fatigue after stroke or traumatic brain injury. *Brain Injury: [BI]*, *26*(13-14), 1621–1628. doi:10.3109/02699052.2012.700082 PMID:22794665

John, A., Sadasivan, A., Sukumaran, B., Bhola, P., David, N. J., & Manickam, L. S. S. (2013). Practice Guidelines: Learning Disabilities. *Indian Journal of Clinical Psychology*, *40*(1), 65–88.

Johnson, C. B., & Deitz, J. C. (1985). Time use of mothers with pre-school children: A pilot study. *The American Journal of Occupational Therapy*, *39*(9), 578–583. doi:10.5014/ajot.39.9.578 PMID:2931990

Johnson, E. S., Humphrey, M., Mellard, D. F., Woods, K., & Swanson, H. L. (2010). Cognitive processing deficits and students with specific learning disabilities: A selective meta-analysis of the literature. *Learning Disability Quarterly*, *33*(1), 3–1. doi:10.1177/073194871003300101

Johnson, K., Walden, T., Conture, E., & Karrass, J. (2010). Spontaneous regulation of emotions in preschool-age children who stutter: Preliminary findings. *Journal of Speech, Language, and Hearing Research: JSLHR*, *53*(6), 1478–1495. doi:10.1044/1092-4388(2010/08-0150) PMID:20643793

Johnson, S. K., DeLuca, J., Diamond, B. J., & Natelson, B. H. (1996). Selective impairment of auditory processing in chronic fatigue syndrome: A comparison with multiple sclerosis and healthy controls. *Perceptual and Motor Skills*, *83*(1), 51–62. doi:10.2466/pms.1996.83.1.51 PMID:8873173

Johnson, S., & Harris, O. (2014). Special educator attitudes toward children with communication disorders in the Caribbean. *Caribbean Educational Research Journal*, *12*(2), 133–148.

Johnson, W. (1934). *Stuttering in the preschool child (Child Welfare Pamphlets No. 37)*. Iowa City, IA: University of Iowa.

Johnson, W. (1942). A study of onset and development of stuttering. *The Journal of Speech Disorders*, *7*(3), 251–257. doi:10.1044/jshd.0703.251

Johnson, W. (1948). Stuttering. In W. Johnson, S. Brown, J. Curtis, C. Edney, & J. Keaster (Eds.), *Speech handicapped school children*. New York, NY: Harper and Row.

Johnson, W., & ... (1959). *The onset of stuttering: Research findings and implications*. Minneapolis, MN: University of Minnesota.

Johnston, J. M. (1993). Phenomenology and treatment of rumination. *Eating and Growth Disorders*, *2*, 93–107.

Jones, G. C., Crews, J. E., & Danielson, M. L. (2010). Health risk profile for older adults with blindness: An application of the International Classification of Functioning, Disability, and Health framework. *Ophthalmic Epidemiology*, *17*(6), 400–410. doi:10.3109/09286586.2010.528137 PMID:21090913

Jones, J. (2002). *Fact sheet: Communication*. Birmingham, UK: British Institute of Learning Disabilities.

Jones, M., Onslow, M., Packman, A., O'Brian, S., Hearne, A., Williams, S., ... Schwarz, I. (2008). Extended follow up of a randomized controlled trial of the Licombe program of early stuttering intervention. *International Journal of Language & Communication Disorders*, *43*(6), 649–661. doi:10.1080/13682820801895599 PMID:18608610

Jones, M., Onslow, M., Packman, A., Williams, S., Ormond, T., Schwarz, I., & Gebski, V. (2005). Randomised controlled trial of the Lidcombe Programme of Early Stuttering Intervention. *British Medical Journal*, *331*(7518), 659–661. doi:10.1136/bmj.38520.451840.E0 PMID:16096286

Jones-Prus, D. (1980). Training fluency as a motor skill in the treatment of dysfluent children. *Human Communication*, *5*, 75–86.

Jones, R. B. (2001). Impairment, disability, and handicap: Old-fashioned concepts? *Journal of Medical Ethics*, *37*(6), 377–379. doi:10.1136/jme.27.6.377 PMID:11731599

Kadambari, N., & Venkatesan, S. (2014). Concurrent use of customized behavioral interventions in skill enhancement and problem behavior reduction in children with autism. *Guru Journal of Behavioral and Social Sciences*, *2*(3), 270–283.

Kadir, S. A., & Jamaluddin, M. (2012). User's satisfaction and perception of the accessibility of public buildings in Putrajaya: Access audit study. *Procedia: Social and Behavioral Sciences*, *50*, 429–441. doi:10.1016/j.sbspro.2012.08.047

Kagan, A. (1999). *Supported conversation for adults with aphasia: Methods and evaluation* (Published doctoral dissertation). Toronto: University of Toronto.

Kagan, A., Black, S., Duchan, J. F., Simmons-Mackie, N., & Square, P. (2001). Training Volunteers as Conversation Partners Using "Supported Conversation for Adults with Aphasia" (SCA): A Controlled Trial. *Journal of Speech, Language, and Hearing Research: JSLHR*, *44*(3), 624–638. doi:10.1044/1092-4388(2001/051) PMID:11407567

Kahol, K., Leyba, M. J., Deka, M., Deka, V., Mayes, S., Smith, M., ... Panchanathan, S. (2008). Effect of fatigue on psychomotor and cognitive skills. *American Journal of Surgery*, *195*(2), 195–204. doi:10.1016/j.amjsurg.2007.10.004 PMID:18194679

Kalia, M. (2003). Dysphagia and aspiration pneumonia in patients with Alzheimer's disease. *Metabolism: Clinical and Experimental*, *52*, 36–38. doi:10.1016/S0026-0495(03)00300-7 PMID:14577062

Kalyanpur, M., Harry, B., & Skrtic, T. (2000). Equity and advocacy expectations of culturally diverse families' participation in special education. *International Journal of Disability Development and Education*, *47*(2), 119–136. doi:10.1080/713671106

Kamala, R., & Ramganesh, E. (2013). Knowledge of Specific Learning Disabilities among Teacher Educators in Puducherry, Union Territory in India. *International Review of Social Sciences and Humanities*, *6*(1), 168–175.

Kamhi, A. G., & Catts, H. W. (Eds.). (1989). *Reading Disabilities: A Developmental language Perspective*. Boston: Allyn & Bacon.

Kanfer, F. H., & Saslow, G. (1969). Behaviour diagnosis. In C. M. Franks (Ed.), *Behaviour therapy: Appraisal and status* (pp. 417–444). New York: McGraw Hill.

Kaplan, S. (2001). Meditation, restoration, and the management of mental fatigue. *Environment and Behavior*, *33*(4), 480–506. doi:10.1177/00139160121973106

Kapur, M., Barnabas, I., Reddy, M. V., Rozario, J., & Uma, H. (1995). Developmental psychopathology checklist for children (DPCL): A preliminary report. *Nimhans Journal*, *13*, 1–9.

Kapur, M., John, A., Rozario, J., & Oommen, A. (2002). *NIMHANS index of specific learning disabilities. In Psychological Assessment of Children in the Clinical Setting* (pp. 88–126). Bangalore: Department of Clinical Psychology, National Institute of Mental Health and Neurosciences.

Karande, S. (2008). Current challenges in managing specific learning disability in Indian children. *Journal of Postgraduate Medicine*, *54*(2), 75. doi:10.4103/0022-3859.40765 PMID:18480515

Karande, S., & Kulkarni, M. (2005). Specific learning disability: The invisible handicap. *Indian Pediatrics*, *42*(4), 315–319. PMID:15876592

Karanth, P. (2003). *Cross-linguistic study of acquired reading disorders: Implications for reading models, disorders, acquisition, and teaching*. New York: Kluwer Academic/Plenum Publishers. doi:10.1007/978-1-4419-8923-9

Karanth, P. (2007). *Communication DEALL Developmental Checklists*. Bangalore: Com DEALL Trust.

Karanth, P. (2008). Learning disability and language learning. In K. Thapa, G. M. Aalsvoort, & J. Pandey (Eds.), *Perspectives on Learning Disabilities in India* (pp. 80–94). New Delhi: Sage Publications.

Kargarfard, M., Etemadifar, M., Baker, P., Mehrabi, M., & Hayatbakhsh, R. (2012). Effect of aquatic exercise training on fatigue and health-related quality of life in patients with multiple sclerosis. *Archives of Physical Medicine and Rehabilitation*, *93*(10), 1701–1708. doi:10.1016/j.apmr.2012.05.006 PMID:22609300

Karibasappa, C. N., Nishanimut, S. P., & Padakannaya, P. (2008). A remedial teaching programme to help children with mathematical disability. *Asia Pacific Disability Rehabilitation Journal*, *19*(2), 76–90.

Kasai, Y., Sakakibara, T., Kyaw, T. A., Soe, Z. W., Han, Z. M., & Htwe, M. M. (2017). Psychological effects of meditation at a Buddhist monastery in Myanmar. *Journal of Mental Health (Abingdon, England)*, *26*(1), 4–7. doi:10.3109/09638237.2015.1124405 PMID:26698922

Kato, Y., Endo, H., & Kizuka, T. (2009). Mental fatigue and impaired response processes: Event-related brain potentials in a Go/NoGo task. *International Journal of Psychophysiology*, *72*(2), 204–211. doi:10.1016/j.ijpsycho.2008.12.008 PMID:19135100

Kaufmann, W. E., & Galaburda, A. M. (1989). Cerebrocortical microdysgenesis in neurologically normal subjects: A histopathologic study. *Neurology*, *39*(2), 238–244. doi:10.1212/WNL.39.2.238 PMID:2915796

Kaushanskaya, M., & Marian, V. (2007). Bilingual language processing and interference in bilinguals: Evidence from eye tracking and picture naming. *Language Learning*, *57*(1), 119–163. doi:10.1111/j.1467-9922.2007.00401.x

Kaushik, S. S. (1981). *Parents are teachers: A study in behavior modification of mental sub-normal*. New Delhi: Northern Book Center.

Kaushik, S. S. (1984). Behavior modification workshop for parents and teachers of mentally retarded: Program evaluation. *The Journal of Rehabilitation in Asia*, *25*(2), 47.

Kawai, N., Healey, E. C., Nagasawa, T., & Vanryckeghem, M. (2012). Communication attitudes of Japanese school-age children who stutter. *Journal of Communication Disorders*, *45*(5), 348–354. doi:10.1016/j.jcomdis.2012.05.004 PMID:22796115

Kaya, K., Unsal-Delialioglu, S., Ordu-Gokkaya, N. K., Ozisler, Z., Ergun, N., Ozel, S., & Ucan, H. (2010). Musculoskeletal pain, quality of life and depression in mothers of children with cerebral palsy. *Disability and Rehabilitation*, *32*(20), 1666–1672. doi:10.3109/09638281003649912 PMID:20170278

Kazak, E., & Marvin, R. S. (1984). Differences, difficulties and adaptation: Stress and social networks in families with a handicapped child. *Family Relations*, *33*(1), 67–77. doi:10.2307/584591

Kazdin, A. E. (2013). *Behavior modification in applied settings*. Long Grove, IL: Waveland Press.

Kearns, K. P. (1985). Response elaboration training of patient initiated utterances. In R. H. Brookshire (Ed.), *Clinical Aphasiology* (p. 15). Minneapolis, MN: BRK Publishers.

Keller, D., & Honig, A. S. (2004). Maternal and paternal stress in families with school-aged children with disabilities. *The American Journal of Orthopsychiatry*, *74*(3), 337–348. doi:10.1037/0002-9432.74.3.337 PMID:15291710

Kelman, E., & Nicholas, A. (2008). *Practical intervention for early childhood stammering: Palin PCI Approach*. Milton Keynes, UK: Speechmark Publishing.

Kennedy, D. (2004). *The dark sides of virtue: Reassessing international humanitarianism*. Princeton, NJ: Princeton University Press. doi:10.1515/9781400840731

Kennedy, J. G. III, & Kent, R. D. (1988). Physiological substrates of normal deglutition. *Dysphagia*, *3*(1), 24–37. doi:10.1007/BF02406277 PMID:3073916

Keogh, B. K., & Sears, S. (1991). Learning disabilities from a developmental perspective: Early identification and prediction. In B. Y. L. Wong (Ed.), *Learning about learning disabilities* (pp. 485–503). San Diego, CA: Academic Press. doi:10.1016/B978-0-12-762530-0.50023-0

Kersten, P., Low, J., Ashburn, A., George, S., & McLellan, D. (2002). The unmet needs of young people who have had a stroke: Results of a national UK survey. *Disability and Rehabilitation*, *24*(16), 860–866. doi:10.1080/09638280210142167 PMID:12450462

Kertesz, A. (1982). *Western aphasia battery test manual*. Psychological Corp.

Kertesz, A. (1982). *Western Aphasia Battery*. New York: Grune and Stratton.

Key, A. P., Gustafson, S. J., Rentmeester, L., Hornsby, B. W. Y., & Bess, F. H. (2017). Speech processing fatigue in children: Auditory event-related potential and behavioral measures. *Journal of Speech, Language, and Hearing Research: JSLHR*, 1–15. PMID:28595261

Khalsa, K. L., Azok, S. D., & Leutenberg, E. A. (1994). *Life management skills III*. Wellness Reproductions, Inc.

Khansa, I., Hall, C., Madhoun, L., Splaingard, M., Baylis, A., Kirschner, R., & Pearson, G. (2016). Prospective evaluation of airway and feeding outcomes of mandibular distraction, tongue-lip adhesion and conservative management in Pierre-robin sequence. *The Cleft Palate-Craniofacial Journal*, *53*(4), E148.

Kientz, M. A., & Dunn, W. (1997). A comparison of the performance of children with and without autism on the sensory profile. *The American Journal of Occupational Therapy*, *51*(7), 530–537. doi:10.5014/ajot.51.7.530 PMID:9242859

Kimble, G. A. (1990). Mother Nature's Bag of tricks is small. *Psychological Science*, *1*(1), 36–41. doi:10.1111/j.1467-9280.1990.tb00062.x

Kim, J. S., Han, Z. A., Song, D. H., Oh, H. M., & Chung, M. E. (2013). Characteristics of dysphagia in children with cerebral palsy, related to gross motor dysfunction. *American Journal of Physical Medicine & Rehabilitation*, *92*(10), 912–919. doi:10.1097/PHM.0b013e318296dd99 PMID:23739271

Kingdon-Ward, W. (1941). Stammering. London: Hamilton.

Kinzl, J., Biebl, W., Rauchegger, H., Weissbacher, S., & Hinterhuber, H. (1988). Funktionelle Aphonie-Ein Konversionssymptom zur Angstabwehr. *Psychosomatik Medizinische Psychologie*, *38*(1), 347–351. PMID:3186903

Kiran, S., & Bassetto, G. (2008). Evaluating the effectiveness of semantic based treatment for naming disorders in aphasia: What works? *Seminars in Speech and Language*, *29*(1), 71–82. doi:10.1055-2008-1061626 PMID:18348093

Kirk, S. A. (1962). *Educating exceptional children*. Boston: Houghton Miffin.

Kirk, S. A., & Weiner, B. B. (1963). *Behavioural Research on Exceptional Children*. Washington, DC: The Council for Exceptional Children.

Kishore, T. M., & Nagar, R. K. (2008). Mountaineering expedition by persons with intellectual disability. *Journal of Intellectual Disabilities*, *12*(3), 183–189. doi:10.1177/1744629508095322 PMID:18728141

Kitzmüller, G., Asplund, K., & Häggström, T. (2012). The long-term experience of family life after stroke. *The Journal of Neuroscience Nursing*, *44*(1), E1–E13. doi:10.1097/JNN.0b013e31823ae4a1 PMID:22210306

Klassen, T. R. (2001). Perceptions of people who stutter: Re-assessing the negative stereotype. *Perceptual and Motor Skills*, *92*(2), 551–559. doi:10.2466/pms.2001.92.2.551 PMID:11361320

Knecht, H. A., Nelson, P. B., Whitelaw, G. M., & Feth, L. L. (2002). Background noise levels and reverberation times in unoccupied classrooms: Predictions and measurements. *American Journal of Audiology*, *11*(2), 65–71. doi:10.1044/1059-0889(2002/009) PMID:12691216

Knight, A., & Oliver, C. (2007). Advocacy for disabled children and young people: Benefits and dilemmas. *Child & Family Social Work*, *12*(4), 417–425. doi:10.1111/j.1365-2206.2007.00500.x

Knudsen, E. I. (2004). Sensitive periods in the development of the brain and behavior. *Journal of Cognitive Neuroscience*, *16*(8), 1412–1425. doi:10.1162/0898929042304796 PMID:15509387

Koch, L., Egbert, N., Coeling, H., & Ayers, D. (2005). Returning to work after the onset of illness: Experiences of right hemisphere stroke survivors. *Rehabilitation Counseling*, *48*(4), 209–218. doi:10.1177/00343552050480040201

Koch, M. B. (1961). Anxiety in preschool children from Broken Homes. *Merrill-Palmer Quarterly of Behavior and Development*, *7*(4), 225–231.

Kohli, A., Malhotra, S., Mohanty, M., Khehra, N., & Kaur, M. (2005). Specific learning disabilities in children: Deficits and neuropsychological profile. *International Journal of Rehabilitation Research. Internationale Zeitschrift fur Rehabilitationsforschung. Revue Internationale de Recherches de Readaptation*, *28*(2), 165–169. doi:10.1097/00004356-200506000-00011 PMID:15900188

Kolvin, I., Trowell, J., Le Couteur, A., Baharaki, S., & Morgan, J. (1997). The origin of selective mutism: Some strategies in attachment and bonding research. *Occasional Papers-Association of Child Psychology and Psychiatry, 14,* 17-26.

Konadath, S., Chatni, S., Lakshmi, M. S., & Saini, J. K. (2017). Prevalence of communication disorders in a group of islands in India. *Clinical Epidemiology and Global Health*, *5*(2), 79–86. doi:10.1016/j.cegh.2016.08.003

Konarski, E. A., Favell, J. E., & Favell, J. E. (1992). *Manual for the assessment and treatment of the behavior disorders of people with mental retardation*. Western Carolina Center Foundation.

Konathambigi, R. J., & Shetty, M. (2008). Teacher identification of learning problems. In K. Thapa, G. M. Aalsvoort, & J. Pandey (Eds.), *Perspectives on Learning Disabilities in India*. New Delhi: Sage Publications.

Koretsky, J. (2007). *The odd one out the Maverick's guide to adult ADD; How to be happy and different*. Plattekill, NY: Vervante.

Korhonen, T. T. (1995). The persistence of rapid naming problems in children with reading disabilities: A nine-year follow-up. *Journal of Learning Disabilities*, *28*(4), 232–239. doi:10.1177/002221949502800405 PMID:7738435

Kotby, M. N., Baraka, M., El Sady, S. R., Ghanem, M., & Shoeib, R. (2003, October). Psychogenic stress as a possible etiological factor in non-organic dysphonia. Elsevier. doi:10.1016/S0531-5131(03)00858-6

Kothari, S., Rohit, V. S., & Jain, S. (2017). Effect of Specific Leaning Disability on Auditory Stream Segregation, Auditory Working Memory and Speech Perception in Noise Abilities in Children. *Proceedings of Indian Speech and Hearing Association Conference.*

Koushik, S., Shenker, R., & Onslow, M. (2009). Follow-up of 6-10 year old stuttering children after Lidcombe Program treatment: A Phase I trial. *Journal of Fluency Disorders*, *34*(4), 279–290. doi:10.1016/j.jfludis.2009.11.001 PMID:20113771

Kovarsky, D. (2014). The ethnography of communication disorders revisited. In M. J. Ball, N. Muller, & R. L. Nelson (Eds.), *Handbook of Qualitative research in communication disorders* (pp. 55–78). New York, NY: Psychology Press.

Kramer, S. E., Kapteyn, T. S., & Houtgast, T. (2006). Occupational performance: Comparing normally-hearing and hearing-impaired employees using the Amsterdam Checklist for Hearing and Work. *International Journal of Audiology*, *45*(9), 503–512. doi:10.1080/14992020600754583 PMID:17005493

Kratchowill, T. (1981). *Selective Mutism: Implications of Research and Treatment*. Hillsdale, NJ: Lawrence Erlbaum.

Kraus, N., Bradlow, A. R., Cheatham, M. A., Cunningham, J., King, C. D., Koch, D. B., ... Wright, B. A. (2000). Consequences of neural asynchrony: A case of auditory neuropathy. *Journal of the Association for Research in Otolaryngology*, *1*(1), 33–45. doi:10.1007101620010004 PMID:11548236

Kraus, N., Ozdamar, O., Stein, L., & Reed, N. (1984). Absent auditory brain stem response: Peripheral hearing loss or brain stem dysfunction? *The Laryngoscope*, *94*(3), 400–406. doi:10.1288/00005537-198403000-00019 PMID:6700356

Krick, J., & Van Duyn, M. A. (1984). The relationship between oral-motor involvement and growth: A pilot study in a pediatric population with cerebral palsy. *Journal of the American Dietetic Association*, *84*(5), 555–559. PMID:6715752

Krishnaswamy, J. (1992). The Upanayana early intervention program (UEIP). *Indian Journal of Pediatrics*, *59*(8), 701–705. doi:10.1007/BF02859404 PMID:1340858

Kristersen, H., & Torgersen, S. (2001). MCMI-II personality traits and symptoms traits in parents of children with selective mutism: A case control study. *Journal of Abnormal Psychology*, *110*(4), 648–652. doi:10.1037/0021-843X.110.4.648

Kroll, J. F., Bobb, S. C., & Wodniecka, Z. (2006). Language selectivity is the exception, not the rule: Arguments against a fixed locus of language selection in bilingual speech. *Bilingualism: Language and Cognition*, *9*(02), 119–135. doi:10.1017/S1366728906002483

Krupanidhi, P., Urs, B., Prateeksha, K., & Jain, S. (2016). Effect of musical training on the perception of instrumental music. Proceedings of Indian Speech and Hearing Association, 2016.

Krupp, L. B., Sliwinski, M., Masur, D. M., Friedberg, F., & Coyle, P. K. (1994). Cognitive functioning and depression in patients with chronic fatigue syndrome and multiple sclerosis. *Archives of Neurology*, *51*(7), 705–710. doi:10.1001/archneur.1994.00540190089021 PMID:8018045

Kully, D., & Boberg, E. (1991). Therapy for school-age children. *Seminars in Speech and Language*, *12*(4), 291–300. doi:10.1055-2008-1064230

Kumar, U. A., & Jayaram, M. (2006). Prevalence and audiological characteristics in individuals with auditory neuropathy/auditory dys-synchrony. *International Journal of Audiology*, *45*(6), 360–366. doi:10.1080/14992020600624893 PMID:16777783

Kumpulainen, K., Rasanen, E., Raaska, H., & Somppi, V. (1998). Selective mutism among second graders in elementary school. *European Child & Adolescent Psychiatry*, *7*(1), 24–29. doi:10.1007007870050041

Kuruvilla, K. (2010). Indian contribution to behavior therapy. *Indian Journal of Psychiatry*, *52*(7S1), S371–S377. doi:10.4103/0019-5545.69271 PMID:21836708

Kutner, L. (2016). When A Sibling Is Disabled. *Psych Central.* Retrieved September 14, 2017, from https://psychcentral.com/lib/when-a-sibling-is-disabled/

La Pointe, L. L. (2005). Foundations: Adaptation, Accomodation, Aristos. In L. L. La Pointe (Ed.), *Aphasia and related neurogenic language disorders* (pp. 1–18). New York: Thieme Medical.

Laborde, P. R., & Seligman, M. (1983). Individual counselling with parents of handicapped children: Rationale and strategies. In M. Seligman (Ed.), *The family with a handicapped child: Understanding and treatment* (pp. 261–284). New York, NY: Grune & Stratton, Inc.

Labounty, D. (2009). *Affluenza*. Denver, CO: Silver Thought Press.

Lakhan, R. (2014). Behavioral management in children with intellectual disabilities in a resource-poor setting in Barwani, India. *Indian Journal of Psychiatry*, *56*(1), 39–45. doi:10.4103/0019-5545.124712 PMID:24574557

Lakhan, R., & Singh, A. (2014). Early intervention tool for children with developmental delay: A pilot study. *The European Health Psychologist*, *16*(1), 18–25.

Lall, A., Hirisavae, U., Kapur, M., & Subbakrisha, D. K. (1997). Perceived peer relations, social competance in children with specific disorders of socialistic skills. *Nimhans Journal*, *15*(2), 133–137.

Lal, S. K., & Craig, A. (2001). A critical review of the psychophysiology of driver fatigue. *Biological Psychology*, *55*(3), 173–194. doi:10.1016/S0301-0511(00)00085-5 PMID:11240213

Langevin, M., & Hagler, P. (2004). Development of a scale to measure peer attitudes toward children who stutter. In A. K. Bothe (Ed.), *Evidence-based treatment of stuttering: Empirical bases and clinical applications* (pp. 139–170). Mahwah, NJ: Erlbaum.

Langevin, M., Packman, A., & Onslow, M. (2009). Peer responses to stuttering in the preschool setting. *American Journal of Speech-Language Pathology*, *18*(3), 264–276. doi:10.1044/1058-0360(2009/07-0087) PMID:19332523

Langevin, M., Packman, A., & Onslow, M. (2010). Parent perceptions of the impact of stuttering on their preschoolers and themselves. *Journal of Communication Disorders*, *43*(5), 407–423. doi:10.1016/j.jcomdis.2010.05.003 PMID:20599207

Langner, R., Steinborn, M. B., Chatterjee, A., Sturm, W., & Willmes, K. (2010). Mental fatigue and temporal preparation in simple reaction-time performance. *Acta Psychologica*, *133*(1), 64–72. doi:10.1016/j.actpsy.2009.10.001 PMID:19878913

Language in India. (2014). *Census of India 2011 towards a bright future.* Retrieved from http://www.languageinindia.com/feb2014/censusofindia2011data.pdf

Latterman, C., Euler, H. A., & Neumann, K. (2008). A randomized control trial to investigate the impact of the Lidcombe program on early stuttering in German-speaking preschoolers. *Journal of Fluency Disorders*, *33*(1), 52–65. doi:10.1016/j.jfludis.2007.12.002 PMID:18280869

Lau, C. (2006). Oral feeding in the preterm infant. *NeoReviews*, *7*(1), e19–e27. doi:10.1542/neo.7-1-e19

Lau, C., Smith, E. O., & Schanler, R. J. (2003). Coordination of suck swallow and swallow respiration in preterm infants. *Acta Paediatrica (Oslo, Norway)*, *92*(6), 721–727. doi:10.1111/j.1651-2227.2003.tb00607.x PMID:12856985

Layton, T. L., & Holmes, D. W. (1985). *Carolina picture vocabulary test for dead and hearing impaired children (CPVT).* PRO-ED Inc.

Le Dorze, G., & Brassard, C. (1995). A description of the consequences of aphasia on aphasic persons and their relatives and friends, based on the WHO model of chronic diseases. *Aphasiology*, *9*(3), 239–255. doi:10.1080/02687039508248198

Leben, N. (n.d.). *Selective Mutism: A Case Study of a 10 Year Old Korean Boy and Applicable Play Therapy Techniques.* Retrieved from http://www.playtherapygames.com/HTML/SelectiveMutism_NormaLeben.pdf

LeComer, L. (2006). *A parent's guide to developmental delays: Recognising and coping with missed milestones in speech, movement, learning and other areas.* Stillwater, OK: New Forums Press Inc.

Ledford, J. R., & Gast, D. L. (2006). Feeding problems in children with autism spectrum disorders: A review. *Focus on Autism and Other Developmental Disabilities*, *21*(3), 153–166. doi:10.1177/10883576060210030401

Lee, D. L., & Axelrod, S. (2005). *Behavior modification: Basic principles.* Austin, TX: Pro-Ed.

Lee, L., Stemple, J. C., Glaze, L., & Kelchner, L. N. (2004). Quick screen for voice and supplementary documents for identifying pediatric voice disorders. *Language, Speech, and Hearing Services in Schools*, *35*(4), 308–319. doi:10.1044/0161-1461(2004/030 PMID:15609634

Leiva, P. B., Inzunza, B. N., Pérez, T. H., Castro, G. V., Jansana, M. J., Toro, D. T., ... Ivanovic, M. D. (2001). The impact of malnutrition on brain development, intelligence and school work performance. *Archivos Latinoamericanos de Nutricion*, *51*(1), 64–71. PMID:11515234

Lenhard, W., Breitenbach, E., Ebert, H., Schindelhaues-Deutscher, H. J., & Henn, W. (2005). Psychological benefit of diagnostic certainty for mothers of children with disabilities: Lessons from Down's syndrome. *American Journal of Medical Genetics. Part A*, *133*(2), 170–175. doi:10.1002/ajmg.a.30571 PMID:15666306

Lennerstrandt, G., Ygge, J., & Jacobsson, C. (1993). Control of binocular eye movements in normals and dyslexics. *Annals of the New York Academy of Sciences*, *682*, 232–239. PMID:8323115

Leonard, R., & Kendall, K. (1997). Dysphagia Assessment and Treatment Planning: A Team Approach. San Diego, CA: Singular Publishing Group, Inc.

Leopold, N. A., & Kagel, M. C. (1996). Prepharyngeal dysphagia in Parkinson's disease. *Dysphagia*, *11*(1), 14–22. doi:10.1007/BF00385794 PMID:8556872

Lewington, W., & Clipson, C. (2004). *Advocating for equality*. London, UK: Independent Advocacy Campaign, Scope.

Lewis, C., Packman, A., Onslow, M., Simpson, J. A., & Jones, M. (2008). A Phase II trial of telehealth delivery of the Lidcombe Program of Early Stuttering Intervention. *American Journal of Speech-Language Pathology*, *17*(2), 139–149. doi:10.1044/1058-0360(2008/014) PMID:18448601

Lewis, D. J. (2010). *Foundations of behavioral therapy*. London: Transaction Publishers.

Lewis, D., Schmid, K., O'Leary, S., Spalding, J., Heinrichs-Graham, E., & High, R. (2016). Effects of noise on speech recognition and listening effort in children with normal hearing and children with mild bilateral or unilateral hearing loss. *Journal of Speech, Language, and Hearing Research: JSLHR*, *59*(5), 1218–1232. doi:10.1044/2016_JSLHR-H-15-0207 PMID:27784030

Li, F., Wang, H., Chen, J., & Liang, R. (2005). Auditory neuropathy in children (analysis of 14 cases). *Journal of Clinical Otorhinolaryngology*, *19*(1), 19–21. PMID:15830698

Lima, A., Mantello, E., & Anastasio, A. (2015). Monitoring the hearing handicap and the recognition threshold of sentences of a patient with unilateral auditory neuropathy spectrum disorder with use of a hearing aid. *International Archives of Otorhinolaryngology*, *20*(2), 185–188. doi:10.1055-0034-1397338 PMID:27096026

Lim, J., Wu, W., Wang, J., Detre, J. A., Dinges, D. F., & Rao, H. (2010). Imaging brain fatigue from sustained mental workload: An ASL perfusion study of the time-on-task effect. *NeuroImage*, *49*(4), 3426–3435. doi:10.1016/j.neuroimage.2009.11.020 PMID:19925871

Lincoln, M., Onslow, M., Lewis, C., & Wilson, L. (1996). A clinical trial of an operant treatment for school-age children who stutter. *American Journal of Speech-Language Pathology*, *5*(2), 73–85. doi:10.1044/1058-0360.0502.73

Linden, P., & Siebens, A. A. (1983). Dysphagia: Predicting laryngeal penetration. *Archives of Physical Medicine and Rehabilitation*, *64*(6), 281–284. PMID:6860100

Lindsay, G., & Dockrell, J. (2000). The behaviour and self-esteem of children with specific speech and language difficulties. *The British Journal of Educational Psychology*, *70*(4), 583–601. doi:10.1348/000709900158317 PMID:11191188

Lindsay, G., Dockrell, J., Desforges, M., Law, J., & Peacey, N. (2010). Meeting the needs of children and young people with speech, language and communication difficulties. *International Journal of Language & Communication Disorders*, *45*(4), 448–460. doi:10.3109/13682820903165693 PMID:20565326

Lindsey, K. A., Manis, F. R., & Bailey, C. E. (2003). Prediction of first-grade reading in Spanish-speaking English-language learners. *Journal of Educational Psychology, 95*(3), 482–494. doi:10.1037/0022-0663.95.3.482

Lingeswaran, A. (2013). Assessing knowledge of primary school teachers on specific learning disabilities in two schools in India. *Journal of Education and Health Promotion, 2*(1), 30. doi:10.4103/2277-9531.115807 PMID:24083280

Linscheid, T. R. (1983). Eating problems in children. In C. E. Walker & M. C. Roberts (Eds.), *Handbook of Clinical Child Psychology* (pp. 616–639). New York: Wiley.

Liu, J., Zhou, G., Wang, Y., Ai, Y., Pinto-Martin, J., & Liu, X. (2012). Sleep problems, fatigue, and cognitive performance in Chinese kindergarten children. *The Journal of Pediatrics, 161*(3), 520–525.e2. doi:10.1016/j.jpeds.2012.03.018 PMID:22521112

Livingstone, M. S., Rosen, G. D., Drislane, F. W., & Galaburda, A. M. (1991). Physiological and anatomical evidence for a magnocellular defect in developmental dyslexia. *Proceedings of the National Academy of Sciences of the United States of America, 88*(18), 7943–7947. doi:10.1073/pnas.88.18.7943 PMID:1896444

Lobato, D. J., & Kao, B. T. (2005). Brief Report: Family-based group intervention for young siblings of children with chronic illnesses and developmental disability. *Journal of Pediatric Psychology, 30*(8), 678–682. doi:10.1093/jpepsy/jsi054 PMID:16260437

Lobstein, T. (1991). *The Nutrition of Women on Low Income*. London: Food Commission.

Locke, A., Ginsberg, J., & Peers, L. (2002). Development and disadvantage: Implications for the early years and beyond. *International Journal of Communication Disorders, 37*(1), 3–15. doi:10.1080/13682820110089911 PMID:11852457

Logan, W. J. (1996). Neuroimaging and functional brain analysis. In J. H. Beitchman, N. J. Cohen, M. M. Konstantareas, & R. Tannock (Eds.), *Language learning and behavior disorders: Developmental, biological and clinical perspectives*. Cambridge, UK: Cambridge University Press.

Logemann, J. A. (1998). The evaluation and treatment of swallowing disorders. *Current Opinion in Otolaryngology & Head & Neck Surgery, 6*(6), 395–400. doi:10.1097/00020840-199812000-00008

Logemann, J. A., & Logemann, J. A. (1983). *Evaluation and Treatment of Swallowing Disorders. National Student Speech Hearing Language Association*. NSSHLA.

Logemann, J., Shanahan, T., Rademaker, A., Kahrilas, P., Lazar, R., & Halper, A. (1993). Oropharyngeal swallowing after stroke in the left basal ganglion/internal capsule. *Dysphagia, 8*(3), 230–234. doi:10.1007/BF01354543 PMID:8359043

Lombe, M. (2007). *Presentation*. In Expert Group Meeting on Creating and Inclusive Society: Practical Strategies to Promote Social Integration, Paris, France.

Longerich, M. C. (1968). *Manual for the Aphasia Patient*. New York: Macmillan Company.

Lopes, R. C. F., & Crenitte, P. A. P. (2013). Analytical study of teacher's knowledge about learning disorders. *Revista CEFAC, 15*(5), 1214–1226. doi:10.1590/S1516-18462012005000091

Lorist, M. M. (2008). Impact of top-down control during mental fatigue. *Brain Research, 1232*, 113–123. doi:10.1016/j.brainres.2008.07.053 PMID:18687317

Lorist, M. M., Boksem, M. A. S., & Ridderinkhof, K. R. (2005). Impaired cognitive control and reduced cingulate activity during mental fatigue. *Brain Research. Cognitive Brain Research, 24*(2), 199–205. doi:10.1016/j.cogbrainres.2005.01.018 PMID:15993758

Lorist, M. M., Klein, M., Nieuwenhuis, S., De Jong, R., Mulder, G., & Meijman, T. F. (2000). Mental fatigue and task control: Planning and preparation. *Psychophysiology, 37*(5), 614–625. doi:10.1111/1469-8986.3750614 PMID:11037038

Luk, G., & Bialystok, E. (2008). Common and distinct cognitive bases for reading in English–Cantonese bilinguals. *Applied Psycholinguistics, 29*(02), 269–289. doi:10.1017/S0142716407080125

Luo, C., Guo, Z., Lai, Y., Liao, W., Liu, Q., Kendrick, K. M., ... Li, H. (2012). Musical training induces functional plasticity in perceptual and motor networks: Insights from resting-state fMRI. *PLoS One, 7*(5), e36568. doi:10.1371/journal.pone.0036568 PMID:22586478

Lustig, D. C. (1997). Families with an adult with mental retardation: Empirical family typologies. *Rehabilitation Counseling Bulletin, 41*(2), 138–157.

Lustig, D. C. (2002). Family coping in families with a child with a disability. *Education and Training in Mental Retardation and Developmental Disabilities, 37*(1), 14–22.

Luthar, S. S. (2003). The culture of affluence: Psychological costs of material wealth. *Child Development, 74*(6), 1581–1593. doi:10.1046/j.1467-8624.2003.00625.x PMID:14669883

Luthar, S. S., & Latendresse, S. J. (2005). Children of the Affluent. *Current Directions in Psychological Science, 14*(1), 49–53. doi:10.1111/j.0963-7214.2005.00333.x PMID:17710193

Lutz, A., McFarlin, D. R., Perlman, D. M., Salomons, T. V., & Davidson, R. J. (2013). Altered anterior insula activation during anticipation and experience of painful stimuli in expert meditators. *NeuroImage, 64*, 538–546. doi:10.1016/j.neuroimage.2012.09.030 PMID:23000783

Lyon, G. R., Fletcher, J. M., Shaywitz, S. E., Shaywitz, B. A., Torgesen, J. K., Wood, F. B., & Olson, R. (2001). Rethinking learning disabilities. In C. E. Finn, A. J. Rotherman, & C. R. Hokanson (Eds.), *Rethinking Education for a New Century* (pp. 259–287). Washington, DC: Thomas B. Fordham Foundation and the Progressive Policy Institute.

MacDonald, R., Parry-Cruwys, D., Dupere, S., & Aheam, W. (2014). Assessing progress and outcome of early intensive behavioral intervention for toddlers with autism. *Research in Developmental Disabilities, 35*(12), 3632–3644. doi:10.1016/j.ridd.2014.08.036 PMID:25241118

Mahalihali, K. (n.d.). *Family influences on the development of a child's behavior*. Retrieved from http://www.kon.org/urc/v5/mahalihali.html

Mahar, A. L., Cobigo, V., & Stuart, H. (2013). Conceptualizing belonging. *Disability and Rehabilitation, 35*(12), 1026–1032. doi:10.3109/09638288.2012.717584 PMID:23020179

Mahoney, S. C. (1958). Observations concerning counselling with parents of mentally retarded children. *American Journal of Mental Deficiency, 63*(1), 81–86. PMID:13559295

Makeig, S., & Jung, T. P. (1995). Changes in alertness are a principal component of variance in the EEG spectrum. *Neuroreport, 7*(1), 213–216. doi:10.1097/00001756-199512000-00051 PMID:8742454

Malec, J. F., Brown, A. W., & Moessner, A. (2010). Two new measures for assessing advocacy activities and perceived control after acquired brain injury. *Disability and Rehabilitation, 32*(1), 33–40. doi:10.3109/09638280902980936 PMID:19925274

Manickam, L. S. S. (2010). Psychotherapy in India. *Indian Journal of Psychiatry, 52*(S), S366-S370. doi: 10.4103/0019-5545.69270

Marchand, W. R. (2014). Neural mechanisms of mindfulness and meditation: Evidence from neuroimaging studies. *World Journal of Radiology*, *6*(7), 471–479. doi:10.4329/wjr.v6.i7.471 PMID:25071887

Marcora, S. M., Staiano, W., & Manning, V. (2009). Mental fatigue impairs physical performance in humans. *Journal of Applied Physiology*, *106*(3), 857–864. doi:10.1152/japplphysiol.91324.2008 PMID:19131473

Marian, V., Spivey, M., & Hirsch, J. (2003). Shared and separate systems in bilingual language processing: Converging evidence from eye tracking and brain imaging. *Brain and Language*, *86*(1), 70–82. doi:10.1016/S0093-934X(02)00535-7 PMID:12821416

Marijcke, W. M., Veltman, B. A., & Browne, K. D. (2001). Identifying childhood abuse through favorite kind of and kinetic family drawing. *The Arts in Psychotherapy*, *28*(4), 251–259. doi:10.1016/S0197-4556(01)00110-1

Marijcke, W., Veltman, M., & Browne, K. D. (2003). Trained raters' evaluation of kinetic family drawings of physically abused children. *The Arts in Psychology*, *30*(1), 3–12. doi:10.1016/S0197-4556(02)00230-7

Marland, P. (1957). Shadowing: A contribution to the treatment of stuttering. *Folia Phoniatrica*, *9*(4), 242–245. doi:10.1159/000262784 PMID:13480408

Marr, J. N. (2010). *Manual of behavior modification: A guide for parents*. Bloomington, IN: Xlibris Corporation.

Martin, D., & Miller, C. (2003). *Speech and language difficulties in the classroom* (2nd ed.). London: David Fulton Publishers.

Martin, G., & Pear, J. J. (2016). *Behavior modification: What it is and how to do it*. New York: Routledge.

Martins, R. H. G., do Amaral, H. A., Tavares, E. L. M., Martins, M. G., Gonçalves, T. M., & Dias, N. H. (2016). Voice disorders: Etiology and diagnosis. *Journal of Voice, 30*(6), 761-e1- e15.

Martirosyan, A. (2013). *Sibling relationships in families with a child with special needs: A case study of a Norwegian family with a child with Down syndrome and her three siblings* (Unpublished Master's dissertation). University of Oslo, Norway.

Mary, R. A., Marslin, G., Franklin, G., & Sheeba, C. J. (2014). Test anxiety levels of board exam going students in Tamil Nadu. India. *BioMed Research International*, *21*, 1–9. doi:10.1155/2014/578323 PMID:25143938

Masarei, A. G., Sell, D., Habel, A., Mars, M., Sommerlad, B. C., & Wade, A. (2007). The nature of feeding in infants with unrepaired cleft lip and/or palate compared with healthy noncleft infants. *The Cleft Palate-Craniofacial Journal*, *44*(3), 321–328. doi:10.1597/05-185 PMID:17477749

Mash, E. J., & Johnston, C. (1983). Parental perceptions of child behaviour problems, parenting self esteem, and mother's reported stress in younger and older hyperactive and normal children. *Journal of Consulting and Clinical Psychology*, *51*(1), 86–99. doi:10.1037/0022-006X.51.1.86 PMID:6826870

Mason, J. C., De Michele, A., Stevens, C., Ruth, R. A., & Hashisaki, G. T. (2003). Cochlear implantation in patients with auditory neuropathy of varied etiologies. *The Laryngoscope*, *113*(1), 45–49. doi:10.1097/00005537-200301000-00009 PMID:12514381

Massoud, F., Chertkow, H., Whitehead, V., Overbury, O., & Bergman, H. (2002). Word-reading thresholds in Alzheimer disease and mild memory loss: A pilot study. *Alzheimer Disease and Associated Disorders*, *16*(1), 31–39. doi:10.1097/00002093-200201000-00005 PMID:11882747

Mather, N., & Greg, N. (2006). Specific learning disabilities: Clarifying, not eliminating a construct. *Professional Psychology, Research and Practice*, *37*(1), 99–106. doi:10.1037/0735-7028.37.1.99

Mathur, R., & Goswami, S. P. (2010). *Protocol to Measure Participation of Persons with Aphasia* (Unpublished dissertation). University of Mysore.

Matos, M. A. C., Jesus, L. M., & Cruice, M. (2014). Consequences of stroke and aphasia according to the ICF domains: Views of Portuguese people with aphasia, family members and professionals. *Aphasiology*, *28*(7), 771–796. doi:10.1080/02687038.2014.906561

Matson, J. L., & Bamburg, J. W. (1999). A descriptive study of pica behavior in persons with mental retardation. *Journal of Developmental and Physical Disabilities*, *11*(4), 353–361. doi:10.1023/A:1021870925227

Matson, J. L., Fodstad, J. C., & Boisjoli, J. A. (2008). Cutoff scores, norms and patterns of feeding problems for the Screening Tool of feeding Problems (STEP) for adults with intellectual disabilities. *Research in Developmental Disabilities*, *29*(4), 363–372. doi:10.1016/j.ridd.2007.06.001 PMID:17662575

Matson, J. L., Gardner, W. I., Coe, D. A., & Sovner, R. (1991). A scale for evaluating emotional disorders in severely and profoundly mentally retarded persons. Development of the Diagnostic Assessment for the Severely Handicapped (DASH) Scale. *The British Journal of Psychiatry*, *159*(03), 404–409. doi:10.1192/bjp.159.3.404 PMID:1958951

Matson, J. L., & Kuhn, D. E. (2001). Identifying feeding problems in mentally retarded persons: Development and reliability of the screening tool of feeding problems (STEP). *Research in Developmental Disabilities*, *22*(2), 165–172. doi:10.1016/S0891-4222(01)00065-8 PMID:11325163

Mayes, S. D., Calhoun, S. L., Bixler, E. O., & Vgontzas, A. N. (2008). Nonsignificance of sleep relative to IQ and neuropsychological scores in predicting academic achievement. *Journal of Developmental and Behavioral Pediatrics*, *29*(3), 206–212. doi:10.1097/DBP.0b013e31816d924f PMID:18480734

Mayes, S. D., Calhoun, S. L., & Crowell, E. W. (2000). Learning disabilities and ADHD: Overlapping spectrumn disorders. *Journal of Learning Disabilities*, *33*(5), 417–424. doi:10.1177/002221940003300502 PMID:15495544

McAllister, J. (2016). Behavioural, emotional and social development of children who stutter. *Journal of Fluency Disorders*, *50*, 23–32. doi:10.1016/j.jfludis.2016.09.003 PMID:27865227

McCabe, H. (2007). Parent advocacy in the face of adversity: Autism and families in the People's Republic of China. *Focus on Autism and Other Developmental Disabilities*, *22*(1), 39–50. doi:10.1177/10883576070220010501

McCauley, R. J. (2001). *Assessment of language disorders in children*. New York: Psychology Press.

McGeown, J. (2012). *Out of the shadows: A qualitative study of parents' and professionals' attitudes and beliefs about children with communication disability in Uganda and how best to help them* (Unpublished master's thesis). University College London, UK.

McHale, S. M., Simeonsson, R. J., & Sloan, J. (1984). Children with handicapped brothers and sisters. In E. Schopler & G. Mesibov (Eds.), *The effect of Autism on the family* (pp. 327–342). New York: Plenum. doi:10.1007/978-1-4899-2293-9_19

McHale, S., Sloan, J., & Simeonsson, J. (1986). Sibling relationships of children with autism, mentally retarded, and nonhandicapped brothers and sisters. *Journal of Autism and Developmental Disorders*, *16*(4), 399–413. doi:10.1007/BF01531707 PMID:3804956

McKeever, P., & Miller, K. L. (2004). Mothering children who have disabilities: A Bourdieusian interpretation of maternal practices. *Social Science & Medicine*, *59*(6), 1177–1191. doi:10.1016/j.socscimed.2003.12.023 PMID:15210090

McKhann, G. M., Knopman, D. S., Chertkow, H., Hyman, B. T., Jack, C. R., Kawas, C. H., & Mohs, R. C. (2011). The diagnosis of dementia due to Alzheimer's disease: Recommendations from the National Institute on Aging-Alzheimer's Association workgroups on diagnostic guidelines for Alzheimer's disease. *Alzheimer's & Dementia*, *7*(3), 263–269. doi:10.1016/j.jalz.2011.03.005 PMID:21514250

McLeod, S., & McKinnon, D. H. (2010). Support required for primary and secondary students with communication disorders and/or other learning needs. *Child Language Teaching and Therapy*, *26*(2), 123–143. doi:10.1177/0265659010368754

Meadow, K. P. (1980). *Meadow/Kendall Social-Emotional Assessment Inventory for Deaf Students: Manual*. Academic Press.

Medin, J., Barajas, J., & Ekberg, K. (2006). Stroke patients' experiences of return to work. *Disability and Rehabilitation*, *28*(17), 1051–1060. doi:10.1080/09638280500494819 PMID:16950735

Mehmood, Z., Bhatti, A. G., & Ali, S. H. (2015). Schools as an agent of socialization for disabled children: A study of disabled children of special education institutes in Jalapur Pirwala. *Journal of Social Sciences*, *9*, 333–342.

Mehta, H. (2000). *A Low Cost Diagnostic Test of Mathematics Disability (TMD) in Children aged 7 to 10 Yrs* (M.Ed Dissertation). Mumbai: SNDT Womens University.

Mehta, M., & Ochaney, M. (1984). Training mental retardation: Involving mothers in the operant conditioning program. *Indian Journal of Clinical Psychology*, *11*, 45–49.

Meltzer, H., Gatward, R., Goodman, R., & Ford, T. (2000). *Mental Health of Children & Adolescents in Great Britain*. London: The Stationary Office. doi:10.1037/e622732007-001

Mendel, L. L., & Widner, H. (2016). Speech perception in noise for bilingual listeners with normal hearing. *International Journal of Audiology*, *55*(2), 126–134. doi:10.3109/14992027.2015.1061710 PMID:26189557

Mendez, L., Friedman, L., & Castell, L. (1991). Swallowing disorders in the elderly. *Clinics in Geriatric Medicine*, *7*, 215–230. PMID:1855155

Menzies, R. G., O'Brian, S., Onslow, M., Packman, A., St. Clare, T., & Block, S. (2008). An experimental clinical trial of a cognitive-behavior therapy package for chronic stuttering. *Journal of Speech, Language, and Hearing Research: JSLHR*, *51*(6), 1451–1464. doi:10.1044/1092-4388(2008/07-0070) PMID:18664696

Menzies, R. G., Onslow, M., Packman, A., & O'Brian, S. (2009). Cognitive-behavior therapy for adults who stutter: A tutorial for the speech-language pathologist. *Journal of Fluency Disorders*, *34*(3), 187–200. doi:10.1016/j.jfludis.2009.09.002 PMID:19948272

Meyer, D. (2001). Meeting the unique concerns of brothers of sisters of children with special needs. *Insights*, *51*, 28–32.

Michallet, B., Tétreault, S., & Le Dorze, G. (2003). The consequences of severe aphasia on the spouses of aphasic people: A description of the adaptation process. *Aphasiology*, *17*(9), 835–859. doi:10.1080/02687030344000238

Mikulas, W. L. (1981). Buddhism and behavior modification. *The Psychological Record*, *31*(3), 331–334. doi:10.1007/BF03394746

Millard, S. K., Edwards, S., & Cook, F. M. (2009). Parent-child interaction therapy: Adding to the evidence. *International Journal of Speech-Language Pathology*, *11*(1), 61–76. doi:10.1080/17549500802603895

Millard, S. K., Nicholas, A., & Cook, F. M. (2008). Is parent-child interaction therapy effective in reducing stuttering? *Journal of Speech, Language, and Hearing Research: JSLHR*, *51*(3), 636–650. doi:10.1044/1092-4388(2008/046) PMID:18506041

Miller, B., & Guitar, B. (2009). Long-term outcome of the Lidcombe program for early stuttering intervention. *American Journal of Speech-Language Pathology, 18*(1), 42–49. doi:10.1044/1058-0360(2008/06-0069) PMID:18845699

Miller, F. P., Vandome, A. F., & Mc Brewster, J. (2010). *The medical model of disability*. VDM Publishing.

Miller, N. B. (1994). *Nobody's perfect*. Baltimore, MD: Paul H. Brooks Publishing Co.

Milovanov, R., Huotilainen, M., Välimäki, V., Esquef, P. A. A., & Tervaniemi, M. (2008). Musical aptitude and second language pronunciation skills in school-aged children: Neural and behavioral evidence. *Brain Research, 1194*, 81–89. doi:10.1016/j.brainres.2007.11.042 PMID:18182165

Miltenberger, R. G. (2012). *Behavior modification: Principles and procedures*. Belmont, CA: Wadsworth Cengage Learning.

Ministry of Urban Development. (2016). *Central public works department guidelines and space standards for barrier-free and accessibility*. New Delhi: Ministry of Urban Development, Government of India.

Mion, L. C., McDowell, J. A., & Heaney, L. K. (1994). Nutritional assessment of the elderly in the ambulatory care setting. *Nurse Practitioner Forum, 5*(1), 46–51. PMID:8148658

Mishra, H. (1998). Cognitive behavior therapy. *Behavior Medicine Journal, 1*(1), 14–19.

Misono, S., Peterson, C. B., Meredith, L., Banks, K., Bandyopadhyay, D., Yueh, B., & Frazier, P. A. (2014). Psychosocial distress in patients presenting with voice concerns. *Journal of Voice, 28*(6), 753–761. doi:10.1016/j.jvoice.2014.02.010 PMID:24930373

Misra, G., & Paranjpe, E. A. C. (2012). Psychology in modern India. In *Encyclopedia of the history of psychological theories* (pp. 881–892). New York: Springer.

Mittler, P. (2000). *Working towards inclusive education: Contexts*. London, UK: David Fulton Publishers.

Mizuno, K., Tanaka, M., Fukuda, S., Imai-Matsumura, K., & Watanabe, Y. (2013). Divided attention of adolescents related to lifestyles and academic and family conditions. *Brain & Development, 35*(5), 435–440. doi:10.1016/j.braindev.2012.07.007 PMID:22877835

Mizuno, K., Tanaka, M., Fukuda, S., Yamano, E., Shigihara, Y., Imai-Matsumura, K., & Watanabe, Y. (2011). Low visual information-processing speed and attention are predictors of fatigue in elementary and junior high school students. *Behavioral and Brain Functions, 7*(1), 20. doi:10.1186/1744-9081-7-20 PMID:21672212

Mizuno, K., & Ueda, A. (2003). The maturation and coordination of sucking, swallowing, and respiration in preterm infants. *The Journal of Pediatrics, 142*(1), 36–40. doi:10.1067/mpd.2003.mpd0312 PMID:12520252

Moes, D. R., & Frea, W. D. (2000). Using family context to inform prevention planning for the treatment of a child with autism. *Journal of Positive Behavior Interventions, 2*(1), 40–46. doi:10.1177/109830070000200106

Monsch, A. U., Foldi, N. S., Ermini-Fünfschillin, D. E., Berres, M., Taylor, K. I., Seifritz, E., & Spiegel, R. (1995). Improving the diagnostic accuracy of the Mini-Mental State Examination. *Acta Neurologica Scandinavica, 92*(2), 145–150. doi:10.1111/j.1600-0404.1995.tb01029.x PMID:7484063

Montague, M., Maddox, C. D., & Dereshiwsky, M. I. (1990). Story grammar and comprehension and production of narrative prose by students with learning disabilities. *Journal of Learning Disabilities, 23*(21), 190–197. doi:10.1177/002221949002300310 PMID:2313193

Mooney, S., & Smith, P. K. (1995). Bullying and the child who stammers. *British Journal of Special Education, 22*(1), 24–27. doi:10.1111/j.1467-8578.1995.tb00907.x

Moore, M., Howard, V., & McLaughlin, T. (2002). Siblings of children with disabilities: A review and analysis. *International Journal of Special Education, 17*, 49–64.

Mophosho, M., Widdows, J., & Taylor Gomez, M. (2010). Relationships between adolescent children and their siblings with cerebral palsy: A Pilot Study. *Journal on Developmental Disabilities, 15*(3), 81–87.

Moreno, S., & Bidelman, G. M. (2014). Examining neural plasticity and cognitive benefit through the unique lens of musical training. *Hearing Research, 308*, 84–97. doi:10.1016/j.heares.2013.09.012 PMID:24079993

Morgan, C. T., King, R. A., Weisz, J. R., & Schopler, J. (1993). Principles of learning. In Introduction to Psychology (7th ed.). New Delhi: Tata McGraw-Hill Publishing Company Limited.

Mori, H., Ohsawa, H., Tanaka, T. H., Taniwaki, E., Leisman, G., & Nishijo, K. (2004). Effect of massage on blood flow and muscle fatigue following isometric lumbar exercise. *Medical Science Monitor, 10*, CR173–CR178. PMID:15114265

Morris, R. G. (1986). Short-term forgetting in senile dementia of the Alzheimer's type. *Cognitive Neuropsychology, 3*(1), 77–97. doi:10.1080/02643298608252670

Morrow, W. R., & Gochros, H. L. (1970). Misconceptions regarding behavior modification. *The Social Service Review, 44*(3), 293–307. doi:10.1086/642579

Mosier, H. D., Grossman, H. J., & Dingman, H. F. (1965). Physical growth in mental defectives. *Pediatrics, 36*(3), 465–519. PMID:5825691

Moss, A. S., Wintering, N., Roggenkamp, H., Khalsa, D. S., Waldman, M. R., Monti, D., & Newberg, A. B. (2012). Effects of an 8-week meditation program on mood and anxiety in patients with memory loss. *Journal of Alternative and Complementary Medicine (New York, N.Y.), 18*(1), 48–53. doi:10.1089/acm.2011.0051 PMID:22268968

MSJE. (2009). *Ministry of Social Justice and Empowerment. Scientific Report on Research Project for Development of Indian Scale for Assessment of Autism.* New Delhi: Government of India.

Mukerjee, S., Hirisave, U., Kapur, M., & Subbakrishna, D. K. (1995). Anxiety, self-esteem in children with specific disorders of scholastic skills. *Nimhans Journal, 17*(2), 117–121.

Mukherjee, S. B., Malhotra, M. K., Aneja, S., Chakraborty, S., & Deshpande, S. (2015). Diagnostic accuracy of Indian scale for assessment of autism (ISAA) in children aged 2-9 years. *Indian Pediatrics, 52*(3), 212–216. doi:10.100713312-015-0608-z PMID:25848996

Mulligan, H., Wilkinson, A., Barclay, A., Whiting, H., Heynike, C., & Snowdon, J. (2016). Evaluation of a fatigue self-management program for people with multiple sclerosis. *International Journal of MS Care, 18*(3), 116–121. doi:10.7224/1537-2073.2015-019 PMID:27252598

Murray, C. J. L., & Lopez, A. D. (1996). *The global burden of disease : A comprehensive assessment of mortality and disability from diseases, injuries, and risk factors in 1990 and projected to 2020.* Boston: Harvard School of Public Health: World Health Organization.

Murta, T., Leite, M., Carmichael, D. W., Figueiredo, P., & Lemieux, L. (2015). Electrophysiological correlates of the BOLD signal for EEG-informed fMRI. *Human Brain Mapping, 36*(1), 391–414. doi:10.1002/hbm.22623 PMID:25277370

Myers, B. J., Mackintosh, V. H., & Goin-Kochel, R. P. (2009). My greatest joy and my greatest heartache: Parents own words on how having a child on the autism spectrum has affected their lives and their families lives. *Research in Autism Spectrum Disorders, 3*(3), 670–684. doi:10.1016/j.rasd.2009.01.004

Myles, W. S. (1985). Sleep deprivation, physical fatigue, and the perception of exercise intensity. *Medicine and Science in Sports and Exercise*, *17*(5), 580–584. doi:10.1249/00005768-198510000-00011 PMID:4068965

Myreddi, V., Narayan, J., Saleem, S., Sumalini, K., & Padma, V. (2004). *Functional assessment checklist for programming of students with profound mental retardation (FACP-PMR)*. National Institute for the Mentally Handicapped.

Nachshen, J. S., Anderson, L., & Jamieson, J. (2001). The parent advocacy scale: Measuring advocacy in parents of children with special needs. *Journal on Developmental Disabilities*, *8*, 93–105.

Nachtegaal, J., Festen, J. M., & Kramer, S. E. (2012). Hearing ability in working life and its relationship with sick leave and self-reported work productivity. *Ear and Hearing*, *33*(1), 94–103. doi:10.1097/AUD.0b013e318228033e PMID:21826005

Nachtegaal, J., Kuik, D. J., Anema, J. R., Goverts, S. T., Festen, J. M., & Kramer, S. E. (2009). Hearing status, need for recovery after work, and psychosocial work characteristics: Results from an internet-based national survey on hearing. *International Journal of Audiology*, *48*(10), 684–691. doi:10.1080/14992020902962421 PMID:19863354

Nagaraja, M. N. (2002). Challenges in Vocational & Technical Education of PWHI. In *Proceeding of Challenges in Vocational & Technical Education to persons with disabilities*. Mumbai: Seminar at Ali Yavar Jung National Institute of Hearing Handicapped.

Nanda, J. L., & Sukla, G. D. (1978). Some probable factors causing mental retardation. *Child Psychiatry Quarterly*, *10*, 4–106.

Naniwadekar, K., & Venkatesan, S. (2014). Impact of behavioral intervention on reduction of problem behaviors in children with autism. *Journal of Disability Management and Special Education*, *4*(2), 1–15.

Narayan, C. L., & John, T. (2017). The Rights of Persons with Disabilities Act, 2016: Does it address the needs of the persons with mental illness and their families. *Indian Journal of Psychiatry*, *59*(1), 17–20. doi:10.4103/psychiatry.IndianJPsychiatry_75_17 PMID:28529356

Nardi, P. M. (2015). *Doing survey research. A guide to quantitative methods* (3rd ed.). London: Routledge.

Nario-Redmond, M. R. (2010). Cultural stereotypes of disabled and non-disabled men and women: Consensus for global category representations and diagnostic domains. *British Journal of Social Psychology*, *49*(3), 471–488. doi:10.1348/014466609X468411 PMID:19793408

Narne, V. K., Prabhu, P., Chandan, H. S., & Deepthi, M. (2014). Audiological profiling of 198 individuals with auditory neuropathy spectrum disorder. *Hearing, Balance and Communication*, *12*(3), 112–120. doi:10.3109/21695717.2014.938481

National Education Association USA. (2008). *Policy brief: Parent, Family, Community Involvement in Education*. Retrieved from www.nea.org/assets/doc/PBII_Parent Involvement08.pdf

Neely-Barnes, S. L., & Dia, D. A. (2008). Families of children with disabilities: A review of literature and recommendations for interventions. *Journal of Early and Intensive Behavior Intervention: JEIBI*, *5*(3), 93–107. doi:10.1037/h0100425

Neher, T., Lunner, T., Hopkins, K., & Moore, B. C. J. (2012). Binaural temporal fine structure sensitivity, cognitive function, and spatial speech recognition of hearing-impaired listeners (L). *The Journal of the Acoustical Society of America*, *131*(4), 2561–2564. doi:10.1121/1.3689850 PMID:22501036

Nehru, R. (2001). *Distorted grapheme representation: A new hypothesis to explain reading disorders*. Poster presentation at the 5th British Dyslexia Association International Conference, York, UK.

Neki, J. S. (1975). Psychotherapy in India: Past, present, and future. *American Journal of Psychotherapy*, *29*(1), 92–100. PMID:1096647

Neu, D., Kajosch, H., Peigneux, P., Verbanck, P., Linkowski, P., & Le Bon, O. (2011). Cognitive impairment in fatigue and sleepiness associated conditions. *Psychiatry Research*, *189*(1), 128–134. doi:10.1016/j.psychres.2010.12.005 PMID:21196050

Ngugi, T. O. (1993). *Moving the center: The struggle for cultural freedoms*. Oxford, UK: James Curry Limited.

Nielsen, K. E. (2012). *A disability history of the United States*. Boston: Beacon Press.

Niemi, M. L., Laaksonen, R., Kotila, M., & Weltimo, O. (1988). Quality of life 4 years after stroke. *Stroke*, *19*(9), 1101–1107. doi:10.1161/01.STR.19.9.1101 PMID:3413807

Nixon, G. M., Charbonneau, I., Kermack, A. S., Brouillette, R. T., & McFarland, D. H. (2008). Respiratory-swallowing interactions during sleep in premature infants at term. *Respiratory Physiology & Neurobiology*, *160*(1), 76–82. doi:10.1016/j.resp.2007.08.010 PMID:17942377

Noelle, T. (2017). *Selective Mutism: Frozen in Silence*. Retrieved from https://www.nami.org/Blogs/NAMI-Blog/January-2017/Selective-Mutism-Frozen-in-Silence

Nulty, D. D. (2008). The adequacy of response rates to online and paper surveys: What can be done? *Assessment & Evaluation in Higher Education*, *33*(3), 301–314. doi:10.1080/02602930701293231

Nunez, B., & Rodriguez, L. (2005). *Los hermanos de persons con discapacidad: una asignatura pendiente*. Buenos Aires: Asociacion AMAR.

O'Brian, S., Iverach, L., Jones, M., Onslow, M., Packman, A., & Menzies, R. (2013). Effectiveness of the Lidcombe program for early stuttering in Australian communities clinics. *International Journal of Speech-Language Pathology*, *15*(6), 593–603. doi:10.3109/17549507.2013.783112 PMID:23691980

O'dowd, H., Gladwell, P., Rogers, C. A., Hollinghurst, S., and Gregory, A. (2006). Cognitive behavioural therapy in chronic fatigue syndrome: A randomised controlled trial of an outpatient group programme. *Health Technology Assessment-Southampton, 10*(37).

Oerbeck, B., Manassis, K., Overgaard, K. R., & Kristensen, H. (2016). Selective Mutism. In IACAPAP e-Textbook of Child and Adolescent Mental Health (pp. 1-23). Geneva: International Association for Child and Adolescent Psychiatry and Allied Professions.

Okogbaa, O. G., Shell, R. L., & Filipusic, D. (1994). On the investigation of the neurophysiological correlates of knowledge worker mental fatigue using the EEG signal. *Applied Ergonomics*, *25*(6), 355–365. doi:10.1016/0003-6870(94)90054-X PMID:15676987

Olichney, J. M., Morris, S. K., Ochoa, C., Salmon, D. P., Thal, L. J., Kutas, M., & Iragui, V. J. (2002). Abnormal verbal event related potentials in mild cognitive impairment and incipient Alzheimer's disease. *Journal of Neurology, Neurosurgery, and Psychiatry*, *73*(4), 377–384. doi:10.1136/jnnp.73.4.377 PMID:12235303

Olika, R. E. L. (2013). *Attitudes hearing impaired children face from hearing people* (Unpublished master's dissertation). University of Oslo, Norway.

Oliver, J. (2007). *Affluenza: How to be successful and stay sane*. London: Vermilion, Ebury Publishing

Oller, J. W., Oller, S. D., & Badon, L. C. (2010). Cases: Introducing Communication Disorders across the lifespan. Oxfordshire, UK: Plural Publishing.

Olusanya, B. O., Ruben, R. J., & Parving, A. (2006). Reducing the burden of communication disorders in the developing world: An opportunity for the Millennium Development Project. *Journal of the American Medical Association, 296*(4), 441–444. doi:10.1001/jama.296.4.441 PMID:16868302

Onslow, M., Jones, M., Menzies, R., O'Brian, S., & Packman, A. (2012). Stuttering. In P. Sturmey & M. Hersen (Eds.), Handbook of evidence-based practice in clinical psychology (pp. 185 – 207). Hoboken, NJ: Wiley.

Onslow, M., Andrews, C., & Lincoln, M. (1994). A control/experimental trial of an operant treatment for early stuttering. *Journal of Speech, Language, and Hearing Research: JSLHR, 37*(6), 1244–1259. doi:10.1044/jshr.3706.1244 PMID:7877284

Onslow, M., Attanasio, J., & Harrison, E. (2003). Parents talk about the Lidcombe Program. In M. Onslow, A. Packman, & E. Harrison (Eds.), *The Lidcombe Program of early stuttering intervention: A clinician's guide* (pp. 193–206). Austin, TX: Pro-Ed.

Onwuegbuzie, A. J., & Leech, N. L. (2006). Linking research questions to mixed methods data analysis procedures. *Qualitative Report, 11*(3), 474–498.

Orgogozo, J. M. (1994). The concepts of impairment, disability, and handicap. *Cerebrovascular Diseases (Basel, Switzerland), 4*(2), 2–6. doi:10.1159/000108531

Ormerod, M. (2005). Understanding access audits and appraisals: An inclusive design approach. *Journal of Building Appraisal, 1*(2), 140–152. doi:10.1057/palgrave.jba.2940013

Orsmond, G. I., & Seltzer, M. M. (2000). Brothers and sisters of adults with mental retardation gendered nature of the sibling relationship. *American Journal of Mental Retardation, 105*(6), 486–508. doi: PMID:11958202

Ortiz, K. Z., & Marinelli, M. R. (2013). Investigation on the complaint of dysphagia in aphasic patients. *Revista CEFAC, 15*(6), 1503–1511. doi:10.1590/S1516-18462013005000043

Ostergren, J. A. (2014). *Speech-language pathology assistants: A resource manual.* San Diego, CA: Plural Publishing.

Owens, R. E. (2017). *Introduction to communication disorders: A lifespan evidence-based perspective.* Content Technologies.

Oyler, M. E. (1996). Vulnerability in stuttering children. *Dissertation Abstracts International, 56*, 3374.

Packman, A., Onslow, M., & Attanasio, J. (2003). The timing of early intervention with the Lidcombe Program. In M. Onslow, A. Packman, & E. Harrison (Eds.), *The Lidcombe Program of early stuttering intervention: A clinician's guide* (pp. 41–55). Austin, TX: Pro-Ed.

Padencheri, S., Swamidhas, P., & Russell, S. (2011). The role of gender of children with intellectual disability and their parents in marital intimacy in southern India. *Journal of Intellectual Disabilities, 15*, 241–251. PMID:22158461

Paes, E. C., de Vries, I. A., Penris, W. M., Hanny, K. H., Lavrijsen, S. W., van Leerdam, E. K., ... Breugem, C. C. (2017). Growth and prevalence of feeding difficulties in children with Robin sequence: A retrospective cohort study. *Clinical Oral Investigations, 21*(6), 2063–2076. doi:10.100700784-016-1996-8 PMID:27868158

Papathanasiou, I., & Coppens, P. (2013). Basic concepts and operational definitions. In I. Papathanasiou, P. Coppens, & C. Potagas (Eds.), *Aphasia and related neurogenic communication disorders* (pp. xx–xxii). Burlington, MA: Jones and Bartlett Learning.

Parrish, J. B., Weinstock-Guttman, B., Smerbeck, A., Benedict, R. H. B., & Yeh, E. A. (2013). Fatigue and depression in children with demyelinating disorders. *Journal of Child Neurology*, *28*(6), 713–718. doi:10.1177/0883073812450750 PMID:22805247

Parr, S. (2007). Living with severe aphasia: Tracking social exclusion. *Aphasiology*, *21*(1), 98–123. doi:10.1080/02687030600798337

Parr, S., & Byng, S. (1998). Breaking new ground in familiar territory: A response to 'Supported conversation for adults with aphasia' by Aura Kagan. *Aphasiology*, *12*(9), 839–844. doi:10.1080/02687039808249579

Partridge, L. (2017). *Siblings of children with special needs*. Retrieved from http://extendedfamilycare.com/pittsburgh/siblings-of-children-with-special-needs/

Patel, M. R., & Piazza, C. C. (2001). Your finicky eater: A guide for parents. *Exceptional Parent*, *31*(6), 82–84.

Patra, S., & Arun, P. (2011). Use of Indian scale for assessment of autism in child guidance clinic: An experience. *Indian Journal of Psychological Medicine*, *33*(2), 217–219. doi:10.4103/0253-7176.92043 PMID:22345858

Paul, D. R., Frattali, C. M., Holland, A. L., Thompson, C. K., Caperton, C. J., & Slater, S. C. (2003). *Quality of communication life scale (QCL)*. Rockville, MD: American Speech-Language-Hearing Association.

Pelchat, D., Levert, M. J., & Bourgeois-Gue'rin, V. (2009). How do mothers and fathers who have a child with a disability describe their adaptation/ transformation process? *Journal of Child Health Care*, *13*(3), 239–259. doi:10.1177/1367493509336684 PMID:19713407

Pennington, B. F., & Bishop, D. V. (2009). Relations among speech, language, and reading disorders. *Annual Review of Psychology*, *60*(1), 283–306. doi:10.1146/annurev.psych.60.110707.163548 PMID:18652545

Perkins, M. (2014). Linguistic recycling in typical and atypical interactions. *Clinical Linguistics & Phonetics*, *28*(6-7), 590–601. doi:10.3109/02699206.2014.926995 PMID:25000380

Perry, R. J., & Hodges, J. R. (1999). Attention and executive deficits in Alzheimer's disease. *Brain*, *122*(3), 383–404. doi:10.1093/brain/122.3.383 PMID:10094249

Perske, R., Clifton, A., McClean, B. M., & Stein, J. I. (1977). *Meal Times for Severely and Profoundly Handicapped Persons: New Concepts and Attitudes*. Baltimore, MD: University Park Press.

Peshawaria, R., Menon, D. K., Bailey, D., Skinner, D., Ganguly, R., & Rajshekar, C. (2000). *Behavior Assessment Scales for Adult Living with Mental Retardation (BASAL-MR)*. National Institute for the Mentally Handicapped.

Peshawaria, R., & Venkatesan, S. (1992a). *Behavioral Assessment Scales for Indian Children with Mentally Retardation (BASIC-MR)*. National Institute for the Mentally Handicapped.

Peshawaria, R., & Venkatesan, S. (1992b). *Behavioral Approaches to training mentally handicapped children: A manual for teachers*. National Institute for the Mentally Handicapped.

Peshawaria, R., Venkatesan, S., & Menon, D. K. (1988). Consumer demand for services by parents of mentally handicapped individuals. *Indian Journal of Disability and Rehabilitation*, *2*(2), 43–57.

Peshawaria, R., Venkatesan, S., & Menon, D. K. (1990). Behavior problems in mentally handicapped persons: An analysis of parent needs. *Indian Journal of Clinical Psychology*, *17*(2), 63–70.

Peshawaria, R., Venkatesan, S., Mohapatra, B., & Menon, D. K. (1990). Teachers' perception of problem behaviors among mentally handicapped persons in special school settings. *Indian Journal of Disability and Rehabilitation*, *4*(1), 23–30.

Petersen, R. C., Doody, R., Kurz, A., Mohs, R. C., Morris, J. C., Rabins, P. V., ... Winblad, B. (2001a). Current concepts in mild cognitive impairment. *Archives of Neurology*, *58*(12), 1985–1992. doi:10.1001/archneur.58.12.1985 PMID:11735772

Petersen, R. C., Stevens, J. C., Ganguli, M., Tangalos, E. G., Cummings, J. L., & DeKosky, S. T. (2001b). Practice parameter: Early detection of dementia: Mild cognitive impairment (an evidence-based review) Report of the Quality Standards Subcommittee of the American Academy of Neurology. *Neurology*, *56*(9), 1133–1142. doi:10.1212/WNL.56.9.1133 PMID:11342677

Peterson, A., Shallop, J., Driscoll, C., Breneman, A., Babb, J., Stoeckel, R., & Fabry, L. (2003). Outcomes of cochlear implantation in children with auditory neuropathy. *Journal of the American Academy of Audiology*, *14*(4), 188–201. PMID:12940703

Phetrasuwan, S., & Miles, M. S. (2009). Parenting stress in mothers of children with autism spectrum disorders. *Journal for Specialists in Pediatric Nursing*, *188*(3), 157–165. doi:10.1111/j.1744-6155.2009.00188.x PMID:19614824

Pichon, E., & Borel-Maisonny, S. (1937). *Stuttering, its nature and treatment*. Paris, France: Masson.

Pierce, S. R., & Patterson, P. J. (1996). Treatment of auditory comprehension impairment. In G. L. Wallace (Ed.), *Adult Aphasia Rehabilitation*. Butterworth-Heinemann.

Pimm, P. L. (1996). Some of the implications of caring for a child or adult with cerebral palsy. *British Journal of Occupational Therapy*, *59*(7), 335–341. doi:10.1177/030802269605900714

Pindzola, R. (1987). *Stuttering intervention program: Age 3 to grade 3*. Austin, TX: Pro-Ed.

Pindzola, R. (1999). *The stuttering intervention program. In The handbook of early stuttering intervention* (pp. 119–138). London: Singular Publishing Inc.

Pinki & Pauranik, A. (2013). The diversity of burden for significant others of person with aphasia. *Journal of All India Institute of Speech and Hearing, 32,* 167-172.

Pisula, E. (2007). A comparative study of stress profiles in mothers of children with autism and those of children with Down's syndrome. *Journal of Applied Research in Intellectual Disabilities*, *20*(3), 274–278. doi:10.1111/j.1468-3148.2006.00342.x

Planning Commission of India. (2013). *Report on 12th Five year Plan*. New Delhi: Government of India.

Poindexter, B. B., & Ehrenkranz, R. A. (2015). Nutrient requirements and provision of nutritional support in the premature neonate. In R. J. Martin, A. A. Fanaroff, & M. C. Walsh (Eds.), *Neonatal-Perinatal Medicine* (10th ed.). Philadelphia, PA: Elsevier.

Porch, B. E. (1971). *The Porch Index of Communicative Ability*. Palo Alto, CA: Consulting Psychologists Press.

Porrazzo, A. S. (1975). *Evaluation and treatment of reading deficits in aphasic patients*. Paper presentation at the fifth conference on clinical aphasiology, Santa Fe, NM.

Portway, S. M., & Johnson, B. (2005). Do you know I have Asperger Syndrome? Risks of a non-obvious disability. *Health Risk & Society*, *7*(1), 73–83. doi:10.1080/09500830500042086

Possl, J., Jurgensmeyer, S., Karlbauer, F., Wenz, C., & Goldenberg, G. (2001). Stability of employment after brain injury: A 7 year follow up study. *Brain Injury: [BI]*, *15*(1), 15–27. doi:10.1080/02699050150209093 PMID:11201311

Pound, C., Parr, S., Lindsay, J., & Woolf, C. (2000). *Beyond Aphasia: Therapies for Living with Communication Disability*. Bicester: Speechmark.

Powel, T. H., & Gallagher, P. A. (1993). *Brothers and sisters: A special part of exceptional families*. Baltimore, MD: Paul H. Brookes.

Power, A. (2013). Making space for belonging: Critical reflections on the implementation of personalized adult social care under the veil of meaningful inclusion. *Social Science & Medicine*, *88*, 68–75. doi:10.1016/j.socscimed.2013.04.008 PMID:23702211

Pozo, P., & Sarriá, E. (2014). Prediction of stress in mothers of children with autism spectrum disorders. *The Spanish Journal of Psychology*, *17*, 1–12. doi:10.1017jp.2014.6 PMID:25012691

Prabhu, P. (2016). Evaluation of depression, anxiety, and stress in adolescents and young adults with auditory neuropathy spectrum disorder. *Scientifica*, *2016*, 1–8. doi:10.1155/2016/4378269 PMID:27579218

Prabhu, P. P., & Sneha, P. (2014). Self report tinnitus handicap in individuals with auditory neuropathy spectrum disorder. *Journal of Hearing Science*, *4*(3), 43–50.

Prabhu, P., Avilala, V. K. Y., & Manjula, P. (2012). Predisposing factors in individuals with late-onset auditory dys-synchrony. *Asia Pacific Journal of Speech, Language and Hearing*, *15*(1), 41–50. doi:10.1179/136132812805253758

Prabhu, P., & Jamuar, P. (2017a). Evaluation of dizziness handicap in adolescents and adults with auditory neuropathy spectrum disorder. *International Archives of Otorhinolaryngology*, *49*(1), 30–43.

Prabhu, P., & Jamuar, P. (2017b). Prevalence of vestibular symptoms in individuals with auditory neuropathy spectrum disorder-A retrospective study. *Intractable & Rare Diseases Research*, *6*(1), 46–49. doi:10.5582/irdr.2016.01098 PMID:28357181

Prakash, P. (2003). Early reading acquisition. In P. Karanth & J. Rozario (Eds.), *Learning disabilities in India: Willing the mind to learn* (pp. 63–65). New Delhi: Sage Publications.

Prakash, P., & Rekha, B. (1992). Phonological awareness and reading acquisition in Kannada. In A. K. Srivastava (Ed.), *Researches in child and adolescent psychology* (pp. 47–52). New Delhi: NCERT.

Prakash, P., Rekha, D., Nigam, R., & Karanath, P. (1993). Phonological awareness, orthography and literary. In R. J. Scholes (Ed.), *Literary and language analysis*. Hillsdale, NJ: Lawrence Erlbaum Associates.

Prasad, L., Varrey, A., & Sisti, G. (2016). Medical students' stress levels and sense of well being after six weeks of yoga and meditation. *Evidence-Based Complementary and Alternative Medicine*, *2016*, 1–7. doi:10.1155/2016/9251849 PMID:28053644

Prasad, M., & Sitholey, P. (1988). Behavior therapy in a retarded adolescent with conduct disorder: A case report. *Indian Journal of Clinical Psychology*, *15*(2), 74–76.

Prema, K. S. (1998). *Reading Acquisition Profile in Kannada* (Doctoral dissertation). Mysore: University of Mysore.

Prince, M., Bryce, R., Albanese, E., Wimo, A., Ribeiro, W., & Ferri, C. P. (2013). The global prevalence of dementia: A systematic review and metaanalysis. *Alzheimer's & Dementia*, *9*(1), 63–75. doi:10.1016/j.jalz.2012.11.007 PMID:23305823

Pueschel, S. M., Bernier, J. C., & Weidenman, L. E. (1988). *The special child*. Baltimore, MD: Paul H. Brooks Publishing, Co.

Purdy, M., & Hindenlang, J. (2005). Educating and training caregivers of persons with aphasia. *Aphasiology*, *19*(3-5), 377–388. doi:10.1080/02687030444000822

Purves, B. A., & Phinney, A. (2012). Family voices: A family systems approach to understanding communication in dementia. *Canadian Journal of Speech-Language Pathology and Audiology*, *36*(4), 284–300.

Qureshi, M. A., Vice, F. L., Taciak, V. L., Bosma, J. F., & Gewolb, I. H. (2002). Changes in rhythmic suckle feeding patterns in term infants in the first month of life. *Developmental Medicine and Child Neurology*, *44*(1), 34–39. doi:10.1017/S0012162201001621 PMID:11811648

Raakhee, A. S., & Aparna, N. (2011). A study on the prevalence of anxiety disorders among higher secondary students. *Education Science and Psychology*, *1*, 33–37.

Radcliffe, D. (2004). *Video and Audio Methods in Qualitative Research* [On-Line Booklet]. Retrieved September 14, 2017, from http://www.don.ratcliffs.net/video/

Radovic, S., & Malmgren, H. (1998). Fatigue and Fatiguability- semantic and etiologic perspectives. *Proceedings of Neural Correlates of Consciousness: Empirical and conceptual issues*. Retrieved from http://www.phil.gu.se/posters/fatigue.html

Raikes, H. A., & Thompson, R. A. (2005). Efficacy and social support as predictors of parenting stress among families in poverty. *Infant Mental Health Journal*, *26*(3), 177–190. doi:10.1002/imhj.20044 PMID:28682501

Raju, S., & Nataraja, N. P. (2016a). Assessment of working memory in bilingual children. *Indian Journal of Positive Psychology*, *7*, 159.

Raju, S., & Nataraja, N. P. (2016b). Lexical-semantic production and inhibitory control skills in monolingual (Kannada) and bilingual (Kannada-English) children. *Journal of All India Institute of Speech and Hearing*, *34*, 90–100.

Ramaa, S. (1984). *Diagnosis and remediation of dyslexia* (Doctoral dissertation). Mysore: University of Mysore.

Ramaa, S., & Gowramma, I. P. (2002). A systematic procedure for identifying and classifying children with dyscalculia among primary school children in India. *Dyslexia (Chichester, England)*, *8*(2), 67–85. doi:10.1002/dys.214 PMID:12067188

Rance, G., Beer, D. E., Cone-Wesson, B., Shepherd, R. K., Dowell, R. C., King, A. M., ... Clark, G. M. (1999). Clinical findings for a group of infants and young children with auditory neuropathy. *Ear and Hearing*, *20*(3), 238–252. doi:10.1097/00003446-199906000-00006 PMID:10386850

Rance, G., McKay, C., & Grayden, D. (2004). Perceptual characterization of children with auditory neuropathy. *Ear and Hearing*, *25*(1), 34–46. doi:10.1097/01.AUD.0000111259.59690.B8 PMID:14770016

Rani, K. R., Chakravarthy, K.N.V.V.S.S.S., & Reddy, D.C.S. (2016). Perceptions and problems of other siblings in a family having mentally retarded children. *IOSR Journal of Humanities and Social Science, 21*(1), 7-12.

Ranjini, A., Natesh, G., & Jain, S. (2017). Auditory stream segregation abilities in musicians and its association with verbal working memory and speech perception in noise. Proceedings of Indian Speech and Hearing Association.

Rao, A. N. (2009). Poverty and disability in India. *Social Change*, *39*(1), 29–45. doi:10.1177/004908570903900102

Rao, I. (2002). *Portage Guide to Early Child Education (PGECE).* Bangalore: CBR Network. *South Asia*.

Rao, K. (2010). Psychological interventions: From theory to practice. In G. Mishra (Ed.), *Psychology in India: Clinical and Health Psychology* (Vol. 3, pp. 317–360). New Delhi: Indian Council of Social Science Research/Dorling Kindersley.

Rao, K., Barnabas, I., & Gopinath, P. S. (1989). Behavior modification in a rehabilitation setting. *Journal of Personality and Clinical Studies*, *5*(1), 23–27.

Rao, T. A. S. (1992). *Manual on developing communication skills in mentally retarded persons*. National Institute for the Mentally Handicapped.

Rapolienė, L., Razbadauskas, A., Sąlyga, J., & Martinkėnas, A. (2016). Stress and fatigue management using balneotherapy in a short-time randomized controlled trial. *Evidence-Based Complementary and Alternative Medicine, 2016*, 1–10. doi:10.1155/2016/9631684 PMID:27051455

Rasch, T., Günther, S., Hoppe, U., Eysholdt, U., & Rosanowski, F. (2005). Voice-related quality of life in organic and functional voice disorders. *Logopedics, Phoniatrics, Vocology*, *30*(1), 9–13. doi:10.1080/14015430510006640 PMID:16040435

Rathna, N. (Ed.). (1968). *Behaviour therapy and speech disorders*. Mysore: All India Institute of Speech and Hearing.

Rautakoski, P. (2011). Partners' self-perceptions of the use of different communication strategies during total communication intervention. *Aphasiology*, *25*(12), 1523–1542. doi:10.1080/02687038.2011.624164

Rautakoski, P. (2011). Training total communication. *Aphasiology*, *25*(3), 344–365. doi:10.1080/02687038.2010.530671

Read, J. (2000). *Disability, the Family and Society: Listening to Mothers*. Buckingham, UK: Open University Press.

Reagon, K., Higbee, T., & Endicott, K. (2006). Teaching pretend play skills to students with autism using video modeling with siblings as model and play partners. *Education & Treatment of Children*, *29*, 517–528.

Reddy, G., Kumari, P. S., & Kusuma, A. (2004). *Language disorders and intervention strategies: A practical guide to the teachers*. New Delhi: Discovery Publishing House.

Reddy, R. P., Sharma, M. P., & Shivashankar, N. (2010). Cognitive behavior therapy for stuttering: A case series. *Indian Journal of Psychological Medicine*, *32*(1), 49–53. doi:10.4103/0253-7176.70533 PMID:21799560

Rehabilitation Council of India. (2009a). *Bachelor of Audiology and speech-language pathology (BASLP): Semester scheme regulations, norms, scheme of exam and curriculum*. New Delhi: Author.

Rehabilitation Council of India. (2009b). *Master of science in audiology/speech-language pathology: Semester scheme regulations, norms, scheme of exam and curriculum*. New Delhi: Author.

Rehabilitation Council of India. (2009c). *Diploma course in the hearing, language, and speech: Course curriculum*. New Delhi: Author.

Rehm, R. S., & Bradley, J. F. (2005). Normalization in families raising a child who is medically fragile, technology dependent and developmentally delayed. *Qualitative Health Research*, *15*(6), 807–821. doi:10.1177/1049732305276754 PMID:15961877

Reid, J., Reilly, S., & Kilpatrick, N. (2007). Sucking performance of babies with cleft conditions. *The Cleft Palate-Craniofacial Journal*, *44*(3), 312–320. doi:10.1597/05-173 PMID:17477747

Reilly, S., Skuse, D., & Poblete, X. (1996). Prevalence of feeding problems and oral motor dysfunction in children with cerebral palsy: A community survey. *The Journal of Pediatrics*, *129*(6), 877–882. doi:10.1016/S0022-3476(96)70032-X PMID:8969730

Reis, A., & Petersson, K. M. (2003). Educational level, socioeconomic status and aphasia research: A comment on Connor et al. (2001)-effect of socioeconomic status on aphasia severity and recovery. *Brain and Language*, *87*(3), 449–452. doi:10.1016/S0093-934X(03)00140-8 PMID:14642547

Reitan, R. M., & Wolfson, D. (1985). *The Halstead-Reitan neuropsychological test battery: Theory and clinical interpretation* (Vol. 4). Reitan Neuropsychology.

Rempel, G. R., Colwell, S. O., & Nelson, R. P. (1988). Growth in children with cerebral palsy fed via gastrostomy. *Pediatrics*, *82*, 857–863. PMID:3186375

Rentschler, G. J. (2012). *Here's how to do stuttering therapy*. San Diego, CA: Plural Publishing.

Resch, J. A., Mireles, G., Benz, M. R., Grenwelge, C., Peterson, R., & Zhang, D. (2010). Giving parents a voice: A qualitative study of the challenges experienced by parents of children with disabilities. *Rehabilitation Psychology*, *55*(2), 139–150. doi:10.1037/a0019473 PMID:20496968

Reynolds, C. R., & Willson, V. L. (1974). Critical measurement issues in learning disabilities. *The Journal of Special Education*, *18*(4), 451–476. doi:10.1177/002246698401800403

Reynolds, W. M. (2001). *Reynolds adolescent adjustment screening inventory: RAASI: Professional manual*. Psychological Assessment Resources.

Rezaei, M., Rashedi, V., Gharib, M., & Lotfi, G. (2011). Prevalence of feeding problems in children with intellectual disability. *Iranian Rehabilitation Journal*, *9*, 56–59.

Richburg, M. L., & Cobia, D. C. (1994). Using behavioral techniques to treat elective mutism: A case study. *Elementary School Guidance & Counselling*, *28*(3), 214–220.

Rights of Persons With Disabilities Act. (2016). Ministry of Law and Justice, Government of India.

Riley, G. D., & Ingham, J. C. (2000). Acoustic duration changes associated with two types of treatment for children who stutter. *Journal of Speech, Language, and Hearing Research: JSLHR*, *43*(4), 965–978. doi:10.1044/jslhr.4304.965 PMID:11386482

Riley, G. D., & Riley, J. (1984). A component model for treating stuttering in children. In M. Peins (Ed.), *Contemporary approaches in stuttering therapy* (pp. 123–172). Boston: Little, Brown.

Riordan, M. M., Iwata, B. A., Finney, J. W., Wohl, M. K., & Stanley, A. E. (1984). Behavioral assessment and treatment of chronic food refusal in handicapped children. *Journal of Applied Behavior Analysis*, *17*(3), 327–341. doi:10.1901/jaba.1984.17-327 PMID:6239853

Riva, S., & Antonietti, A. (2010). The application of the ICF-CY model in specific learning difficulties: A case study. *Psychology of Language and Communication*, *14*(2), 37–58. doi:10.2478/v10057-010-0009-2

Rodriguez-Fornells, A., Rotte, M., Heinze, H.-J., Nösselt, T., & Münte, T. F. (2002). Brain potential and functional MRI evidence for how to handle two languages with one brain. *Nature*, *415*(6875), 1026–1029. doi:10.1038/4151026a PMID:11875570

Rodriguez-Fornells, A., van der Lugt, A., Rotte, M., Britti, B., Heinze, H.-J., & Münte, T. F. (2005). Second language interferes with word production in fluent bilinguals: Brain potential and functional imaging evidence. *Journal of Cognitive Neuroscience*, *17*(3), 422–433. doi:10.1162/0898929053279559 PMID:15814002

Roeltgen, D. P., Sevush, S., & Heilman, K. M. (1983). Phonological agraphia: Writing by the lexical-semantic route. *Neurology*, *33*(6), 755–765. doi:10.1212/WNL.33.6.755 PMID:6682519

Rogers, B., Arvedson, J., Buck, G., Smart, P., & Msall, M. (1994). Characteristics of dysphagia in children with cerebral palsy. *Dysphagia*, *9*(1), 69–73. doi:10.1007/BF00262762 PMID:8131428

Roid, G. H., & Miller, L. J. (1997). *Leiter international performance scale-revised: Examiners manual*. Wood Dale, IL: Stoelting.

Ross, D., & Spencer, S. (1980). *Aphasia Rehabilitation-An Auditory and Verbal Task Hierarchy*. Charles C. Thomas.

Rosselli, M., Matute, E., Pinto, N., & Ardila, A. (2006). Memory abilities in children with subtypes of dyscalculia. *Developmental Neuropsychology*, *30*(3), 801–818. doi:10.120715326942dn3003_3 PMID:17083294

Rossetti, H. C., Lacritz, L. H., Cullum, C. M., & Weiner, M. F. (2011). Normative data for the Montreal Cognitive Assessment (MoCA) in a population-based sample. *Neurology, 77*(13), 1272–1275. doi:10.1212/WNL.0b013e318230208a PMID:21917776

Ross, K. B., & Wertz, R. T. (2002). Relationships between language-based disability and quality of life in chronically aphasic adults. *Aphasiology, 16*(8), 791–800. doi:10.1080/02687030244000130

Ross, K., & Wertz, R. (2003). Quality of life with and without aphasia. *Aphasiology, 17*(4), 355–364. doi:10.1080/02687030244000716

Roush, P., Frymark, T., Venediktov, R., & Wang, B. (2011). Audiologic management of auditory neuropathy spectrum disorder in children: A systematic review of the literature. *American Journal of Audiology, 20*(2), 159–170. doi:10.1044/1059-0889(2011/10-0032) PMID:21940978

Roy, N. (2011). Personality and voice disorders. *SIG 3 Perspectives on Voice and Voice Disorders, 21*(1), 17- 23.

Royal College of Speech and Language Therapists (RCSLT). (2009). Resource manual for commissioning and planning services for SLCN: Speech and language impairment. London, UK: RCSLT.

Roy, N., & Bless, D. M. (2000). Toward a theory of the dispositional bases of functional dysphonia and vocal nodules: Exploring the role of personality and emotional adjustment. In R. D. Kent & M. J. Ball (Eds.), *The handbook of voice quality measurement* (pp. 461–480). San Diego, CA: Singular Publishing Group.

Roy, N., & Leeper, H. A. (1993). Effects of the manual laryngeal musculoskeletal tension reduction technique as a treatment for functional voice disorders: Perceptual and acoustic measures. *Journal of Voice, 7*(3), 242–249. doi:10.1016/S0892-1997(05)80333-9 PMID:8353642

Rozario, J. (2003). Assessment of Learning Disabilities. In P. Karanth & J. Rozario (Eds.), *Learning Disabilities in India: Willing the Mind to Learn* (pp. 51–61). New Delhi: Sage Publications.

Ruby, D. O., & Matheny, W. D. (1962). Comments on growth of cerebral palsied children. *Journal of the American Dietetic Association, 40*, 525–527. PMID:14494972

Runyan, C. M., & Runyan, S. E. (1986). A fluency rules therapy program for young children in the public schools. *Language, Speech, and Hearing Services in Schools, 17*(4), 276–284. doi:10.1044/0161-1461.1704.276

Ruotsalainen, J. H., Sellman, J., Lehto, L., Jauhiainen, M., & Verbeek, J. H. (2007). Interventions for treating functional dysphonia in adults. *Cochrane Database of Systematic Reviews*, 3. PMID:17636842

Rupured, M., & Quick, S. (1989). *Family vitality: Characteristics of strong families. Publication H.E. 7-138.* University of Kentucky Cooperative Extension Service.

Russell, C., Russell, C., & Russell, M. (2003). We're here too: Supporting 'sibs' of children with special needs. *Exceptional Parent, 33*, 36–39.

Rustin, L., Botterill, W., & Kelman, E. (1996). *Assessment and therapy for young dysfluent children: Family interaction.* London: Whurr.

Ryan, B. P., & Ryan, B. V. K. (1983). Programmed stuttering therapy for children: Comparison of four establishment programs. *Journal of Fluency Disorders, 8*(4), 291–321. doi:10.1016/0094-730X(83)90011-6

Ryan, B. P., & Ryan, B. V. K. (1995). Programmed stuttering treatment for children: Comparison of two establishment programs through transfer, maintenance, and follow-up. *Journal of Speech and Hearing Research, 38*(1), 61–75. doi:10.1044/jshr.3801.61 PMID:7731220

Ryan, S. (2005). "People don't do odd, do they?" Mothers making sense of the reactions of others towards their learning-disabled children in public places. *Children's Geographies*, *3*(3), 291–306. doi:10.1080/14733280500352920

Ryan, S. (2010). 'Meltdowns', surveillance and managing emotions; going out with children with autism. *Health & Place*, *16*(5), 868–875. doi:10.1016/j.healthplace.2010.04.012 PMID:20462783

Ryan, S., & Cole, K. R. (2009). From Advocate to Activist? Mapping the Experiences of Mothers of Children on the Autism Spectrum. *Journal of Applied Research in Intellectual Disabilities*, *22*(1), 43–53. doi:10.1111/j.1468-3148.2008.00438.x

Sacks, H., Schegloff, E. A., & Jefferson, G. (1974). A simplest systematics for the organization of turn-taking for conversation. *Language*, *50*(4), 696–735. doi:10.1353/lan.1974.0010

Sadock, B. J., Kaplan, H. I., & Sadock, V. A. (2007). Selective Mutism. *Annals of Clinical Psychiatry*, *10*, 4475–4483.

Saika, N., Bora, J. K., Jasilionis, D., & Shkolnikov, V. M. (2016). Disability divides India: Evidence from the 2011 census. *PLoS One*, *11*(8), E0159809. doi:10.1371/journal.pone.0159809 PMID:27490469

Sakalidis, V. S., Kent, J. C., Garbin, C. P., Hepworth, A. R., Hartmann, P. E., & Geddes, D. T. (2013). Longitudinal changes in suck-swallow-breathe, oxygen saturation, and heart rate patterns in term breastfeeding infants. *Journal of Human Lactation*, *29*(2), 236–245. doi:10.1177/0890334412474864 PMID:23492760

Saludes, M. C., & Artenita, D. (2009). *The knowledge and perceptions on learning disabilities in the cities of region XI of the Philippines and a region in New York City, N.Y., U.S.A.* The 19th Asian Conference on Mental Retardation, Singapore. Retrieved from www.gtid.net/acmr19/pdf/11.pdf

Sanders, M. R., Markie-Dadds, C., Tully, L. A., & Bor, W. (2000). The Triple P-Positive Parenting Program: A comparison of enhanced, standard, and self-directed behavioral family intervention for parents of children with early onset conduct problems. *Journal of Consulting and Clinical Psychology*, *68*(4), 624–640. doi:10.1037/0022-006X.68.4.624 PMID:10965638

Sapir, E. (1921). *Language: An introduction to the study of speech*. New York: Harcout, Brace and Company.

Saravanabhavan, S., & Saravanabhavan, R. C. (2001). Attitudes toward disabilities across cultures. *Educational Theory and Practice*, *23*(2), 49–60. doi:10.7459/ept/23.2.04

Saravanabhavan, S., & Saravanabhavan, R. C. (2010). Knowledge of learning disability among pre-and in-service teachers in India. *International Journal of Special Education*, *25*(3), 133–139.

Saunders, N. L., & Summers, M. J. (2011). Longitudinal deficits to attention, executive, and working memory in subtypes of mild cognitive impairment. *Neuropsychology*, *25*(2), 237–248. doi:10.1037/a0021134 PMID:21381828

Sawyer, J., Matteson, C., Ou, H., & Nagase, T. (2017). The effects of parent-focused slow relaxed speech intervention on articulation rate, response time latency, and fluency in preschool children who stutter. *Journal of Speech, Language, and Hearing Research: JSLHR*, *60*(4), 794–809. doi:10.1044/2016_JSLHR-S-16-0002 PMID:28289751

Scarborough, H. S. (1990). Very early language deficits in dyslexic children. *Child Development*, *61*(6), 1728–1743. doi:10.2307/1130834 PMID:2083495

Schaff, R. C., Toth-Cohen, S., Johnson, S. L., Outenn, G., & Benevides, T. W. (2011). The everyday routines of families of children with autism: Examining the impact of sensory processing difficulties on the family. *Autism*, *15*(3), 373–389. doi:10.1177/1362361310386505 PMID:21430016

Scherz, N. (2015). Mindfulness meditation improves sleep quality in the elderly. *Praxis (Bern)*, *104*, 591–592. doi:10.1024/1661-8157/a002018 PMID:26098158

Schindler, A., Ruoppolo, G., & Barillari, U. (2010). Communication and its disorders: Definition and taxonomy from a phoniatric perspective. *Audiological Medicine*, *8*(4), 163–170. doi:10.3109/1651386X.2010.530023

Schleichkorn, J. (1993). *Coping with Cerebral Palsy. Answers to Questions Parents Often Ask* (2nd ed.). PRO-ED, Inc.

Schneier, F. R. (2003). Social anxiety disorder is common, underdiagnosed, impairing and treatable. *British Medical Journal*, *327*(7414), 515–516. doi:10.1136/bmj.327.7414.515

Schor, E. L. (2003). Family pediatrics report of the task force on the family. *Pediatrics*, *111*(6), 1541–1571. PMID:12777595

Schreck, K. A., Williams, K., & Smith, A. F. (2004). A comparison of eating behaviors between children with and without autism. *Journal of Autism and Developmental Disorders*, *34*(4), 433–438. doi:10.1023/B:JADD.0000037419.78531.86 PMID:15449518

Schreibman, L. (2000). Intensive behavioural/educational treatments for autism: Research needs and future directions. *Journal of Autism and Developmental Disorders*, *30*(5), 373–378. doi:10.1023/A:1005535120023 PMID:11098871

Schuell, H. (1949). Working with parents of stuttering children. *The Journal of Speech and Hearing Disorders*, *14*(3), 251–254. doi:10.1044/jshd.1403.251 PMID:18137760

Schuell, H. (1965). *Differential diagnosis of aphasia with the Minnesota Test*. Minneapolis, MN: University of Minnesota Press.

Schwartz, R. H., Freedy, A. S., & Sheridan, M. J. (2006). Selective mutism: Are primary care physicians missing the silence? *Clinical Pediatrics*, *45*(1), 43–48. doi:10.1177/000992280604500107

Scorgie, K., & Sobsey, D. (2000). Transformational outcomes associated with parenting children who have disabilities. *Mental Retardation*, *38*(3), 195–206. doi: PMID:10900927

Scorgie, K., Wilgosh, L., & McDonald, L. (1998). Parent's experiences managing life when a child has a disability. *International Journal of Special Education*, *13*, 102–110.

Sebastian, S., Varghese, A., & Gowri, M. (2015). The impact of hearing loss in the life of adults: A comparison between congenital versus late onset hearing loss. *Indian Journal of Otology*, *21*(1), 29. doi:10.4103/0971-7749.152857

Seifert, E., & Kollbrunner, J. (2005). Stress and distress in non-organic voice disorders. *Swiss Medical Weekly*, *135*(27-28), 387–397. PMID:16220409

Seifert, E., & Kollbrunner, J. (2006). An update in thinking about nonorganic voice disorders. *Archives of Otolaryngology--Head & Neck Surgery*, *132*(10), 1128–1132. doi:10.1001/archotol.132.10.1128 PMID:17043264

Seligman, M. (1983). Siblings of handicapped persons. In M. Seligman (Ed.), *The family with a handicapped child: Understanding and treatment* (pp. 147–174). New York: Grune & Stratton Inc.

Selley, W. G., Ellis, R. E., Flack, F. C., & Brooks, W. A. (1990). Coordination of sucking, swallowing and breathing in the newborn: Its relationship to infant feeding and normal development. *International Journal of Language & Communication Disorders*, *25*(3), 311–327. doi:10.3109/13682829009011980 PMID:2095838

Sen, A. (1988). *Psychosocial Integration of the Handicapped*. New Delhi: Mittal Publications.

Sethi, P. K. (2002). Stroke-incidence in India and management of ischemic stroke. *Neurosciences*, *4*(3), 139–141.

Shakespeare, T. (2006). *Disability rights and wrongs*. London: Routledge.

Shakespeare, T. (2013). *Disability rights and wrongs revisited*. London: Routledge.

Shalev, R. S., Manor, O., Auerbach, J., & Gross-Tsur, V. (1998). Persistence of developmental dyscalculia: What counts? Results from a three year prospective follow up study. *The Journal of Pediatrics*, *133*(3), 358–362. doi:10.1016/S0022-3476(98)70269-0 PMID:9738716

Shallop, J. (2002). Auditory neuropathy/dys-synchrony in adults and children. *Seminars in Hearing*, *23*(3), 215–223. doi:10.1055-2002-34474

Shallop, J., Peterson, A., Facer, G. W., Fabry, L. B., & Driscoll, C. L. (2001). Cochlear implants in five cases of auditory neuropathy: Postoperative findings and progress. *The Laryngoscope*, *111*(4), 555–562. doi:10.1097/00005537-200104000-00001 PMID:11359119

Shanks, L., Jason, L. A., Evans, M., & Brown, A. (2013). Cognitive impairments associated with CFS and POTS. *Frontiers in Physiology*, *4*. doi:10.3389/fphys.2013.00113 PMID:23720636

Shapiro, B. K., Green, P., Krick, J., Allen, D., & Capute, A. J. (1986). Growth of severely impaired children: Neurological versus nutritional factors. *Developmental Medicine and Child Neurology*, *28*(6), 729–733. doi:10.1111/j.1469-8749.1986.tb03924.x PMID:3817311

Shari, M., & Vranda, M. N. (2015). Knowledge of primary school teachers in identifying children with learning disabilities. *Disability, CBR and Inclusive Development*, *26*(3), 68–76. doi:10.5463/DCID.v26i3.443

Sharkey, L., & McNicholas, F. (2008). 'More than a 100 years of silence', elective mutism: A review of the literature. *European Child & Adolescent Psychiatry*, *17*(5), 255–263. doi:10.100700787-007-0658-4

Sharma, A. (2000). *Language Skills in Children with Learning Disability* (Unpublished Masters Dissertation). Mangalore University.

Sharma, R., Dhaliwal, L. K., Suri, V., Kaushal, P., Singhal, N., Rana, A. K., & Singh, A. (2017). Implementing a life cycle approach through the establishment of multipurpose behavior therapy room in PGIMER, Chandigarh for enhancing the fitness level of women. *Journal of Postgraduate Medicine Education, and Research*, *51*(3), 115–122.

Sharma, R., Kumar, M., & Singh, A. (2013). Evaluation of disable friendliness of a railway transport facility in Ludhiana city of Punjab, India. *International Journal on Disability and Human Development: IJDHD*, *12*(3), 333–339. doi:10.1515/ijdhd-2012-0117

Sharpe, D., & Rossiter, L. (2002). Siblings of Children with a Chronic Illness: A Meta-Analysis. *Journal of Pediatric Psychology*, *2*(8), 699–710. doi:10.1093/jpepsy/27.8.699 PMID:12403860

Shaywitz, S. E. (1998). Dyslexia. *The New England Journal of Medicine*, *338*(5), 307–312. doi:10.1056/NEJM199801293380507 PMID:9445412

Shearn, J., & Todd, S. (2000). Maternal employment and family responsibilities: The perspectives of mothers of children with intellectual disabilities. *Journal of Applied Research in Intellectual Disabilities*, *13*(3), 109–131. doi:10.1046/j.1468-3148.2000.00021.x

Shenoy, M. (2011). *Persons with disability and the India labour market: Challenges and Opportunities Geneva*. International Labour Organization.

Shield, B., & Dockrell, J. (2003). The effects of noise on children at school: A review. *Building Acoustics*, *10*(2), 97–116. doi:10.1260/135101003768965960

Shine, R. E. (1984). Assessment and fluency training and the young stutterer. In M. Peins (Ed.), *Contemporary approaches in stuttering therapy* (pp. 173–216). Boston: Little, Brown.

Shipon-Blum, E. (2009). *What can we do to assess and treat selective mutism.* Retrieved from www.asha.org/Events/convention/handouts/2009/2296_Shipon-Blum_Elisa/

Shipon-Blum, E. (2007). *When the words just won't come out: Understanding selective mutism.* Jenkintown, PA: Selective Mutism Group-Childhood Anxiety Network.

Shivashankar, N., Satishchandra, P., Shashikala, H. R., & Gore, M. (2003). Primary auditory neuropathy-An enigma. *Acta Neurologica Scandinavica, 108*(2), 130–135. doi:10.1034/j.1600-0404.2003.00104.x PMID:12859291

Short, C., DeOrnellas, K., & Walrath, R. (2011). Draw-A-Person Test. In S. Goldstein & J. A. Naglieri (Eds.), *Encyclopedia of Child Behavior and Development* (pp. 523–524). New York: Springer.

Shriver, M. D., Segool, N., & Gortmaker, V. (2011). Behavior Observation for linking assessment to treatment for selective mutism. *Education & Treatment of Children, 34*(3), 389–411. doi:10.1353/etc.2011.0023

Shumow, L., & Lomax, R. (2001). *Parental efficacy: Predictor of parenting behavior and adolescent outcomes.* Paper presented at the Annual Meeting of the American Educational Research Association, Seattle, WA.

Silvers, A. (2010). An essay on modeling: Their social model of disability. In D. C. Ralston & H. O. Justin (Eds.), *Philosophical reflections on disability* (pp. 19–36). London: Springer.

Simeonsson, R. J., Leornardi, M., Lollar, D., Bjorck-Akesson, E., Hollenwerger, J., & Martinuzzi, A. (2003). Applying the International Classification of Functioning, Disability, and Health (ICF) to measure childhood disability. *Disability and Rehabilitation, 25*(11-12), 602–610. doi:10.1080/0963828031000137117 PMID:12959334

Simmons-Mackie, N. (1998a). A solution to the discharge dilemma in aphasia: Social approaches to aphasia management. *Aphasiology, 12*(3), 231–239. doi:10.1080/02687039808249451

Simmons-Mackie, N. (1998b). In support of supported conversation for adults with aphasia. *Aphasiology, 12*(9), 831–838. doi:10.1080/02687039808249576

Simmons-Mackie, N., & Kagan, A. (1999). Communication strategies used by "good" versus "poor" speaking partners of individuals with aphasia. *Aphasiology, 13*(9-11), 807–820. doi:10.1080/026870399401894

Simmons-Mackie, N., & Kagan, A. (2007). Application of the ICF in aphasia. *Seminars in Speech and Language, 28*(4), 244–253. doi:10.1055-2007-986521 PMID:17935009

Simmons-Mackie, N., Kearns, K., & Potechin, G. (2005). Treatment of aphasia through family member training. *Aphasiology, 19*(6), 583–593. doi:10.1080/02687030444000408

Simmons, R. (2002). *Odd girl out: The hidden culture of aggression in girls.* Boston: Mariner Books Houghton Mifflin Harcourt.

Simplican, S. C. (2015). *The capacity contract: Intellectual disability and the question of citizenship.* Minneapolis, MN: University of Minnesota Press. doi:10.5749/minnesota/9780816693979.001.0001

Sinanović, O., Mrkonjić, Z., & Zečić, S. (2012). Quality of life and post-stroke aphasic syndromes. *Periodicum Biologorum, 114*(3), 435–440.

Singh, A. N. (1973). Behavior problems of the mentally retarded deaf. *Social Welfare, 19*, 4.

Singh, H. G. (1977). *Psychotherapy in India: From Vedic to modern times.* Agra: National Psychological Corporation.

Singh, M. V., & Dagar, B. (1982). Sociological aspects of behavior problems in a community child guidance center. *Child Psychiatry Quarterly, 15*(2), 43–49.

Singh, P., & Pauranik, A. (2014). Supportive conversational strategies for person with aphasia (PWA) and their significant others (SO). *Proceedings of 8th World Congress for Neuro Rehabilitation (WCNR).*

Singh, R., & Kaushik, S. S. (1982). Parent training techniques in acquisition and generalization of behavior modification skill to train the retarded. *Indian Journal of Clinical Psychology*, *9*(2), 193–201.

Singh, S. (2017). Perseverance pays. In S. Halder & L. C. Assaf (Eds.), *Inclusion, disability, and culture: An ethnographic perspective traversing abilities and challenges* (pp. 41–59). New York: Springer International Publishing. doi:10.1007/978-3-319-55224-8_4

Singh, V. (2015). Hearing in India: All aspects. *Online Journal of Otolaryngology*, *5*(1), 39–70.

Sinha, S. K., Shivaswamy, J., Barman, A., Seth, D., Seshadri, D., & Savithri, S. R. (2017). Prevalence of communication disorders in a rural population at taluq level of Gujarat, India. *Clinical Epidemiology and Global Health*, *5*(2), 73–78. doi:10.1016/j.cegh.2016.08.006

Sininger, Y., & Oba, S. (2001). Patients with auditory neuropathy: Who are they and what can they hear? In Y. Sininger & A. Starr (Eds.), *Auditory neuropathy: A new perspective on hearing disorder* (pp. 15–36). Singular Publishing Group.

Siraj-Blatchford, I. (2004). Quality teaching in the early years. In A. Anning, J. Cullen, & M. Fleer (Eds.), *Early childhood education: Society and culture* (pp. 137–148). London, UK: SAGE Publications Ltd.

Sisson, L. A., & Van Hasselt, V. B. (1989). Feeding Disorders. In J. K. Luiselli (Ed.), *Behavioral Medicine and Developmental Disabilities. Disorders of Human Learning, Behavior, and Communication* (pp. 45–73). New York, NY: Springer. doi:10.1007/978-1-4613-8844-9_3

Skill Development Initiative. (2008). *Modular Employable Skills Scheme*. Ministry of Labour and Employment, Government of India.

Skuse, D., Pickles, A., Wolke, D., & Reilly, S. (1994). Postnatal growth and mental development: Evidence for a "sensitive period". *Journal of Child Psychology and Psychiatry, and Allied Disciplines*, *35*(3), 521–545. doi:10.1111/j.1469-7610.1994.tb01738.x PMID:7515070

Slee, R. (2004). Inclusive education: A framework for reform? In V. Heung & M. Ainscow (Eds.), *Inclusive education: A framework for reform* (pp. 58–66). Hong Kong: Hong Kong Institute of Education.

Slee, R. (2011). *The irregular school: Exclusion, schooling and inclusive education*. New York, NY: Routledge.

Smith, J. D. (2016). *On parenting: Eight things siblings of children with special needs struggle with*. Retrieved from https://www.washingtonpost.com/news/parenting/wp/2016/12/20/8-things-siblings-of-children-with-special-needs-struggle-with/?utm_term=.faaa29548765

Smith, A., & Kelly, E. (1997). Stuttering: A dynamic, multifactorial model. In R. F. Curlee & G. M. Siegel (Eds.), *Nature and treatment of stuttering: New directions* (pp. 97–127). Boston, MA: Allyn and Bacon.

Smith, J. A., Flowers, P., & Larkin, M. (2009). *Interpretative Phenomenological Analysis: Theory, Method and Research*. London: Sage.

Snow, C. E., Burns, M. S., & Griffin, P. (Eds.). (2000). *Preventing Reading Difficulties in Young Children. US National Research Council Report*. Washington, DC: National Academy Press.

Sparrow, S. S. (2011). Vineland adaptive behavior scales. In *Encyclopedia of clinical neuropsychology* (pp. 2618–2621). New York: Springer. doi:10.1007/978-0-387-79948-3_1602

Spencer, L., Ritchie, J., Lewis, J., & Dillon, L. (2003). *Quality in qualitative evaluation: A framework for assessing research evidence*. London, UK: National Center for Social Research.

Spiegler, M. D. (2016). *Contemporary behavior therapy*. Boston, MA: Cengage Learning.

Srikanth, N., & Karanth, P. (2003). Speech language pathologists and remediation of reading disabilities. In P. Karanth & J. Rozario (Eds.), *Learning Disabilities in India: Willing the Mind to Learn* (pp. 150–165). New Delhi: Sage Publications.

Sroufe, L. A., & Rutter, M. (1984). The domain of developmental psychopathology. *Child Development*, *55*(1), 17–29. doi:10.2307/1129832 PMID:6705619

Stahmer, A. C., Akshoomoff, N., & Cunningham, A. B. (2011). Inclusion for toddlers with autism spectrum disorders. *Autism*, *15*(5), 625–641. doi:10.1177/1362361310392253 PMID:21486899

Stamos, D. N. (2013). *The myth of universal human rights: Its origin, history, and explanation, along with a more humane way*. New York: Routledge.

Stanovich, K. E. (1991). Discrepancy definitions of reading disability: Has intelligence led us astray? *Reading Research Quarterly*, *26*(1), 7–29. doi:10.2307/747729

Stanovich, K. E. (1993). A model for studies of reading disability. *Developmental Review*, *13*(3), 225–245. doi:10.1006/drev.1993.1010

Stanovich, K. E., Siegel, L. S., & Linda, S. (1994). Phenotypic performance profile of children with reading disabilities: A regression-based test of the phonological-core variable-difference model. *Journal of Educational Psychology*, *86*(1), 24–53. doi:10.1037/0022-0663.86.1.24

Stark, R., Gordon-Burns, D., Purdue, K., Rarere-Briggs, B., & Turncock, K. (2011). Other parents' perceptions of disability and inclusion in early childhood education: Implications for the teachers' role in creating inclusive communities. *He Kupu*, *2*(4), 4–18.

Starkweather, C. (1997). Therapy for younger children. In R. F. Curlee & G. M. Siegel (Eds.), *Nature and treatment of stuttering: New directions* (pp. 257–292). Boston, MA: Allyn and Bacon.

Starr, A., Zeng, F. G., Michalewski, H. J., & Moser, T. (2010). Perspectives on auditory neuropathy: Disorders of inner hair Cell, auditory nerve, and their synapse. In The Senses: A Comprehensive Reference, (3), 397–412.

Starr, A., McPherson, D., Patterson, J., Don, M., Luxford, W., Shannon, R., ... Waring, M. (1991). Absence of both auditory evoked potentials and auditory percepts dependent on timing cues. *Brain*, *114*(3), 1157–1180. doi:10.1093/brain/114.3.1157 PMID:2065245

Starr, A., Picton, T. W., & Kim, R. (2001). Pathophysiology of auditory neuropathy. In Y. Sininger & A. Starr (Eds.), *Auditory neuropathy: A new perspective on hearing disorder* (pp. 67–82). Singular Publishing Group.

Starr, A., Picton, T. W., Sininger, Y., Hood, L. J., & Berlin, C. I. (1996). Auditory neuropathy. *Brain*, *119*(3), 741–753. doi:10.1093/brain/119.3.741 PMID:8673487

Starr, A., Sininger, Y. S., & Pratt, H. (2000). The varieties of auditory neuropathy. *Journal of Basic and Clinical Physiology and Pharmacology*, *11*(3), 215–230. doi:10.1515/JBCPP.2000.11.3.215 PMID:11041385

Steinhausen, H., & Juzi, C. (1996). Elective Mutism: An analysis of 100 cases. *Journal of the American Academy of Child and Adolescent Psychiatry*, *35*(5), 606–614. doi:10.1097/00004583-199605000-00015

Stemple, J. C., Glaze, L. E., & Klaben, B. K. (2010). *Clinical voice pathology: Theory and management* (4th ed.). San Diego, CA: Plural.

Stevenson, J., Kreppner, J., Pimperton, H., Worsfold, S., & Kennedy, C. (2015). Emotional and behavioural difficulties in children and adolescents with hearing impairment: A systematic review and meta-analysis. *European Child & Adolescent Psychiatry*, *24*(5), 477–496. doi:10.100700787-015-0697-1 PMID:25758233

Stokoe, E. (2013). Overcoming barriers to mediation in intake calls to services: Research-based strategies for mediators. *Negotiation Journal*, *29*(3), 289–314. doi:10.1111/nejo.12026

Stoneman, Z. (2005). Siblings of children with disability: Research themes. *Mental Retardation*, *43*(5), 339–350. PMID:16131231

Stores, G., & Stores, R. (2013). Sleep disorders in children with traumatic brain injury: A case of serious neglect. *Developmental Medicine and Child Neurology*, *55*(9), 797–805. doi:10.1111/dmcn.12163 PMID:23662906

Strauss, A., & Corbin, J. (1990). *Basics of qualitative research. Grounded theory procedures and techniques*. Sage.

Stress [Def.1]. (n.d.). In *Merriam-Webster*. Retrieved from https://www.merriam-webster.com/dictionary/stress

Strohm, K. (2008). Too important to ignore: Siblings of children with special needs. *Australian e-Journal for the Advancement of Mental Health*, *7*(2), 1–6. doi:10.5172/jamh.7.2.78

Stroman, D. (2003). *The disability rights movement: From deinstitutionalization to self-determination*. University Press of America.

Strong, C. J., Mayer, M., & Mayer, M. (1998). *The strong narrative assessment procedure (SNAP)*. Thinking Publications.

Stuntzner, S., & Hartley, M. T. (2015). Balancing self- compassion with self-advocacy: A new approach for persons with disabilities. *Annals of Psychotherapy and Integrative Health*, 12-28. Retrieved from http://www.annalsofpsychotherapy.com/

Suarez, P. A., Gollan, T. H., Heaton, R., Grant, I., & Cherner, M. (2014). Second-language fluency predicts native language stroop effects: Evidence from Spanish-English bilinguals. *Journal of the International Neuropsychological Society*, *20*(03), 342–348. doi:10.1017/S1355617714000058 PMID:24622502

Su, B. H. (2014). Optimizing nutrition in preterm infants. *Pediatrics and Neonatology*, *55*(1), 5–13. doi:10.1016/j.pedneo.2013.07.003 PMID:24050843

Sudlow, C. L. M., & Warlow, C. P. (1997). Comparable studies of the incidence of stroke and its pathological types. *Stroke*, *28*(3), 491–499. doi:10.1161/01.STR.28.3.491 PMID:9056601

Suh, M. K., Kim, H., & Na, D. L. (2009). Dysphagia in patients with dementia: Alzheimer versus vascular. *Alzheimer Disease and Associated Disorders*, *23*(2), 178–184. doi:10.1097/WAD.0b013e318192a539 PMID:19474573

Sulheim, D., Fagermoen, E., Sivertsen, Ø. S., Winger, A., Wyller, V. B., & Øie, M. G. (2015). Cognitive dysfunction in adolescents with chronic fatigue: A cross-sectional study. *Archives of Disease in Childhood*, *100*(9), 838–844. doi:10.1136/archdischild-2014-306764 PMID:25791841

Sulkowski, M. L., Pence, S. L., Carlson, J. S., & Storch, E. A. (2014). Treating Selective mutism with exposure therapy: A Case Study. *Annals of Psychotherapy*.

Sumiya, H., & Healy, A. F. (2004). Phonology in the bilingual Stroop effect. *Memory & Cognition*, *32*(5), 752–758. doi:10.3758/BF03195865 PMID:15552352

Sun, I. Y. I., & Fernandes, F. D. M. (2014). Communication difficulties perceived by parents of children with developmental disorders. *Communication and Developmental Disorders*, *26*(4), 270–275. PMID:25211685

Sunil, R., & Shyamala, K. C. (2009). Dementia assessment battery (Part B, VII, pp. 262-275). Mysore: Students Research at All India Institute of Speech and Hearing.

Suresh, P. A., & Sebastian, S. (2003). Epidemiological and neurological aspects of learning disabilities. In P. Karanth & J. Rozario (Eds.), *Learning Disabilities in India: Willing the Mind to Learn* (pp. 30–43). New Delhi: Sage Publications.

Swanson, H. L., & Jerman, O. (2006). Math disabilities: A selective meta-analysis of the literature. *Review of Educational Research*, *76*(2), 249–274. doi:10.3102/00346543076002249

Swanson, H. L., Zheng, X., & Jerman, O. (2009). Working memory, short-term memory, and reading disabilities: A selective meta-analysis of the literature. *Journal of Learning Disabilities*, *42*(3), 260–287. doi:10.1177/0022219409331958 PMID:19255286

Swarup, S., & Mehta, D. H. (1991). *Behavioural Checklist for Screening Learning Disabled*. Mumbai: SNDT Women's University.

Swindoll, C. R. (n.d.). *Characteristics of a healthy family*. Retrieved from http://www.lifeway.com/Article/eight-characteristics-of-a-healthy-family

Taanila, A., Syrjala, L., Kokkonen, J., & Jarvelin, M.-R. (2002). Coping of parents with physically and/or intellectually disabled children. *Child: Care, Health and Development*, *28*(1), 73–86. doi:10.1046/j.1365-2214.2002.00244.x PMID:11856190

Tabri, D., Chacra, A., Smith, K. M., & Pring, T. (2011). Speech perception in noise by monolingual, bilingual and trilingual listeners. *International Journal of Language & Communication Disorders*, *46*, 411–422. PMID:21771217

Taillefer, S. S., Kirmayer, L. J., Robbins, J. M., & Lasry, J. C. (2002). Psychological correlates of functional status in chronic fatigue syndrome. *Journal of Psychosomatic Research*, *53*(6), 1097–1106. doi:10.1016/S0022-3999(02)00566-4 PMID:12479992

Taillefer, S. S., Kirmayer, L. J., Robbins, J. M., & Lasry, J. C. (2003). Correlates of illness worry in chronic fatigue syndrome. *Journal of Psychosomatic Research*, *54*(4), 331–337. doi:10.1016/S0022-3999(02)00332-X PMID:12670610

Taler, V., & Jarema, G. (2006). On-line lexical processing in AD and MCI: An early measure of cognitive impairment? *Journal of Neurolinguistics*, *19*(1), 38–55. doi:10.1016/j.jneuroling.2005.07.002

Tallal, P., Miller, S., & Fitch, R. H. (1993). Neurobiological basis of speech: A case for the prominence of mental processing. *Annals of the New York Academy of Sciences*, *682*(1 Temporal Info), 27–47. doi:10.1111/j.1749-6632.1993.tb22957.x PMID:7686725

Tanaka, M. (2015). Effects of mental fatigue on brain activity and cognitive performance: A magnetoencephalography study. *Anatomy & Physiology*, *s4*. doi:10.4172/2161-0940.S4-002

Tanaka, M., Shigihara, Y., Ishii, A., Funakura, M., Kanai, E., & Watanabe, Y. (2012). Effect of mental fatigue on the central nervous system: An electroencephalography study. *Behavioral and Brain Functions*, *8*(1), 48. doi:10.1186/1744-9081-8-48 PMID:22954020

Tang, Y., McPherson, B., Yuen, K. C. P., Wong, L. L. N., & Lee, J. S. M. (2004). Auditory neuropathy/auditory dys-synchrony in school children with hearing loss: Frequency of occurrence. *International Journal of Pediatric Otorhinolaryngology*, *68*(2), 175–183. doi:10.1016/j.ijporl.2003.10.004 PMID:14725984

Tang, Y.-Y., Ma, Y., Wang, J., Fan, Y., Feng, S., Lu, Q., ... Posner, M. I. (2007). Short-term meditation training improves attention and self-regulation. *Proceedings of the National Academy of Sciences of the United States of America*, *104*(43), 17152–17156. doi:10.1073/pnas.0707678104 PMID:17940025

Tannock, R. (2013). Rethinking ADHD and LD in DSM-5: Proposed changes in diagnostic criteria. *Journal of Learning Disabilities*, *46*(1), 5–25. doi:10.1177/0022219412464341 PMID:23144062

Taylor, P. (2007). *UNESCO and IUAV EGM on cosmopolitan urbanism: Urban policies for the social and spatial integration of international migrants.* Retrieved from http://www.unescochair-iuav.it/wp-content/uploads/2007/09/sarah-toner_paul-taylor.pdf

Teasell, R. W., Bach, D., & McRae, M. (1994). Prevalence and recovery of aspiration post stroke: A retrospective analysis. *Dysphagia*, *9*(1), 35–39. doi:10.1007/BF00262757 PMID:8131423

Teassell, R., McRae, M., & Finestone, H. (2000). Social issues in the rehabilitation of younger stroke patients. *Archives of Physical Medicine and Rehabilitation*, *81*(2), 205–209. doi:10.1016/S0003-9993(00)90142-4 PMID:10668776

Thackeray, R., & Hunter, M. (2010). Empowering youth: Use of technology in advocacy to affect social change. *Journal of Computer-Mediated Communication*, *15*(4), 575–591. doi:10.1111/j.1083-6101.2009.01503.x

The Persons with Disability (Equal Opportunities, Protection of Rights, and Full Participations) Act. (1995). Ministry of Law, Justice and Company Affairs, Government of India.

Therborn, G. (2007). *Final report the expert group meeting on creating an inclusive society: Practical strategies to promote social integration.* Paris, France: DESA.

Theunissen, S. C. P. M., Rieffe, C., Netten, A. P., Briaire, J. J., Soede, W., Kouwenberg, M., & Frijns, J. H. M. (2014). Self-esteem in hearing-impaired children: The influence of communication, education, and audiological characteristics. *PLoS One*, *9*(4), e94521. doi:10.1371/journal.pone.0094521 PMID:24722329

Thomas, C. (2004). Developing the social relational in the social model of disability: A theoretical agenda. In M. Corker & T. Shakespeare (Eds.), *Implementing the social model of disability: Theory and research* (pp. 32–47). London: Continuum.

Thomas, D. M. (2009). Culture and disability: A Cape Verdean perspective. *Journal of Cultural Diversity*, *16*(4), 178–186. PMID:20069806

Thomas, R. M. (2003). *Blending qualitative and quantitative research methods in theses and dissertations.* London, UK: SAGE Publications. doi:10.4135/9781412983525

Thomas, S., Bhanutej, K., & John, S. (2003). Dealing with Dyslexia. *The Week*, *21*, 36–42.

Thompson, C. E. (2000). *Raising a handicapped child.* New York: Oxford University Press Inc.

Thressiakutty, A. T. (1998). *NIMH Vocational Assessment and Programming System (NIMH-VAPS).* National Institute for the Mentally Handicapped.

Tobis, J. S., Saturen, P., Larios, G., & Posnaik, A. O. (1961). Study of growth patterns in cerebral palsy. *Archives of Physical Medicine and Rehabilitation*, *42*, 475–481. PMID:13777130

Tomanik, S., Harris, G. E., & Hawkins, J. (2004). The relationship between behaviors exhibited by children with autism and maternal stress. *Journal of Intellectual & Developmental Disability*, *29*(1), 16–26. doi:10.1080/13668250410001662892

Trajkovski, N., Andrews, C., Onslow, M., Packman, A., O'Brian, S., & Menzies, R. (2009). Using syllable-timed speech to treat preschool children who stutter: A multiple baseline experiment. *Journal of Fluency Disorders*, *34*(1), 1–10. doi:10.1016/j.jfludis.2009.01.001 PMID:19500711

Trajkovski, N., Andrews, C., Onslow, M., Packman, A., O'Brian, S., & Menzies, R. (2011). A phase II trial of the Westmead Program: Syllable-timed speech treatment for pre-school children who stutter. *International Journal of Speech-Language Pathology*, *13*(6), 500–509. doi:10.3109/17549507.2011.578660 PMID:22070727

Travis, L. E. (1931). *Speech Pathology*. New York: Appleton-Century.

Tregaskis, C. (2004). *Constructions of disability: Researching the interface between disabled and non-disabled people*. London, UK: Routledge. doi:10.4324/9780203299517

Tuch, B. E., & Nielson, J. M. (1941). Apraxia of swallowing. *Bulletin of the Los Angeles Neurological Society*, *6*, 52–54.

Turnbull, A. P., & Ruef, M. (1996). Family perspectives on problem behavior. *Mental Retardation*, *34*, 280–293. PMID:8908993

United Nations Department of Economic and Social Affairs (UNDESA). (1995). *Report of the world summit for social development*. New York, NY: UNDESA.

United Nations Department of Economic and Social Affairs (UNDESA). (2000). *Millennium declaration*. Retrieved from http://www.un.org/millennium/declaration/ares552e.pdf

United Nations Department of Economic and Social Affairs (UNDESA). (2009). *Creating an inclusive society: Practical strategies to promote social integration*. New York, NY: UNDESA.

United Nations Department of Economic and Social Affairs (UNDESA). (2010). *Analysing and measuring social inclusion in a global context*. New York, NY: UNDESA.

United Nations Department of Economic and Social Affairs (UNDESA). (2016). *Leaving no one behind: The imperative of inclusive development (Report on the world social situation 2016)*. New York, NY: UNDESA.

United Nations. (2006). *Convention on the rights of persons with disabilities*. New York: United Nations.

Unruh, A. (1992). Siblings of children with special needs. *School of Occupational Therapy*, *59*(3), 151–158. PMID:10120258

Upadhyaya, G. R., & Havalappanavar, N. B. (2008). Stress in parents of the mentally challenged. *Journal of the Indian Academy of Applied Psychology*, *34*, 53–59.

Urion, D. K., Huff, H. V., & Carullo, M. P. (2015). MRI in assessing children with learning disability, focal findings, and reduced automaticity. *Neurology*, *85*(7), 604–609. doi:10.1212/WNL.0000000000001849 PMID:26180142

Vahia, N. S. (1969). A therapy based on some concepts prevalent in India. *Indian Journal of Psychiatry*, *11*, 7–14.

Valtolina, G. G. (2004). *L'altro fratello. Relazione fraternal e disabilita*. Milano: FrancoAngeli.

van den Engel-Hoek, L., Erasmus, C. E., Hendriks, J. C., Geurts, A. C., Klein, W. M., Pillen, S., ... de Groot, I. J. (2013). Oral muscles are progressively affected in Duchenne muscular dystrophy: Implications for dysphagia treatment. *Journal of Neurology*, *260*(5), 1295–1303. doi:10.100700415-012-6793-y PMID:23263593

van der Linden, D., & Eling, P. (2006). Mental fatigue disturbs local processing more than global processing. *Psychological Research*, *70*(5), 395–402. doi:10.100700426-005-0228-7 PMID:15968553

van der Linden, D., Frese, M., & Meijman, T. F. (2003). Mental fatigue and the control of cognitive processes: Effects on perseveration and planning. *Acta Psychologica*, *113*(1), 45–65. doi:10.1016/S0001-6918(02)00150-6 PMID:12679043

Van Riper, C. (1971). *The nature of stuttering*. Englewood Cliffs, NJ: Prentice-Hall.

Van Straten, A., deHaan, R. J., Limburg, M., Schuling, J., Bossuyt, P. M., & van den Bos, G. A. M. (1997). A stroke-adapted 30-item version of the Sickness Impact Profile to assess quality of life (SA-SIP30). *Stroke*, *28*(11), 2155–2161. doi:10.1161/01.STR.28.11.2155 PMID:9368557

Vanryckeghem, M. (1995). The Communication Attitude Test: A concordancy investigation of stuttering and non-stuttering children and their parents. *Journal of Fluency Disorders*, *26*(2), 191–203. doi:10.1016/0094-730X(94)00021-K

Vanryckeghem, M., & Brutten, G. J. (1996). The relationship between communication attitude and fluency failure of stuttering and non-stuttering children. *Journal of Fluency Disorders*, *21*(2), 109–118. doi:10.1016/0094-730X(96)00015-0

Vanryckeghem, M., & Brutten, G. J. (2007). *Communication attitude test for preschool and kindergarten children who stutter*. San Diego, CA: Plural Publishing.

Vanryckeghem, M., Hylebos, C., Brutten, G. J., & Peleman, M. (2001). The relationship between communication attitude and emotion of children who stutter. *Journal of Fluency Disorders*, *26*(1), 1–15. doi:10.1016/S0094-730X(00)00090-5

Vanryckeghem, M., Vanrobayes, S., & De Niels, T. (2015). The KiddyCAT: A test-retest reliability investigation. *Cross-Cultural Communication*, *11*(4), 10–16.

Vecchio, J., & Kearney, C. A. (2007). Assessment and treatment of a Hispanic youth with Selective Mutism. *Clinical Case Studies*, *6*(1), 34–43. doi:10.1177/1534650106290393

Veeraraghavan, V. (1998). Behavior medicine: Its relevance to the 21st century. *Behavior Medicine Journal*, *1*(1), 1–9.

Veeraraghavan, V., & Malik, S. C. (Eds.). (1994). *Readings in behavior medicine*. New Delhi: Phoenix Publishing.

Veereshwar, P. (2002). *Indian systems of psychotherapy*. New Delhi: Kalpaz Publications.

Veisson, M. (1999). Depression symptoms and emotional states in parents of disabled and non-disabled children. *Social Behavior and Personality*, *27*(1), 87–98. doi:10.2224bp.1999.27.1.87

Vellutino, F. R., Scanlon, D. M., & Lyon, G. R. (2000). Differentiating between difficult-to-remediate and readily re-mediated poor readers: More evidence against the IQ-achievement discrepancy definition of reading disability. *Journal of Learning Disabilities*, *33*(3), 223–238. doi:10.1177/002221940003300302 PMID:15505962

Venkatesan, S. (1994). Recent trends and issues in the behavioral assessment of individuals with mental handicap in India. *The Creative Psychologist*, *6*(1), 1–7.

Venkatesan, S. (2004). *Children with Developmental Disabilities: A Training Guide for Parents, Teachers and Caregivers*. New Delhi: Sage Publications.

Venkatesan, S. (2004). *Children with developmental disabilities: A training guide for parents, teachers and caregivers*. Thousand Oaks, CA: Sage Publications.

Venkatesan, S. (2006). *Mimeograph on Development and Standardisation of Appraisal of Kids with Specific Handicaps in Arithmetic and Reasoning Activities (AKSHARA)*. Mysore: All India Institute of Speech and Hearing.

Venkatesan, S. (2010a). Book Review; Portage Guide to Early Childhood Education. *Journal of All India Institute of Speech and Hearing*, *29*(1), 128–130.

Venkatesan, S. (2010b). Cultural factors in clinical assessment: The Indian perspective. *Indian Journal of Clinical Psychology*, *37*(1), 75–85.

Venkatesan, S. (2013). Preliminary try out and validation of problem behavior survey schedule for children with developmental disabilities. *Journal of Disability Management and Special Education*, *3*(2), 9–22.

Venkatesan, S. (2015a). Socio-cultural dimensions of cleft lip and palate in India. *Global Journal of Interdisciplinary Social Sciences*, *4*(3), 72–77.

Venkatesan, S. (2015a). Socio-Cultural dimensions of cleft lip and palate in India. *Global Journal of Interdisciplinary Social Sciences*, *4*(3), 72–77.

Venkatesan, S. (2015b). A growing trend in pseudo-diagnosis: A field study on children frequently mistaken for autism in India. *Psychological Studies*, *60*(1), 91–100. doi:10.100712646-015-0302-1

Venkatesan, S. (2015c). Engagement between justice system vis-à-vis persons with intellectual and developmental disabilities. *International Journal of Psychology and Psychiatry*, *3*(1), 30–56. doi:10.5958/2320-6233.2015.00003.6

Venkatesan, S. (2015c). *Problem Behavior Survey Schedule*. Bangalore: Psychotronics.

Venkatesan, S. (2015d). Evaluation of teaching objectives earmarked for children with developmental disabilities. *Disabilities and Impairments*, *29*(2), 85–96.

Venkatesan, S. (2015e). Revisiting goal setting for children with developmental disabilities. *Journal of Disability Management and Special Education*, *5*(2), 19–27.

Venkatesan, S. (2016a). Themes of intrapsychic conflict in communication disorders having a psychogenic origin. *Global Journal of Interdisciplinary Social Sciences*, *5*(2), 20–26.

Venkatesan, S. (2016b). Some cultural aspects of clinical counseling in Indian Context. *Global Journal of Interdisciplinary Social Sciences*, *5*(6), 21–26.

Venkatesan, S. (2017). Analysis of attributes in the official definitions for learning disability. *The International Journal of Indian Psychology*, *4*(2), 46–57.

Venkatesan, S., Jayakaran, G. T., Purusotham, P., & Rafi, M. (2012). Disability access audit of public service facilities. *Journal of All India Institute of Speech and Hearing*, *31*, 190–201.

Venkatesan, S., & Lokesh, L. (2016). Differential perception of problem behaviors between parents, teachers, and therapists. *The International Journal of Indian Psychology*, *3*(4), 21–33.

Venkatesan, S., & Lokesh, L. (2017). Consequence mapping of problem behaviors in children with developmental delays. *Disabilities and Impairments*, *31*(3), 47–64.

Venkatesan, S., Peshawaria, R., & Anuradha, M. P. (1996). Reward preferences in parents/caregivers of children with mental handicaps. *Indian Journal of Applied Psychology*, *33*(1), 11–17.

Venkatesan, S., & Purusotham, P. (2007). Historical analysis on course and clinical presentations of children with learning disabilities in India. *Disabilities and Impairments*, *21*(2), 99–107.

Venkatesan, S., Pushpavathi, M., & Purushotham, K. (2011). Adjustment patterns in voice disorders. *Journal of Indian Speech. Language and Hearing Association*, *25*(1), 21–30.

Venkatesan, S., & Ravindran, N. (2011). Attitudes of well siblings of children with developmental disabilities. *Journal of Disability Management and Special Education*, *1*(2), 1–23.

Venkatesan, S., & Ravindran, N. (2015). Autism behavior checklist for disability estimation: A preliminary field tryout. *Psychological Studies*, *60*(2), 215–225. doi:10.100712646-015-0304-z

Venkatesan, S., & Vepuri, V. G. D. (1993). Parental perceptions of causes and management of problem behaviors in individuals with a mental handicap. *Disabilities and Impairments*, *7*(2), 29–37.

Venkatesan, S., Yashodharakumar, G. Y., Gupta, S. K., & Vasudha, H. H. (2015). Gap analysis for evaluation of individualized education programs for children with developmental disabilities. *International Journal of Psychology and Psychiatry*, *3*(2), 64–76. doi:10.5958/2320-6233.2015.00017.6

Venugopal, M. B., & Goswami, S. P. (2008). *Manual for Adult Non-fluent Aphasia Therapy-in Kannada. In Student Research* (Vol. 3, pp. 181–189). Mysore: All India Institute of Speech and Hearing.

Vernon-Feagans, L., Pancsofar, N., Willoughby, M., Odom, E., Quade, A., & Cox, M. (2008). Predictors of maternal language to infants during a picture book task in the home: Family SES, child characteristics and the parenting environment. *Journal of Applied Developmental Psychology*, *29*(3), 213–226. doi:10.1016/j.appdev.2008.02.007 PMID:18618023

Viana, G. A., Biedel, D. C., & Rabian, B. (2009). Selective Mutism: A review and integration of the last 15 years. *Clinical Psychology Review*, *29*(1), 57–67. doi:10.1016/j.cpr.2008.09.009

Viner, R., & Christie, D. (2005). Fatigue and somatic symptoms. *British Medical Journal*, *330*(7498), 1012–1015. doi:10.1136/bmj.330.7498.1012 PMID:15860829

Vismara, L. A., & Rogers, S. L. (2010). Behavioral treatments for autism spectrum disorder: What do we know? *Annual Review of Clinical Psychology*, *6*(1), 447–468. doi:10.1146/annurev.clinpsy.121208.131151 PMID:20192785

Vitaliano, P. P., Zhang, J., & Scanlan, J. M. (2003). Is caregiving hazardous to one's physical health? A meta-analysis. *Psychological Bulletin*, *129*(6), 946–972. doi:10.1037/0033-2909.129.6.946 PMID:14599289

Vocational Rehabilitation - the way forward: Report of a working party. (2000). London: British Society of Rehabilitation Medicine.

Vocational Rehabilitation and Employment (Disabled Persons) Convention. (1983). (*No. 159*). International Labour Organization.

Vohr, B. R., Coll, C. G., Lobato, D., Yunis, K. A., O'Dea, C., & Oh, W. (1991). Neurodevelopmental and medical status of low-birthweight survivors of bronchopulmonary dysplasia at 10 to 12 years of age. *Developmental Medicine and Child Neurology*, *33*(8), 690–697. doi:10.1111/j.1469-8749.1991.tb14946.x PMID:1717327

Volkert, V. M., & Vaz, P. (2010). Recent studies on feeding problems in children with autism. *Journal of Applied Behavior Analysis*, *43*(1), 155–159. doi:10.1901/jaba.2010.43-155 PMID:20808508

Vong, E., Wilson, L., & Lincoln, M. (2016). The Lidcombe program of early stuttering intervention for Malaysian families: Four case studies. *Journal of Fluency Disorders*, *49*, 29–39. doi:10.1016/j.jfludis.2016.07.003 PMID:27638190

Voss, S. E., & Bullock, R. A. (2004). Executive function: The core feature of dementia? *Dementia and Geriatric Cognitive Disorders*, *18*(2), 207–216. doi:10.1159/000079202 PMID:15211077

Wakaba, Y. Y. (1983). Group play therapy for Japanese children who stutter. *Journal of Fluency Disorders*, *8*(2), 93–118. doi:10.1016/0094-730X(83)90023-2

Wakelin, M. M. (2008). Challenging disparities in special education: Moving parents from disempowered team members to ardent advocates. *Northwestern Journal of Law and Social Policy*, *3*(2), 263–288.

Walenski, M., Tager-Flusberg, H., & Ullman, M. T. (2006). Language in autism. In S. O. Moldin & J. L. Rubenstein (Eds.), *Understanding autism: From basic neuroscience to treatment* (pp. 175–203). Florida: CRC Press.

Walinder, R., Gunnarsson, K., Runeson, R., & Smedje, G. (2007). Physiological and psychological stress reactions in relation to classroom noise. *Scandinavian Journal of Work, Environment & Health*, *33*(4), 260–266. doi:10.5271jweh.1141 PMID:17717617

Wang, M., Mannan, H., Poston, D., Turnbull, A. P., & Summers, J. A. (2004). Parents' perceptions of advocacy activities and their impact on family quality of life. *Research and Practice for Persons with Severe Disabilities*, *29*(2), 144–155. doi:10.2511/rpsd.29.2.144

Ware, J. E., Snow, K. K., Kosinski, M., & Gandek, B. (1993). *SF-36 Health Survey Manual and Interpretation Guide*. Boston, MA: The Health Institute.

Weatherby, A. M. (2006). Understanding and measuring social communication in children with autism spectrum disorders. In T. Charman & W. Stone (Eds.), *Social and communication development in autism spectrum disorders: Early identification, diagnosis, and intervention* (pp. 3–34). New York: Guilford Press.

Weatherley-White, R. C. A., Eiserman, W., Beddoe, M., & Vanderberg, R. (2005). Perceptions, expectations, and reactions to cleft lip and palate surgeries in native populations: A pilot study in rural India. *The Cleft Palate-Craniofacial Journal*, *42*(5), 550–564. doi:10.1597/04-003.1 PMID:16149840

Webster, A., Cumming, J., & Rowland, S. (2016). *Empowering parents of children with autism spectrum disorder: Critical decision-making for quality outcomes*. Singapore: Springer.

Wechsler, D. (1991). *Wechsler Intelligence Scale for Children* (3rd ed.). San Antonio, TX: Psychological Corp.

Wechsler, D. (1992). *Wechsler Individual Achievement Tests*. San Antonio, TX: Psychological Corp.

Wegner, J. R., Grosche, K., & Edmister, E. (2003). Students with speech and language disorders. In F. E. Obiakor, C. A. R. Utley, & A. F. Rotari (Eds.), *Effective education for learners with exceptionalities* (Vol. 15, pp. 181–193). Oxford, UK: Elsevier Sciences. doi:10.1016/S0270-4013(03)80039-9

Weinberger, N. M. (2004). Specific long-term memory traces in primary auditory cortex. *Nature Reviews. Neuroscience*, *5*(4), 279–290. doi:10.1038/nrn1366 PMID:15034553

Weiner, H. (1977). *Psychobiology and Human diseases*. New York: Elsevier.

Weir, K., McMahon, S., Barry, L., Ware, R., Masters, I. B., & Chang, A. B. (2007). Oropharyngeal aspiration and pneumonia in children. *Pediatric Pulmonology*, *42*(11), 1024–1031. doi:10.1002/ppul.20687 PMID:17893917

Weiss, M. J. (2002). Hardiness and social support as predictors of stress in mothers of typical children, children with autism and children with mental retardation. *Autism*, *6*(1), 115–130. doi:10.1177/1362361302006001009 PMID:11918107

Wellington, J., & Szczerbinski, M. (2007). *Research methods for the social sciences*. London: Continuum.

Wenke, R. J., Stabler, P., Walton, C., Coman, L., Lawrie, M., O'Neill, J., ... & Cardell, E. (2014). Is more intensive better? Client and service provider outcomes for intensive versus standard therapy schedules for functional voice disorders. *Journal of Voice, 28*(5), 652-e31-e43.

Wessely, S., Hotopf, M., & Sharpe, M. (1999). *Chronic fatigue and its syndromes (Repr)*. Oxford, UK: Oxford University Press.

Westwood, P., & Graham, L. (2000). How many children with special needs in regular classes? Official predictions vs teachers' perceptions in South Australia and New South Wales. *Australian Journal of Learning Disabilities*, *5*(3), 24–35. doi:10.1080/19404150009546632

Whithworth, A., Webster, J., & Howard, D. (2005). *A cognitive neuropsychological approach to assessment and treatment of aphasia. A clinicians guide*. East Sussex, UK: Psychology Press.

Whoqol Group. (1995). The World Health Organization quality of life assessment (WHOQOL): Position paper from the World Health Organization. *Social Science & Medicine*, *41*(10), 1403–1409. doi:10.1016/0277-9536(95)00112-K PMID:8560308

Whoqol Group. (1998). Development of the World Health Organization WHOQOL-BREF quality of life assessment. *Psychological Medicine*, *28*(3), 551–558. doi:10.1017/S0033291798006667 PMID:9626712

Wickremesooriya, S. F. (2012). *Talking is fun: Enhancing oral language development of students with learning difficulties, in a hard-to-reach area of Sri Lanka* (Unpublished doctoral dissertation). University of Sheffield, Sheffield, UK.

Wicks-Nelson, R., & Israel, A. C. (2013). Anxiety and related disorders. In Abnormal Child and Adolescent Psychology with DSM-V Updates (8th ed.; pp. 114-117). Pearson Education Inc.

Wijesuriya, N., Tran, Y., Thuraisingham, R. A., Nguyen, H. T., & Craig, A. (2008). Effects of mental fatigue on 8-13Hz brain activity in people with spinal cord injury. *Conference Proceedings: ... Annual International Conference of the IEEE Engineering in Medicine and Biology Society. IEEE Engineering in Medicine and Biology Society. Annual Conference, 2008*, 5716–5719.

Williams, L. S., Weinberger, M., Harris, L. E., Clark, D. O., & Biller, J. (1999). Development of a stroke-specific quality of life scale. *Stroke*, *30*(7), 1362–1369. doi:10.1161/01.STR.30.7.1362 PMID:10390308

Williams, P. G., Dalrymple, N., & Neal, J. (2000). Eating habits of children with autism. *Pediatric Nursing*, *26*(3), 259–264. PMID:12026389

Williams, S. (2001). *Emotion and Social Theory*. London: Sage.

Wilson, A. J., & Dehaene, S. (2007). Number sense and developmental dyscalculia. In D. Coch, G. Dawson, & K. Fischer (Eds.), *Human behavior, learning and the developing brain: Atypical development*. New York: Guilford Press.

Wilson, L., Onslow, M., & Lincoln, M. (2004). Telehealth adaptation of the Lidcombe program of early stuttering intervention: Five case studies. *American Journal of Speech-Language Pathology*, *13*(1), 81–93. doi:10.1044/1058-0360(2004/009) PMID:15101816

Wingate, M. (1976). *Stuttering: Theory and treatment*. New York, NY: Wiley.

Witteman, C. L. M., Harries, C., Bekker, H. L., & Van Aarle, E. J. M. (2007). Evaluating psychodiagnostic decisions. *Journal of Evaluation in Clinical Practice*, *13*(1), 10–15. doi:10.1111/j.1365-2753.2006.00689.x PMID:17286717

Wolf, D. F. (1991). *The effects of task, language of assessment, and target language experience on foreign language learners performance on reading comprehension tests* (Doctoral dissertation). University of Illinois at Urbana-Champaign.

Wolf, L., & Glass, R. (1992). *Feeding and Swallowing Disorders in Infancy: Assessment and Management*. Tucson, AZ: Therapy Skill Builders.

Wong, K. L., Ong, S. F., & Kuek, T. Y. (2012). Constructing a survey questionnaire to collect data on service quality of business academics. *European Journal of Soil Science*, *29*, 209–221.

Woodcock, S. (2013). Trainee teachers attitudes towards students with specific learning disabilities. *Australian Journal of Teachers Education*, *38*(8), 16–29.

Woodgate, R. L., Ateah, C., & Secco, L. (2008). Living in a world of our own: The experience of parents who have children with autism. *Qualitative Health Research*, *18*(8), 1075–1083. doi:10.1177/1049732308320112 PMID:18650563

Wood, N., & Dockrell, J. (2010). Psychological assessment procedures for assessing deaf or hard-of-hearing children. *Educational and Child Psychology*, *27*(2), 11.

World Health Organisation. (2001). *Classification of Functioning, Disability and Health. Retrieved from* http://www.who.int/classifications/icf/en/

World Health Organization (WHO). (2007). *The world health report 2007 - A safer future: Global public health security in the 21st century.* Geneva, Switzerland: World Health Organization.

World Health Organization. (1992). *The ICD-10 classification of mental and behavioural disorders: Clinical descriptions and diagnostic guidelines.* Geneva: World Health Organization.

World Health Organization. (2001). *International Classification of Functioning, Disability and Health: ICF.* Geneva, Switzerland: World Health Organization.

World Health Organization. (2007). *International Classification of Functioning, Disability, and Health: Children and Youth Version.* Geneva: Author.

World Health Organization. (2008). *The ICD-10 classification of mental and behavioral disorders descriptions and diagnostic guidelines.* Geneva: World Health Organization.

World Health Organization. (2012). *WHO global estimates on prevalence of hearing loss.* Geneva: World Health Organization.

World Health Organization. (2012). *World Stroke Day.* Retrieved from http://www.who.int/cardiovascular_diseases/media/events/stroke_day/en/

World Health Organization. (2013). *The ICD-10-CM codes and criteria.* Retrieved from http://www.icd10data.com/search?s=autism%20

Worrall, L., & Holland, A. (2003). Quality of life in aphasia. *Aphasiology, 17*(4), 329–332. doi:10.1080/02687030244000699 PMID:27005901

Wright, A. C., & Taylor, S. (2014). Advocacy by parents of young children with special needs: Activities, processes, and perceived effectiveness. *Journal of Social Service Research, 40*(5), 591–605. doi:10.1080/01488376.2014.896850

Wright, K. B. (2005). Researching internet-based populations: Advantages and disadvantages of online survey research, online questionnaire authoring software packages, and web survey services. *Journal of Computer-Mediated Communication, 10*(3). Retrieved from http://onlinelibrary.wiley.com/doi/10.1111/j.1083-6101.2005.tb00259.x/full

Wyatt, G. L. (1969). *Language learning and communication disorders in children.* New York: Free Press.

Yadav, D., & Agarwal, V. (2008). A baseline study of learning disabilities: Its prevalence, teacher awareness and classroom practices. In K. Thapa, G. M. Aalsvoort, & J. Pandey (Eds.), *Perspectives on Learning Disabilities in India* (pp. 221–238). New Delhi: Sage Publication.

Yairi, E. (1983). The onset of stuttering in two- and three-year-old children: A preliminary report. *The Journal of Speech and Hearing Disorders, 48*(2), 171–177. doi:10.1044/jshd.4802.171 PMID:6621009

Yairi, E., & Ambrose, N. (1992a). Onset of stuttering in preschool children: Selected factors. *Journal of Speech and Hearing Research, 35*(4), 782–788. doi:10.1044/jshr.3504.782 PMID:1405533

Yairi, E., & Ambrose, N. (1992b). A longitudinal study of stuttering in children: A preliminary report. *Journal of Speech and Hearing Research, 35*(4), 755–760. doi:10.1044/jshr.3504.755 PMID:1405530

Yairi, E., & Ambrose, N. (2005). *Early childhood suttering.* Austin, TX: Pro-Ed.

Yairi, E., & Ambrose, N. (2013). Epidemiology of stuttering: 21st century advancements. *Journal of Fluency Disorders*, *38*(2), 66–87. doi:10.1016/j.jfludis.2012.11.002 PMID:23773662

Yairi, E., & Seery, C. H. (2015). *Stuttering: Foundations and Clinical Applications* (2nd ed.). Upper Saddle River, NJ: Pearson Education, Inc.

Yaruss, J. S., Coleman, C., & Hammer, D. (2006). Treating preschool children who stutter: Description and preliminary evaluation of a family-focused treatment approach. *Language, Speech, and Hearing Services in Schools*, *37*(2), 118–136. doi:10.1044/0161-1461(2006/014) PMID:16646215

Yeganeh, R., Biedel, D. C., Turner, S. M., Pina, A. A., & Silverman, W. K. (2003). Clinical distinctions between selective mutism and social phobia: An investigation of childhood psychopathology. *Journal of Adolescent and Child Psychiatry*, *43*, 605–612.

Ylvisaker, M., Turkstra, L. S., & Coelho, C. (2005). Behavioral and social interventions for individuals with traumatic brain injury: A summary of the research with clinical implications. *Seminars in Speech and Language*, *26*(4), 256–267. doi:10.1055-2005-922104 PMID:16278797

Young, E., & Hawk, S. (1955). *Moto-kinesthetic speech training*. Standford, CA: Stanford University.

Young, R. (1999). Sociolinguistic approaches to SLA. *Annual Review of Applied Linguistics*, *19*, 105–132. doi:10.1017/S0267190599190068

Young, S. (2007). The forgotten sibling. *Australian and New Zealand Journal of Family Therapy*, *28*(01), 21–27. doi:10.1375/anft.28.1.21

Yun, G. W., & Trumbo, C. W. (2000). Comparative response to a survey executed by post, e-mail, and web form. *Journal of Computer-Mediated Communication*, *6*(1). Retrieved from http://onlinelibrary.wiley.com/doi/10.1111/j.1083-6101.2000.tb00112.x/full

Yuvaraj, P., & Jayaram, M. (2016). Audiological profile of adult persons with auditory neuropathy spectrum disorders. *Journal of Audiology & Otology*, *20*(3), 158–167. doi:10.7874/jao.2016.20.3.158 PMID:27942602

Zebrowski, P., & Kelly, E. (2002). Manual of stuttering intervention. Singular Publishing Group, Thomson Learning.

Zebrowski, P., & Conture, E. G. (1998). Influence of nontreatment variables on treatment effectiveness for school age children who stutter. In A. Cordes & R. Ingham (Eds.), *Treatment efficacy for stuttering: A search for empirical bases* (pp. 293–310). San Diego, CA: Singular.

Zeidan, F., Johnson, S. K., Diamond, B. J., David, Z., & Goolkasian, P. (2010). Mindfulness meditation improves cognition: Evidence of brief mental training. *Consciousness and Cognition*, *19*(2), 597–605. doi:10.1016/j.concog.2010.03.014 PMID:20363650

Zeidan, F., Martucci, K. T., Kraft, R. A., Gordon, N. S., McHaffie, J. G., & Coghill, R. C. (2011). Brain mechanisms supporting the modulation of pain by mindfulness meditation. *The Journal of Neuroscience*, *31*(14), 5540–5548. doi:10.1523/JNEUROSCI.5791-10.2011 PMID:21471390

Zeidan, F., Martucci, K. T., Kraft, R. A., McHaffie, J. G., & Coghill, R. C. (2014). Neural correlates of mindfulness meditation-related anxiety relief. *Social Cognitive and Affective Neuroscience*, *9*(6), 751–759. doi:10.1093can/nst041 PMID:23615765

Zeng, F., Kong, Y., Michalewski, H. J., & Starr, A. (2005). Perceptual consequences of disrupted auditory nerve activity. *Journal of Neurophysiology*, *93*(6), 3050–3063. doi:10.1152/jn.00985.2004 PMID:15615831

Zeng, F., Oba, S., Garde, S., Sininger, Y., & Starr, A. (1999). Temporal and speech processing deficits in auditory neuropathy. *Neuroreport*, *10*(16), 3429–3435. doi:10.1097/00001756-199911080-00031 PMID:10599857

Zetlin, A. G. (1986). Mentally retarded adults and their siblings. *American Journal of Mental Deficiency*, *91*(3), 217–225. PMID:3799727

Zigmond, N. (1993). Learning disabilities from an educational perspective. In G. R. Lyon, D. B. Gray, J. F. Kavanaugh, & N. A. Krasnegor (Eds.), *Better understanding learning disabilities: New views from research and their implications for education and public policies* (pp. 251–272). Baltimore, MD: Brookes.

Zikmund, W. G. (2003). *Business Research Methods* (7th ed.). Thompson/South-Western.

About the Contributors

Sanjeev Kumar Gupta is currently working as a Clinical Psychologist at All India Institute of Speech and Hearing, India. He has completed PhD in Psychology from the University of Mysore and has more than 10 years of experience in the field of Clinical Psychology. His areas of interest include cognitive retraining for neurodevelopmental disorders; cognitive behaviour therapy for stuttering, mindfulness meditation, telerehabilitation, and electrophysiology. He has contributed two chapters in books and published 15 articles in various national and international peer-reviewed and indexed journals. He has presented several research papers both at National and International conferences such as 31st International Congress of Psychology, Japan and also conducted several workshops/symposiums and training programs for professionals and caregivers of children with neurodevelopmental disorders. Currently, he is busy in editing a forthcoming publication entitled "Handbook of Research on Trends in the Diagnosis and Intervention of Neurodevelopmental Disorders" to be published by IGI Global, Hershey, PA.

Srinivasan Venkatesan is Professor & Head, Department of Clinical Psychology, AIISH, Mysore, Karnataka. He has earlier served at NIMH, Secunderabad-Hyderabad. He has authored 26 books, contributed 24 chapters in books, another 35 varieties of technical literature, published 135 research papers, served as resource person for workshops for different target groups He has completed projects through collaboration with national/international agencies, guided students for Ph.D., been on editorial board for journals and peer-reviewed research articles, presented papers in conferences and served as examiner for adjudication of doctoral thesess. A consistently first class and university rank holder from school to pre-doctoral courses at NIMHANS, Bangalore, in 1987; he was awarded doctorate in 1993. A Fellow of the Society for Advanced Studies in Medical Sciences, New Delhi, in psychiatry, he was decorated with Gold Medal from former President of India, Sri Giani Zail Singh in 1994, NN Sen Memorial Award for 'Best Research Paper' by Indian Association of Clinical Psychologists in 2002, 'Psycho Oration Award' in January 2009, and Prof. Anima Sen Memorial Award in 2012.

* * *

Divya Baveja, Assistant Professor in Department of Clinical Psychology, Amity Institute of Behavioral and Allied Sciences, Amity University, Lucknow Campus. She is a licensed Clinical Psychologist and involved in teaching and training of M. Phil in Clinical Psychology. Her area of interest lies in parent's counseling of children with disabilities.

Shyamala K. Chengappa is a senior most professor in Language Pathology and chairperson of the special clinic on Autism Spectrum disorders at the Department of Speech-Language Pathology at All India Institute of Speech and Hearing at Mysore, India. With her vast experience of 33 years at various esteemed organizations such as CIIL, Mysore, NIMHANS, Bangalore and AIISH at various positions, she has worked & published books, book chapters, and research articles widely on child language and adult language disorders and bi/multilingualism. She was a postdoctoral fellow at Texas A & M University at the college station, Texas, USA in 2000-2001. She was an invited key note speaker at the 7th International Symposium on Bilingualism held at Utrecht, Netherlands (2009). She has been the recipient of a visiting professorship (Postdoctoral) at EMCL, Potsdam, Germany from May-August, 2008. She had represented India in the panel on childhood bilingualism- International perspectives in the International conference at Hong Kong in December 2008. She has published over twelve books and 160 papers in national and International Journals. She has successfully guided over 10 Ph.D. theses and 80 MSc dissertations, besides managing over 38 projects with funding from Indian Council of Medical Research, Department of Science and Technology, ICSSR, UGC, and ARF. She has over 36 years of research, clinical and teaching experience besides administrative experience. She is a recognized guide for not only speech and hearing but also Speech language pathology and Linguistics. She has also received Dr. N. Rathna Oration Award in 2012 from Indian Speech and Hearing Association and Best AIISHIAN award in 2015.

Anusha Chilakalapudi has done her B.Sc (ASLP) from AYJNIHH,SRC and M.Sc (ASLP) from Helen Keller's Institute, Hyderabad, certified as Specialist in Laryngectomy Rehabilitation (SLR). Her areas of interest include: Voice disorders, Laryngectomy rehabilitation, adult language disorders and craniofacial anomalies. Currently working in the area of Cleft Lip & Palate. She has two invited presentations in the area of laryngectomy rehabilitation, 2 research publications and poster presentations. She has attended national conferences, workshops, seminars and webinars.

Malar G. has been working in the field of special education for more than fifteen years and has gained experience in educational management of children with communication disorders. This expertise in handling children has paved way to many evidence based research. In the area of research, the co-author has authored, co-authored, written and edited chapters in many journals and books respectively. Inclusive education, adapting new teaching techniques, cross disability study has been her area of research interest.

Krupa Saira George has completed her Bachelors and Masters in Audiology & Speech Language Pathology in India. She had worked as Assistant Professor at Naseema Institute of Speech and Hearing, Bangalore till recently and currently, she is working as Assistant Professor at Samvaad Institute of Speech and Hearing, Bangalore, Karnataka, India. Her areas of interest include maxillofacial anomalies, language disorders, and diagnostic audiology. She has presented several research papers at national and international conferences such as 9th Asia Pacific Conference on Speech, Language, and Hearing held at Guangzhou, China.

Dilani Gopi is Co-Founder of Cerebral Palsy Lanka Foundation and Director of the National Center for Cerebral Palsy and Developmental Disorders in Sri Lanka. She is an Arts graduate from the University of Colombo and a trained Special Education teacher having followed a Diploma in Special Education at the National Institute of Education, Sri Lanka.

S. P. Goswami holds Ph. D in Speech and Hearing and also PGDHRM and MBA in Health Care Management. He is the first Speech and Hearing professional to receive the prestigious CV Raman fellowship from UGC, Government of India as Visiting Scholar at College of Applied Health Sciences, Department of Speech & Hearing Science, University of Illinois at Urbana-Champaign under CV Raman fellowship, UGC, GOI, New Delhi (August, 2013 to July, 2014). Presently he is working as Professor and Head Department of Speech-Language Pathology and Academic coordinator and formerly worked as Head Department of Clinical services, Speech-Language Pathology at AIISH, Mysore. Dr. Goswami has more than 18 years of academic, clinical, research and administrative experience. He works in the area of Aphasia, ageing and neuro-cognitive communication disorders in adults and elderly. He has published more than 31 research articles in national and international journals, 20 in-house publication and 19 Books/ chapters/tools/tests with ISBN numbers. Two candidates have been awarded Ph.D and four are presently pursuing for their doctorate program under his guidance.

Raju Hanumanthaiah has done his Post graduation in Psychology from the Department of Psychology, University of Mysore, India. He is working as Clinical assistant in the Department of Clinical Psychology, All India Institute of Speech and Hearing for more than 20 years. He has immense professional experience working with individuals having functional voice disorder. He has successfully treated more than 150 cases with functional voice therapy.

Shyamani Hettiarachchi is a Speech & Language Therapist, and Senior Lecturer at the Department of Disability Studies, Faculty of Medicine, University of Kelaniya in Sri Lanka. She graduated from the University of Kelaniya and completed her postgraduate studies in the UK, at the Universities of London and Oxford and trained as a Dramatherapist at the University of Roehampton. Her special research interests include speech sound disorders, dysphagia, and the intersectionality between culture, poverty, gender and disability.

Shyam H. R. has done his post graduation in Psychology and pursuing his doctoral degree from the Department of Psychology, University of Mysore, India. He has done his M.Phil in Clinical psychology from National Institute of Mental Health and Neuro Sciences, Bengaluru, India. He is working as Clinical Psychologist Grade-II in All India Institute of Speech and Hearing, India for more than 3 years. He has experience in the management of individuals with communication disorders and intellectual disabilities.

Mary Iype, MD, DM. FRCPCH (London), is currently working as Additional Professor of Pediatric Neurology, Government Medical College, Trivandrum and Visiting Faculty of Institute for Communicative & Cognitive Neurosciences, Trivandrum. Has 21 years of experience in Pediatric Neurology. Areas of research interest include Pediatric epilepsies, demyelinating disorders and Autism. Has many International and national peer reviewed publications. Is a reviewer for several national and international journals.

Saransh Jain is presently working as Lecturer in Audiology at JSS institute of Speech and Hearing, Mysuru, India. His research interest is in understanding the physiology of human auditory system, psychoacoustic characteristics of speech and influence of cognition on human performances.

Nandini Jayachandran is currently working as Lecturer in Clinical Psychology at the Institute for Communicative & Cognitive Neurosciences (ICCONS), Trivandrum, Kerala, India. Has completed M.A. (Applied Psychology), followed by Ph.D in the topic 'Developmental dyscalculia: Identification & Remediation' from the Department of Psychology, University of Kerala. Has been involved in regular psychological evaluation, diagnostic testing and therapeutic management of disorders of cognition & language such as Specific Learning Disorders, Autism Spectrum Disorders, Developmental Language disorders, Cerebral Palsy, Epilepsies, Intellectual Disabilities, Aphasias, and other neurological disorders, primarily in the 0-18 age group, over the past 17 years. Areas of research interest are SLD & ASD (specifically in developing evidence based practices), currently the Principal Investigator of two research projects funded by the Department of Science & Technology, Government of India. Has organized and actively participated in Conferences and Continuing Rehabilitation Education programs in the area of cognitive disorders. Has published and presented several research papers in National & International Conferences. Has been involved in teaching at Graduate, Post-graduate and M.Phil courses and also served as Examiner and Subject Expert for Kerala University of Health Sciences and Universities of Calicut and Kerala.Is a member of accredited professional bodies such as The Rehabilitation Council of India (Rehabilitation Psychologist) and The British Psychological Society (Chartered Psychologist).

Gopi Kitnasamy is Founder/Director of Cerebral Palsy Lanka Foundation. He is a Bobath-trained physiotherapist. His research interests include evidence-based local early interventions for children with cerebral palsy and children on the autism spectrum.

Gayathri Krishnan is a post graduate in Speech-Language Pathology working in All India Institute of Speech and Hearing since 2012. Introduced to dysphagia in her student training period, she developed keen interest in this field and has been passionate towards learning and practicing swallowing therapy. Currently, she is one of the members of the Dysphagia Unit Team and is also pursuing her Doctoral Degree in this innovative science.

Charu Kriti is the teaching faculty of Psychology at National University of Study and Research in Law, Nagri, P.O Bukru, Kanke-Pithoria Road, Kanke, Ranchi. She has done her B.A and M.A. in Psychology from Banaras Hindu University. She has also done her LL.B. from the University of Delhi.

Santosh Maruthy, Ph.D., is Reader in the Department of Speech-Language Sciences at the All India Institute of Speech and Hearing, Mysore, India. His research focuses on the mechanisms underlying stuttering as well as bilingualism and stuttering, speech science, speech perception, and voice disorders in professional voice users.

Sharon Mathews is working as a Research Officer at All India Institute of Speech and Hearing, Mysore, and has worked in various research projects since 2014. Her areas of interest are aphasia and cognitive communicative disorders in the elderly.

Prithi Mondreti works in the field of special education for more than ten years, has enriched my knowledge and experience in dealing with children special needs. This experience in special education has helped to conduct evidence based research on children with special needs, especially hearing impaired. Conducting research in the area of mathematics which includes error identification, developing arithmetic diagnostic test, identification of difficulties, development of appropriate remedial instructional material has been my area of research interest. However, research has also been conducted in the area of identification of stress among teachers and parents of children with special needs.

Kadambari Naniwadekar has done B.Sc. Home Science, M.Sc. Applied Psychology, B.Ed., P.G. Diploma in Developmental Therapy, and Ph.D. in Psychology. Currently, she is working as a Special Educator at All India Institute of Speech and Hearing, Mysuru. She has published 9 research papers and received three best paper awards.

Fathima Shamra Nizar is a Speech & Language Therapist attached to the National Center for Cerebral Palsy and Developmental Disorders, Sri Lanka. She has a BSc in Speech and Hearing Sciences (specializing in Speech and Language Therapy) from the University of Kelaniya, Sri Lanka.

Divya P. has completed her Masters degree in Speech Language Pathology from All India Institute of Speech and Hearing, Mysore and she has been working at Naseema Institute of Speech and Hearing, Bangalore for several years. Her major areas of interest include neurogenic communication disorders. She has presented and published several research papers at national conferences on Speech Language Pathology.

Apoorva Pauranik received MBBS in 1975, M.D Medicine in 1979, and D.M. Neurology in 1985 from AIIMS New Delhi. Currently working as a professor in Neurology, MGM Medical College & Hospital, India. His area of interest is teaching, clinical neurology, aphasia, advocacy, evidence-based practice, public health education and patient education in Hindi. He is a co-chair of Special Interest Group on Communication Disorders at World Federation of Neuro-Rehabilitation.

Prashanth Prabhu received his Masters in Audiology from University of Mysuru in 2010. In 2010, he was hired as a clinical audiologist at the Department of Audiology, AIISH, Mysuru and currently working as Lecturer in Audiology at AIISH, Mysuru. His major interest is in auditory neuropathy spectrum disorder (ANSD). He has published several research articles, conference presentations in the area. He is currently working on developing hearing aid modification strategies to help individuals with ANSD.

Brajesh Priyadarshi is a Reader in Linguistics at All India Institute of Speech and Hearing, Mysore and has been working in this Institute for the last eleven years. He previously held a teaching position at Ali Yavar Jung National Institute for Hearing Handicapped (AYJNIHH), New Delhi. He completed M.Phil in linguistics in 2002 from the Jawaharlal Nehru University, New Delhi, and was awarded his Ph.D in Linguistics from the same University in 2014. He presently also holds the position of Head, Department of Material Development at All India Institute of Speech and Hearing, Mysore. His areas of interest are research in clinical linguistics and psycho-linguistics. He has completed three research projects as the principal investigator and two projects as the co-investigator. He also has three ongoing projects. He has over 20 publications to his credit., including journal articles, a book and book chapter.

Suma Raju is working as reader in Speech Language Pathology at JSS Institute of Speech and Hearing, Mysuru, India. Her research interest is in understanding language processing in the human brain, bilingualism and cognition.

Sunil Kumar Ravi is currently working as Associate Professor & Principal at Shravana Institute of Speech & Hearing, Ballari, India. He has also served as the Faculty Consultant for Bachelors of Health Sciences (Majors in Speech & Hearing) at Gulf Medical University, Ajman, United Arab Emirates. He had done his M.Sc (Speech-Language Pathology) & Ph.D. (SLP) at AIISH, Mysore. His areas of interest include but are not limited to aphasia, electrophysiology, bilingualism, dementia and child language disorders. He had written a book chapter on 'Fast mapping of novel words in multilingual context' in the book "Handbook of South & Southeast Asian Psycholinguistics", Cambridge University Press, New York. He has published several research papers in national & international journals (Asia Pacific Journal of SLH, International Journal of Multilingualism). He has presented research papers at both International and national level conferences. He has also delivered guest lectures at various conferences and seminars in India. He has been the chair, co-chair, and reviewer for scientific sessions on language for various conferences.

Divya Seth is a Junior Research Fellow (JRF) in the Department of Speech-Language Sciences at All India Institute of Speech and Hearing, Mysuru. She completed both her graduation and post graduation at AIISH, Mysuru. She received Manohar Gold Medal, Smt. Jayalakshmi Gold Medal and FRIENDS United Organization Endowment Scholarship for securing highest marks in M.Sc (Speech-Language Pathology) for the academic year 2013-2015. She served as a Research Officer at AIISH, Mysuru in 2015-2016. Her areas of interest include Fluency Disorders, Child Language Disorders, Neurobiology of speech and language.

Pinki Singh did MASLP from AYJNIHH, Mumbai. Currently, working as a Speech-Language Pathologist at the All India Institute of Medical Sciences-Bhopal, India. Earlier worked as an Assist. Professor, SAIMS, Indore. She has received the best poster award at aphasia workshop and Manohar memorial award for best speech-language research paper at the national conference, ISHACON at Kochi. She has 8 research publications, 7 presentations, and organised 2 workshops related to dysphagia and autism. Her area of Interest is Neuro speech & language disorders, Dysphagia, and childhood developmental disorders

Poovathinal Azhakan Suresh, MD., DM., MBA is the Founder Director and present Executive Director of Institute for Communicative and Cognitive Neurosciences (ICCONS), Trivandrum & Shoranur, Kerala. He has more than 30 years of clinical, research and teaching experience in the field of Behavioural Neurology, specifically in the area of Neurodevelopmental disorders. He started his career as a faculty at the prestigious Sree Chithra Tirunal Institute for Medical Sciences & Technology, Trivandrum in 1992, after attaining DM from the same. Being a pioneer in his field, he has presented more than 50 papers in National and International forums and has published widely in national and international, peer reviewed journals. His areas of research interest include Cognitive Neuroscience, Neurodevelopmental disorders, Neurogenetics, Aphasia, Neurocytobiology, Developmental Neurobiology, Neuroscience Engineering and computation, Human robotics and Neurocognitive Kinesiology. He has headed over 13 research projects, funded by Government of Kerala, Government of India and the UNDP. He is a recipient of many awards including Save India National award, 2011 for contribution to Medical Sciences and the Lions International Excellence award in 2014. He is also an expert committee member in bodies like the Cognitive Science Research Initiative (CSRI), Department of Science and Technology (DST), New Delhi and Research Advisory Board Member of Jubilee Centre for Medical Research, Thrissur.

Rachel V. has a Master's degree in Audiology and Speech Language Pathology. She has been awarded Sri MPC Shetty Gold Medal for securing highest marks in MASLP course for the academic year 2012-13. Since then, she has worked as a school based Speech Language Pathologist, Research Associate and SLP-Grade 1 for various research project. Presently she is working as a Research Officer at All India Institute of Speech and Hearing.

Reuben Thomas Varghese has completed his under graduation from AYJNIHH, Mumbai and his post graduation from All India Institute of Speech & Hearing, Mysuru. He is presently doing his Ph.D (SLP) in the field of dementia. He has won numerous awards like the best clinician award, best paper in Phonocon etc. He has presented papers both at the international and national levels and has research articles to his credit in both national and international journals.

Divya Vinod is a Lecturer in Speech, Language Pathology, Institute for Communicative & Cognitive Neurosciences, Trivandrum. Has completed Bachelors in Speech & Language Pathology from NISH, Trivandrum & Masters in Audiology & Speech Language Pathology (MASLP) from Dr.M.V.Shetty College of Speech and Hearing, Mangalore. Has 9 years of clinical experience and teaching experience in the field of Audiology & Speech Language Pathology.Is a life memeber of Indian Speech and Hearing Association (ISHA) and a Rehabilitation Council of India (RCI) registered practitioner.

Shalini Felicity Wickremesooriya is a qualified Speech and Language Pathologist and a Counseling Psychologist. She is a certified member of The Royal College of Speech & Language Therapists (UK). She is also a Speech and Language Therapist licensed by the Sri Lanka Medical Council and a licensed member of the Sri Lankan Association of Psychology, Counseling and Psychotherapy. Shalini Wickremesooriya completed her Doctoral Studies in Human Communication Sciences at the University of Sheffield, UK in 2012. Her Master's thesis which focused at empowering children with disabilities in rural Sri Lanka, was heralded as a work of high distinction at the University of Birmingham UK in 2004. She has also contributed to the global understanding of disability with journal articles, a chapter contribution in the book titled – "Embedding evidence-based practice in speech and language therapy – International Perspectives, and published her own book – Invincible: Stories of hope and courage by individuals with disabilities- endorsing her belief that individuals with disabilities have right to be heard. Shalini Wickremesooriya has worked predominantly in Sri Lanka, in varied contexts and with clients from varied economic strata, in the city, suburbs and in rural villages and among people of different races and religions. She also has international experience working with children who communicate through alternative communication devices and experience working on summer camps for children who stutter. Shalini Wickremesooriya's research interests revolve around the philosophy of Inclusion and the action research methodology to bring about lasting change. She believes that when people are not coerced but empowered through the cyclical process of action research, social change will take place.

S. Z. H. Zaidi is Professor and Head of the Department, Department of Clinical Psychology, Amity University, Lucknow Campus. He is a Clinical Psychologist with over 40 years of experience in teaching and clinical practice. He has worked in the area of Rehabilitation in various parts of India, under the Government of India. He has had the honour of being bestowed the National Award for his outstanding work and contribution toward the Empowerment of Persons with Disabilities.

Index

A

B

C

D

E

F

G

H

I

Q

R

S

T

V

W

www.ingramcontent.com/pod-product-compliance
Lightning Source LLC
LaVergne TN
LVHW060353300926
849162LV00006B/1258